Antibiotic Resistance: Mechanisms and Antimicrobial Approaches

Antibiotic Resistance: Mechanisms and Antimicrobial Approaches

Edited by Cooper Smith

STATES
ACADEMIC PRESS
www.statesacademicpress.com

States Academic Press,
109 South 5th Street,
Brooklyn, NY 11249, USA

Visit us on the World Wide Web at:
www.statesacademicpress.com

ISBN: 978-1-63989-050-7

Cataloging-in-Publication Data

Antibiotic resistance : mechanisms and antimicrobial approaches / edited by Cooper Smith.
p. cm.
Includes bibliographical references and index.
ISBN 978-1-63989-050-7
1. Drug resistance in microorganisms. 2. Antibiotics. 3. Microorganisms--Effect of drugs on.
4. Anti-infective agents. I. Smith, Cooper.

QR177 .A58 2022
616.904 1--dc23

Table of Contents

Preface

Over the recent decade, advancements and applications have progressed exponentially. This has led to the increased interest in this field and projects are being conducted to enhance knowledge. The main objective of this book is to present some of the critical challenges and provide insights into possible solutions. This book will answer the varied questions that arise in the field and also provide an increased scope for furthering studies.

Antimicrobial resistance develops when micro-organisms evolve different mechanisms to protect themselves from the effects of antimicrobials. Such micro-organisms that develop antimicrobial resistance are difficult to treat and require higher doses or alternative medications that are more toxic to them. When micro-organisms are resistant to multiple antimicrobials, then they are called multidrug resistant. All classes of microbes, such as bacteria, fungi, protozoa and viruses, can develop resistance. The bacteria that are resistant to a wide range of antibiotics are known as extensively drug resistant or superbugs. Antibiotic resistance can be spontaneous, as a result of random mutations, or can be caused by extensive use of anti-microbials, which encourage the selection of mutants that are resistant to them. This book is a valuable compilation of topics, ranging from the basic to the most complex advancements in the field of antibiotic resistance. It covers in detail some existent theories and innovative concepts revolving around antibiotic resistance. This book is a vital tool for all researching and studying this field.

I hope that this book, with its visionary approach, will be a valuable addition and will promote interest among readers. Each of the authors has provided their extraordinary competence in their specific fields by providing different perspectives as they come from diverse nations and regions. I thank them for their contributions.

Editor

1

Effect of antimicrobial exposure on AcrAB expression in *Salmonella enterica* subspecies *enterica* serovar Choleraesuis

Masaru Usui[1,2], Hidetaka Nagai[1], Mototaka Hiki[1], Yutaka Tamura[2] and Tetsuo Asai[1]*

[1] National Veterinary Assay Laboratory, Ministry of Agriculture, Forestry and Fisheries, Kokubunji, Tokyo, Japan
[2] School of Veterinary Medicine, Rakuno Gakuen University, Ebetsu, Hokkaido, Japan

Edited by:
Kunihiko Nishino, Osaka University, Japan

Reviewed by:
Julie Zilles, University of Illinois Urbana Champaign, USA
Glenn Kaatz, John D. Dingell VA Medical Center, USA

***Correspondence:**
Tetsuo Asai, National Veterinary Assay Laboratory, Ministry of Agriculture, Forestry and Fisheries, 1-15-1 Tokura, Kokubunji, Tokyo 185-8511, Japan.
e-mail: asai-t@nval.maff.go.jp

Understanding the impact of antimicrobial use on the emergence of resistant bacteria is imperative to prevent its emergence. For instance, activation of the AcrAB efflux pumps is responsible for the emergence of antimicrobial-resistant *Salmonella* strains. Here, we examined the expression levels of *acrB* and its multiple regulator genes (RamA, SoxS, MarA, and Rob) in 17 field isolates of *S.* Choleraesuis by using quantitative PCR methods. The expression of *acrB* increased in eight of the field isolates ($P < 0.05$). The expression of *acrB* was associated with that of *ramA* in one isolate, *soxS* in one isolate, and both these genes in six isolates. Thereafter, to examine the effect of selected antimicrobials (enrofloxacin, ampicillin, oxytetracycline, kanamycin, and spectinomycin) on the expression of *acrB* and its regulator genes, mutants derived from five isolates of *S.* Choleraesuis were selected by culture on antimicrobial-containing plates. The expression of *acrB* and *ramA* was higher in the mutants selected using enrofloxacin (3.3–6.3- and 24.5–37.7-fold, respectively), ampicillin (1.8–7.7- and 16.1–55.9-fold, respectively), oxytetracycline (1.7–3.3- and 3.2–31.1-fold, respectively), and kanamycin (1.6–2.2- and 5.6–26.4-fold, respectively), which are AcrAB substrates, than in each of the parental strains ($P < 0.05$). In contrast, in AcrAB substrate-selected mutants, the expression of *soxS*, *marA*, and *rob* remained similar to that in parental strains. Of the four antimicrobials, the level of *ramA* expression was significantly higher in the enrofloxacin- and ampicillin-selected mutants than in the oxytetracycline- and kanamycin-selected mutants ($P < 0.05$), whereas the expression levels of *acrB* and multiple regulator genes in spectinomycin-selected mutants were similar to those in each parental strain. These data suggest that exposure to antimicrobials that are AcrAB substrates enhance the activation of the AcrAB efflux pump *via* RamA, but not *via* SoxS, MarA, or Rob in *S.* Choleraesuis.

Keywords: AcrAB efflux pump, antimicrobial resistance, RamA, *Salmonella* Choleraesuis, SoxS

INTRODUCTION

Salmonella enterica subspecies *enterica* serovar Choleraesuis is a bacterial pathogen that causes severe diarrhea, pneumonia, and septicemia in pigs and in elderly and immunocompromised humans (Chiu et al., 2004). These bacteria sometimes cause severe infections, necessitating antimicrobial treatment of affected patients. A high rate of multidrug resistance among *S.* Choleraesuis has been reported in several countries (Lee et al., 2009; Asai et al., 2010), raising a concern for public and animal health.

Activation of an efflux system that removes the drug from the cell is one antimicrobial resistance mechanism in bacteria (Chen et al., 2007; Li and Nikaido, 2009). The AcrAB-TolC system is the main multidrug efflux system in Gram-negative bacteria (Giraud et al., 2000). The expression level of *acrAB* mRNAs correlates with efflux activities and is regulated by global regulatory proteins and local repressors (Rosenberg et al., 2003; Li and Nikaido, 2004; Olliver et al., 2004; Abouzeed et al., 2008). In particular, the expression of *acrAB* is regulated by the global regulators, RamA, SoxS, MarA, and Rob (Rosenberg et al., 2003; Abouzeed et al., 2008). Moreover, mutations within the local repressor AcrR contribute to the overexpression of *acrAB* (Olliver et al., 2004). In *S.* Typhimurium and *S.* Haardt, RamA mainly regulates the expression of *acrAB* (**Figure 1**; Nikaido et al., 2008; Zheng et al., 2009; Kim and Woo, 2011). Other regulators, SoxS and MarA, are also known to regulate *acrAB* expression, but the contributions of SoxS and MarA to antimicrobial susceptibilities are lower than that of RamA (Abouzeed et al., 2008). Little is known about Rob and its contribution to the enhancement of AcrAB in *Salmonella* (Rosenberg et al., 2003). In *S.* Pullorum, the expression of *acrB*, which shifts from sensitivity to resistance against bile salt (deoxycholate, an AcrAB substrate), was independent of *ramA*, *soxS*, *marA*, and *rob* expression (Usui et al., 2011).

We have previously recorded the various efflux activity levels of *S.* Choleraesuis under field conditions, suggesting that elevated efflux activities are related to the emergence of fluoroquinolone resistance (Usui et al., 2009). In fluoroquinolone-selected *S.* Choleraesuis, efflux pumps including AcrAB were enhanced and resulted in decreasing susceptibilities to several antimicrobials (Usui et al., 2010). However, little is known about roles of regulator genes for efflux pumps in S. Choleraesuis. In this study, we examined the expression levels of *acrAB* and multiple regulator genes in 17 clinical swine isolates of S. Choleraesuis and antimicrobial-selected mutants in order to understand the impact of antimicrobial exposure on the efflux activities in this organism.

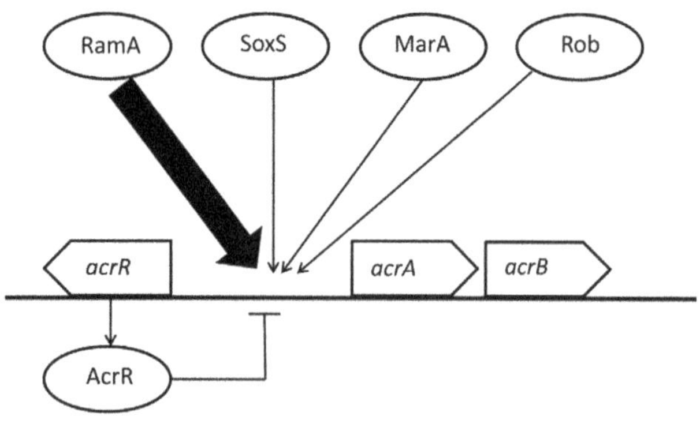

FIGURE 1 | Regulation of *acrAB* expression by multiple regulators in *Salmonella* Typhimurium and *S.* Haardt. This figure was produced using data from the literature (see main text). Functional interactions are represented as arrows for activation/induction and as "⊣" for repression. The size of arrows indicates the estimated impact.

MATERIALS AND METHODS

BACTERIAL STRAINS

Seventeen strains of S. Choleraesuis, obtained from different diseased pigs between 2001 and 2005 (Asai et al., 2010), were used in this study (**Table 1**). These strains comprised 6 nalidixic acid-resistant strains (low enrofloxacin-accumulation), and 11 nalidixic acid-susceptible strains (two strains: low enrofloxacin-accumulation; three strains: intermediate enrofloxacin-accumulation; six strains: high enrofloxacin-accumulation) as previously recorded (Usui et al., 2009). The intracellular concentration of enrofloxacin was significantly lower in nalidixic acid-resistant isolates, and the nalidixic acid-susceptible isolates ZSC-8 and 582 as compared to other susceptible isolates with the exception of isolates 143, ZSC-12, and 1002 ($P < 0.1$; Usui et al., 2009). The intracellular enrofloxacin concentrations of isolates 143, ZSC-12, and 1002 were at an intermediate level. Minimum inhibitory concentrations (MIC) of enrofloxacin, ampicillin, oxytetracycline, and kanamycin had been determined in our previous study (Asai et al., 2010). MIC of spectinomycin was

Table 1 | Characterization of *Salmonella* Choleraesuis used in this study.

Strain no.	Susceptibility to nalidixic acid[a]		Enrofloxacin-accumulation		mRNA expression		Mutations	
	Category[b]	MIC (mg/L)[b]	Category[c]	(ng/10^5 cfu)[c]	*acrA*[d]	*acrB*[d]	AcrR[e]	Binding site
13-PLS-6	Resistance	256	Low	8.2	1.6±0.2*	1.8±0.2*	WT	WT
14-PLS-21	Resistance	>512	Low	8.7	3.9±0.3*	2.7±0.2*	WT	WT
16-PLS-45	Resistance	>512	Low	6.5	1.5±0.1*	1.9±0.3*	Q78ter	WT
16-PLS-46	Resistance	>512	Low	6.6	2.4±0.2*	2.4±0.4*	Q78ter	WT
sal-1372	Resistance	>512	Low	6.3	1.8±0.1*	2.2±0.2*	WT	WT
16-PLS-33	Resistance	>512	Low	5.1	1.5±0.1*	1.9±0.2*	Q78ter	WT
ZSC-8	Susceptible	8	Low	8.1	1.7±0.1*	1.8±0.2*	Q78ter	WT
582	Susceptible	8	Low	7.2	1.4±0.1*	1.4±0.2*	Q78ter	WT
143	Susceptible	8	Intermediate	9.1	1.1±0.1	1.3±0.1	Q78ter	WT
ZSC-12	Susceptible	4	Intermediate	9.5	1.0±0.1	1.0±0.1	Q78ter	WT
1002	Susceptible	4	Intermediate	9.8	1.1±0.2	1.2±0.2	Q78ter	WT
916	Susceptible	4	High	10.7	1.1±0.1	1.1±0.1	Q78ter	WT
03-197-1	Susceptible	2	High	11.4	0.9±0.1	0.8±0.1	Q78ter	WT
03-228-1	Susceptible	2	High	10.7	1.0±0.2	1.1±0.1	Q78ter	WT
ZSC-14-1	Susceptible	4	High	11.0	0.9±0.1	1.1±0.1	Q78ter	WT
ZSC-40	Susceptible	4	High	10.5	0.9±0.2	0.9±0.2	WT	WT
419	Susceptible	4	High	12.7	1.0±0.2	0.9±0.1	Q78ter	WT

MIC, minimum inhibitory concentration; WT, wild-type sequence.

[a] *MIC break point of nalidixic acid is 32 mg/L.*

[b] *Data from a previous report (Asai et al., 2010).*

[c] *Data from a previous report (Usui et al., 2009).*

[d] *Relative expression level compared to the average for six high enrofloxacin-accumulating nalidixic acid-susceptible strains.*

[e] *Q78ter, stop codon mutation, glutamine-78-termination.*

**Indicates mRNA expression is significantly higher than mRNA expression of six high enrofloxacin-accumulating nalidixic acid-susceptible strains ($P < 0.05$).*

determined by the broth microdilution method according to CLSI guidelines (Clinical and Laboratory Standard Institute, 2008).

LABORATORY-SELECTED MUTANTS

Five strains (582, 143, 916, 1002, and 419), susceptible to all of the antimicrobial agents evaluated in this study, were selected as parent strains from which mutants were isolated. Cultures grown on agar containing various agents was employed, including three AcrAB substrates (ampicillin, oxytetracycline, and kanamycin) and one non-substrate (spectinomycin; Bailey et al., 2008; Ricci and Piddock, 2009a,b). For selection of mutants, 0.1 mL of each strain, adjusted to 10^8–10^9cfu/mL were exposed to 4 × MIC of the respective substance for each strain in the agar medium, as described previously (Ricci and Piddock, 2009b). A single strain was selected for each combination. In addition, as fluoroquinolone is an AcrAB substrates, enrofloxacin-selected mutants obtained in our previous report were used as control (Usui et al., 2010). MICs of antimicrobials for mutants were determined as described above.

QUANTITATIVE PCR ANALYSIS OF EXPRESSION OF 16S rRNA, *acrAB*, AND MULTIPLE GLOBAL REGULATORS

To evaluate the genes conferring efflux pump activity and their multiple global regulators, quantitative PCR was applied to the detection and quantification of mRNAs (Usui et al., 2010, 2011). The preparation of cDNA was performed as described by Zheng et al. (2009), with slight modifications. In brief, extraction of total RNA from 5 mL of bacterial suspensions was carried out with an ISOGEN kit (Nippon Gene, Tokyo, Japan). cDNA was synthesized from these RNA samples using the PrimeScript RT reagent kit (TaKaRa, Shiga, Japan). Quantitative PCR was performed with SYBR premix EX TaqII (TaKaRa) on a One Step real-time system (Applied Biosystems, Foster City, CA, USA) according to the manufacturer's instructions. The oligonucleotide primers used for the detection of cDNA are listed in **Table 2**. The yields of amplicons from *acrA*, *acrB*, *ramA*, *soxS*, *marA*, and *rob* were normalized to those originating from 16S rRNA. Within bacterial cells, 16S rRNA was assumed to be transcribed at a constant rate throughout the growth conditions used in this study.

After normalization to the levels of 16S rRNA, gene expression was compared with the average values for the six high enrofloxacin-accumulating susceptible strains.

acrR DNA SEQUENCE ANALYSIS

Mutations in the local repressor gene, *acrR*, and the regulator-binding site were detected by direct DNA sequencing, using previously reported primer sets (Zheng et al., 2009). Amplification of the gene and purification of the resulting amplicon were performed as described before (Zheng et al., 2009). Nucleotide

Table 2 | Primers used in this study.

Primer name	Sequence (5′–3′)	Reference
acrA-F	AAAACGGCAAAGCGAAGGT	Usui et al. (2011)
acrA-R	GTACCGGACTGCGGGAATT	Usui et al. (2011)
acrB-rt1	GGCATTGGGTATGACTGGAC	Zheng et al. (2009)
acrB-rt2	GCATTACGGAGAACGGGATAG	Zheng et al. (2009)
ramA-rt1	TTTCCGCTCAGGTTATCGAC	Zheng et al. (2009)
ramA-rt2	CGGGCAATATCATCAATACG	Zheng et al. (2009)
soxS-rt1	AAATCGGGCTACTCCAAG	Zheng et al. (2009)
soxS-rt2	TACTCGCCTAATGTTTGATG	Zheng et al. (2009)
marA-rt1	ATTCTCTATCTGGCGGAAC	Zheng et al. (2009)
marA-rt2	CGGGTCAATGTTTGCTGTG	Zheng et al. (2009)
robA-rt1	TATTCCGCCAGTGCTTTATG	Zheng et al. (2009)
robA-rt2	CCTGCTCATCGTCTTTCTCC	Zheng et al. (2009)
16S rRNA-F	CCAGCAGCCGCGGTAAT	Usui et al. (2010)
16S rRNA-R	TTTACGCCCAGTAATTCCGATT	Usui et al. (2010)

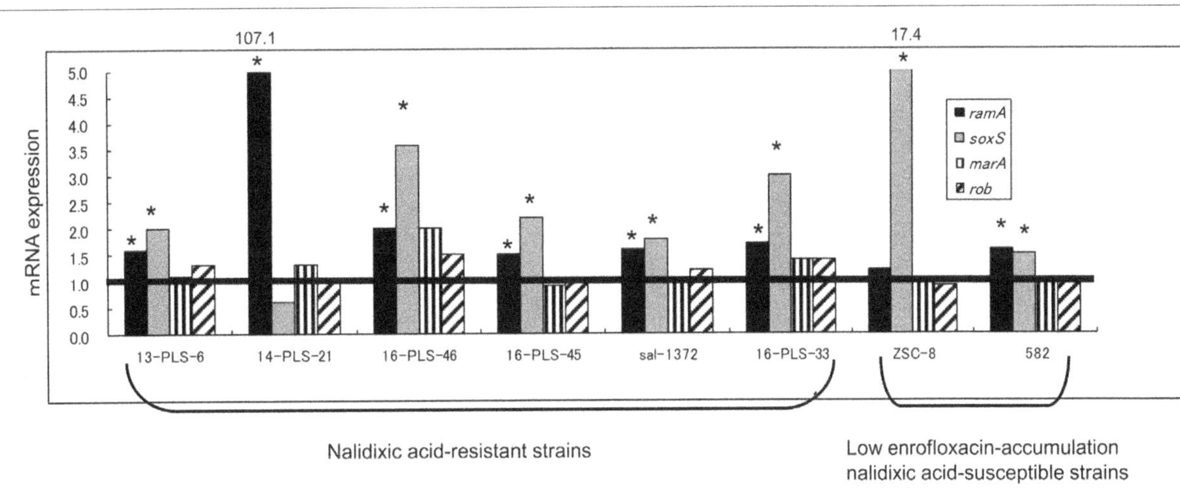

FIGURE 2 | Expression of multiple regulator genes in field isolates of *S.* Choleraesuis. The expression of multiple regulator genes in resistant strains and low enrofloxacin-accumulating nalidixic acid-susceptible strains was compared to the average expression of the corresponding genes in high enrofloxacin-accumulating nalidixic acid-susceptible strains ($n = 6$). Horizontal line indicates the average gene expression in the six susceptible strains, which expressions were set to be 1.0. *Indicates that mRNA expression is significantly higher in a strain compared to mRNA expression in the six susceptible strains ($P < 0.05$).

Table 3 | The MICs of several antimicrobials and gene expressions of *acrB* and multiple regulator genes in laboratory-selected mutants.

Strain no.	Selecting agent[a]	MIC (mg/L)					mRNA expression[c]				
		Enrofloxacin (2)[b]	Ampicillin (32)[b]	Oxytetracycline (16)[b]	Kanamycin (64)[b]	Spectinomycin (128)[b]	*acrB*	*ramA*	*soxS*	*marA*	*rob*
582		0.0625	1	2	2	32	1.4	1.6	1.5	1.1	1.0
582/E	Enrofloxacin	0.25	4	4	2	32	6.9	39.2	0.8	1.2	0.6
582/A	Ampicillin	0.25	4	8	2	32	7.7	89.5	0.3	1.2	0.8
582/O	Oxytetracycline	0.125	4	4	2	32	4.2	9.5	0.3	1.1	0.9
582/K	Kanamycin	0.125	2	4	4	32	3.1	9.0	0.5	1.3	0.6
582/S	Spectinomycin	0.0625	1	2	2	128	1.7	1.4	1.5	1.2	0.8
143		0.0625	1	2	2	32	1.3	1.2	1.2	1.1	1.0
143E	Enrofloxacin	0.25	4	4	2	32	4.3	45.2	0.6	0.9	0.7
143/A	Ampicillin	0.125	4	4	2	32	2.9	38.8	0.1	0.7	0.5
143/O	Oxytetracycline	0.0625	2	8	2	32	2.2	10.2	1.3	1.2	0.3
143/K	Kanamycin	0.0625	2	4	8	32	2.1	9.3	1.1	1.2	0.4
143/S	Spectinomycin	0.0625	1	2	2	128	1.6	0.9	0.9	0.7	0.7
1002		0.0625	1	2	2	32	1.2	1.0	0.8	1.0	1.0
1002/E	Enrofloxacin	0.25	4	4	2	32	8.0	29.8	0.1	1.2	1.0
1002/A	Ampicillin	0.125	4	2	2	32	2.4	16.1	0.1	0.3	0.5
1002/O	Oxytetracycline	0.125	2	8	2	32	2.2	14.7	0.2	1.2	0.9
1002/K	Kanamycin	0.125	2	4	4	32	2.4	14.2	0.3	1.0	0.9
1002/S	Spectinomycin	0.0625	1	2	2	128	1.1	1.4	0.4	1.1	0.9
916*		0.0625	1	2	2	32	1.1	1.1	0.8	0.9	0.9
916/E	Enrofloxacin	0.5	4	4	2	32	7.4	34.2	0.4	0.8	0.9
916/A	Ampicillin	0.25	4	4	2	32	8.5	58.2	0.1	0.9	0.8
916/O	Oxytetracycline	0.0625	1	4	2	32	2.2	3.5	0.2	1.0	0.9
916/K	Kanamycin	0.0625	1	4	8	32	2.2	6.5	0.1	1.0	0.6
916/S	Spectinomycin	0.0625	1	2	2	128	1.2	0.6	0.2	0.7	0.6
419*		0.0625	4	2	2	32	0.9	0.7	1.0	1.0	1.0
419/E	Enrofloxacin	0.25	16	4	2	32	5.7	24.2	0.2	1.7	0.8
419/A	Ampicillin	0.0625	8	2	2	32	1.6	32.5	0.3	0.7	0.9
419/O	Oxytetracycline	0.125	8	8	2	32	3.0	21.8	0.8	3.4	1.6
419/K	Kanamycin	0.0625	8	4	8	32	1.5	18.5	0.3	1.1	0.9
419/S	Spectinomycin	0.0625	4	2	2	128	0.9	1.1	0.4	2.1	1.2
03-197-1*		0.0625	>128	256	2	32	0.8	1.1	1.3	1.2	1.2
03-228-1*		0.0625	1	256	8	32	1.1	1.1	1.0	0.9	0.9
ZSC-14-1*		0.0625	1	256	2	32	1.1	1.0	1.0	1.0	0.8
ZSC-40*		0.0625	>128	256	2	32	0.9	0.8	0.8	1.1	0.9

MIC, minimum inhibitory concentration.

[a]Mutants were selected by exposing to fourth the MIC of the antimicrobials for each susceptible strain.

[b]MIC data of antimicrobials except for spectinomycin in parental strains from a previous report (Asai et al., 2010). Parenthesis indicates break points.

[c]Relative expression level of acrB and multiple regulator genes compared to average of six high accumulation susceptible strains represented as asterisks.

sequences were determined using a BigDye Terminator v3.1 Cycle Sequencing Kit (Applied Biosystems) with a 3130 Genetic Analyzer (Applied Biosystems).

STATISTICAL ANALYSIS

Student's t-test was used to compare results between and within experiments. P-values < 0.05 were considered significant.

RESULTS

RELATIONSHIP BETWEEN THE ENHANCEMENT OF EFFLUX PUMPS AND THE EXPRESSION OF *acrAB*

Expression of *acrA* and *acrB* in the six resistant strains and in the two low enrofloxacin-accumulation nalidixic acid-susceptible strains was significantly higher than that in the other susceptible strains ($P < 0.05$; **Table 1**). Expression levels of *acrB* correlated significantly with those of *acrA* in this study (correlation coefficient: 0.89).

RELATIONSHIP BETWEEN INCREASED EXPRESSION OF *acrB* AND GLOBAL REGULATORS

Of the eight strains with a high *acrB* expression level, six strains showed higher levels of both *ramA* and *soxS* expression compared with the average values for the six high accumulating susceptible strains ($P < 0.05$; **Figure 2**). The remaining strains showed a higher level of *ramA* or *soxS* expression ($P < 0.05$): the 14-PLS-21 strain showed only a higher expression level of *ramA* (107.1-fold ± 42.0-fold), while the ZSC-8 strain showed only a higher expression level of *soxS* (17.4-fold ± 2.7-fold). Neither the expression of *marA* nor that of *rob* changed in any of the strains tested.

SEQUENCING OF THE LOCAL REPRESSOR GENE *acrR* AND OF THE REGULATOR-BINDING SITE

A stop codon mutation in AcrR (glutamine-78-to-terminal; Q78ter) was found in 13 strains (**Table 1**). No significant relationship was found between the Q78ter stop codon mutation in AcrR and the expression of *acrB*. None of the strains tested had a point mutation in the regulator-binding site, which affects the *acrB* expression, previously determined using the *S.* serovar Typhimurium strain BN18 (Olliver et al., 2004).

GENE EXPRESSION IN LABORATORY-SELECTED MUTANTS

Expression levels of both *acrB* and *ramA* increased significantly in AcrAB substrate-selected mutants compared to these levels in parental strains ($P < 0.05$; **Table 3**). Among four AcrAB substrates, a higher level of *ramA* expression was observed in the enrofloxacin- and ampicillin-selected mutants than in the oxytetracycline- and kanamycin-selected mutants ($P < 0.05$). In contrast, the expression of *soxS* decreased significantly in AcrAB substrate-selected mutants compared to that in parental strains ($P < 0.05$; **Table 3**). MICs of AcrAB substrates were increased in AcrAB substrate-selected mutants as compared with those in the parental strains (**Table 3**).

Expression of *acrB* and multiple regulator genes remained stable in spectinomycin-selected mutants. In spectinomycin-selected mutants, MICs of AcrAB substrates were of the same level as compared with those in the parental strains (**Table 3**).

DISCUSSION

The current study showed that the expression of *ramA* and/or *soxS* was associated with *acrAB* overexpression in field isolates of *S.* Choleraesuis. In this study, expression of *ramA*, but not *soxS*, *marA*, or *rob*, was enhanced in laboratory-derived *S.* Choleraesuis mutants selected using antimicrobials that are AcrAB substrates. Several previous studies have reported that *ramA*, but not *soxS*, is involved in activation of the AcrAB-TolC system in *S.* Typhimurium (Ricci et al., 2006; Bailey et al., 2008; Zheng et al., 2009). Interestingly, in this study, *soxS* expression was downregulated in AcrAB substrate-selected mutants of *S.* Choleraesuis. In addition, enrofloxacin- and ampicillin-selected mutants derived from the ZSC-8 strain with a high level of *soxS* expression, showed increased expression of *ramA*, but not of *soxS* (data not shown). Several studies have suggested that increased expression of *ramA* downregulates *soxS* expression (Nikaido et al., 2008; O'Regan et al., 2009). These results suggest that the *acrA* and *acrB* expression in antimicrobial-selected mutants of *S.* Choleraesuis were dependent on *ramA* expression.

The present study showed that increased levels of both *ramA* and *soxS* expression were demonstrated by some field isolates of *S.* Choleraesuis upon activation of the AcrAB-TolC system. There was a marked difference in *soxS* expression between the field isolates and the laboratory-derived strains. As all of the strains used in this study were isolated from diseased pigs, these isolates would have been exposed to antimicrobials and disinfectants used in disease treatment and hygiene management. This suggests that the resistance in some field isolates was mediated through a different mechanism, and therefore could have arisen from a different selective pressure.

Activation of the AcrAB efflux pump is responsible for the emergence of fluoroquinolone-resistant *Salmonella* strains (Ricci et al., 2006; Usui et al., 2009). In Japan, the description of veterinary fluoroquinolone drugs includes an explanation that the drug is considered as a second-line drug. In the AcrAB substrate-selected mutants, the level of *acrB* expression generally increased, depending on *ramA* expression. It is possible that the use of an AcrAB substrate as a first-line drug crucially selects strains of *S.* Choleraesuis with activated AcrAB efflux systems. Among AcrAB substrates used in this study, the degree of *acrB* expression may be different due to exposure to the various antimicrobial agents. Therefore, the antimicrobial class used as first-line drugs may be associated with the frequency of fluoroquinolone resistance in bacterial strains. Further studies are needed in order to clarify the effects of each antimicrobial on *acrB* expression in these bacteria.

In conclusion, the AcrAB-TolC efflux system in field isolates of *S.* Choleraesuis is likely regulated by external factors in the environment, such as antimicrobials and drug residues *via ramA* and *soxS*. In particular, exposure of AcrAB substrates enhances activation of AcrAB *via* RamA in *S.* Choleraesuis.

ACKNOWLEDGMENTS

We would like to thank the staff at the Prefectural Livestock Hygiene Service Center for providing *S.* Choleraesuis isolates. This work was supported in part by a Grant-in Aid from the Ministry of Health, Labor and Welfare of Japan (H21-Shokuhin-Ippan-013).

REFERENCES

Abouzeed, Y. M., Baucheron, S., and Cloeckaert, A. (2008). ramR mutations involved in efflux-mediated multidrug resistance in *Salmonella enterica* serovar Typhimurium. *Antimicrob. Agents Chemother.* 52,2428–2434.

Asai, T., Namimatsu, T., Osumi, T., Kojima, A., Harada, K., Aoki, H., et al. (2010). Molecular typing and antimicrobial resistance of *Salmonella enterica* subspecies *enterica* serovar Choleraesuis isolates from diseased pigs in Japan. *Comp. Immunol. Microbiol. Infect. Dis.* 33, 109–119.

Bailey, A. M., Paulsen, I. T., and Piddock, L. J. (2008). RamA confers multidrug resistance in *Salmonella enterica* via increased expression of *acrB*, which is inhibited by chlorpromazine. *Antimicrob. Agents Chemother.* 52, 3604–3611.

Chen, S., Cui, S., McDermott, P. F., Zhao, S., White, D. G., Paulsen, I., et al. (2007). Contribution of target gene mutations and efflux to decreased susceptibility of *Salmonella enterica* serovar Typhimurium to fluoroquinolones and other antimicrobials. *Antimicrob. Agents Chemother.* 51, 535–542.

Chiu, C. H., Su, L. H., and Chu, C. (2004). *Salmonella enterica* serotype Choleraesuis: epidemiology, pathogenesis, clinical disease, and treatment. *Clin. Microbiol. Rev.* 17, 311–322.

Clinical and Laboratory Standard Institute. (2008). *Performance Standards for Antimicrobial Disk and Dilution Susceptibility Tests for Bacteria Isolated from Animals, Third Edition: Approved Standard M31-A3.* Wayne, PA: Clinical and Laboratory Standard Institute.

Giraud, E., Cloeckaert, A., Kerboeuf, D., and Chaslus-Dancla, E. (2000). Evidence for active efflux as the primary mechanism of resistance to ciprofloxacin in *Salmonella enterica* serovar Typhimurium. *Antimicrob. Agents Chemother.* 44, 1223–1228.

Kim, K. Y., and Woo, G. J. (2011). Expression of *acrB* and *ramA* in fluoroquinolone resistant mutants from multi-drug resistant *Salmonella enterica* serovar Haardt. *Lett. Appl. Microbiol.* 52, 484–490.

Lee, H. Y., Su, L. H., Tsai, M. H., Kim, S. W., Chang, H. H., Jung, S. I., et al. (2009). High rate of reduced susceptibility to ciprofloxacin and ceftriaxone among nontyphoid *Salmonella* clinical isolates in Asia. *Antimicrob. Agents Chemother.* 53, 2696–2699.

Li, X. Z., and Nikaido, H. (2004). Efflux-mediated drug resistance in bacteria. *Drugs* 64, 159–204.

Li, X. Z., and Nikaido, H. (2009). Efflux-mediated drug resistance in bacteria: an update. *Drugs* 69, 1555–1623.

Nikaido, E., Yamaguchi, A., and Nishino, K. (2008). AcrAB multidrug efflux pump regulation in *Salmonella enterica* serovar Typhimurium by RamA in response to environmental signals. *J. Biol. Chem.* 283, 24245–24253.

Olliver, A., Valle, M., Chaslus-Dancla, E., and Cloeckaert, A. (2004). Role of an *acrR* mutation in multidrug resistance of in vitro-selected fluoroquinolone-resistant mutants of *Salmonella enterica* serovar Typhimurium. *FEMS Microbiol. Lett.* 238, 267–272.

O'Regan, E., Quinn, T., Pages, J. M., McCusker, M., Piddock, L., and Fanning, S. (2009). Multiple regulatory pathways associated with high-level ciprofloxacin and multidrug resistance in *Salmonella enterica* serovar enteritidis: involvement of RamA and other global regulators. *Antimicrob. Agents Chemother.* 53, 1080–1087.

Ricci, V., and Piddock, L. J. (2009a). Ciprofloxacin selects for multidrug resistance in *Salmonella enterica* serovar Typhimurium mediated by at least two different pathways. *J. Antimicrob. Chemother.* 63, 909–916.

Ricci, V., and Piddock, L. J. (2009b). Only for substrate antibiotics are a functional AcrAB-TolC efflux pump and RamA required to select multidrug-resistant *Salmonella* Typhimurium. *J. Antimicrob. Chemother.* 64, 654–657.

Ricci, V., Tzakas, P., Buckley, A., and Piddock, L. J. (2006). Ciprofloxacin-resistant *Salmonella enterica* serovar Typhimurium strains are difficult to select in the absence of AcrB and TolC. *Antimicrob. Agents Chemother.* 50, 38–42.

Rosenberg, E. Y., Bertenthal, D., Nilles, M. L., Bertrand, K. P., and Nikaido, H. (2003). Bile salts and fatty acids induce the expression of *Escherichia coli* AcrAB multidrug efflux pump through their interaction with Rob regulatory protein. *Mol. Microbiol.* 48, 1609–1619.

Usui, M., Asai, T., and Sato, S. (2011). Low expression of *acrB* in the deoxycholate-sensitive strains of *Salmonella enterica* subspecies *enterica* serovar Pullorum. *Microbiol. Immunol.* 55, 366–368.

Usui, M., Uchiyama, M., Baba, K., Nagai, H., Yamamoto, Y., and Asai, T. (2010). Contribution of enhanced efflux to reduced susceptibility of *Salmonella enterica* serovar Choleraesuis to fluoroquinolone and other antimicrobials. *J. Vet. Med. Sci.* 73, 279–282.

Usui, M., Uchiyama, M., Iwanaka, M., Nagai, H., Yamamoto, Y., and Asai, T. (2009). Intracellular concentrations of enrofloxacin in quinolone-resistant *Salmonella enterica* subspecies *enterica* serovar Choleraesuis. *Int. J. Antimicrob. Agents* 34, 592–595.

Zheng, J., Cui, S., and Meng, J. (2009). Effect of transcriptional activators RamA and SoxS on expression of multidrug efflux pumps AcrAB and AcrEF in fluoroquinolone-resistant *Salmonella* Typhimurium. *J. Antimicrob. Chemother.* 63, 95–102.

2

Origin and evolution of antibiotic resistance: the common mechanisms of emergence and spread in water bodies

Agnese Lupo[1]*, Sébastien Coyne[2] and Thomas Ulrich Berendonk[1]

[1] Institute of Hydrobiology, Department of Hydrosciences, Technical University Dresden, Dresden, Germany
[2] Department of Biomolecular Chemistry, Leibniz Institute for Natural Product Research and Infection Biology – Hans Knöll Institute, Jena, Germany

Edited by:
Stefania Stefani, University of Catania, Italy

Reviewed by:
Fernando Baquero, Ramón y Cajal Institute for Health Research, Spain
Manuela Coci, National Research Council, Italy

***Correspondence:**
Agnese Lupo, Institute of Hydrobiology, Department of Hydrosciences, Technical University Dresden, Zellescher Weg 40, 01217 Dresden, Germany.
e-mail: agnese.lupo@tu-dresden.de

The environment, and especially freshwater, constitutes a reactor where the evolution and the rise of new resistances occur. In water bodies such as waste water effluents, lakes, and rivers or streams, bacteria from different sources, e.g., urban, industrial, and agricultural waste, probably selected by intensive antibiotic usage, are collected and mixed with environmental species. This may cause two effects on the development of antibiotic resistances: first, the contamination of water by antibiotics or other pollutants lead to the rise of resistances due to selection processes, for instance, of strains over-expressing broad range defensive mechanisms, such as efflux pumps. Second, since environmental species are provided with intrinsic antibiotic resistance mechanisms, the mixture with allochthonous species is likely to cause genetic exchange. In this context, the role of phages and integrons for the spread of resistance mechanisms appears significant. Allochthonous species could acquire new resistances from environmental donors and introduce the newly acquired resistance mechanisms into the clinics. This is illustrated by clinically relevant resistance mechanisms, such as the fluoroquinolones resistance genes *qnr*. Freshwater appears to play an important role in the emergence and in the spread of antibiotic resistances, highlighting the necessity for strategies of water quality improvement. We assume that further knowledge is needed to better understand the role of the environment as reservoir of antibiotic resistances and to elucidate the link between environmental pollution by anthropogenic pressures and emergence of antibiotic resistances. Only an integrated vision of these two aspects can provide elements to assess the risk of spread of antibiotic resistances via water bodies and suggest, in this context, solutions for this urgent health issue.

Keywords: water, freshwater, antibiotic resistance, environment, gene transfer

INTRODUCTION

Evolution of bacterial antibiotic resistances, and its spread and emergence, represent one of the most threatening health care problems with worldwide proportions (Hawkey, 2008). The rise of new resistances and of multi-drug resistances urgently asks for a better understanding of the factors and hot spots involved in its diffusion and development. All the known antibiotic resistance mechanisms, acquired by opportunistic and pathogenic bacteria, evolve by means of Darwinian forces, i.e., mutations occurring in pre-existing genes of the bacterial chromosome positively selected by environmental forces (Gullberg et al., 2011; Zhang et al., 2011). Mutations within the chromosome can be responsible for the decreased affinity of antibiotics to their targets. Furthermore, some resistance mechanisms (e.g., efflux pumps, chromosomal AmpC β-lactamases) are finely regulated in their expression and at a basal level confer a naturally reduced susceptibility to the drugs. Mutations in the genomic architectures regulating such mechanisms result in their over-expression and high level of antibiotic resistance (Jacoby, 2009; Coyne et al., 2011). However, adaptation to the selective pressure of antibiotics accelerates acquisition of antibiotic resistance genes by lateral transfer from donor species (Wiedenbeck and Cohan, 2011). Aminov (2011) has reviewed the role of horizontal gene transfer mechanisms in environmental microbiota. Although many more studies are necessary to completely understand the role of horizontal gene transfer in the environment, experimental evidences have demonstrated that transduction has an important role in genetic exchanges among environmental microbiota, especially in freshwater. Horizontal gene transfer events are responsible for the acquisition of heterologous resistance mechanisms among species and from antibiotic producers to commensal and pathogen bacteria. Hospitals, human community, farms, aquacultures, and agriculture are reactors where the usage of antibiotics selects for resistant bacteria and promotes the gene exchange. Recently, much more attention has focused on the role of the environment and of connected ecological habitats, water bodies such as rivers, streams, waste water effluents, and lakes, that have been suggested to be important in facilitating the transport and transfer of the antibiotic resistance genes (Aminov and Mackie, 2007; Baquero et al., 2008). Low-cost pharmaceuticals, preventative medication with broad spectrum antibiotics together with the overuse of those drugs contribute significantly to the emergence of bacterial drug resistances (Depledge, 2011). The combination of all these factors together with an inadequate waste-management of the pharmaceuticals seem to be responsible for the alarming pollution of the environmental habitats such as agricultural soils and rivers, which probably contribute to the selection of antibiotic resistant bacteria and speed up the emergence of new resistances. Furthermore, rivers often receive bacteria from different sources, e.g., waste water treatment plants or water originating from urban effluent, industrial, or agricultural activities, thus constituting potential compartments where environmental, human, and/or animal related bacteria can coexist, at least temporally (Baquero et al., 2008). This mixing can result in two main risks: (i) many environmental bacterial species are provided with intrinsic antibiotic resistance genes, constituting part of the so-called resistome. These bacteria represent a reservoir of drug resistance mechanisms and may act as donors for human related bacteria which, in turn, could introduce new acquired resistance mechanisms in the clinics (Wright, 2010); (ii) due to the intensive usage of antibiotics in medicine, agriculture, and aquaculture, human or animal related bacteria are more likely to be selected for antibiotic resistances within polluted environments directly by the presence of antibiotics and indirectly through co-selection by other pollutants (Martinez, 2009). Thus, when antibiotic resistant bacteria contaminate rivers, their resistance mechanisms can spread in the environment through bacteria, and/or mobile genetic elements. The localization of antibiotic resistance genes on diverse genetic structures such as integrons, which are platforms for gene aggregation, and mobile genetic elements (e.g., transposons and plasmids), together with the presence of phages, enhance their spread, influencing the course of their evolution (Wright et al., 2008). In particular, integrons are supposed to have a crucial role in the development of multi-drug resistances (Cambray et al., 2010). Recent studies suggest that the spread of resistant bacteria in natural fresh water systems can reach drinking water supplies and thus enter the human food chain (Walsh et al., 2011). These factors lead to an unlimited spread of antibiotic resistances and indicate that water sanitation or a better management of the respective water quality is crucial for a better control of the spread of antibiotic resistances.

This review aims to describe the current knowledge on the origins of antibiotic resistances mechanisms and environmental reservoirs of antibiotic resistances. Mechanisms, originating and spreading in bacterial populations naturally occurring in the water habitats, will be highlighted. The consequences of horizontal gene transfer by transduction and gene recombination events mediated by integrons in water habitats will be underlined. The **Table 1** summarizes the mechanisms of resistances cited in the review.

MUTATIONS AND THE RISE OF ANTIBIOTIC RESISTANCES IN FRESH WATER HABITATS

Mutations in environmental habitats occur frequently and usually depend on evolutionary or demographic factors such as population size etc. Generally, the rate of mutations can be increased due to anthropogenic impacts. However, especially antibiotics in the environment are more likely to select for specific mutations within bacteria. We summarize which mutations are most relevant in the context of antibiotic resistance in water habitats and might therefore be selected to a higher frequency due to the presence of antibiotics in water bodies.

In the clinics it has often been observed that the onset of spontaneous mutations in chromosomal bacterial genes may lead to the emergence of resistances affecting from one antibiotic to several drug classes of antibiotics. For instance, different point mutations in ribosomal proteins confer aminoglycosides, tetracyclines, and macrolides resistance; or in the RNA polymerase confer rifampicin resistance. To the best of our knowledge, these mechanisms have never been reported in bacteria of environmental origin, most likely because they have been overlooked.

Mutations in the penicillin binding proteins (PBPs) can lead to a decreased affinity for β-lactams drugs establishing bacterial resistance (Lambert, 2005). This mechanism has been extensively reported from clinical species. Although no direct reports exist from environmental sources, bacterial species such as *Enterococcus faecium* and *Proteus mirabilis* have been described to resist to β-lactams by mutations in PBP5 and PBP2 respectively. *E. faecium* has been frequently reported as contaminant of water body and *P. mirabilis* has been described as shuttle species between human or animal guts and water bodies (Sosa et al., 2006). The risk associated with the spread of organisms harboring such mechanisms is probably low. However, investigations to understand the link between PBP modification and fitness in terms of survival in water could yield significant information, to better assess the risk of spread for these species and antibiotic resistances. Probably, the role of mutations in the propagation and emergence of antibiotic resistant bacteria is minor compared to the acquisition of heterologous determinants. However, it seems that also very low concentrations of antibiotics can select for less susceptible bacteria (Gullberg et al., 2011). In environmental habitats this could result in an ecological imbalance with a higher prevalence of resistant microorganisms.

CHROMOSOMALLY ENCODED CEPHALOSPORINASE

Bacteria, especially Gram-negative, can also resist to β-lactams by the production of hydrolytic enzymes, β-lactamases. Detection of antibiotic resistant bacteria, in freshwater, harboring β-lactamases has been reported from several geographical areas. Clinical occurrence of β-lactamases encoding genes has been extensively reviewed (Bonnet, 2004; Pitout et al., 2005; Coque et al., 2008; Bush, 2010) and recently much attention to their propagation in the environment has been paid (see hereafter the section on acquired β-lactamases). According to Ambler (1980) β-lactamases are classified in four classes, simplistically ranging from A to D. Bush and Jacoby have proposed a categorization of the β-lactamases according to their hydrolytic and inhibitory profiles. For an exhaustive knowledge of β-lactamases nomenclature and biochemical characteristics, we suggest the recent review by Bush and Fisher (2011). Jacoby (2009) has reviewed the distribution, origins, and enzymatic action of AmpC β-lactamases, belonging to the class C. The author has observed that *amp*C genes are located on the chromosome of bacteria belonging to different and phylogenetically distant species. *amp*C genes are widely distributed in bacterial species of environmental origins. Water borne species such as *Aeromonas* spp., *Pseudomonas aeruginosa*, *Pseudomonas fluorescens*, *Ochrobactrum anthropi*, as well as several Enterobacteriaceae, commonly found in water habitats, like *Enterobacter* spp., *Morganella morganii*, and *Hafnia alvei* harbor chromosomal *amp*C genes. Typically, *amp*C genes are regulated

Table 1 | Overview of some mechanisms of bacterial antibiotic resistances occurring in water habitats.

Antibiotic	Resistance mechanism	Host	Source
β-Lactams	PBP2 mutations	*Proteus mirabilis*	–[a]
	PBP5 mutations	*Enterococcus faecium*	–[a]
	*amp*C regulators mutations	Gram-negative species	–[a]
	*amp*C promoter region mutations	*Escherichia coli*	Recreational beaches, drinking water
	Acquired AmpC	*E. coli*	Recreational beaches, drinking water, river, biofilm of water supplies
	Acquired CTX-M	*E. coli*	River, sediment, birds
	Acquired KPC	*Klebsiella pneumoniae*	Hospital waste water effluent
	Acquired VIM	*Brevundimonas diminuta, Rhizobium radiobacter, Pseudomonas monteilii, Pseudomonas aeruginosa, Ochrobactrum anthropi, Enterobacter ludwigii, Pseudomonas pseudoalcaligenes*	Hospital waste water effluent
	Acquired IMP	*Pseudomonas fluorescens*	Waste water
	Acquired OXA-23	*Acinetobacter baumannii*	River, hospital waste water effluent
	Acquired OXA-48	*Serratia marcescens*	River
	Acquired NDM-1	*P. aeruginosa, Achromobacter* spp., *Kingella denitrificans*	Tap water
Fluoroquinolones	QRDR (quinolones resistance determining region) mutations	*P. aeruginosa*	Hospital and urban waste water effluent
		Aeromonas spp., *E. coli*	River and lake, urban effluent
	QnrS	*Aeromonas allosaccarophila*	Lake
		E. coli	River
	QnrS2	*Aeromonas punctata, Aeromonas media*	Lake
	QnrVC4	*A. punctata*	Waste water effluent
	QepA efflux	Metagenome	River sediment, water from farm environment
	OqxAB efflux	*E. coli*	Farm water
Vancomycin	modification of the peptidoglycan	*Enterococci* spp.	Waste water effluents, biofilm
Chloramphenicol and florfenicol	FloR efflux	Gram-negative species *Aeromonas bestiarium*	Aquacultures streams
Tetracyclines	Tet efflux	Several species	Farms, sediment
MDR[b]	Over-expression of RND efflux pumps	Gram-negative	–[a]

[a] Observed in clinics but likely occurring in environmental and water habitats.
[b] MDR, multi-drug resistance.

and their expression is induced in the presence of β-lactams. The regulation of *amp*C expression is quite complex and has been reviewed for *P. aeruginosa* by Lister et al. (2009). Mutations in the transcription factor AmpR, a LysR-type transcriptional regulator, in the inner membrane permease AmpG, or in the cytosolic amidase AmpD, have been found to confer a constitutive expression of the cephalosporinase gene, even in the absence of antibiotics.

Mataseje et al. (2009) described the over-expression of *amp*C, by mutations in the promoter region, in *Escherichia coli* strains isolated from recreational beaches and drinking water (**Table 1**). As for other β-lactamases, chromosomal cephalosporinases have been described to evolve by point mutation, hydrolyzing a broader spectrum of β-lactams (Jacoby, 2009). Of particular concern is the plasmidic location of several *amp*C genes, which likely originated from the chromosomal cephalosporinase of environmental species. Details will be discussed in the section on acquired β-lactamases. AmpC enzymes are indistinguishable from the D-peptidases, involved in the cell wall biosynthesis (Jacoby, 2009). Thus, these enzymes probably adapted to confer β-lactams resistance from the natural physiological function, likely by gene duplication and mutation events (Sandegren and Andersson, 2009). Genes encoding AmpC enzymes are largely distributed on the chromosomes of many bacterial species of environmental origins. The intrinsic function of AmpC remains unknown, but the conservation of this enzyme in several unrelated species and the complex regulation of its structural gene highly suggests a physiological role. Deciphering this role could provide useful information on the evolutionary processes and driving forces that have lead to the selection of β-lactamases.

DNA GYRASE AND TOPO-ISOMERASE

Generally, mutations in the quinolone resistance determining region (QRDR) of *gyr*A, *gyr*B, *par*C, and *par*E genes coding for the bacterial DNA gyrase and the topo-isomerase IV respectively, are responsible for the onset of bacterial resistance to fluoroquinolones. This mechanism is known to occur in water environments. Schwartz et al. (2006) have detected ciprofloxacin resistant *P. aeruginosa* in six different treatment plants from four cities in Germany receiving the waste water from hospitals and cities. Molecular investigations demonstrated the occurrence of mutations in *gyr*A and *par*C genes. Further, the study demonstrated the spread of the ciprofloxacin resistant *P. aeruginosa* also in the waste water receiving river (**Table 1**). Alcaide et al. (2010) have reported about the *gyr*A and *par*C mutation conferring fluoroquinolones resistances in a variety of *Aeromonas* spp. isolated from freshwater. The authors found that the mutations in *gyr*A and *par*C, which are responsible for fluoroquinolones resistance, in recently described *Aeromonas* spp. such as *Aeromonas media, Aeromonas veronii,* and *Aeromonas popoffi* are similar to the one described in *Aeromonas hydrophila, Aeromonas sobria, Aeromonas caviae,* and *Aeromonas salmonicida.* In Portugal, Figueira et al. (2011) reported about mutations in *gyr*A and *par*C mostly linked to *Aeromonas punctata* and *A. media* isolated from an urban effluent. The same authors have recently characterized *E. coli* strains, isolated from a waste water effluent, that harbored mutations in *gyr*A and *par*C genes, likely responsible for the observed ciprofloxacin resistance (**Table 1**).

EFFLUX PUMPS

The role of efflux pumps in conferring antibiotic resistance and multi-drug resistances in bacteria has been extensively studied and reviewed (Poole, 2004; Piddock, 2006; Martinez, 2009; Nikaido and Pages, 2011). Efflux systems conferring drug resistance typically belong to five main families: the ATP-binding cassette (ABC) transporter, the major facilitator superfamily (MFS), the small multi-drug resistance (SMR), the multi-drug and toxic-compound extrusion (MATE), and the resistance nodulation division (RND) families, the latter present only in Gram-negative bacteria and chromosomally located. The structural genes for these systems can be located on transferable genetic elements and constitute the main acquired mechanisms for drug resistance (e.g., the Tet and the CmlA/FloR efflux systems families for tetracycline and chloramphenicol resistance, respectively). However, bacteria are intrinsically provided with chromosomally encoded efflux systems that are believed to participate in the cell homeostasy, by extruding endo and/or exogenous toxic compounds, heavy metals, virulence factors, quorum sensing signal, etc. In Gram-negative bacteria, RND systems exhibit a wide substrate spectrum, which usually includes drugs of different classes. Nikaido and Pages (2011) have recently reviewed the role of these efflux pumps in a wide range of pathogenic and opportunistic bacterial species such as *E. coli, Klebsiella pneumoniae, Enterobacter* spp., *P. aeruginosa, Acinetobacter baumannii,* and the emergent opportunistic *Stenotrophomonas maltophilia.* Typically, the expression of RND efflux pumps is finely regulated by a dedicated regulator (Coyne et al., 2011). A more complex regulation network, linking efflux to membrane permeability and other cellular functions, is likely to occur in these bacteria, as described for the *mar* regulon in *E. coli* (reviewed by Grkovic et al., 2002). Some RND efflux genes are not expressed in absence of inducing signal, whereas others exhibit a basal level of expression, and therefore contribute to intrinsic resistance (Coyne et al., 2011). Point mutations in a regulator or in the promoter sequence of RND efflux genes can be responsible for their over-expression and, in turn, for enhanced resistance. Similarly, the acquisition of an insertion sequence, carrying a strong and constitutive promoter, upstream of the regulator or the promoter sequence of RND efflux genes, can also mediate their over-expression and cause drug resistance. These systems have been mostly studied in the context of antibiotic resistance; therefore only little information concerning the natural and physiological mechanisms inducing the expression of RND efflux genes exist. Recently, studies have identified the role of oxidative and nitrosative stress in the activation of MexXY and MexEF–OprN, respectively (Fetar et al., 2011; Fraud and Poole, 2011). These stress signals are likely to occur in the environment and might represent natural inducers of the efflux systems expression. The natural role of efflux systems has been extensively reviewed by Martinez et al. (2009) who concluded that the intrinsic role of efflux in the bacterial physiology has lead to the conservation of the genes coding for efflux pumps among species of the same genus. For example, if the over-expression of *mdf*A confers MDR to *E. coli,* a basal expression is involved in the $Na^+(K^+)/H^+$ antiport, that allows the pH homeostasis of the cell (Lewinson and Bibi, 2001). Efflux pumps conferring resistance to antibiotics, such as the AcrAB–TolC from *Salmonella* spp. has also been shown to efflux bile salts, therefore conferring a selective advantage which allowed colonizing and surviving in human or animal intestines (Lacroix et al., 1996). Mosqueda and Ramos (2000) described the contribution of efflux pumps in the cellular extrusion of toluene, an organic solvent, in *Pseudomonas putida.* This species, able to grow on the liquid interface of water and toluene and to survive in highly contaminated environments, extrudes the solvent by the TtgABC pump. The genes coding for this RND efflux pump usually exhibit a basal expression level but are induced by the presence of toluene in the medium. In water sediment, Groh et al. (2007) demonstrated that a MexF-like pump from *Shewanella oneidensis,* further than contributing to resistance to tetracycline and chloramphenicol, confers an increased fitness in anoxic environments. The underlying mechanism is unclear but could involve the extrusion of toxic compounds. A well documented role, for some efflux pumps, is their involvement in the cell to cell communication. This function has been demonstrated for MexAB–OprM in *P. aeruginosa* (Evans et al., 1998), BpeAB–OprB in *Burkholderia pseudomallei* (Chan and Chua, 2005) and AcrAB–TolC in Enterobacteriaceae (Rahmati et al., 2002). These RND pumps, further than extruding homoserine lactones, are also able to confer MDR. Moreover, several reports have shown that efflux pumps, notably from the RND family, are involved in mechanisms leading to bacterial virulence. For example, Piddock (2006) highlighted the crucial role of efflux pumps in extruding abiotic substances such as flavonoids during plant colonization and in establishing virulence. In antibiotic producing bacteria, efflux pumps play a crucial role as a self defense mechanism by extruding the bioactive secondary metabolites. For instance, an efflux-mediated self-resistance has been developed in the oxytetracycline-producing *Streptomyces rimosus* (Petkovic et al., 2006). Bacteria living in the same habitat, being exposed to the produced antibiotics, could either adapt their intrinsic mechanisms, e.g., by the over-expression of an efflux pump, or acquire by horizontal gene transfer the resistance mechanism from the producers. The first option would require a point mutation to over-express a pre-existing efflux system able to pump out the toxic compound, whereas the second pathway would involve the mobilization and transfer of the gene coding for the self-protecting mechanism. Thus, efflux pumps had an ecological role much before they conferred drug resistances in clinics, as they constitute a selective advantage in presence of competing microorganisms. The massive usage of these drugs has further selected optimized mechanisms and enhanced their spread. The role of mobile and mobilizing genetic elements, such as insertion sequences, integrons, transposons, and plasmids, were critical for a successful and rapid spread. Nikaido and Pages (2011) have observed that the rise of resistance due to efflux pumps mechanisms in clinics is tightly linked to the sub-inhibitory concentration of the antibiotics during clinical therapies. Consequently, the appearance of this kind of resistance favors the emergence of other mechanisms such as reduced membrane permeability to drugs, increase of point mutation in the drug target genes or activation of enzymatic resistance mechanisms. It would be of interest to investigate this aspect of resistance development in environmental habitats, where the concentration of antibiotics varies dependent on the degree of pollution and where other selective forces are present. Especially, heavy metals, naturally present in the soil, and solvents produced as consequences of metabolic activities, have been demonstrated to be substrates of several efflux pumps conferring multi-drug resistance (Silver and Phung, 1996; Moken et al., 1997). Concerning heavy metals, pumps have the additional role to defend bacteria from a toxic excess and to maintain the proper intra-cellular concentration for co-factors and enzymes (Teitzel et al., 2006). The presence of these compounds in freshwater could therefore select for the over-expression of an intrinsic efflux pump. Some heavy metals efflux genes, notably from the SMR family, are located on R plasmids containing antibiotic resistance genes, and heavy metals may favor the co-selection of these two features. In the environment, maintenance and propagation of antibiotic resistance genes might have been promoted by heavy metals selection (Martinez et al., 2009). Moreover, a causal relationship between pollution of the water environment by antibiotics or other pollutants agents and the selection of bacteria expressing or over-expressing efflux pumps appears conceivable. Hernandez et al. (2011a) have recently demonstrated *in vitro* how triclosan, a detergent antibiotic used in cosmetic, binds the regulator SmeT of the SmeDEF pump in *S. maltophilia*, leading to the over-expression of the pump and consequent multi-drug resistance. This observation is of major concern since *S. maltophilia* is an aquatic species that can be responsible for nosocomial infection.

Until now, it remains unclear how the efflux pumps contribute to the emergence of resistant bacteria in the environment. It has been demonstrated that an efflux pump over-expression could be coupled with a reduced bacterial fitness. However, this is not a general rule. Sanchez et al. (2002) investigated the fitness of two *P. aeruginosa* mutants over-expressing the MexAB–OprM and MexCD–OprJ efflux pumps, both conferring multi-drug resistance. The authors demonstrated *in vitro* that the MexAB–OprM over-expressing mutant showed a significantly decreased survival in water compared to the wild type strain, while no significant differences were observed for the second efflux pump mutant. In addition, the production of biofilm in both mutants was not affected if not promoted in the MexCD–OprJ mutant. Production of biofilm implies a higher probability of survival in natural water ecosystem and would thus constitute a beneficial characteristic. Selection in polluted environments of opportunistic species such as *P. aeruginosa*, *S. maltophilia*, or *A. baumannii*, over-expressing efflux systems could contribute to the spread of these bacteria and their introduction into clinics. It would be interesting to focus on the above described mechanisms also in water environments, to gain a better understanding of their physiological function and their role in the emergence of bacterial drug resistance.

ACQUISITION OF GENES IN WATER HABITATS AND DEVELOPMENT OF ANTIBIOTIC RESISTANCES

Acquisition of heterologous genes by lateral transfer largely facilitate the adaptive evolution of bacteria, especially under strong selective pressures. Transfer of exogenous DNA in bacteria may be mediated by plasmids, phages, transposons, genomic islands, or captation of free DNA by transformation. Sengelov and Sorensen (1998) have found that in environments such as bulk water, plasmid transfer from a donor to a recipient cell occur, even at a low frequency. Taylor et al. (2011) have observed that several factors could, not only influence, but also promote gene transfer among bacteria in water environment. One such factor is filter feeding organisms that collect bacteria belonging to different species and concentrate them at high density in a reduced space, facilitating gene exchange. Biofilm matrix in water habitats also creates favorable conditions both for plasmid exchange and transformation process (Molin and Tolker-Nielsen, 2003). Interestingly, Meibom et al. (2005) have demonstrated how chitin present in the crustacean exoskeletons is able to activate the competence status of *Vibrio cholerae*, and thus enhance transformation by acquisition of exogenous DNA. Although they are not classified as mobile genetic elements, integrons are platforms for genes aggregation, and thus contribute to MDR development. Furthermore, the abundance of integrons in bacterial communities of water habitats seems to be associated with the degree of water bodies' pollution (Wright et al., 2008). Many findings support the crucial role of genetic transfer in water habitats mediated by phages (Ripp and Miller, 1995).

INTEGRONS

Several studies have highlighted the crucial role of integrons, particularly class 1 integrons, in the evolution of antibiotic resistances in clinics (Cambray et al., 2010). Indeed, class 1 integrons are not only platforms for genes aggregation, leading to the establishment of multi-drug resistance, but their localization on mobile genetic elements such as plasmids and transposons favor the spread of several genes in a unique transfer event. Recently, studies on environmental microbial communities have demonstrated that integrons of class 1 are largely present in the environment. Gillings et al. (2008) have provided evidences that the clinical class 1 integrons originated from environmental bacterial communities. The authors observed that class 1 integrons isolated from environmental samples do not carry any antibiotic resistance gene and harbored the *qac* gene cassettes, which is responsible for the bacterial resistance to quaternary ammoniums by efflux. Clinical class 1 integrons would have arisen from environmental ones by integration on a *Tn*402-like transposon, which then disseminated in human commensals and pathogens. The presence of the *qac* gene has conferred a selective advantage to adapt in clinical environments, where bacteria are often challenged by disinfectants. The establishment of class 1 integrons in clinical strains has later on enabled the acquisition of antibiotic resistances positively selected by the usage of drugs. This hypothesis is also supported by the fact that clinical class 1 integrons demonstrated similar structures among them, in terms of integrases and recombination site, inferring a common ancestor. Gaze et al. (2005) have demonstrated how pollution of water bodies and their sediments with quaternary ammonium compounds, directly select for bacteria harboring *qac*E gene cassettes, located on the class 1 integrons. Furthermore, evidence of selection of bacteria harboring class 1 integrons in water bodies contaminated by industrial waste has been provided by Wright et al. (2008). The authors demonstrated that the contamination of freshwater with heavy metals correlated positively with a higher abundance of class 1 integrons in the bacterial community. More recently, Gaze et al. (2011) showed in sewage sludge and pig slurry that the prevalence of class 1 integrons and of *qac* genes was higher in bacteria exposed to detergents and/or antibiotic residues. All these studies demonstrate that pollution of water bodies with different agents increases the risk of selection and spread of integron structures. These genetic structures may be acquired by bacterial species that play role as shuttle between environment and clinics, constituting gene vectors for further dissemination in nosocomial bacteria.

PHAGES

Phages are major constituents of environmental ecosystems, in particular freshwater (Weinbauer, 2004; Srinivasiah et al., 2008). Their abundance is usually higher than bacterial abundance and, since a significant fraction of the prokaryotic community is infected with phages in aquatic systems, phages are likely to play an important role in horizontal gene transfer. Parsley et al. (2010) have proven the presence of β-lactamases genes in the viral metagenome of an activated sludge, confirming that transduction events may be responsible for the propagation of antibiotic resistance genes in these environments. Interestingly, Colomer-Lluch et al. (2011) demonstrated the presence of bla_{TEM} and $bla_{\text{CTX-M}}$, the most common genes conferring β-lactams resistance in Enterobacteriaceae, and *mec*A, responsible for methicillin resistance in *Staphylococcus aureus*, in phage DNA isolated from a waste water treatment plant and the natural water of the receiving river.

The presence of *mec*A in the phage fraction of natural freshwater is of great sanitary concern because of the threat represented by methicillin resistant *Staphylococcus aureus* (MRSA) infections, both in hospitals and communities (Campanile et al., 2011). This finding is also of interest for the understanding of the propagation of this gene. *mec*A codes for a protein with a low affinity to penicillin (PBP2a), conferring methicillin resistance. This gene is located on a mobile genomic element, the staphylococcal cassette chromosome (SCC*mec*), and has been reported only from the *Staphylococcus* genus from clinics. Baba et al. (2009) have characterized a methicillin resistance gene complex, $mecIRA_m$, which could be the progenitor of SCC*mec* observed in clinical MRSA, from a strain of *Macrococcus caseolyticus* (closely related to *S. aureus*), isolated from animal meat. Interestingly, Tsubakishita et al. (2010) found a *mec*A gene in *S. fleurettii* chromosomally located and not associated to the SCC*mec* element. Thus, the authors advanced the hypothesis that *S. fleurettii*, an animal related species, is the progenitor of this resistance mechanism. The *mec*A gene has been reported rarely from natural water, but Schwartz et al. (2003) detected *mec*A in hospital waste waters. Later, Bockelmann et al. (2009) have reported the sporadic presence of *mec*A in a ground water recharge system. Kassem et al. (2008) described the presence of the *mec*A gene in 18 *Proteus vulgaris*, four *M. morganii*, and three *Enterococcus faecalis* isolated from surface water. A ca. 250 bp-sequence of *mec*A from one representative isolate of *P. vulgaris*, *M. morganii*, and *E. faecalis* was found to exhibit 100% similarity with the *S. aureus mec*A gene. However, this result, which is the first report of *MecA* in non-staphylococcal organisms, has never been confirmed by other studies or investigated further. Acquisition by transduction of heterologous genes, particularly of antibiotic resistance genes, might represent an important mechanism of horizontal gene transfer in water bodies. Considering the high concentration of phages in such environments (Weinbauer, 2004; Srinivasiah et al., 2008), transduction constitutes probably one of the main gene transfer mechanisms and of genome evolution for bacteria in water habitats. More studies are needed to understand the impact of phage communities on bacterial evolution and antibiotic resistance spread within the water bodies.

ORIGINS OF ACQUIRED ANTIBIOTIC RESISTANCE MECHANISMS

Recently, D'Costa et al. (2011) have reported a metagenomic analysis of the Beringian permafrost, which is 30,000 years old. They showed molecular evidences of the ancient origins of antibiotic resistances, detecting β-lactamases genes, *van*X-like, component of the vancomycin resistance operon, and *tet*M, coding for a protein protecting the ribosomal target from tetracycline. Sequence analysis revealed that the β-lactamases genes recovered from the permafrost demonstrated an amino-acid homology (53–84%) to known β-lactamases from β-lactams producing *Streptomyces*. The *tet*M sequences revealed a high similarity to the genes coding for the ribosomal protection protein of actinomycetes. The *van*X sequence showed a similarity to the *van*X gene recovered in pathogenic vancomycin resistant enterococci (VRE) and to the *van*X gene from *Amycolatopsis orientalis*. This environmental species, belonging to the actinobacteria phylum, is a natural producer of vancomycin, and very likely the progenitor of the *van* genes operons, responsible for resistance to vancomycin. The integration of the *van* operons on transposons and on conjugative plasmids has enhanced their spread (Courvalin, 2006). Reports of VRE in freshwater have been provided by several authors (Talebi et al., 2008; Lata et al., 2009; Luczkiewicz et al., 2010). Interestingly, Schwartz et al. (2003) detected *van*A genes in the biofilm of drinking water supplies, in the absence of enterococci, demonstrating the lateral transfer of this gene. Notably, the progenitors of these resistance genes are soil bacteria thus most likely, a shuttle has been responsible for the introduction of these genes into the commensal bacterial community and afterward into the pathogenic species.

FLUOROQUINOLONES RESISTANCE BY TARGET PROTECTION

Resistance mechanisms originating from bacterial population of water bodies are less well documented than from soil organisms. However, the significance of water bodies as natural source for resistance mechanisms is similar compared to the soil. For example, a well known example is provided by the acquired fluoroquinolones resistance genes of the *qnr* family. *qnr* genes encode proteins binding the bacterial DNA gyrase, thus preventing the interaction of the antibiotic with its target. Generally, the presence of these acquired genes does not confer a high level of fluoroquinolones resistance, but provides a selective advantage in the presence of these drugs, even at low concentrations (Rodriguez-Martinez et al., 2011). Further, this protecting mechanism and the associated low level resistance may favor the emergence of strains with higher resistances to fluoroquinolones by mutations in the QRDR, quinolones resistance determining region, and/or by over-expressing efflux systems. Several aquatic bacterial species have been proposed as progenitors for these genes families. Poirel et al. (2005b) reported evidences that the *qnr*A gene located on plasmids and found in clinical isolates of fluoroquinolones resistant Enterobacteriaceae, is derived from the chromosome of *Shewanella algae*, a bacterial species present in marine and freshwater. The authors advanced the hypothesis that the gene jumped from the environmental species to Enterobacteriaceae probably under pressure of antibiotic usage. Beaber et al. (2004) have demonstrated that the presence of fluoroquinolones induces the SOS bacterial repair system, which in turn promotes horizontal gene transfer. Poirel et al. (2005a) conducted further investigations in order to understand the origin of this antibiotic resistance mechanism. Their study highlighted that the chromosomes of water borne bacteria, *Vibrio vulnificus*, *Vibrio parahaemolyticus*, and *Photobacterium profundum* harbored *qnr*-like genes with homology (40–67% identity) to the plasmidic *qnr*A, *qnr*B, and *qnr*S genes described in clinical Enterobacteriaceae.

Interestingly, *qnr*A has been observed frequently associated with the insertion sequence IS*CR1*, a genetic element able to mobilize adjacent genes. Toleman et al. (2006) hypothesized that the IS*CR1* mediated mobilization of *qnr*A, as well as a further localization on a class 1 integron to form a so-called complex integron structure. The authors formulated that this complex integron structure is responsible for the successful dissemination of *qnr*A gene. Arsène and Leclercq (2007) investigated the intrinsic resistance of *E. faecalis* to fluoroquinolones and found that this species is provided with a chromosomal *qnr*-like gene, which contributes to resistance against fluoroquinolones. Soon afterward, Sánchez et al. (2008) discovered that the aquatic bacterium *S. maltophilia* is a sink of *qnr* genes and the chromosomally located *Sm*qnr gene identified in this species is able to confer resistance to fluoroquinolones in heterologous species. In 2010, Velasco et al. (2010) reported *qnr*-like genes from *Serratia marcescens*, an environmental species. These genes, called *Sma*qnr, were largely present in the chromosome of the genus. Recently, Jacoby et al. (2011) have highlighted that the *Citrobacter* spp. chromosome constitutes a reservoir for the *qnr*B fluoroquinolones resistance gene. The presence of *qnr* genes on the chromosome of phylogenetically distant bacterial species (*Shewanella*, *Stenotrophomonas*, *Vibrio*, *Enterococcus*, *Serratia*, *Citrobacter*), suggests an ancestral role of this antibiotic resistance mechanism. Hernandez et al. (2011b) postulated a regulatory role for the Qnr proteins. Indeed, by interacting with the DNA gyrase, Qnr may protect the DNA gyrase against toxic DNA substances and indirectly modulate gene expression in response to environmental changes. Moreover, a beneficial role of these protecting mechanisms has been shown for *qnr*A3, which confers a fitness advantage to the bacteria, favoring its dissemination. The fitness advantage was found abolished when *qnr*A3 was carried by large multi-drug resistance plasmids (Michon et al., 2011). The activation of *qnr*B expression by the SOS-response system could also have an implication in the conservation of such mechanism. As ciprofloxacin induces the SOS-response system, it activates its corresponding resistance mechanisms (Da Re et al., 2009). Several studies have reported *qnr* genes in heterologous species from water habitats. Cattoir et al. (2008) recovered from the Seine River *A. punctata* and *A. media* harboring *qnr*S2. Similarly, Picao et al. (2008) detected *qnr*S genes in *Aeromonas allosaccarophila* from the Lugano Lake, in Switzerland. A *qnr*VC4 allele was isolated from aquatic environments in *A. punctata* by Xia et al. (2010). All these reports demonstrate that the *Aeromonas* genus represents a reservoir for fluoroquinolones resistance mediated by Qnr. Our own studies characterized a *qnr*S determinant in *E. coli* belonging to ST131 isolated from freshwater of a Ukrainian River (Lupo et al., submitted). Similarly, Dhanji et al. (2011) isolated *E. coli* strains belonging to ST131 harboring a *qnr*S allele from the Thames River (**Table 1**). These findings reflect a spread of these resistance mechanisms by geographical and clonal means and highlight the potential of rivers in the dissemination of international resistant clones.

ACQUIRED EFFLUX MECHANISMS

Another acquired fluoroquinolones resistance mechanisms is represented by efflux mechanisms. The *qep*A gene, initially characterized on a conjugative plasmid from a clinical isolate of *E. coli* (Perichon et al., 2007), encodes a MFS efflux pump. It has been recently recovered from the metagenome of river sediments impacted by improperly managed urban waste waters (Cummings et al., 2011). Environmental reports of this gene are rare; however, Deng et al. (2011) have highlighted the possible spread of this gene by animal and human related bacterial strains in water compartments. Similarly, the detection of the OqxAB efflux pump, conferring resistance to fluoroquinolones, olaquindox, and chloramphenicol, remains rare in environmental samples. The *oqx*AB, found on a conjugative plasmid in *E. coli* strains, represents the only example of transferable RND efflux pumps, so far (Hansen et al., 2004). Recently, Zhao et al. (2010) have reported an *E. coli* strain, isolated from a water pond in a farm environment, harboring the *oqx*AB gene (**Table 1**).

Resistance by acquired efflux mechanisms to other drug classes than fluoroquinolones has been extensively reported in the literature (Poole, 2004; Piddock, 2006; Nikaido and Pages, 2011). Studies conducted in water habitats such as aquaculture, impacted by anthropogenic activities, and notably by the application of antibiotics, demonstrated the risk of selection of acquired efflux pumps. Fernandez-Alarcon et al. (2010) reported the presence of different Gram-negative species from aquacultures in Chile expressing the *flo*R gene, which codes for a chloramphenicol and florfenicol exporter, drugs intensively used in veterinary medicine. Alarmingly, those strains resistant to florfenicol also demonstrated a multi-drug resistance, suggesting a process of co-selection. Gordon et al. (2008) characterized the *flo*R gene, in *Aeromonas bestiarum* strains from freshwater streams in France, located on a 25-kb-plasmid harboring also the tetracycline efflux gene *tet*(Y), *str*B-*str*A, conferring resistance to streptomycin, and *sul*2 conferring resistance to sulfonamides (**Table 1**). Interestingly, this plasmid contained sequences with high nucleotide homologies to other genetic elements recognized in different aquatic bacterial species such as *V. cholerae* and *Photobacterium damselae*. This demonstrated the contribution of horizontal gene transfer in the spread of these resistances in aquatic habitats. Furthermore, genes encoding tetracycline efflux mechanisms have been found to circulate between farm environments and ground water (Aminov et al., 2002). Propagation of tetracycline resistance genes, by efflux or by ribosomal protection, has been linked to the extensive usage of this drug class in animal feeding, and although the usage of this antibiotic has been restricted, tetracycline resistance genes seem to persist in the food chain and in the environment.

THE ENZYMATIC β-LACTAMS RESISTANCE

Resistance to β-lactams has spread worldwide. The low toxicity of these molecules and the broad spectrum of action of some of them make β-lactams the most prescribed antibiotic drug class and propagation of resistance constitutes therefore a major clinical concern. Studies have highlighted that the rise of the bacterial resistance against β-lactams is related to the usage of the drug in clinics, both because of selection of resistant bacteria and by promoting the mobilization of the genes responsible for such resistances (Bush and Fisher, 2011). Similarly, the presence of antibiotics in water environments could promote the selection of antibiotic resistant strains. Detecting and measuring the concentration of antibiotics or intermediary products from their metabolization and degradation in water medium is difficult, mainly because of the lack of standardized methods (Pérez-Parada et al., 2011). However, different studies described analytical methods to investigate pollution of freshwater by antibiotic compounds (Bailon-Perez et al., 2009; Ibanez et al., 2009) and antibiotics, including β-lactams, have been found to contaminate significantly several rivers (Pei et al., 2006; Jiang et al., 2011; Yang et al., 2011). A recent report from Pérez-Parada et al. (2011) has demonstrated the presence of compounds derived from amoxicillin in river effluent water. Although a selection due to these compounds has not been demonstrated, a corresponding risk cannot be excluded.

The most prevalent mechanism of β-lactams resistance in Gram-negative bacteria has been, for a long time, the enzymatic inactivation mediated by penicillinases such as TEM, SHV, and the extended spectrum β-lactamases (ESBLs) derived from these families (Coque et al., 2008). In the last decade, bla_{TEM} and bla_{SHV} genes have become less frequently detected in clinics and have been replaced by the more recently described $bla_{\text{CTX-M}}$ (Bonnet, 2004). CTX-M enzymes represent a special concern in clinics due to the extended spectrum of action and to its global, successful spread that has occurred in bacteria responsible for nosocomial and community acquired infections (Pitout et al., 2005). In 1963, bla_{TEM} has been reported for the first time, located on a plasmid. All the currently known bla_{TEM} genes have been documented to derive from the first characterized allele (Barlow and Hall, 2002). However, the origin of this mechanism has not been elucidated until now. The *K. pneumoniae* chromosome is thought to be the origin of bla_{SHV}, even if the physiological role of this mechanism remains unknown (Haeggman et al., 2004). CTX-M enzymes have been extensively investigated in clinics and more recently reported from environmental samples. Presence of $bla_{\text{CTX-M}}$ in bacteria from freshwater (Dhanji et al., 2011; Lupo et al., submitted), water sediment (Lu et al., 2010), or water-associated birds (Randall et al., 2011) constitutes further reservoirs and shuttles for these resistance determinants (**Table 1**). Based on aminoacidic homology, the $bla_{\text{CTX-M}}$ genes are sorted in four groups: $bla_{\text{CTX-M-1}}$, $bla_{\text{CTX-M-2}}$, $bla_{\text{CTX-M-8}}$, $bla_{\text{CTX-M-9}}$ (Pitout et al., 2005). The progenitor of each gene group has been found located on the chromosome of *Kluyvera* spp., of the Enterobacteriaceae family. Mobilization events from the ancestor genes have given rise to the clinically relevant mechanisms. In detail, $bla_{\text{CTX-M-1}}$ and $bla_{\text{CTX-M-2}}$ derived from *Kluyvera ascorbata* (Humeniuk et al., 2002; Rodriguez et al., 2004), $bla_{\text{CTX-M-8}}$ and $bla_{\text{CTX-M-9}}$ from *Kluyvera georgiana* (Poirel et al., 2002; Canton and Coque, 2006). The *Kluyvera* genus seems to be a sink of $bla_{\text{CTX-M}}$. Indeed, *Kluyvera cryocrescens* harbors a chromosomal β-lactamase, KLUC-1, which shares ca. 85% identity with CTX-M-1 (Bonnet, 2004). To the best of our knowledge, KLUC-1 has not been encountered in clinical isolates, but this species represents a reservoir of a new potential clinical ESBL. Although *Kluyvera* spp. are considered environmental bacteria and have been found also in water, elucidating the natural habitat of this species may help to evaluate the risk of the propagation of their β-lactamases. The CTX-M enzymes have been extensively investigated because of the clinical consequences that their spread has caused. However, many class A β-lactamases are chromosomally located in several members of Enterobacteriaceae and could constitute, if integrated on mobile elements, future mechanisms emerging in clinics. Bellais et al. (2001) discovered a chromosomal β-lactamase in *Rahnella aquatilis* (RAHN-1), which had similarities to $bla_{\text{CTX-M-1}}$ and $bla_{\text{CTX-M-2}}$; Arakawa et al. (1989) characterized KOXY from *Klebsiella oxytoca*; Perilli et al. (1991) MAL-1 in *Citrobacter diversus*; Peduzzi et al. (1994) CUM-A in *P. vulgaris*; Liassine et al. (2002) HUG-A from *Proteus penneri*; Peduzzi et al. (1997) SFO-1 from *Serratia fonticola*; Seoane and Garcia Lobo (1991) YENT from *Yersinia enterocolitica*; Vimont et al. (2002) ERP-1 from *Erwinia persicina*; Walckenaer et al. (2004) PLA-1 and ORN-1A from *Raoultella planticola* and *Raoultella ornithinolytica*, respectively. The above mentioned list provides only some examples: Bush and Fisher (2011) have reviewed that almost 600 class A β-lactamases naturally occur and have been reported in 2011. Worryingly, mechanisms exhibiting a spectrum of activity extended to carbapenems are emerging in clinics (Rossolini, 2005; Queenan and Bush, 2007). VIM, IMP, KPC, some OXA, and the newly described NDM-1 represent examples of these enzymes. The emergence of KPC (*K. pneumoniae* carbapenemase) was described in 2001 (Yigit et al., 2001) and this enzyme has been found to spread worldwide and among several bacterial species such as Enterobacteriaceae, *P. aeruginosa*, and *A. baumannii* (Bush and Fisher, 2011). The crucial molecular vector of its spread has been recognized by Naas et al. (2008), who characterized the location of bla_{KPC} gene on a Tn-*3-like* transposon, the Tn*4401*, probably responsible for the original mobilization of this gene. The transposon contains several sequences encoding transposases or insertion sequences derived from environmental bacterial species, but the ancestral host of this enzyme has not been identified, so far. Recently Chagas et al. (2011) have detected *K. pneumoniae* producing KPC in an effluent receiving hospital waste water, highlighting an environmental vector for the dissemination of these enzymes (**Table 1**). VIM enzymes have been rarely reported from environmental isolates. Scotta et al. (2011) isolated *Brevundimonas diminuta, Rhizobium radiobacter, Pseudomonas monteilii, P. aeruginosa, O. anthropi*, and *Enterobacter ludwigii* strains producing VIM enzymes, again from an effluent receiving the waste water of a hospital. Previously, Quinteira et al. (2005) isolated a strain of *Pseudomonas pseudoalcaligenes* harboring bla_{VIM} from a hospital wastewater effluent (**Table 1**). Probably, the presence of VIM producer species in the environment is due to nosocomial selective conditions and contamination by wastewater from hospitals. However, the detection of bla_{VIM} in different environmental species from freshwater highlights the potential of water as a reservoir for these genes and as a vector facilitating their spread. Concerning IMP enzymes, so far, a unique report has been provided by Pellegrini et al. (2009), in a strain of *P. fluorescens* recovered from waste water (**Table 1**). A carbapenemase activity is also exhibited by several class D β-lactamases, among which the families of OXA-23, OXA-40, OXA-58, and OXA-51 are associated to *A. baumannii* (Poirel et al., 2010). This opportunistic pathogen, provided with an intrinsic but silent $bla_{OXA51\text{-}like}$ gene, is widely distributed in nature. The origin of $bla_{OXA\text{-}40}$ and $bla_{OXA\text{-}58\text{-}like}$ genes remains unknown but Poirel et al. (2008) have characterized a $bla_{OXA\text{-}23\text{-}like}$ chromosomally located in *Acinetobacter radioresistens*, suggesting that this species is the progenitor for OXA-23. Moreover, *A. baumannii* isolates carrying $bla_{OXA\text{-}23}$ have been detected in river (Girlich et al., 2010) and wastewater from hospitals (Ferreira et al., 2011, **Table 1**). OXA-48 represents another class D carbapenemase that dramatically spreads among Enterobacteriaceae. This latter enzyme is supposed to originate from the chromosome of the water borne species *S. oneidensis* (Poirel et al., 2004). Recently, *S. marcescens* strains harboring $bla_{OXA\text{-}48}$ have been isolated from a river in Morocco (Potron et al., 2011), demonstrating the risks for their dissemination in water habitats (**Table 1**). The recent emergence and dramatic spread of NDM-1 enzyme in clinical isolates of *A. baumannii* and Enterobacteriaceae, has focused major attentions. Usually, strains harboring this broad spectrum carbapenemase gene demonstrate a multi-drug resistant phenotype and a wide set of virulence genes (Walsh et al., 2011). The carriage of bacteria harboring $bla_{NDM\text{-}1}$ by healthy individuals has lead researchers to investigate the source of this gene. Walsh et al. (2011) recently demonstrated the presence of different bacterial species (*P. aeruginosa, Achromobacter* spp., and *Kingella denitrificans*) harboring $bla_{NDM\text{-}1}$ in tap water used as drinking water in India (**Table 1**). This finding is closing the transmission circle and explains the fast and successful dissemination of this gene. Several genes encoding carbapenemase enzymes have been found chromosomally located in bacterial species of environmental origin and water related, for instance the *sme* gene on the chromosome of *S. marcescens*, and the *sfc* gene on the *S. fonticola* chromosome (Naas and Nordmann, 1994; Henriques et al., 2004). The water borne *S. maltophilia* also harbors a gene coding for the L1 carbapenemase. Avison et al. (2001) have elucidated that this gene is located on a plasmid-like element considered intrinsic to *S. maltophilia*.

Class C β-lactamases located on plasmids (CMY, MIR, DHA, and ACT) have been found worldwide from several sources (Jacoby, 2009). Water borne bacteria, such as *A. hydrophila, M. morganii, H. alvei*, and shuttle species between water and gut such as *Citrobacter freundii, Enterobacter asburiae*, have been proposed to be the progenitors of the most commonly encountered plasmidic *amp*C genes detected in clinical isolates. These genes have been reported from Canadian and Korean water bodies (Kim et al., 2008; Mataseje et al., 2009). Schwartz et al. (2003) detected *amp*C in waste, surface, and drinking water biofilms (**Table 1**). The presence of antibiotic resistance genes in biofilm matrices, especially in those located in drinking water supplies is of particular concern. Indeed, such biofilm matrices can be a long lasting source of antibiotic resistance genes that can directly spread via the food chain.

CONCLUSION

The emergence of antibiotic resistance is the consequence of a complex interaction of factors involved in the evolution and spread of resistance mechanisms. The over-usage of antibiotics in clinics has been believed to be the principal element involved in the rise of new resistances. Recently, many more evidences suggest that environmental habitats especially water bodies such as rivers and streams are ideal vectors for the antibiotic resistance dissemination. Here, the propagation of bacteria harboring antibiotic resistance genes can occur spatially along the river. Furthermore, the dispersion of these bacteria in the environment favors the interaction with the autochthonous microbiota, creating new scenarios for the evolution of antibiotic resistances.

In strong contrast to clinics, there are no data available on the epidemiology of antibiotic resistances in the environment, especially for geographically based data. This in turn makes extremely difficult to make any predictions on the risk of spread and emergence of new antibiotic resistances. For this reason we assume that a better knowledge on the environmental reservoir of resistances is fundamental to predict the emergences of new resistances of clinical concern.

It should be noticed that the pollution of water can select antibiotic resistant bacteria. This process, involving notably co-selection events, could cause an ecological imbalance leading to the dominance of resistant bacteria and global disturbance of the ecosystems. This latter point highlights the necessity of collecting information and data on the status of the sampling sites when performing a study on antibiotic resistance in freshwater. The development of antibiotic resistances occurs very likely naturally in the environment, but factors like pollution, especially of water bodies, could force the speed of its evolution. A good status of water quality could limit this phenomenon. Despite this, the status of the surface water quality in many countries is still poor. We argue for the implementation of feasible methodologies to characterize quality parameters and detect antibiotic resistance in water bodies, and thus to establish adapted and pragmatic measures to improve water resources. Amelioration of water status is of major concern: it can contribute to a direct and local decreased risk for the health of populations living in the vicinity of the freshwater, and lead to more global effects by avoiding that water bodies could constitute reactors for antibiotic resistance emergence and evolution.

ACKNOWLEDGMENTS

Authors' research is financed by the German Federal Ministry of Education and Research (Grant No.: FKZ 02WM1028). We thank the members of the Cost Action TD0803 "Detecting evolutionary hot spots of antibiotic resistances in Europe" for helpful discussion.

REFERENCES

Alcaide, E., Blasco, M. D., and Esteve, C. (2010). Mechanisms of quinolone resistance in *Aeromonas* species isolated from humans, water and eels. *Res. Microbiol.* 161, 40–45.

Ambler, R. P. (1980). The structure of beta-lactamases. *Philos. Trans. R. Soc. Lond. B Biol. Sci.* 289, 321–331.

Aminov, R. I. (2011). Horizontal gene exchange in environmental microbiota. *Front. Microbiol.* 2:158. doi:10.3389/fmicb.2011.00158

Aminov, R. I., Chee-Sanford, J. C., Garrigues, N., Teferedegne, B., Krapac, I. J., White, B. A., and Mackie, R. I. (2002). Development, validation, and application of PCR primers for detection of tetracycline efflux genes of gram-negative bacteria. *Appl. Environ. Microbiol.* 68, 1786–1793.

Aminov, R. I., and Mackie, R. I. (2007). Evolution and ecology of antibiotic resistance genes. *FEMS Microbiol. Lett.* 271, 147–161.

Arakawa, Y., Ohta, M., Kido, N., Mori, M., Ito, H., Komatsu, T., Fujii, Y., and Kato, N. (1989). Chromosomal beta-lactamase of *Klebsiella oxytoca*, a new class A enzyme that hydrolyzes broad-spectrum beta-lactam antibiotics. *Antimicrob. Agents Chemother.* 33, 63–70.

Arsène, S., and Leclercq, R. (2007). Role of a *qnr*-like gene in the intrinsic resistance of *Enterococcus faecalis* to fluoroquinolones. *Antimicrob. Agents Chemother.* 51, 3254–3258.

Avison, M. B., Higgins, C. S., Von Heldreich, C. J., Bennett, P. M., and Walsh, T. R. (2001). Plasmid location and molecular heterogeneity of the L1 and L2 beta-lactamase genes of *Stenotrophomonas maltophilia*. *Antimicrob. Agents Chemother.* 45, 413–419.

Baba, T., Kuwahara-Arai, K., Uchiyama, I., Takeuchi, F., Ito, T., and Hiramatsu, K. (2009). Complete genome sequence of *Macrococcus caseolyticus* strain JCSCS5402, reflecting the ancestral genome of the human-pathogenic staphylococci. *J. Bacteriol.* 191, 1180–1190.

Bailon-Perez, M. I., Garcia-Campana, A. M., Del Olmo-Iruela, M., Gamiz-Gracia, L., and Cruces-Blanco, C. (2009). Trace determination of 10 beta-lactam antibiotics in environmental and food samples by capillary liquid chromatography. *J. Chromatogr. A* 1216, 8355–8361.

Baquero, F., Martinez, J. L., and Canton, R. (2008). Antibiotics and antibiotic resistance in water environments. *Curr. Opin. Biotechnol.* 19, 260–265.

Barlow, M., and Hall, B. G. (2002). Predicting evolutionary potential: in vitro evolution accurately reproduces natural evolution of the tem beta-lactamase. *Genetics* 160, 823–832.

Beaber, J. W., Hochhut, B., and Waldor, M. K. (2004). SOS response promotes horizontal dissemination of antibiotic resistance genes. *Nature* 427, 72–74.

Bellais, S., Poirel, L., Fortineau, N., Decousser, J. W., and Nordmann, P. (2001). Biochemical-genetic characterization of the chromosomally encoded extended-spectrum class A beta-lactamase from *Rahnella aquatilis*. *Antimicrob. Agents Chemother.* 45, 2965–2968.

Bockelmann, U., Dorries, H. H., Ayuso-Gabella, M. N., Salgot De Marcay, M., Tandoi, V., Levantesi, C., Masciopinto, C., Van Houtte, E., Szewzyk, U., Wintgens, T., and Grohmann, E. (2009). Quantitative PCR monitoring of antibiotic resistance genes and bacterial pathogens in three European artificial groundwater recharge systems. *Appl. Environ. Microbiol.* 75, 154–163.

Bonnet, R. (2004). Growing group of extended-spectrum beta-lactamases: the CTX-M enzymes. *Antimicrob. Agents Chemother.* 48, 1–14.

Bush, K. (2010). Alarming beta-lactamase-mediated resistance in multidrug-resistant Enterobacteriaceae. *Curr. Opin. Microbiol.* 13, 558–564.

Bush, K., and Fisher, J. F. (2011). Epidemiological expansion, structural studies, and clinical challenges of new beta-lactamases from gram-negative bacteria. *Annu. Rev. Microbiol.* 65, 455–478.

Cambray, G., Guerout, A. M., and Mazel, D. (2010). Integrons. *Annu. Rev. Genet.* 44, 141–166.

Campanile, F., Bongiorno, D., Falcone, M., Vailati, F., Pasticci, M. B., Perez, M., Raglio, A., Rumpianesi, F., Scuderi, C., Suter, F., Venditti, M., Venturelli, C., Ravasio, V., Codeluppi, M., and Stefani, S. (2011). Changing Italian nosocomial-community trends and heteroresistance in *Staphylococcus aureus* from bacteremia and endocarditis. *Eur. J. Clin. Microbiol. Infect. Dis.* PMID: 21822974. [Epub ahead of print].

Canton, R., and Coque, T. M. (2006). The CTX-M beta-lactamase pandemic. *Curr. Opin. Microbiol.* 9, 466–475.

Cattoir, V., Poirel, L., Aubert, C., Soussy, C. J., and Nordmann, P. (2008). Unexpected occurrence of plasmid-mediated quinolone resistance determinants in environmental *Aeromonas* spp. *Emerging Infect. Dis.* 14, 231–237.

Chagas, T. P., Seki, L. M., Da Silva, D. M., and Asensi, M. D. (2011). Occurrence of KPC-2-producing *Klebsiella pneumoniae* strains in hospital wastewater. *J. Hosp. Infect.* 77, 281.

Chan, Y. Y., and Chua, K. L. (2005). The *Burkholderia pseudomallei* BpeAB-OprB efflux pump: expression and impact on quorum sensing and virulence. *J. Bacteriol.* 187, 4707–4719.

Colomer-Lluch, M., Jofre, J., and Muniesa, M. (2011). Antibiotic resistance genes in the bacteriophage DNA fraction of environmental samples. *PLoS ONE* 6, e17549. doi:10.1371/journal.pone.0017549

Coque, T. M., Baquero, F., and Canton, R. (2008). Increasing prevalence of ESBL-producing Enterobacteriaceae in Europe. *Euro Surveill.* 13, 1–11.

Courvalin, P. (2006). Vancomycin resistance in Gram-positive cocci. *Clin. Infect. Dis.* 42(Suppl. 1), S25–S34.

Coyne, S., Courvalin, P., and Perichon, B. (2011). Efflux-mediated antibiotic resistance in *Acinetobacter* spp. *Antimicrob. Agents Chemother.* 55, 947–953.

Cummings, D. E., Archer, K. F., Arriola, D. J., Baker, P. A., Faucett, K. G., Laroya, J. B., Pfeil, K. L., Ryan, C. R., Ryan, K. R., and Zuill, D. E. (2011). Broad dissemination of plasmid-mediated quinolone resistance genes in sediments of two urban coastal wetlands. *Environ. Sci. Technol.* 45, 447–454.

Da Re, S., Garnier, F., Guerin, E., Campoy, S., Denis, F., and Ploy, M. C. (2009). The SOS response promotes qnrB quinolone-resistance determinant expression. *EMBO Rep.* 10, 929–933.

D'Costa, V. M., King, C. E., Kalan, L., Morar, M., Sung, W. W., Schwarz, C., Froese, D., Zazula, G., Calmels, F., Debruyne, R., Golding, G. B., Poinar, H. N., and Wright, G. D. (2011). Antibiotic resistance is ancient. *Nature* 477, 457–461.

Deng, Y., Zeng, Z., Chen, S., He, L., Liu, Y., Wu, C., Chen, Z., Yao, Q., Hou, J., Yang, T., and Liu, J. H. (2011). Dissemination of IncFII plasmids carrying *rmt*B and *qep*A in *Escherichia coli* from pigs, farm workers and the environment. *Clin. Microbiol. Infect.* 17, 1740–1745.

Depledge, M. (2011). Pharmaceuticals: reduce drug waste in the environment. *Nature* 478, 36.

Dhanji, H., Murphy, N. M., Akhigbe, C., Doumith, M., Hope, R., Livermore, D. M., and Woodford, N. (2011). Isolation of fluoroquinolone-resistant O25b:H4-ST131 *Escherichia coli* with CTX-M-14 extended-spectrum beta-lactamase from UK river water. *J. Antimicrob. Chemother.* 66, 512–516.

Evans, K., Passador, L., Srikumar, R., Tsang, E., Nezezon, J., and Poole, K. (1998). Influence of the MexAB-OprM multidrug efflux system on quorum sensing in *Pseudomonas aeruginosa*. *J. Bacteriol.* 180, 5443–5447.

Fernandez-Alarcon, C., Miranda, C. D., Singer, R. S., Lopez, Y., Rojas, R., Bello, H., Dominguez, M., and Gonzalez-Rocha, G. (2010). Detection of the *flo*R gene in a diversity of florfenicol resistant Gram-negative bacilli from freshwater salmon farms in Chile. *Zoonoses Public Health* 57, 181–188.

Ferreira, A. E., Marchetti, D. P., De Oliveira, L. M., Gusatti, C. S., Fuentefria, D. B., and Corcao, G. (2011). Presence of OXA-23-producing isolates of *Acinetobacter baumannii* in wastewater from hospitals in southern Brazil. *Microb. Drug Resist.* 17, 221–227.

Fetar, H., Gilmour, C., Klinoski, R., Daigle, D. M., Dean, C. R., and Poole, K. (2011). mexEF-oprN multidrug efflux operon of *Pseudomonas aeruginosa*: regulation by the MexT activator in response to nitrosative stress and chloramphenicol. *Antimicrob. Agents Chemother.* 55, 508–514.

Figueira, V., Vaz-Moreira, I., Silva, M., and Manaia, C. M. (2011). Diversity and antibiotic resistance of *Aeromonas* spp. in drinking and waste water treatment plants. *Water Res.* 45, 5599–5611.

Fraud, S., and Poole, K. (2011). Oxidative stress induction of the MexXY multidrug efflux genes and promotion of aminoglycoside resistance development in *Pseudomonas aeruginosa. Antimicrob. Agents Chemother.* 55, 1068–1074.

Gaze, W. H., Abdouslam, N., Hawkey, P. M., and Wellington, E. M. (2005). Incidence of class 1 integrons in a quaternary ammonium compound-polluted environment. *Antimicrob. Agents Chemother.* 49, 1802–1807.

Gaze, W. H., Zhang, L., Abdouslam, N. A., Hawkey, P. M., Calvo-Bado, L., Royle, J., Brown, H., Davis, S., Kay, P., Boxall, A. B., and Wellington, E. M. (2011). Impacts of anthropogenic activity on the ecology of class 1 integrons and integron-associated genes in the environment. *ISME J.* 5, 1253–1261.

Gillings, M., Boucher, Y., Labbate, M., Holmes, A., Krishnan, S., Holley, M., and Stokes, H. W. (2008). The evolution of class 1 integrons and the rise of antibiotic resistance. *J. Bacteriol.* 190, 5095–5100.

Girlich, D., Poirel, L., and Nordmann, P. (2010). First isolation of the *bla*$_{OXA-23}$ carbapenemase gene from an environmental *Acinetobacter baumannii* isolate. *Antimicrob. Agents Chemother.* 54, 578–579.

Gordon, L., Cloeckaert, A., Doublet, B., Schwarz, S., Bouju-Albert, A., Ganiere, J. P., Le Bris, H., Le Fleche-Mateos, A., and Giraud, E. (2008). Complete sequence of the *flo*R-carrying multiresistance plasmid pAB5S9 from freshwater *Aeromonas bestiarum. J. Antimicrob. Chemother.* 62, 65–71.

Grkovic, S., Brown, M. H., and Skurray, R. A. (2002). Regulation of bacterial drug export systems. *Microbiol. Mol. Biol. Rev.* 66, 671–701.

Groh, J. L., Luo, Q., Ballard, J. D., and Krumholz, L. R. (2007). Genes that enhance the ecological fitness of *Shewanella oneidensis* MR-1 in sediments reveal the value of antibiotic resistance. *Appl. Environ. Microbiol.* 73, 492–498.

Gullberg, E., Cao, S., Berg, O. G., Ilback, C., Sandegren, L., Hughes, D., and Andersson, D. I. (2011). Selection of resistant bacteria at very low antibiotic concentrations. *PLoS Pathog.* 7, e1002158. doi:10.1371/journal.ppat.1002158

Haeggman, S., Lofdahl, S., Paauw, A., Verhoef, J., and Brisse, S. (2004). Diversity and evolution of the class A chromosomal β-lactamase gene in *Klebsiella pneumoniae. Antimicrob. Agents Chemother.* 48, 2400–2408.

Hansen, L. H., Johannesen, E., Burmolle, M., Sorensen, A. H., and Sorensen, S. J. (2004). Plasmid-encoded multidrug efflux pump conferring resistance to olaquindox in *Escherichia coli. Antimicrob. Agents Chemother.* 48, 3332–3337.

Hawkey, P. M. (2008). The growing burden of antimicrobial resistance. *J. Antimicrob. Chemother.* 62(Suppl. 1), i1–i9.

Henriques, I., Moura, A., Alves, A., Saavedra, M. J., and Correia, A. (2004). Molecular characterization of a carbapenem-hydrolyzing class A beta-lactamase, SFC-1, from *Serratia fonticola* UTAD54. *Antimicrob. Agents Chemother.* 48, 2321–2324.

Hernandez, A., Ruiz, F. M., Romero, A., and Martinez, J. L. (2011a). The binding of triclosan to SmeT, the repressor of the multidrug efflux pump SmeDEF, induces antibiotic resistance in *Stenotrophomonas maltophilia. PLoS Pathog.* 7, e1002103. doi:10.1371/journal.ppat.1002103

Hernandez, A., Sanchez, M. B., and Martinez, J. L. (2011b). Quinolone resistance: much more than predicted. *Front. Microbiol.* 2:22. doi:10.3389/fmicb.2011.00022

Humeniuk, C., Arlet, G., Gautier, V., Grimont, P., Labia, R., and Philippon, A. (2002). Beta-lactamases of *Kluyvera ascorbata*, probable progenitors of some plasmid-encoded CTX-M types. *Antimicrob. Agents Chemother.* 46, 3045–3049.

Ibanez, M., Guerrero, C., Sancho, J. V., and Hernandez, F. (2009). Screening of antibiotics in surface and wastewater samples by ultra-high-pressure liquid chromatography coupled to hybrid quadrupole time-of-flight mass spectrometry. *J. Chromatogr. A* 1216, 2529–2539.

Jacoby, G. A. (2009). AmpC beta-lactamases. *Clin. Microbiol. Rev.* 22, 161–182.

Jacoby, G. A., Griffin, C. M., and Hooper, D. C. (2011). *Citrobacter* spp. as a source of *qnr*B alleles. *Antimicrob. Agents Chemother.* 55, 4979–4984.

Jiang, L., Hu, X., Yin, D., Zhang, H., and Yu, Z. (2011). Occurrence, distribution and seasonal variation of antibiotics in the Huangpu River, Shanghai, China. *Chemosphere* 82, 822–828.

Kassem, II, Esseili, M. A., and Sigler, V. (2008). Occurrence of *mec*A in nonstaphylococcal pathogens in surface waters. *J. Clin. Microbiol.* 46, 3868–3869.

Kim, J., Kang, H. Y., and Lee, Y. (2008). The identification of CTX-M-14, TEM-52, and CMY-1 enzymes in *Escherichia coli* isolated from the Han River in Korea. *J. Microbiol.* 46, 478–481.

Lacroix, F. J., Cloeckaert, A., Grepinet, O., Pinault, C., Popoff, M. Y., Waxin, H., and Pardon, P. (1996). *Salmonella typhimurium acr*B-like gene: identification and role in resistance to biliary salts and detergents and in murine infection. *FEMS Microbiol. Lett.* 135, 161–167.

Lambert, P. A. (2005). Bacterial resistance to antibiotics: modified target sites. *Adv. Drug Deliv. Rev.* 57, 1471–1485.

Lata, P., Ram, S., Agrawal, M., and Shanker, R. (2009). Enterococci in river Ganga surface waters: propensity of species distribution, dissemination of antimicrobial-resistance and virulence-markers among species along landscape. *BMC Microbiol.* 9, 140. doi:10.1186/1471-2180-9-140

Lewinson, O., and Bibi, E. (2001). Evidence for simultaneous binding of dissimilar substrates by the *Escherichia coli* multidrug transporter MdfA. *Biochemistry* 40, 12612–12618.

Liassine, N., Madec, S., Ninet, B., Metral, C., Fouchereau-Peron, M., Labia, R., and Auckenthaler, R. (2002). Postneurosurgical meningitis due to *Proteus penneri* with selection of a ceftriaxone-resistant isolate: analysis of chromosomal class A beta-lactamase HugA and its LysR-type regulatory protein HugR. *Antimicrob. Agents Chemother.* 46, 216–219.

Lister, P. D., Wolter, D. J., and Hanson, N. D. (2009). Antibacterial-resistant *Pseudomonas aeruginosa*: clinical impact and complex regulation of chromosomally encoded resistance mechanisms. *Clin. Microbiol. Rev.* 22, 582–610.

Lu, S. Y., Zhang, Y. L., Geng, S. N., Li, T. Y., Ye, Z. M., Zhang, D. S., Zou, F., and Zhou, H. W. (2010). High diversity of extended-spectrum beta-lactamase-producing bacteria in an urban river sediment habitat. *Appl. Environ. Microbiol.* 76, 5972–5976.

Luczkiewicz, A., Jankowska, K., Kurlenda, J., and Olanczuk-Neyman, K. (2010). Identification and antimicrobial resistance of *Enterococcus* spp. isolated from surface water. *Water Sci. Technol.* 62, 466–473.

Martinez, J. L. (2009). Environmental pollution by antibiotics and by antibiotic resistance determinants. *Environ. Pollut.* 157, 2893–2902.

Martinez, J. L., Sanchez, M. B., Martinez-Solano, L., Hernandez, A., Garmendia, L., Fajardo, A., and Alvarez-Ortega, C. (2009). Functional role of bacterial multidrug efflux pumps in microbial natural ecosystems. *FEMS Microbiol. Rev.* 33, 430–449.

Mataseje, L. F., Neumann, N., Crago, B., Baudry, P., Zhanel, G. G., Louie, M., and Mulvey, M. R. (2009). Characterization of cefoxitin-resistant *Escherichia coli* isolates from recreational beaches and private drinking water in Canada between 2004 and 2006. *Antimicrob. Agents Chemother.* 53, 3126–3130.

Meibom, K. L., Blokesch, M., Dolganov, N. A., Wu, C. Y., and Schoolnik, G. K. (2005). Chitin induces natural competence in *Vibrio cholerae. Science* 310, 1824–1827.

Michon, A., Allou, N., Chau, F., Podglajen, I., Fantin, B., and Cambau, E. (2011). Plasmidic *qnr*A3 enhances *Escherichia coli* fitness in absence of antibiotic exposure. *PLoS ONE* 6, e24552. doi:10.1371/journal.pone.0024552

Moken, M. C., Mcmurry, L. M., and Levy, S. B. (1997). Selection of multiple-antibiotic-resistant (mar) mutants of *Escherichia coli* by using the disinfectant pine oil: roles of the *mar* and *acr*AB loci. *Antimicrob. Agents Chemother.* 41, 2770–2772.

Molin, S., and Tolker-Nielsen, T. (2003). Gene transfer occurs with enhanced efficiency in biofilms and induces enhanced stabilisation of the biofilm structure. *Curr. Opin. Biotechnol.* 14, 255–261.

Mosqueda, G., and Ramos, J. L. (2000). A set of genes encoding a second toluene efflux system in *Pseudomonas putida* DOT-T1E is linked to the tod genes for toluene metabolism. *J. Bacteriol.* 182, 937–943.

Naas, T., Cuzon, G., Villegas, M. V., Lartigue, M. F., Quinn, J. P., and Nordmann, P. (2008). Genetic structures at the origin of acquisition of the beta-lactamase *bla*$_{KPC}$ gene.

Antimicrob. Agents Chemother. 52, 1257–1263.

Naas, T., and Nordmann, P. (1994). Analysis of a carbapenem-hydrolyzing class A beta-lactamase from *Enterobacter cloacae* and of its LysR-type regulatory protein. *Proc. Natl. Acad. Sci. U.S.A.* 91, 7693–7697.

Nikaido, H., and Pages, J. M. (2011). Broad-specificity efflux pumps and their role in multidrug resistance of Gram-negative bacteria. *FEMS Microbiol. Rev.* doi: 10.1111/j.1574-6976.2011.00290.x

Parsley, L. C., Consuegra, E. J., Kakirde, K. S., Land, A. M., Harper, W. F. Jr., and Liles, M. R. (2010). Identification of diverse antimicrobial resistance determinants carried on bacterial, plasmid, or viral metagenomes from an activated sludge microbial assemblage. *Appl. Environ. Microbiol.* 76, 3753–3757.

Peduzzi, J., Farzaneh, S., Reynaud, A., Barthelemy, M., and Labia, R. (1997). Characterization and amino acid sequence analysis of a new oxyimino cephalosporin-hydrolyzing class A beta-lactamase from *Serratia fonticola* CUV. *Biochim. Biophys. Acta* 1341, 58–70.

Peduzzi, J., Reynaud, A., Baron, P., Barthelemy, M., and Labia, R. (1994). Chromosomally encoded cephalosporin-hydrolyzing beta-lactamase of *Proteus vulgaris* RO104 belongs to Ambler's class A. *Biochim. Biophys. Acta* 1207, 31–39.

Pei, R., Kim, S. C., Carlson, K. H., and Pruden, A. (2006). Effect of river landscape on the sediment concentrations of antibiotics and corresponding antibiotic resistance genes (ARG). *Water Res.* 40, 2427–2435.

Pellegrini, C., Mercuri, P. S., Celenza, G., Galleni, M., Segatore, B., Sacchetti, E., Volpe, R., Amicosante, G., and Perilli, M. (2009). Identification of *bla*$_{IMP-22}$ in *Pseudomonas* spp. in urban wastewater and nosocomial environments: biochemical characterization of a new IMP metallo-enzyme variant and its genetic location. *J. Antimicrob. Chemother.* 63, 901–908.

Pérez-Parada, A., Aguera, A., Gomez-Ramos Mdel, M., Garcia-Reyes, J. F., Heinzen, H., and Fernandez-Alba, A. R. (2011). Behavior of amoxicillin in wastewater and river water: identification of its main transformation products by liquid chromatography/electrospray quadrupole time-of-flight mass spectrometry. *Rapid Commun. Mass Spectrom.* 25, 731–742.

Perichon, B., Courvalin, P., and Galimand, M. (2007). Transferable resistance to aminoglycosides by methylation of G1405 in 16S rRNA and to hydrophilic fluoroquinolones by QepA-mediated efflux in *Escherichia coli*. *Antimicrob. Agents Chemother.* 51, 2464–2469.

Perilli, M., Franceschini, N., Segatore, B., Amicosante, G., Oratore, A., Duez, C., Joris, B., and Frere, J. M. (1991). Cloning and nucleotide sequencing of the gene encoding the beta-lactamase from *Citrobacter diversus*. *FEMS Microbiol. Lett.* 67, 79–84.

Petkovic, H., Cullum, J., Hranueli, D., Hunter, I. S., Peric-Concha, N., Pigac, J., Thamchaipenet, A., Vujaklija, D., and Long, P. F. (2006). Genetics of *Streptomyces rimosus*, the oxytetracycline producer. *Microbiol. Mol. Biol. Rev.* 70, 704–728.

Picao, R. C., Poirel, L., Demarta, A., Silva, C. S., Corvaglia, A. R., Petrini, O., and Nordmann, P. (2008). Plasmid-mediated quinolone resistance in *Aeromonas allosaccharophila* recovered from a Swiss lake. *J. Antimicrob. Chemother.* 62, 948–950.

Piddock, L. J. (2006). Multidrug-resistance efflux pumps – not just for resistance. *Nat. Rev. Microbiol.* 4, 629–636.

Pitout, J. D., Nordmann, P., Laupland, K. B., and Poirel, L. (2005). Emergence of Enterobacteriaceae producing extended-spectrum beta-lactamases (ESBLs) in the community. *J. Antimicrob. Chemother.* 56, 52–59.

Poirel, L., Figueiredo, S., Cattoir, V., Carattoli, A., and Nordmann, P. (2008). *Acinetobacter radioresistens* as a silent source of carbapenem resistance for *Acinetobacter* spp. *Antimicrob. Agents Chemother.* 52, 1252–1256.

Poirel, L., Heritier, C., and Nordmann, P. (2004). Chromosome-encoded ambler class D beta-lactamase of *Shewanella oneidensis* as a progenitor of carbapenem-hydrolyzing oxacillinase. *Antimicrob. Agents Chemother.* 48, 348–351.

Poirel, L., Kampfer, P., and Nordmann, P. (2002). Chromosome-encoded Ambler class A beta-lactamase of *Kluyvera georgiana*, a probable progenitor of a subgroup of CTX-M extended-spectrum beta-lactamases. *Antimicrob. Agents Chemother.* 46, 4038–4040.

Poirel, L., Liard, A., Rodriguez-Martinez, J. M., and Nordmann, P. (2005a). Vibrionaceae as a possible source of Qnr-like quinolone resistance determinants. *J. Antimicrob. Chemother.* 56, 1118–1121.

Poirel, L., Rodriguez-Martinez, J. M., Mammeri, H., Liard, A., and Nordmann, P. (2005b). Origin of plasmid-mediated quinolone resistance determinant QnrA. *Antimicrob. Agents Chemother.* 49, 3523–3525.

Poirel, L., Naas, T., and Nordmann, P. (2010). Diversity, epidemiology, and genetics of class D beta-lactamases. *Antimicrob. Agents Chemother.* 54, 24–38.

Poole, K. (2004). Efflux-mediated multiresistance in Gram-negative bacteria. *Clin. Microbiol. Infect.* 10, 12–26.

Potron, A., Poirel, L., Bussy, F., and Nordmann, P. (2011). Occurrence of the carbapenem-hydrolyzing beta-lactamase gene *bla*$_{OXA-48}$ in the environment in Morocco. *Antimicrob. Agents Chemother.* 55, 5413–5414.

Queenan, A. M., and Bush, K. (2007). Carbapenemases: the versatile beta-lactamases. *Clin. Microbiol. Rev.* 20, 440–458.

Quinteira, S., Ferreira, H., and Peixe, L. (2005). First isolation of *bla*$_{VIM-2}$ in an environmental isolate of *Pseudomonas pseudoalcaligenes*. *Antimicrob. Agents Chemother.* 49, 2140–2141.

Rahmati, S., Yang, S., Davidson, A. L., and Zechiedrich, E. L. (2002). Control of the AcrAB multidrug efflux pump by quorum-sensing regulator SdiA. *Mol. Microbiol.* 43, 677–685.

Randall, L. P., Clouting, C., Horton, R. A., Coldham, N. G., Wu, G., Clifton-Hadley, F. A., Davies, R. H., and Teale, C. J. (2011). Prevalence of *Escherichia coli* carrying extended-spectrum beta-lactamases (CTX-M and TEM-52) from broiler chickens and turkeys in Great Britain between 2006 and 2009. *J. Antimicrob. Chemother.* 66, 86–95.

Ripp, S., and Miller, R. V. (1995). Effects of suspended particulates on the frequency of transduction among *Pseudomonas aeruginosa* in a freshwater environment. *Appl. Environ. Microbiol.* 61, 1214–1219.

Rodriguez, M. M., Power, P., Radice, M., Vay, C., Famiglietti, A., Galleni, M., Ayala, J. A., and Gutkind, G. (2004). Chromosome-encoded CTX-M-3 from *Kluyvera ascorbata*: a possible origin of plasmid-borne CTX-M-1-derived cefotaximases. *Antimicrob. Agents Chemother.* 48, 4895–4897.

Rodriguez-Martinez, J. M., Cano, M. E., Velasco, C., Martinez-Martinez, L., and Pascual, A. (2011). Plasmid-mediated quinolone resistance: an update. *J. Infect. Chemother.* 17, 149–182.

Rossolini, G. M. (2005). Acquired metallo-beta-lactamases: an increasing clinical threat. *Clin. Infect. Dis.* 41, 1557–1558.

Sánchez, M. B., Hernandez, A., Rodriguez-Martinez, J. M., Martinez-Martinez, L., and Martinez, J. L. (2008). Predictive analysis of transmissible quinolone resistance indicates *Stenotrophomonas maltophilia* as a potential source of a novel family of Qnr determinants. *BMC Microbiol.* 8, 148. doi:10.1186/1471-2180-8-148

Sanchez, P., Linares, J. F., Ruiz-Diez, B., Campanario, E., Navas, A., Baquero, F., and Martinez, J. L. (2002). Fitness of in vitro selected *Pseudomonas aeruginosa nal*B and *nfx*B multidrug resistant mutants. *J. Antimicrob. Chemother.* 50, 657–664.

Sandegren, L., and Andersson, D. I. (2009). Bacterial gene amplification: implications for the evolution of antibiotic resistance. *Nat. Rev. Microbiol.* 7, 578–588.

Schwartz, T., Kohnen, W., Jansen, B., and Obst, U. (2003). Detection of antibiotic-resistant bacteria and their resistance genes in wastewater, surface water, and drinking water biofilms. *FEMS Microbiol. Ecol.* 43, 325–335.

Schwartz, T., Volkmann, H., Kirchen, S., Kohnen, W., Schon-Holz, K., Jansen, B., and Obst, U. (2006). Real-time PCR detection of *Pseudomonas aeruginosa* in clinical and municipal wastewater and genotyping of the ciprofloxacin-resistant isolates. *FEMS Microbiol. Ecol.* 57, 158–167.

Scotta, C., Juan, C., Cabot, G., Oliver, A., Lalucat, J., Bennasar, A., and Alberti, S. (2011). Environmental microbiota represents a natural reservoir for dissemination of clinically relevant metallo-beta-lactamases. *Antimicrob. Agents Chemother.* 55, 5376–5379.

Sengelov, G., and Sorensen, S. J. (1998). Methods for detection of conjugative plasmid transfer in aquatic environments. *Curr. Microbiol.* 37, 274–280.

Seoane, A., and Garcia Lobo, J. M. (1991). Nucleotide sequence of a new class A beta-lactamase gene from the chromosome of *Yersinia enterocolitica*: implications for the evolution of class A beta-lactamases. *Mol. Gen. Genet.* 228, 215–220.

Silver, S., and Phung, L. T. (1996). Bacterial heavy metal resistance: new surprises. *Annu. Rev. Microbiol.* 50, 753–789.

Sosa, V., Schlapp, G., and Zunino, P. (2006). *Proteus mirabilis* isolates of different origins do not show correlation with virulence attributes and can colonize the urinary tract of mice. *Microbiology* 152, 2149–2157.

Srinivasiah, S., Bhavsar, J., Thapar, K., Liles, M., Schoenfeld, T., and Wommack, K. E. (2008). Phages across the biosphere: contrasts of viruses in soil and aquatic environments. *Res. Microbiol.* 159, 349–357.

Talebi, M., Pourshafie, M. R., Katouli, M., and Mollby, R. (2008). Molecular structure and transferability of Tn*1546-like* elements in *Enterococcus faecium* isolates from clinical, sewage, and surface water samples in Iran. *Appl. Environ. Microbiol.* 74, 1350–1356.

Taylor, N. G., Verner-Jeffreys, D. W., and Baker-Austin, C. (2011). Aquatic systems: maintaining, mixing and mobilising antimicrobial resistance? *Trends Ecol. Evol. (Amst.)* 26, 278–284.

Teitzel, G. M., Geddie, A., De Long, S. K., Kirisits, M. J., Whiteley, M., and Parsek, M. R. (2006). Survival and growth in the presence of elevated copper: transcriptional profiling of copper-stressed *Pseudomonas aeruginosa*. *J. Bacteriol.* 188, 7242–7256.

Toleman, M. A., Bennett, P. M., and Walsh, T. R. (2006). Common regions e.g. *orf*513 and antibiotic resistance: IS*91-like* elements evolving complex class 1 integrons. *J. Antimicrob. Chemother.* 58, 1–6.

Tsubakishita, S., Kuwahara-Arai, K., Sasaki, T., and Hiramatsu, K. (2010). Origin and molecular evolution of the determinant of methicillin resistance in staphylococci. *Antimicrob. Agents Chemother.* 54, 4352–4359.

Velasco, C., Rodriguez-Martinez, J. M., Briales, A., Diaz De Alba, P., Calvo, J., and Pascual, A. (2010). *Smaq*nr, a new chromosome-encoded quinolone resistance determinant in *Serratia marcescens*. *J. Antimicrob. Chemother.* 65, 239–242.

Vimont, S., Poirel, L., Naas, T., and Nordmann, P. (2002). Identification of a chromosome-borne expanded-spectrum class a beta-lactamase from *Erwinia persicina*. *Antimicrob. Agents Chemother.* 46, 3401–3405.

Walckenaer, E., Poirel, L., Leflon-Guibout, V., Nordmann, P., and Nicolas-Chanoine, M. H. (2004). Genetic and biochemical characterization of the chromosomal class A beta-lactamases of *Raoultella* (formerly *Klebsiella*) *planticola* and *Raoultella ornithinolytica*. *Antimicrob. Agents Chemother.* 48, 305–312.

Walsh, T. R., Weeks, J., Livermore, D. M., and Toleman, M. A. (2011). Dissemination of NDM-1 positive bacteria in the New Delhi environment and its implications for human health: an environmental point prevalence study. *Lancet Infect. Dis.* 11, 355–362.

Weinbauer, M. G. (2004). Ecology of prokaryotic viruses. *FEMS Microbiol. Rev.* 28, 127–181.

Wiedenbeck, J., and Cohan, F. M. (2011). Origins of bacterial diversity through horizontal genetic transfer and adaptation to new ecological niches. *FEMS Microbiol. Rev.* 35, 957–976.

Wright, G. D. (2010). Antibiotic resistance in the environment: a link to the clinic? *Curr. Opin. Microbiol.* 13, 589–594.

Wright, M. S., Baker-Austin, C., Lindell, A. H., Stepanauskas, R., Stokes, H. W., and Mcarthur, J. V. (2008). Influence of industrial contamination on mobile genetic elements: class 1 integron abundance and gene cassette structure in aquatic bacterial communities. *ISME J.* 2, 417–428.

Xia, R., Guo, X., Zhang, Y., and Xu, H. (2010). *qnr*VC-like gene located in a novel complex class 1 integron harboring the IS*CR1* element in an *Aeromonas punctata* strain from an aquatic environment in Shandong Province, China. *Antimicrob. Agents Chemother.* 54, 3471–3474.

Yang, J. F., Ying, G. G., Zhao, J. L., Tao, R., Su, H. C., and Liu, Y. S. (2011). Spatial and seasonal distribution of selected antibiotics in surface waters of the Pearl Rivers, China. *J. Environ. Sci. Health B* 46, 272–280.

Yigit, H., Queenan, A. M., Anderson, G. J., Domenech-Sanchez, A., Biddle, J. W., Steward, C. D., Alberti, S., Bush, K., and Tenover, F. C. (2001). Novel carbapenem-hydrolyzing beta-lactamase, KPC-1, from a carbapenem-resistant strain of *Klebsiella pneumoniae*. *Antimicrob. Agents Chemother.* 45, 1151–1161.

Zhang, Q., Lambert, G., Liao, D., Kim, H., Robin, K., Tung, C. K., Pourmand, N., and Austin, R. H. (2011). Acceleration of emergence of bacterial antibiotic resistance in connected microenvironments. *Science* 333, 1764–1767.

Zhao, J., Chen, Z., Chen, S., Deng, Y., Liu, Y., Tian, W., Huang, X., Wu, C., Sun, Y., Zeng, Z., and Liu, J. H. (2010). Prevalence and dissemination of *oqx*AB in *Escherichia coli* isolates from animals, farmworkers, and the environment. *Antimicrob. Agents Chemother.* 54, 4219–4224.

3

MexXY multidrug efflux system of *Pseudomonas aeruginosa*

Yuji Morita*, Junko Tomida and Yoshiaki Kawamura

Department of Microbiology, School of Pharmacy, Aichi Gakuin University, Nagoya, Japan

Edited by:
Kunihiko Nishino, Institute of Scientific and Industrial Research, Osaka University, Japan

Reviewed by:
Herbert P. Schweizer, Colorado State University, USA
Aixin Yan, The University of Hong Kong, Hong Kong

***Correspondence:**
Yuji Morita, Department of Microbiology, School of Pharmacy, Aichi Gakuin University, 1-100 Kusumoto, Chikusa, Nagoya, Aichi 464-8650, Japan.
e-mail: yujmor@dpc.agu.ac.jp

Anti-pseudomonas aminoglycosides, such as amikacin and tobramycin, are used in the treatment of *Pseudomonas aeruginosa* infections. However, their use is linked to the development of resistance. During the last decade, the MexXY multidrug efflux system has been comprehensively studied, and numerous reports of laboratory and clinical isolates have been published. This system has been increasingly recognized as one of the primary determinants of aminoglycoside resistance in *P. aeruginosa*. In *P. aeruginosa* cystic fibrosis isolates, upregulation of the pump is considered the most common mechanism of aminoglycoside resistance. Non-fermentative Gram-negative pathogens possessing very close MexXY orthologs such as *Achromobacter xylosoxidans* and various *Burkholderia* species (e.g., *Burkholderia pseudomallei* and *B. cepacia* complexes), but not *B. gladioli*, are intrinsically resistant to aminoglycosides. Here, we summarize the properties (e.g., discovery, mechanism, gene expression, clinical significance) of the *P. aeruginosa* MexXY pump and other aminoglycoside efflux pumps such as AcrD of *Escherichia coli*, AmrAB-OprA of *B. pseudomallei*, and AdeABC of *Acinetobacter baumannii*. MexXY inducibility of the PA5471 gene product, which is dependent on ribosome inhibition or oxidative stress, is noteworthy. Moreover, the discovery of the cognate outer membrane component (OprA) of MexXY in the multidrug-resistant clinical isolate PA7, serotype O12 deserves special attention.

Keywords: aminoglycoside resistance, *Pseudomonas aeruginosa*, efflux, MexXY, PA5471, OprA

INTRODUCTION

Pseudomonas aeruginosa has been recognized as an increasingly important and worrisome species in health care-associated infections (Poole, 2011). This bacterium possesses intrinsic resistance to many antimicrobials because of the low permeability of its outer membrane barrier and the presence of multidrug efflux transporters (Nikaido, 1994; Hancock, 1998). Although fluoroquinolones (e.g., ciprofloxacin), broad-spectrum β-lactams (e.g., imipenem), and anti-pseudomonas aminoglycosides (e.g., amikacin) are often available for treatment, *P. aeruginosa* readily acquires resistance to these anti-pseudomonas agents via chromosomal mutations and lateral gene transfer (Poole, 2011). The emergence and spread of multidrug-, extensive drug-, and pandrug-resistant *P. aeruginosa* infections is of great concern as very few agents are effective against these strains (Fischbach and Walsh, 2009; Poole, 2011). The problem of increasing antimicrobial resistance is even more threatening when considering the very limited number of new antimicrobial agents in development (Fischbach and Walsh, 2009). In particular, the prospects of finding new antibiotics for Gram-negative pathogens are poor because of the low permeability of their outer membrane barriers and the presence of multidrug efflux transporters (Fischbach and Walsh, 2009). To combat these bacteria efficiently, it is necessary to understand the molecular basis of the efflux mechanisms involved in limiting the intracellular (or periplasmic) concentration of many antibiotics (Nikaido and Pages, 2012).

The most clinically relevant multidrug efflux systems in Gram-negative bacteria are those of the resistance-nodulation-cell division (RND) family (Poole, 2004, 2012; Piddock, 2006; Lister et al., 2009). *P. aeruginosa* expresses several RND-type multidrug efflux systems, of which MexAB-OprM, MexCD-OprJ, MexEF-OprN, and MexXY are significant determinants of multidrug resistance in laboratory and clinical isolates (Poole, 2004, 2012; Piddock, 2006; Lister et al., 2009). These pumps are three-component systems comprising antiporters of the RND family driven by proton motive force (MexB, MexD, MexF, and MexY), outer membrane factors (OMF; OprM, OprJ, and OprN), and periplasmic membrane fusion proteins (MFP; MexA, MexC, MexF, and MexX; Piddock, 2006; Lister et al., 2009). These pumps probably function in a similar manner with AcrAB-TolC, which is the best-studied RND-type multidrug pump of *Escherichia coli* (Nakashima et al., 2011; Nikaido, 2011).

Among them, the MexXY system is intriguing in that it is a significant determinant of aminoglycoside resistance only in *P. aeruginosa*, with numerous reports of clinical isolates during the last decade (Nikaido and Pages, 2012; Poole, 2012). Relatively few bacterial drug efflux systems are known to accommodate aminoglycosides (Poole, 2012). In addition to MexXY, AmrAB-OprA of *B. pseudomallei* is noteworthy for its contribution to this organism's intrinsic aminoglycoside resistance, while AdeABC of *Acinetobacter baumannii* is implicated in acquired aminoglycoside resistance (Poole, 2012). The upregulation of the MexXY pump is considered the most common mechanism of resistance (Armstrong and Miller, 2010) and appears to be the major determinant of aminoglycoside resistance in cystic fibrosis (CF) lung isolates of *P. aeruginosa* (Poole, 2011). Here, we summarize the properties of these pumps and discuss how to combat efflux-mediated aminoglycoside resistance.

PRE-MexXY DISCOVERY ERA: RND MULTIDRUG EFFLUX PUMPS AS DETERMINANTS OF RESISTANT TO A WIDE RANGE OF ANTIMICROBIALS, BUT NOT AMINOGLYCOSIDES

In 1993, the first RND-type multidrug efflux system of *P. aeruginosa*, MexAB-OprM (OprM was called OprK at that time), was discovered at approximately the same time as the AcrAB (AcrB was called AcrE at that time) system of *E. coli* (Poole et al., 1993b). It was the first genetic evidence that an efflux operon was involved in multiple antibiotic resistance in *P. aeruginosa* (Poole et al., 1993b). The following year, the efflux activity of tetracycline, chloramphenicol, norfloxacin, and benzylpenicillin was shown using antibiotic accumulation assays in intact cells, which was the first biochemical evidence of the role of efflux in intrinsic multidrug resistance in *P. aeruginosa* (Li et al., 1994a,b; Li et al., 1995). Taken together, the MexAB-OprM system was shown to contribute to the intrinsic resistance of *P. aeruginosa* to a wide range of antimicrobial compounds including fluoroquinolones, tetracycline, chloramphenicol, and β-lactams such as carbenicillin (Poole et al., 1993b; Li et al., 1995). Its homologs (MexCD-OprJ and MexEF-OprN) were then discovered as determinants of *nfxB* and *nfxC* fluoroquinolone-resistant (e.g., norfloxacin) mutants from *P. aeruginosa* (Poole et al., 1996; Kohler et al., 1997). Incidentally, these two pumps are not expressed in normal laboratory growth conditions, but are induced under some conditions in wild-type *P. aeruginosa* (e.g., Morita et al., 2003; Fetar et al., 2011). An unidentified efflux system that requires OprM was shown to contribute to resistance to quinolones and cephalosporins, such as cefpirome, erythromycin, and tetracycline, but not β-lactams, such as cefoperazone and carbenicillin, in the *P. aeruginosa* PAO1 background (Zhao et al., 1998). More details on these three pumps can be found in recent reviews (e.g., Li and Nikaido, 2004, 2009; Lister et al., 2009).

In those days, RND multidrug efflux systems such as MexAB-OprM and AcrAB-TolC, which can handle a wide variety of drugs that appear to contain hydrophobic domains of significant sizes (Nikaido, 1996), were considered to be similar to the P-glycoprotein multidrug efflux pump of mammalian cells, which extrudes not only basic compounds but also neutral and weakly acidic compounds (Nikaido, 1994). However, there was no evidence for the efflux of aminoglycosides, which are very hydrophilic compounds, among the antibiotics used to treat *P. aeruginosa* infections (Li et al., 1994a; Nikaido, 1996).

MexXY SYSTEM OF *P. aeruginosa* WAS IDENTIFIED BY THREE DIFFERENT GROUPS

The MexXY system was discovered in 1999 in Japan as the fourth RND-type multidrug efflux system of *P. aeruginosa* PAO1 (Mine et al., 1999). This system was functionally expressed and conferred resistance to fluoroquinolones, tetracycline, erythromycin, etc. in the *E. coli* KAM3 mutant (Morita et al., 1998) lacking the *acrB* gene, which is an RND transporter component of the major multidrug efflux pump (AcrAB-TolC) in *E. coli*. Interestingly, unlike the other three already known systems, no open-reading frame encoding the outer membrane component, such as OprM, was found in the region downstream from the *mexY* gene (Mine et al., 1999). However, this system was found to function cooperatively with OprM of *P. aeruginosa* and TolC of *E. coli* (Mine et al., 1999).

Nine months after the discovery described above, a French group showed that MexXY was involved in the natural resistance of *P. aeruginosa* PAO1 to aminoglycosides as well as tetracycline and erythromycin (Aires et al., 1999). Although the overexpression of MexXY increased the level of resistance to fluoroquinolones in *P. aeruginosa* PAO1 cells, disruption of *mexXY* from PAO1 had no detectable effect on susceptibility to these agents (Aires et al., 1999). *mexZ*, which is located upstream of but transcribed separately from *mexXY*, was identified (Aires et al., 1999). Its product, MexZ, contains a helix-turn-helix motif, which is characteristic of DNA-binding proteins, at its N-terminus, similar to the repressors of RND-type multidrug efflux genes (e.g., AcrR, a repressor of *acrAB* in *E. coli*), supporting the notion that *mexZ* negatively controls the expression of the operon (Aires et al., 1999).

The following month (10 months after the first discovery), a group in the USA showed that MexXY, which they called AmrAB, was an aminoglycoside impermeability factor in spontaneous aminoglycoside-resistant mutants of the impermeability phenotype from *P. aeruginosa* PAO1 (Westbrock-Wadman et al., 1999). Interestingly, a dramatic decrease in the amount of OprM was observed in the mutants compared to wild-type PAO1, indicating that OprM is unlikely to be the outer membrane component associated with this efflux system in the mutants (Westbrock-Wadman et al., 1999). In addition, MexXY was shown to be upregulated in clinical *P. aeruginosa* isolates displaying aminoglycoside impermeability, suggesting that the pump is a clinically relevant mechanism of aminoglycoside resistance in *P. aeruginosa* (Westbrock-Wadman et al., 1999).

The following year, the complete genomic sequence of *P. aeruginosa* strain PAO1 (PAO1-UW) was published in *Nature* (Stover et al., 2000). Although the locus IDs PA2019-18 of the PAO1-UW genome sequence correspond to the *mexXY* genes, the nucleotide sequences of PA2019-18 were not identical with those of previously published *mexXY* (Aires et al., 1999; Mine et al., 1999) findings. This is probably because the DNA sequencing technology at that time was unable to analyze GC-rich bacteria such as *P. aeruginosa* (66–67% GC content; Winsor et al., 2011). Therefore, we analyzed MexXY using the nucleotide sequences from the PAO1-UW complete genome (Winsor et al., 2011) because we live in the post-genome era.

STRUCTURE AND FUNCTION OF MexY

The RND components of RND-type tripartite multidrug efflux pumps determine substrate specificity (e.g., Srikumar et al., 1997; Eda et al., 2003); therefore, we focused on the structure and function of MexY rather than MexX or OprM. Very recently, the crystal structure of the RND-type multidrug efflux pump AcrB of *E. coli* revealed the presence of two discrete, high-volume multisite binding pockets that contribute to the remarkably broad substrate recognition of AcrB and its homologs (Nakashima et al., 2011). Although we basically assume that MexY pumps out antimicrobials in a similar manner as AcrB, it will be intriguing to uncover the molecular basis of how MexY accommodates aminoglycosides because they are strongly hydrophilic molecules that are completely different from the relatively hydrophobic compounds (e.g., minocycline, doxorubicin, rifampicin, and erythromycin) used as substrates of AcrB (Nakashima et al., 2011).

Generally speaking, the function of a transporter (e.g., substrate specificity and energy coupling) should be determined by its time course efflux assay and evaluated using kinetic constants (e.g., Yerushalmi et al., 1995; Edgar and Bibi, 1997; Mine et al., 1998; Morita et al., 2000). However, it is difficult to conduct such an assessment in a small bacteriology laboratory. The reconstitution of proteoliposomes revealed that AcrB, AcrD, and MdtBC of *E. coli* were H^+/drug antiporters (Zgurskaya and Nikaido, 1999; Aires and Nikaido, 2005; Kim et al., 2010), and we assume that MexY pumps out antimicrobials coupled with the same energy. In addition, five charged and polar amino acid residues that are involved in the proton translocation pathway are conserved between MexY and AcrB of *E. coli* (Takatsuka and Nikaido, 2006). Unfortunately, the purification, reconstitution, and characterization of the MexXY pump remain to be established, and the energy coupling and substrate specificity of MexXY has not been examined through its efflux activity. On the other hand, the MexXY-mediated energy-dependent efflux activity of ethidium (Mine et al., 1999), aminoglycosides (Aires et al., 1999; Vogne et al., 2004), tetracycline (Aires et al., 1999), Ala-Nap (MC-005,556) (Mao et al., 2001), and fluorescein-di-β-D-galactopyranoside (Matsumoto et al., 2011) has been measured in whole cells.

It is conventional to use differences in minimum inhibitory concentrations (MICs) between bacterial cells with and without a multidrug efflux transporter to estimate substrate specificity (e.g., Nishino and Yamaguchi, 2001; Nishino et al., 2003). Although the comparison of MICs can sometimes be a misleading indicator of pump function (e.g., Nagano and Nikaido, 2009), it can still indicate the possible clinical relevance of a pump (e.g., Poole, 2004, 2012; Piddock, 2006). Mutant strains lacking major multidrug efflux pump(s) have been used to determine substrate specificity (e.g., Nishino and Yamaguchi, 2001; Morita et al., 2001b). The substrate specificity of MexXY-OprM was determined using a mutant from PAO1 that overproduced MexXY-OprM, but not MexAB (and AmpC in the case of β-lactams), and were compared with a mutant lacking MexXY/MexAB-OprM (and AmpC in the case of β-lactams; Masuda et al., 2000b). MexXY-OprM-mediated resistance was then observed for quinolones, macrolides, tetracyclines, aminoglycosides, chloramphenicol, lincomycin, and most β-lactams, but not for novobiocin, polymyxin B, and some β-lactams (carbenicillin, sulbenicillin, cefsulodin, ceftazidime, oxacephem, imipenem, and aztreonam) among a wide variety of antimicrobial agents (Masuda et al., 2000b). In conclusion, MexXY-OprM is a multidrug efflux transporter whose specificity is extraordinary broad, but different compared with MexAB-OprM, MexCD-OprJ, MexEF-OprN, and other RND efflux transporters in *P. aeruginosa*. In addition, MexXY-OprM was the only pump to mediate aminoglycoside resistance and was thus considered to recognize aminoglycosides as substrates (Masuda et al., 2000b).

Basic local alignment search tool (BLAST) analysis showed that MexY was highly conserved in *P. aeruginosa* strains: more than 99% (99%) identity (positive) for most strains and 97% (98%) identity (positive) for PA7 (Morita et al., 2012). There was no functional difference between the MexYs of PAO1 and PA7 when they were expressed in either *E. coli* or *P. aeruginosa* (Morita et al., 2012). MexY was more similar [70–73% (83–86%) identity (positive)] to orthologs of *B. pseudomallei* and various *B. cepacia* complexes than other RND pumps of *P. aeruginosa* and other *Pseudomonas* species (Morita et al., 2012). These *Burkholderia* species, except for *B. mallei*, are intrinsically resistant to aminoglycosides (e.g., Kenny et al., 1999; Thibault et al., 2004; Vermis et al., 2003; Jassem et al., 2011). *B. gladioli* is also known to be involved in human infections (Segonds et al., 2009); however, no MexY (AmrB) ortholog exists in *B. gladioli* BSR3 (Seo et al., 2011), consistent with the fact that all isolates tested were susceptible to aminoglycosides (Segonds et al., 2009). Interestingly, the most similar functional ortholog to MexY exists in *Achromobacter xylosoxidans* and has a 74% identity (86% positive); this pump was named AxyY in strain AXX-A (Bador et al., 2012). *A. xylosoxidans* is also an opportunistic human pathogen capable of causing a wide range of infections (Glupczynski et al., 1988; Bador et al., 2011). Most *A. xylosoxidans* clinical isolates were resistant to the tested aminoglycosides, including amikacin (Ngeow and Puthucheary, 1985; Glupczynski et al., 1988). The AxyY pump contributes to aminoglycoside resistance in a similar manner to MexY and AmrBs (Bador et al., 2012).

COBALT analysis is a multiple sequence alignment tool for finding a collection of pairwise constraints. Such constraints are derived from data of the conserved domain database, protein motif database, and sequence similarity of RND pumps (Papadopoulos and Agarwala, 2007), including all pumps from *P. aeruginosa* PAO1-UW and *E. coli* K12 (MG1655). The exception is heavy metal efflux pumps, which are characterized by their relationships. Therefore, we focused on the four branches containing the four Mex pumps in *P. aeruginosa* (**Figure 1**). The MexY branch is located next to the MexD branch and includes the AmrBs of *Burkholderia* species (e.g., Mima and Schweizer, 2010) and AxyY of *A. xylosoxidans* (Bador et al., 2012). The MexD branch includes the AdeB pump of *A. baumannii* (Magnet et al., 2001), MtrD of *Neisseria gonorrhoeae* (Hagman et al., 1997), and BdeB of *Bradyrhizobium japonicum* (Lindemann et al., 2010). The SmeZ pump of *S. maltophilia*, which can mediate aminoglycoside resistance (Crossman et al., 2008), also belongs to the MexD branch. Many pumps in the MexY/MexD branches can mediate aminoglycoside resistance (e.g., Magnet et al., 2001; Crossman et al., 2008; Lindemann et al., 2010; Mima and Schweizer, 2010), which hints at the structure-function relationship of pumps involved in aminoglycoside resistance. MexB is located in the branch that contains the AcrB/D/F and MdtF pumps of *E. coli* (Nishino and Yamaguchi, 2001; Nishino et al., 2003), AdeJ of *A. baumannii* (Damier-Piolle et al., 2008), BpeB of *B. pseudomallei* (Mima and Schweizer, 2010), AxyB of *A. xylosoxidans* (Bador et al., 2011), and VmeB of *Vibrio parahaemolyticus* (Matsuo et al., 2007). Among them, some pumps (e.g., AcrD and MexB) were reported to be involved in aminoglycoside resistance under some conditions (Li et al., 2003; Aires and Nikaido, 2005). The MexF branch includes AdeG of *A. baumannii* (Coyne et al., 2010) and MdsB of *Salmonella enterica* (Nishino et al., 2006).

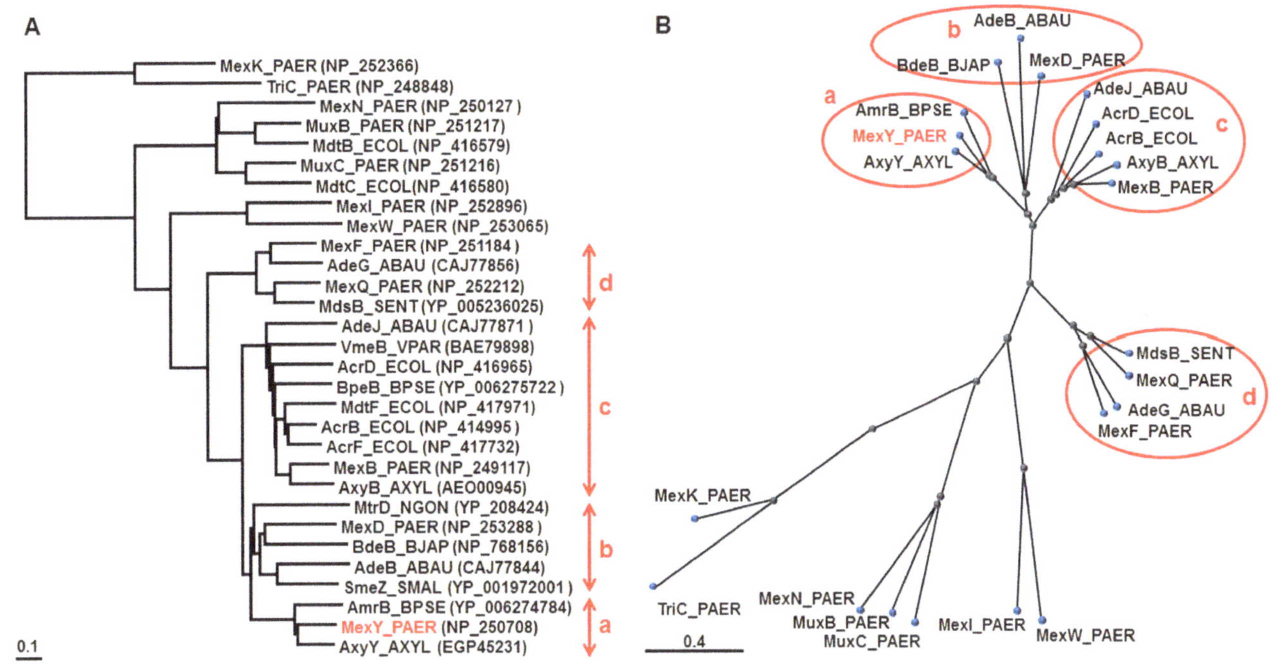

FIGURE 1 | Phylogenetic trees for representative RND transporters. According to the COBALT program, the trees were constructed using the Fast evolution method and rendered with **(A)** Rectangle and **(B)** Radical. Protein names are abbreviated; for example, "MexY_PAER" stands for "MexY of *P. aeruginosa*." Accession numbers are shown in parentheses. The four branches shown in red are: (a) MexY, (b) MexD, (c) MexB, and (d) MexF.

Substrate specificity is determined almost entirely by the periplasmic domain (i.e., two large extramembrane loops that largely protrude toward the periplasmic space) of MexY (and MexB; Eda et al., 2003). $MexY_{F1018L}$ (the F1018L mutation is located in TMS-12 of MexY base on the structure of AcrB; Murakami et al., 2002), enhanced the function of MexY, presumably by increasing the efflux of aminoglycosides, cefepime, and fluoroquinolones, which was the first example of an improved efflux pump *in vivo* (Vettoretti et al., 2009b).

GENE EXPRESSION OF THE MexXY SYSTEM

MexXY was shown to be induced by sub-inhibitory concentrations of tetracycline, erythromycin, aminoglycosides, tigecycline, and LMB415 (a peptide deformylase inhibitor), but not ofloxacin in *P. aeruginosa* PAO1 (Masuda et al., 2000a; Dean et al., 2003; Caughlan et al., 2009). Moreover, ofloxacin and cefpirome were also shown to be inducers, but only in a PAO1 mutant lacking MexAB (and AmpC in the case of cefpirome; Masuda et al., 2000a,b). MexZ was shown to bind an inverted repeat region located in the *mexZ-mexX* intergenic region directly as a homodimer, which encompasses the putative *mexXY* promoter, but the inducers failed to alter the MexZ-operator interactions (Matsuo et al., 2004). The crystal structure of MexZ has since been solved (Alguel et al., 2010). Induction of the MexXY efflux pump in *P. aeruginosa* PAO1 was shown to be dependent on drug–ribosome interactions (Jeannot et al., 2005), and the pump remained inducible, but to a lesser degree, by ribosomal inhibitors, even in the *mexZ* mutant (Jeannot et al., 2005). These data demonstrate the physiological interactions between MexXY and the ribosome and are suggestive of an alternative function for MexXY beyond the efflux of antibiotics (Jeannot et al., 2005). Microarray analysis showed that *mexXY* were the most highly upregulated genes in *P. aeruginosa* PAO1 after 4 h of interaction with primary normal human airway epithelial cells (Frisk et al., 2004) and in response to sub-inhibitory concentrations of tobramycin under normal aerobic conditions, but not under lethal aerobic conditions or anaerobic conditions (Kindrachuk et al., 2011).

The antibiotic inducibility of the MexXY multidrug efflux system of *P. aeruginosa* was shown to be involved in the modulation of MexZ activity by the antibiotic-inducible PA5471 gene product (Morita et al., 2006; **Table 1**). PA5471 encodes a predicted product of 43.5 kDa, which was identified as a hypothetical protein conserved between bacteria and archaea, and is a representative of the uncharacterized protein family UPF0027 in the Pfam protein families database (Morita et al., 2006) or the PRK09588 cluster in ProtClustDB (NCBI Protein Clusters Database; Klimke et al., 2009). Recently, it was demonstrated that RctB of *E. coli*, which is related to members of this family, is a novel RNA ligase and functions as a *bona fide* RNA repair protein *in vivo* (Tanaka and Shuman, 2011). PA5471 is found upstream of and in a possible operon with an open-reading frame dubbed PA5470; RT-PCR confirmed both the drug inducibility of PA5470 and its expression from a polycistronic message that also contains PA5471 (Morita et al., 2006). PA5470 is predicted to encode a peptide chain release factor of 22.3 kDa (Morita et al., 2006). A homolog of PA5471 from *E. coli* K12, *ykfJ* (b0235), which was, however, C-terminally truncated (approximately 1 kb; Baranov et al., 2006), was also shown to be inducible by 4-azaleucine, which is known to interfere with translation, and it too is linked to a putative peptide release factor gene (Morita et al., 2006). *P. aeruginosa* senses antibiotic-mediated ribosomal disruption and links it to PA5471 gene expression by monitoring the translation of a 13-amino-acid-leader peptide region (PA5471.1) found ~250 bp upstream of the PA5471 coding sequence on PA5471 mRNA (Morita et al., 2009). The antimicrobial-inducible PA5471 gene product has been shown to interact with the repressor MexZ and interfere with its DNA binding activity *in vitro* (Yamamoto et al., 2009), and this finding contributed to elucidating the molecular mechanisms of the MexXY induction. However, PA5471 is not sufficient for MexXY recruitment in response to antibiotic exposure, and additional antibiotic-dependent effects are needed in *P. aeruginosa* (Morita et al., 2009). Exposure to reactive oxygen species (ROS; e.g., peroxide) induces the expression of the PA5471 gene, leading to MexXY-dependent aminoglycoside resistance (Fraud and Poole, 2011). Moreover, long-term (8-day) exposure of *P. aeruginosa* to peroxide (mimicking chronic *in vivo* ROS exposure) increased the frequency of PA5471- and *mexXY*-dependent aminoglycoside resistance (Fraud and Poole, 2011). Recently, reduced (approximately twofold) expression of the *rplU-rpmA* operon (encoding the 50S ribosomal proteins L21 and L27) was shown to promote *mexXY* expression via the PA5471 gene in pan-aminoglycoside resistant mutants from PAO1 and a CF clinical isolate (Lau et al., 2012). Such expression was in the form of ribosomal protein mutations that influence *mexXY* expression, including *rplY* (encoding ribosomal protein L25; El'Garch et al., 2007) and *rplA* (encoding ribosomal protein L1; Westbrock-Wadman et al., 1999). Transcriptome profiling revealed that significantly increased expression was observed for the *mexXY* and PA5471 genes in both the PA2572 and PA2573 mutants compared with the wild-type PAO1 strain during exponential growth in Luria–Bertani media (McLaughlin et al., 2012). PA2572 encodes a putative response regulator of a two-component system required for full virulence to *Galleria mellonella* (Wax moth) and PA2573 also encodes an ophan chemotaxis sensor which seems to function in part through signal transduction involving PA2572 (McLaughlin et al., 2012).

A recent study identified a gene, *parR*, encoding the response regulator of a two-component system, ParRS, which promotes either induced or constitutive *mexXY* upregulation, thereby activating the MexXY efflux system as well as OprD porin loss and lipopolysaccharide modification in a MexZ-independent manner (Muller et al., 2011). Overexpression of PaeIII, a small non-coding RNA between PA3505 and PA3536 in the genome of *P. aeruginosa* PAO1, in the stationary phase increased the expression of the *mexXY* and *mexZ* genes as well as type III secretion genes, while reducing the expression of genes for arginine metabolism (Goldberg et al., 2008).

MexXY SYSTEM AS AN ANTIMICROBIAL RESISTANCE DETERMINANT IN *P. aeruginosa*

Pseudomonas aeruginosa shows intrinsic resistance against many antimicrobials because of the low permeability of its outer membrane and the presence of efflux systems (Nikaido, 1994; Hancock, 1998). MexXY was shown to be involved in natural resistance to aminoglycosides, tetracycline, tigecycline, erythromycin, and LBM415 in *P. aeruginosa* PAO1 (Aires et al., 1999; Masuda et al., 2000a; Morita et al., 2001a; Dean et al., 2003; Caughlan et al., 2009). MexXY was also shown to be necessary for the adaptive resistance of *P. aeruginosa* PAO1 to aminoglycosides (Hocquet et al., 2003). It is of note that MexXY is the only pump of the 12 identified RND systems that mediates aminoglycoside resistance in *P. aeruginosa* PAO1 (Poole, 2011). The antagonism of aminoglycosides by the divalent cations Mg^{2+} and Ca^{2+} is well documented (Medeiros et al., 1971), and culture in cation-adjusted Mueller–Hinton broth is recommended as a susceptibility test to ensure acceptable results when *P. aeruginosa* isolates are tested (Barry et al., 1992). MexXY was shown to be required for the antagonism of aminoglycosides by divalent cations in *P. aeruginosa* PAO1 (Mao et al., 2001). Although Phe-Arg-β-naphthylamide (PAβN, MC-207,110) is known as a non-specific inhibitor against RND-type multidrug efflux pumps (Lomovskaya et al., 2001), this inhibitor, as observed for divalent cations, antagonized the activity of aminoglycosides (amikacin and netilmicin) in a MexXY-dependent manner, even though it also inhibited MexXY-dependent fluoroquinolone (levofloxacin) resistance (Mao et al., 2001). Conversely, PAβN inhibited MexXY-mediated aminoglycoside (gentamicin) resistance (Mesaros et al., 2007). The reason for the discrepancy between these two results remains unknown. Increased susceptibility to aminoglycosides in *nfxB* mutants, which upregulate *mexCD-oprJ* expression, was correlated with increased resistance to fluoroquinolones and some β-lactams, such as cefepime, concomitant with a higher susceptibility to aminoglycosides and some β-lactams, such as ticarcillin, aztreonam, and imipenem. This was shown to be partly due to the impaired activity of MexXY-OprM because of major changes in cell physiology, but not the expression/production of *mexY*/MexY and *oprM*/OprM (Jeannot et al., 2008; Mulet et al., 2011). The increased susceptibility to aminoglycosides in MexEF-OprN-overproducing *nfxC* mutants was also observed, apparently owing to impairment of the MexXY system (Sobel et al., 2005). *mexXY* expression (and so MexXY-mediated resistance) was independent of the AmgRS two-component system in which mutations enhanced aminoglycoside action to control an adaptive response to membrane stress (Lee et al., 2009).

Multidrug resistant *P. aeruginosa* clinical isolates have often been reported to be MexXY overproducers (e.g., Llanes et al., 2004, 2006; Wolter et al., 2004; Deplano et al., 2005; Henrichfreise et al., 2007; Hocquet et al., 2007; Maniati et al., 2007; Vettoretti et al., 2009a; Beaudoin et al., 2010; Xavier et al., 2010; Fehlberg et al., 2012; Pasca et al., 2012). Time series analysis (January 1999 to January 2005) revealed a significant relationship between antibiotic use (aminoglycosides, fluoroquinolones, and cefepime, but not carbapenems) and the incidence of MexXY-overproducing *P. aeruginosa* in a French hospital (Hocquet et al., 2008). MexXY ($n = 39$) and MexAB ($n = 31$) were the most frequently overproduced pumps in 85 non-CF *P. aeruginosa* strains with low-level ciprofloxacin resistance (MICs ranging from 0.25 to 2 μg/mL, which are still susceptible or intermediate according to the CLSI breakpoints; Llanes et al., 2011). A large proportion of the strains were MexXY overproducers in genotypically distinct *P. aeruginosa* clinical isolates that were less susceptible to cefepime than to ceftazidime, and these were identified in Europe (Hocquet et al., 2006; Pena et al., 2009; Campo Esquisabel et al., 2011) and the USA (Laohavaleeson et al., 2008). In contrast, both cefepime and ceftazidime are potent β-lactam antibiotics with similar MICs (1–2 μg/mL) for wild-type *P. aeruginosa* strains. Moreover, ceftobiprole, similar to cefepime, selected MexXY overproducers in clinical studies (Baum et al., 2009). Actually, a single step MexXY overproducer was selected *in vitro* by cefepime and ceftobiprole, but not ceftazidime (Queenan et al., 2010). MexXY contributed very significantly to the development of high-level (100–1000 μg/mL MIC) aminoglycoside resistance via a combination of aminoglycoside-modifying enzymes (AMEs) in multidrug resistant *P. aeruginosa* non-CF clinical isolates (Morita et al., 2012). However, AMEs are common determinants of aminoglycoside resistance in *P. aeruginosa*, except for CF isolates (Poole, 2011). In clinical CF isolates, MexXY has been primarily implicated in pan-aminoglycoside resistance (e.g., Sobel et al., 2003; Vogne et al., 2004; Islam et al., 2004, 2009). MexXY was also shown to be necessary in subpopulations of *P. aeruginosa* CF isolates that are hypersensitive to ticarcillin (called Tic^{hs}; Vettoretti et al., 2009b). *mexZ* was shown to be one of the most frequently mutated genes during chronic infection by *P. aeruginosa* in CF patients (Smith et al., 2006; Feliziani et al., 2010). However, a number of studies highlighted the absence of mutations in *mexZ* or the *mexXY* promoter region in MexXY-overproducing *P. aeruginosa* CF isolates (Sobel et al., 2003; Vogne et al., 2004; Islam et al., 2009). To date, three kinds of mutants (*agrZ*, *agrW1*, and *agrW2*) have been recognized as MexXY overproducers as a result of genetic mechanisms: mutants with impaired binding or unbinding of MexZ due to alterations in the *mexZ* or *mexZ-mexX* intergenic region (type *agrZ*); mutants with impaired protein synthesis (type *agrW1*); and mutants with alterations in *parRS* (type *agrW2*; de Bentzmann and Plesiat, 2011). Oxidative stress, a component of the host's immune system in the CF lung, induced *mexXY* expression via PA5471 and promoted aminoglycoside resistance (Fraud and Poole, 2011). Under conditions of oxidative stress, *P. aeruginosa* can develop aminoglycoside resistance, even in the absence of aminoglycosides (Poole, 2012). It is also very plausible that the routine use of aminoglycosides (e.g., tobramycin) might simply select for MexXY-overproducing *P. aeruginosa* in the CF lung (Smith et al., 2006).

Although it is obvious that MexXY is one of the determinants of antimicrobial resistance in *P. aeruginosa* in the clinical setting (Poole, 2011), only a few reports have assessed the *in vivo* impact of the MexXY system on antibiotic therapy for *P. aeruginosa* infections (e.g., Martha et al., 2006).

COGNATE OUTER-MEMBRANE COMPONENT OprA OF THE MexXY PUMP IS FOUND IN SEROTYPE O12 BUT IS LOST IN OTHERS

The *mexXY* operon lacks a gene coding for the outer membrane protein in *P. aeruginosa* PAO1 (Mine et al., 1999). OprM is necessary for the function of MexXY and MexAB in *P. aeruginosa* PAO1 (Aires et al., 1999; Masuda et al., 2000a; Morita et al., 2001a), although overproduced OpmB (PA2525) can function as an outer membrane component of MexXY, MexAB, and MexCD (Murata et al., 2002). Intriguingly, the multidrug resistant taxonomic outlier *P. aeruginosa* PA7 possesses a unique gene (*oprA*) downstream of *mexXY* encoding an outer membrane channel that is absent in most *P. aeruginosa* strains (Roy et al., 2010). MexXY in this strain utilizes either the OprA or OprM outer membrane channel (Morita et al., 2012; **Table 1**). While OprM is functional with both MexXY and MexAB, OprA did not associate as strongly with MexAB as it did with MexXY (Morita et al., 2012). We compared the OprA of *P. aeruginosa* PA7 with the OprM family (Remans et al., 2010) from *P. aeruginosa* PAO1 as well as TolC of *E. coli* K12 (Mine et al., 1999), OprA of *B. pseudomallei* 1026b (Mima and Schweizer, 2010), OprZ of *A. xylosoxidans* AXX-A (Bador et al., 2012), and AdeC *of A. baumannii* AYE (Magnet et al., 2001; **Figure 2**). COBALT analysis showed that OprA of *P. aeruginosa* PA7 and its close orthologs (OprA of *B. pseudomallei* 1026b and OprZ of *A. xylosoxidans* AXX-A) is located close to OprJ and is followed by OprM of the OprM outer membrane family of *P. aeruginosa* PAO1 (**Figure 2**).

Interestingly, a small portion of the *oprA* gene immediately downstream of the *mexY* gene in PAO1 was identified, suggesting that non-PA7 *P. aeruginosa* strains might have possessed, but lost, the intact *mexXY-oprA* efflux pump locus (Morita et al., 2012; **Table 1**). Consistent with this, the majority of a panel of serotype strains possessed the truncated *oprA*, but the serotype O12 isolate had an intact *mexXY-oprA* locus, similar to PA7 and the related strain DSM 1128 (Morita et al., 2012). O12 is a predominant serotype associated with multidrug resistance to a number of antibiotic classes, including aminoglycosides and β-lactams, although it represents a minor serotype in the environment (Pirnay et al., 2009; Roy et al., 2010). O12 might be more dominant due, in part, to the presence of *oprA* in hospitals in which antimicrobials promoting MexXY-OprA-mediated multidrug resistance, such as aminoglycosides, were used. *P. aeruginosa* PA7 isolated before 1984 from a wound infection in Buenos Aires, Argentina (Pirnay et al., 2009; Roy et al., 2010), might also have acquired multidrug resistance via the heavy use of antibiotics, including gentamicin or tobramycin, to treat wounds at that time. Apparently, a slightly increased resistance (two- to fourfold) to amikacin, ciprofloxacin, and cefpirome was shown in the presence and absence of *oprA* (Morita et al., 2012). Such a small difference might be significant during antibiotic treatment or in the presence of sub-inhibitory concentrations of antibiotics.

AcrD IS AN AMINOGLYCOSIDE EFFLUX PUMP THAT IS THE MOST SIMILAR TO MexY AMONG THE RND PUMPS IN *E. coli* K12

AcrD has the highest similarity score at the amino acid level to MexY of the *E. coli* K12 RND pumps and was shown to be an aminoglycoside efflux pump as judged by MIC determination and the aminoglycoside efflux assay (Rosenberg et al., 2000). However, differences in aminoglycoside resistance (uptake) between the parent strain JC7623 and its *acrD*-deletion mutant JZM320 was possibly not limited to AcrD function because JZM320 was constructed by inserting the *tet* gene from pBR322 into *acrD* (Rosenberg et al., 2000). The increased aminoglycoside uptake might be due to not only AcrD deficiency but also to the production of an aberrant cytoplasmic membrane protein (the product of *acrD* with the inserted *tet*) and/or the tetracycline/H^+ antiporter itself (Merlin et al., 1989a,b; Wyka and St John, 1990). While disruption of *tolC* or *acrA* did not increase the susceptibility of K12 to aminoglycosides (Rosenberg et al., 2000), both of them were

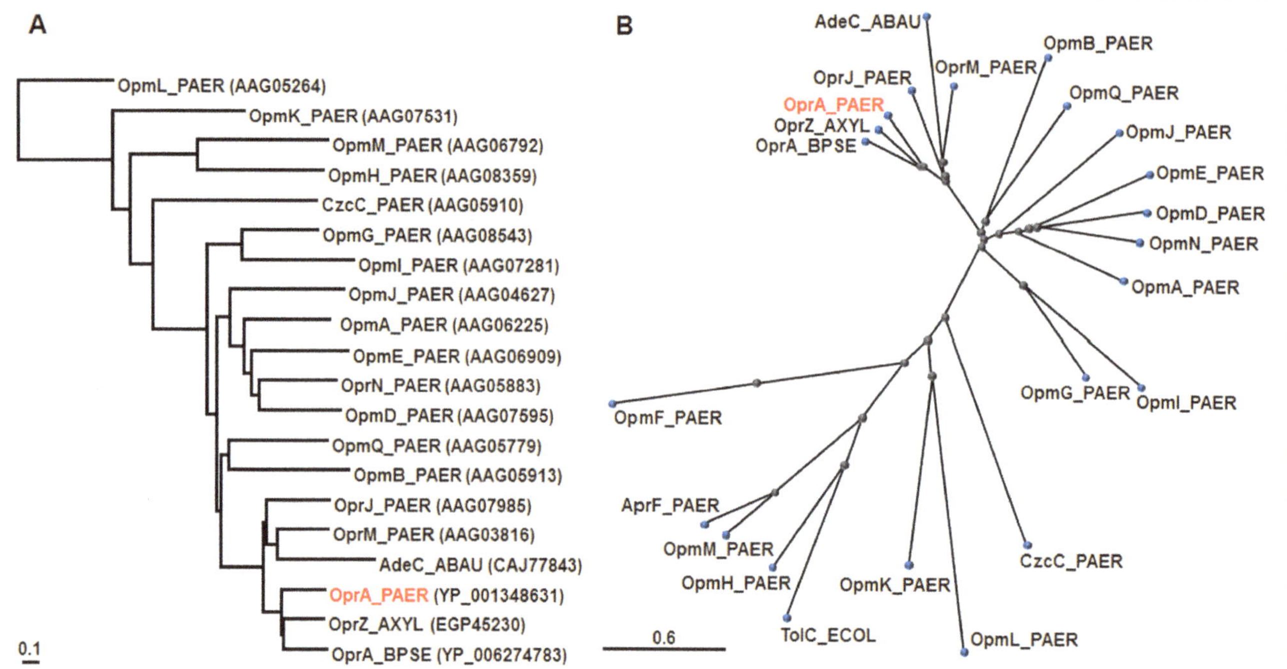

FIGURE 2 | Phylogenetic trees for representative OMPs. According to the COBALT program, the trees were constructed using the Fast evolution method and rendered with **(A)** Rectangle and **(B)** Radical. Protein names are abbreviated; for example, "OprA_PAER" stands for "OprA of *P. aeruginosa*." Accession numbers are shown in parentheses.

necessary for the function of *acrD* against various antimicrobials; however, no aminoglycosides were used in the study (Hirakawa et al., 2003). We do not rule out the hypothesis of Rosenberg et al. (2000) that AcrD protein can perhaps function without the participation of AcrA and TolC in the case of aminoglycoside efflux.

It is evident that purified AcrD can function as an H^+-driven aminoglycoside efflux pump (Aires and Nikaido, 2005). Especially, strong stimulation of proton efflux was observed when aminoglycosides (e.g., streptomycin) were added to the more acidic intra-vesicular space of reconstituted AcrD proteoliposomes containing AcrA and Mg^{2+} (Aires and Nikaido, 2005), indicating that AcrD captures aminoglycosides exclusively from the periplasm in *E. coli* (Nikaido, 2011). The difference in the MICs of amikacin and gentamicin between a parent strain and its in-frame *acrD*-deletion mutant or between an *acrBD*-deletion mutant and its *acrD*-overexpressing complementation mutant was approximately twofold (Elkins and Nikaido, 2002; Aires and Nikaido, 2005). There was no significant difference in kanamycin resistance in the case of an in-frame deletion (Hirakawa et al., 2003), and a twofold difference was observed in the case of overproduction (Nishino and Yamaguchi, 2001; Nishino et al., 2010). An *acrA* in-frame deletion mutant also showed an approximately twofold increased susceptibility to aminoglycosides (Aires and Nikaido, 2005). However, similar observations were not seen for AcrB (Nishino and Yamaguchi, 2001; Elkins and Nikaido, 2002; Aires and Nikaido, 2005). A comparison of the entrances of the vestibules, which are found in the central cavities (Murakami et al., 2002) of AcrD (which transports aminoglycosides) and AcrB (which does not) crystal structures, shows that this area in AcrD is in line with many more acidic residues that may attract polycationic substrates (Yu et al., 2003). Treatment with sub-inhibitory concentrations of kanamycin induced adaptive resistance to aminoglycosides, which was dependent on *acrD* (Sidhu et al., 2012). Aminoglycosides are very hydrophilic and polycationic and assumingly permeate through the porin channel in *E. coli*, unlike *P. aeruginosa* (Nikaido and Pages, 2012) in addition to so called "self-promoted" aminoglycoside uptake across the outer membrane of both of *E. coli* and *P. aeruginosa* (Hancock et al., 1991; Hancock, 1998). The MICs of aminoglycosides on *E. coli*, unlike *P. aeruginosa*, might be poor indicators of aminoglycoside efflux. There are numerous AcrD homologs in other Enterobacteriaceae (Poole, 2004). Although the AcrD of *S. enterica* serovar Typhimurium ATCC 14028s was studied comprehensively, no significant difference between the AcrDs of *E. coli* and *S. enterica* has been observed so far (Nishino et al., 2009; Horiyama et al., 2011; Yamasaki et al., 2011). Interestingly, AcrD pumps mediate resistance to the substrates of MexAB (e.g., carbenicillin, aztreonam, and novobiocin). However, AcrD pumps did not mediate resistance to the substrates of MexXY (e.g., cefpirome, erythromycin, and tetraphenylphosphonium) or shared substrates of both MexAB and MexXY (e.g., fluoroquinolone and tetracycline) when differences of the MICs were compared between a parent strain and its transformant overproducing the pump (Srikumar et al., 1997; Mine et al., 1999; Morita et al., 2001a; Nishino et al., 2003, 2009; Horiyama et al., 2011; Yamasaki et al., 2011). MexAB-OprM was also shown to contribute to aminoglycoside resistance, presumably via active efflux in the low-ionic-strength medium used in this particular study (Li et al., 2003). AcrD and the MdtABC pump were iron-regulated, induced in low-iron conditions, and export the siderophore enterobactin (Bochner et al., 2008), which reminds us that MexAB-OprM was inducible under conditions of iron limitation and compensated for a growth defect in an iron-deficient medium in the presence of the non-metabolizable iron chelator 2,2′-dipyridyl (Poole et al., 1993a,b). AcrD seems to be a functional homolog of MexB rather than MexY, as determined from substrate specificity and physiological function, consistent with the fact that phylogenetic analysis showed that AcrD is closer to MexB than to MexY (**Figure 1**).

AmrAB-OprA IS A MULTIDRUG EFFLUX SYSTEM THAT MEDIATES AMINOGLYCOSIDE RESISTANCE IN *B. pseudomallei*

Burkholderia pseudomallei is the etiologic agent of melioidosis, a rare but serious disease endemic to South Asia, Northern Australia, and other parts of the tropics (Mima and Schweizer, 2010). Melioidosis is very difficult to treat because of the intrinsic resistance to many antimicrobial agents including aminoglycosides, macrolides, polymyxins, and some β-lactams (Mima and Schweizer, 2010). AmrAB-OprA was identified as an efflux determinant of resistance to aminoglycosides and macrolides in the *B. pseudomallei* 1026b clinical isolate (Moore et al., 1999). This pump was actually the first to be demonstrated responsible for the aminoglycoside resistance of RND pumps in Gram-negative bacteria. The gene product of *amrR*, which is located immediately upstream and divergently transcribed from *amrAB-oprA* in *B. pseudomallei* 1026b (Moore et al., 1999), showed strong homology [60% (73%) identity (positive)] to MexZ, which acts as a transcriptional repressor of the *mexXY* operon of *P. aeruginosa* PAO1 (Matsuo et al., 2004; Alguel et al., 2010; **Table 1**).

While the majority of *B. pseudomallei* clinical isolates exhibit high levels of aminoglycoside and macrolide resistance, rare isolates are susceptible to these antibiotics (Simpson et al., 1999; Trunck et al., 2009). While it is noted that the resistance profile of those isolates matches that of the *amrAB-oprA* mutants (Simpson et al., 1999), it was shown experimentally that *amrAB-oprA* was missing in *B. pseudomallei* 708a, an aminoglycoside- and macrolide-susceptible clinical isolate, and this loss was associated with the deletion of >130 kb of genetic material (Trunck et al., 2009). The expression of *amrAB-oprA* increased resistance to not only aminoglycosides and macrolides but also fluoroquinolones and tetracyclines in a BpeAB-OprA pump-deficient mutant of 1026b (Mima and Schweizer, 2010). Judging from the substrate specificity and sequence similarity (Mima and Schweizer, 2010), we have no doubt that AmrAB is a functional ortholog of MexXY in *B. pseudomallei*. BpeAB-OprB of *B. pseudomallei* also reportedly mediates aminoglycoside resistance in strain KHW (Chan et al., 2004), while this pump did not confer aminoglycoside resistance in 1026b (Mima and Schweizer, 2010). In addition, the BpeB RND transporter was also shown to be closely related to MexB of *P. aeruginosa*, both functionally and phylogenetically (Mima and Schweizer, 2010), consistent with our phylogenetic analysis (**Figure 1**).

Table 1 | Genetic organization of aminoglycoside efflux operons of clinical significance and their regulators in non-fermentative Gram-negative pathogens.

Organism	Efflux operon	Product	Function	Regulator	
				Cognate	Other
P. aeruginosa	*mexXY* (*-oprA*)[a]	MexX	MFP	MexZ	PA5471
		MexY	RND		ParRS
		(OprA)[a]	OMF		
		OprM			
A. xylosoxidans	*axyXY-oprZ*	AxyX	MFP	AxyR	
		AxyY	RND		
		OprZ	OMF		
B. pseudomallei (*B. cepacia* complex)	*amrAB-oprA*	AmrA	MFP	AmrR	
		AmrB	RND		
		OprA	OMF		
A. baumannii	*adeAB* (*-adeC*)[b]	AdeA	MFP	AdeRS	?[c]
		AdeB	RND		
		(AdeC)[b]	OMF		
		?[b]			

The genetic organization of genes involved in aminoglycoside efflux and their regulation of expression is summarized. No obvious significant differences on substrate specificities were observed among the pumps. TetR-type negative regulators are encoded by genes located upstream of the operons in P. aeruginosa, A. xylosoxydans, and B. pseudomallei, while the AdeRS two-component regulatory proteins are encoded by genes located upstream of the adeAB (-adeC) operon.

[a]*oprA gene found in the multidrug-resistant clinical isolate PA7 and relatives, all of which are serotype O12, is absent and often OprM encoded by the mexAB-oprM multidrug efflux operon is associated with the MexXY component in most P. aeruginosa strains (Morita et al., 2012). MexXY can utilize OprA or OprM as an outer membrane channel (Morita et al., 2012).*

[b]*AdeC is not essential for AdeAB-mediated resistance (Marchand et al., 2004), suggesting that AdeAB recruits another yet unknown outer membrane protein as indicated by the question mark.*

[c]*The question mark signifies other unknown regulatory mechanism(s) involved in adeABC overexpression (Sun et al., 2010).*

As described above, AmrB orthologs are conserved among various human pathogens belonging to *Burkholderia* species, but not *B. gladioli*. Actually, an AmrAB-OprA ortholog was shown to be a major aminoglycoside resistance contributor in *B. cenocepacia*, a member of the *B. cepacia* complex (Hamad et al., 2010).

AdeABC IS A MULTIDRUG EFFLUX SYSTEM THAT MEDIATES AMINOGLYCOSIDE RESISTANCE IN *A. baumannii*

Acinetobacter baumannii is the most frequently implicated species in nosocomial infections among *Acinetobacter* spp. (Coyne et al., 2011). AdeABC was identified as an RND-type efflux pump involved in resistance to multiple antimicrobials including aminoglycosides, fluoroquinolones, tetracycline, erythromycin, cefotaxime, trimethoprim, and chloramphenicol in *A. baumannii* BM4454, a low-level pan-aminoglycoside resistant clinical isolate

(Magnet et al., 2001). The polycistronic *adeABC* transcript was confirmed experimentally to encode AdeA (MFP), AdeB (RND transporter), and AdeC (OMF; Magnet et al., 2001; Marchand et al., 2004). Because the substrate specificity of AdeAB is very similar to that of MexXY, we have no doubt that AdeAB is a functional homolog of MexXY in *A. baumannii.* AdeC is not essential for AdeAB-mediated resistance (Marchand et al., 2004), indicating that AdeAB recruits another outer membrane protein to form a functional tripartite complex, as observed for the MexXY pump with OprM in *P. aeruginosa* (Aires et al., 1999; Mine et al., 1999). We do not rule out the possibility that AdeAB is functional with AdeC, as observed for the MexXY pump with its linked outer-membrane channel OprA, which was not essential in *P. aeruginosa* PA7 (Morita et al., 2012). The *adeAB* genes are usually present, but the *adeC* gene was not found in ~40% of clinical isolates (Nemec et al., 2007). Our phylogenetic analysis showed that AdeC is more closely related to OprM and OprJ than to OprA in the OprM outer membrane family of *P. aeruginosa* (**Figure 2**).

The *adeABC* operon is expressed at low levels in natural isolates of *A. baumannii* due to stringent control by the AdeRS two-component system, which is encoded adjacent to *adeABC,* but transcribed in the opposite direction (Marchand et al., 2004; **Table 1**). Mutations (e.g., $AdeR_{Pro116Leu}$, $AdeS_{Thr153Met}$, or $AdeS_{Gly30Asp}$) in AdeRS have been shown to be responsible for the constitutive expression of AdeABC (Marchand et al., 2004), which reminds us that mutations (e.g., $ParR_{Met59Ile}$) in the ParRS two-component system are responsible for the constitutive expression of MexXY in *P. aeruginosa* (Muller et al., 2011). Overexpression of the AdeABC system in a tigecycline non-susceptible clinical isolate was due to the transposition of a copy of IS*Aba1* into *adeS* (Ruzin et al., 2007). Very recently, a truncated AdeS kinase protein generated by an IS*Aba1* insertion was shown to be correlated with enhanced *adeABC* expression in *A. baumannii* (Sun et al., 2012). Other regulatory mechanism(s) were shown to be involved in *adeABC* overexpression without any previously known mutation (Sun et al., 2010). Recently the AdeABC ortholog was shown to be a contributor to multiple antimicrobials, including aminoglycosides, in *Acinetobacter* genomospecies 13TU, a non-*A. baumannii* species (Roca et al., 2011).

FUTURE PERSPECTIVES

MexXY is one of the potential targets for novel anti-pseudomonas agents. Its inhibitor is able to not only potentiate previously used ineffective antimicrobial agents (e.g., aminoglycosides against aminoglycoside-resistant *P. aeruginosa* and *B. cepacia* complex), but also to speed up the development of novel anti-pseudomonas agents. Because there are a significant number of potential drug targets encoded by the genome of *P. aeruginosa* (e.g., products of essential genes; Morita et al., 2010), it is the most promising therapeutic strategy to conquer the impermeability barriers of these bacteria. The efflux inhibitor MP 601384, which has specificity toward aminoglycoside-accommodating RND efflux systems and is not toxic to bacteria, is the only MexXY inhibitor reported so far (Jassem et al., 2011). Uncultured bacteria and plants are predicted to be a significant reservoir of novel antimicrobial agents (Stavri et al., 2007; Piel, 2011). Screening novel antibacterial agents, including a MexXY inhibitor, is currently in progress in our laboratory (e.g., Shiota et al., 2004).

ACKNOWLEDGMENTS

This work was supported in part by a Grant-in-Aid for Young Scientists (B) (Kakenhi 23790106) from the Japan Society for the Promotion of Science and a research grant from the Institute of Pharmaceutical Life Sciences, Aichi Gakuin University.

REFERENCES

Aires, J. R., Kohler, T., Nikaido, H., and Plesiat, P. (1999). Involvement of an active efflux system in the natural resistance of *Pseudomonas aeruginosa* to aminoglycosides. *Antimicrob. Agents Chemother.* 43, 2624–2628.

Aires, J. R., and Nikaido, H. (2005). Aminoglycosides are captured from both periplasm and cytoplasm by the AcrD multidrug efflux transporter of *Escherichia coli. J. Bacteriol.* 187, 1923–1929.

Alguel, Y., Lu, D., Quade, N., Sauter, S., and Zhang, X. (2010). Crystal structure of MexZ, a key repressor responsible for antibiotic resistance in *Pseudomonas aeruginosa. J. Struct. Biol.* 172, 305–310.

Armstrong, E. S., and Miller, G. H. (2010). Combating evolution with intelligent design: the neoglycoside ACHN-490. *Curr. Opin. Microbiol.* 13, 565–573.

Bador, J., Amoureux, L., Duez, J. M., Drabowicz, A., Siebor, E., Llanes, C., et al. (2011). First description of an RND-type multidrug efflux pump in *Achromobacter* xylosoxidans, AxyABM. *Antimicrob. Agents Chemother.* 55, 4912–4914.

Bador, J., Amoureux, L., Blanc, E. and Neuwirth, C. (2012). The innate aminoglycoside resistance of *Achromobacter xylosoxidans* is due to AxyXY- OprZ, an RND-type multidrug efflux pump. *Antimicrob. Agents Chemother.* doi: 10.1128/AAC.01243-12 [Epub ahead of print].

Baranov, P. V., Vestergaard, B., Hamelryck, T., Gesteland, R. F., Nyborg, J., and Atkins, J. F. (2006). Diverse bacterial genomes encode an operon of two genes, one of which is an unusual class-I release factor that potentially recognizes atypical mRNA signals other than normal stop codons. *Biol. Direct* 1, 28.

Barry, A. L., Reller, L. B., Miller, G. H., Washington, J. A., Schoenknect, F. D., Peterson, L. R., et al. (1992). Revision of standards for adjusting the cation content of Mueller-Hinton broth for testing susceptibility of *Pseudomonas aeruginosa* to aminoglycosides. *J. Clin. Microbiol.* 30, 585–589.

Baum, E. Z., Crespo-Carbone, S. M., Morrow, B. J., Davies, T. A., Foleno, B. D., He, W., et al. (2009). Effect of MexXY overexpression on ceftobiprole susceptibility in *Pseudomonas aeruginosa. Antimicrob. Agents Chemother.* 53, 2785–2790.

Beaudoin, T., Aaron, S. D., Giesbrecht-Lewis, T., Vandemheen, K., and Mah, T. F. (2010). Characterization of clonal strains of *Pseudomonas aeruginosa* isolated from cystic fibrosis patients in Ontario, Canada. *Can. J. Microbiol.* 56, 548–557.

Bochner, B. R., Giovannetti, L., and Viti, C. (2008). Important discoveries from analysing bacterial phenotypes. *Mol. Microbiol.* 70, 274–280.

Campo Esquisabel, A. B., Rodriguez, M. C., Campo-Sosa, A. O., Rodriguez, C., and Martinez-Martinez, L. (2011). Mechanisms of resistance in clinical isolates of *Pseudomonas aeruginosa* less susceptible to cefepime than to ceftazidime. *Clin. Microbiol. Infect.* 17, 1817–1822.

Chan, Y. Y., Tan, T. M., Ong, Y. M., and Chua, K. L. (2004). BpeAB-OprB, a multidrug efflux pump in *Burkholderia pseudomallei. Antimicrob. Agents Chemother.* 48, 1128–1135.

Caughlan, R. E., Sriram, S., Daigle, D. M., Woods, A. L., Buco, J., Peterson, R. L., et al. (2009). Fmt bypass in *Pseudomonas aeruginosa* causes induction of MexXY efflux pump expression. *Antimicrob. Agents Chemother.* 53, 5015–5021.

Coyne, S., Rosenfeld, N., Lambert, T., Courvalin, P., and Perichon, B. (2010). Overexpression of resistance-nodulation-cell division pump AdeFGH confers multidrug resistance in *Acinetobacter baumannii. Antimicrob. Agents Chemother.* 54, 4389–4393.

Coyne, S., Courvalin, P., and Perichon, B. (2011). Efflux-mediated antibiotic resistance in *Acinetobacter* spp. *Antimicrob. Agents Chemother.* 55, 947–953.

Crossman, L. C., Gould, V. C., Dow, J. M., Vernikos, G. S., Okazaki, A., Sebaihia, M., et al. (2008). The complete genome, comparative and functional analysis of *Stenotrophomonas maltophilia* reveals an organism heavily shielded by drug resistance determinants. *Genome Biol.* 9, R74.

Damier-Piolle, L., Magnet, S., Bremont, S., Lambert, T., and Courvalin, P. (2008). AdeIJK, a resistance-nodulation-cell division pump effluxing multiple antibiotics in *Acinetobacter baumannii*. *Antimicrob. Agents Chemother.* 52, 557–562.

de Bentzmann, S., and Plesiat, P. (2011). The *Pseudomonas aeruginosa* opportunistic pathogen and human infections. *Environ. Microbiol.* 13, 1655–1665.

Dean, C. R., Visalli, M. A., Projan, S. J., Sum, P. E., and Bradford, P. A. (2003). Efflux-mediated resistance to tigecycline (GAR-936) in *Pseudomonas aeruginosa* PAO1. *Antimicrob. Agents Chemother.* 47, 972–978.

Deplano, A., Denis, O., Poirel, L., Hocquet, D., Nonhoff, C., Byl, B., et al. (2005). Molecular characterization of an epidemic clone of panantibiotic-resistant *Pseudomonas aeruginosa*. *J. Clin. Microbiol.* 43, 1198–1204.

Eda, S., Maseda, H., and Nakae, T. (2003). An elegant means of self-protection in gram-negative bacteria by recognizing and extruding xenobiotics from the periplasmic space. *J. Biol. Chem.* 278, 2085–2088.

Edgar, R., and Bibi, E. (1997). MdfA, an *Escherichia coli* multidrug resistance protein with an extraordinarily broad spectrum of drug recognition. *J. Bacteriol.* 179, 2274–2280.

El'Garch, F., Jeannot, K., Hocquet, D., Llanes-Barakat, C., and Plesiat, P. (2007). Cumulative effects of several nonenzymatic mechanisms on the resistance of *Pseudomonas aeruginosa* to aminoglycosides. *Antimicrob. Agents Chemother.* 51, 1016–1021.

Elkins, C. A., and Nikaido, H. (2002). Substrate specificity of the RND-type multidrug efflux pumps AcrB and AcrD of *Escherichia coli* is determined predominantly by two large periplasmic loops. *J. Bacteriol.* 184, 6490–6498.

Fehlberg, L. C., Xavier, D. E., Peraro, P. P., Marra, A. R., Edmond, M. B., and Gales, A. C. (2012). Beta-lactam resistance mechanisms in *Pseudomonas aeruginosa* strains causing bloodstream infections: comparative results between Brazilian and American isolates. *Microb. Drug Resist.* 18, 402–407.

Feliziani, S., Lujan, A. M., Moyano, A. J., Sola, C., Bocco, J. L., Montanaro, P., et al. (2010). Mucoidy, quorum sensing, mismatch repair and antibiotic resistance in *Pseudomonas aeruginosa* from cystic fibrosis chronic airways infections. *PLoS ONE* 5, e12669. doi: 10.1371/journal.pone.0012669

Fetar, H., Gilmour, C., Klinoski, R., Daigle, D. M., Dean, C. R., and Poole, K. (2011). mexEF-oprN multidrug efflux operon of *Pseudomonas aeruginosa*: regulation by the MexT activator in response to nitrosative stress and chloramphenicol. *Antimicrob. Agents Chemother.* 55, 508–514.

Fischbach, M. A., and Walsh, C. T. (2009). Antibiotics for emerging pathogens. *Science* 325, 1089–1093.

Fraud, S., and Poole, K. (2011). Oxidative stress induction of the MexXY multidrug efflux genes and promotion of aminoglycoside resistance development in *Pseudomonas aeruginosa*. *Antimicrob. Agents Chemother.* 55, 1068–1074.

Frisk, A., Schurr, J. R., Wang, G., Bertucci, D. C., Marrero, L., Hwang, S. H., et al. (2004). Transcriptome analysis of *Pseudomonas aeruginosa* after interaction with human airway epithelial cells. *Infect. Immun.* 72, 5433–5438.

Glupczynski, Y., Hansen, W., Freney, J., and Yourassowsky, E. (1988). *In vitro* susceptibility of *Alcaligenes denitrificans* subsp. *xylosoxidans* to 24 antimicrobial agents. *Antimicrob. Agents Chemother.* 32, 276–278.

Goldberg, J. B., Hancock, R. E., Parales, R. E., Loper, J., and Cornelis, P. (2008). *Pseudomonas* 2007. *J. Bacteriol.* 190, 2649–2662.

Hagman, K. E., Lucas, C. E., Balthazar, J. T., Snyder, L., Nilles, M., Judd, R. C., et al. (1997). The MtrD protein of *Neisseria gonorrhoeae* is a member of the resistance/nodulation/division protein family constituting part of an efflux system. *Microbiology* 143 (Pt 7), 2117–2125.

Hamad, M. A., Skeldon, A. M., and Valvano, M. A. (2010). Construction of aminoglycoside-sensitive *Burkholderia cenocepacia* strains for use in studies of intracellular bacteria with the gentamicin protection assay. *Appl. Environ. Microbiol.* 76, 3170–3176.

Hancock, R. E., Farmer, S. W., Li, Z. S., and Poole, K. (1991). Interaction of aminoglycosides with the outer membranes and purified lipopolysaccharide and OmpF porin of *Escherichia coli*. *Antimicrob. Agents Chemother.* 35, 1309–1314.

Hancock, R. E. (1998). Resistance mechanisms in *Pseudomonas aeruginosa* and other nonfermentative gram-negative bacteria. *Clin. Infect. Dis.* 27(Suppl. 1), S93–S99.

Henrichfreise, B., Wiegand, I., Pfister, W., and Wiedemann, B. (2007). Resistance mechanisms of multiresistant *Pseudomonas aeruginosa* strains from Germany and correlation with hypermutation. *Antimicrob. Agents Chemother.* 51, 4062–4070.

Hirakawa, H., Nishino, K., Hirata, T., and Yamaguchi, A. (2003). Comprehensive studies of drug resistance mediated by overexpression of response regulators of two-component signal transduction systems in *Escherichia coli*. *J. Bacteriol.* 185, 1851–1856.

Hocquet, D., Vogne, C., El Garch, F., Vejux, A., Gotoh, N., Lee, A., et al. (2003). MexXY-OprM efflux pump is necessary for a adaptive resistance of *Pseudomonas aeruginosa* to aminoglycosides. *Antimicrob. Agents Chemother.* 47, 1371–1375.

Hocquet, D., Nordmann, P., El Garch, F., Cabanne, L., and Plesiat, P. (2006). Involvement of the MexXY-OprM efflux system in emergence of cefepime resistance in clinical strains of *Pseudomonas aeruginosa*. *Antimicrob. Agents Chemother.* 50, 1347–1351.

Hocquet, D., Berthelot, P., Roussel-Delvallez, M., Favre, R., Jeannot, K., Bajolet, O., et al. (2007). *Pseudomonas aeruginosa* may accumulate drug resistance mechanisms without losing its ability to cause bloodstream infections. *Antimicrob. Agents Chemother.* 51, 3531–3536.

Hocquet, D., Muller, A., Blanc, K., Plesiat, P., Talon, D., Monnet, D. L., et al. (2008). Relationship between antibiotic use and incidence of MexXY-OprM overproducers among clinical isolates of *Pseudomonas aeruginosa*. *Antimicrob. Agents Chemother.* 52, 1173–1175.

Horiyama, T., Yamaguchi, A., and Nishino, K. (2011). TolC dependency of multidrug efflux systems in *Salmonella enterica* serovar Typhimurium. *J. Antimicrob. Chemother.* 65, 1372–1376.

Islam, S., Jalal, S., and Wretlind, B. (2004). Expression of the MexXY efflux pump in amikacin-resistant isolates of *Pseudomonas aeruginosa*. *Clin. Microbiol. Infect.* 10, 877–883.

Islam, S., Oh, H., Jalal, S., Karpati, F., Ciofu, O., Hoiby, N., et al. (2009). Chromosomal mechanisms of aminoglycoside resistance in *Pseudomonas aeruginosa* isolates from cystic fibrosis patients. *Clin. Microbiol. Infect.* 15, 60–66.

Jassem, A. N., Zlosnik, J. E., Henry, D. A., Hancock, R. E., Ernst, R. K., and Speert, D. P. (2011). In vitro susceptibility of *Burkholderia vietnamiensis* to aminoglycosides. *Antimicrob. Agents Chemother.* 55, 2256–2264.

Jeannot, K., Sobel, M. L., El Garch, F., Poole, K., and Plesiat, P. (2005). Induction of the MexXY efflux pump in *Pseudomonas aeruginosa* is dependent on drug-ribosome interaction. *J. Bacteriol.* 187, 5341–5346.

Jeannot, K., Elsen, S., Kohler, T., Attree, I., van Delden, C., and Plesiat, P. (2008). Resistance and virulence of *Pseudomonas aeruginosa* clinical strains overproducing the MexCD-OprJ efflux pump. *Antimicrob. Agents Chemother.* 52, 2455–2462.

Kenny, D. J., Russell, P., Rogers, D., Eley, S. M., and Titball, R. W. (1999). *In vitro* susceptibilities of *Burkholderia mallei* in comparison to those of other pathogenic Burkholderia spp. *Antimicrob. Agents Chemother.* 43, 2773–2775.

Kim, H. S., Nagore, D., and Nikaido, H. (2010). Multidrug efflux pump MdtBC of *Escherichia coli* is active only as a B2C heterotrimer. *J. Bacteriol.* 192, 1377–1386.

Kindrachuk, K. N., Fernandez, L., Bains, M., and Hancock, R. E. (2011). Involvement of an ATP-dependent protease, PA0779/AsrA, in inducing heat shock in response to tobramycin in *Pseudomonas aeruginosa*. *Antimicrob. Agents Chemother.* 55, 1874–1882.

Klimke, W., Agarwala, R., Badretdin, A., Chetvernin, S., Ciufo, S., Fedorov, B., et al. (2009). The National Center for Biotechnology Information's Protein Clusters Database. *Nucleic Acids Res.* 37, D216–D223.

Kohler, T., Michea-Hamzehpour, M., Henze, U., Gotoh, N., Curty, L. K., and Pechere, J. C. (1997). Characterization of MexE-MexF-OprN, a positively regulated multidrug efflux system of *Pseudomonas aeruginosa*. *Mol. Microbiol.* 23, 345–354.

Laohavaleeson, S., Lolans, K., Quinn, J. P., Kuti, J. L., and Nicolau, D. P. (2008). Expression of the MexXY-OprM efflux system in *Pseudomonas aeruginosa* with discordant cefepime/ceftazidime susceptibility profiles. *Infect. Drug Resist.* 1, 51–55.

Lau, C. H., Fraud, S., Jones, M., Peterson, S. N., and Poole, K. (2012). Reduced expression of the rplU-rpmA ribosomal protein operon in mexXY-expressing pan-aminoglycoside-resistant mutants of *Pseudomonas aeruginosa*. *Antimicrob. Agents Chemother.* 56, 5171–5179.

Lee, S., Hinz, A., Bauerle, E., Angermeyer, A., Juhaszova, K., Kaneko, Y., et al. (2009). Targeting a bacterial stress response to enhance antibiotic action. *Proc. Natl. Acad. Sci. U.S.A.* 106, 14570–14575.

Li, X. Z., Livermore, D. M., and Nikaido, H. (1994a). Role of efflux pump(s) in intrinsic resistance of *Pseudomonas aeruginosa*: resistance to tetracycline, chloramphenicol, and norfloxacin. *Antimicrob. Agents Chemother.* 38, 1732–1741.

Li, X. Z., Ma, D., Livermore, D. M., and Nikaido, H. (1994b). Role of efflux pump(s) in intrinsic resistance of *Pseudomonas aeruginosa*: active efflux as a contributing factor to beta-lactam resistance. *Antimicrob. Agents Chemother.* 38, 1742–1752.

Li, X. Z., Nikaido, H., and Poole, K. (1995). Role of mexA-mexB-oprM in antibiotic efflux in *Pseudomonas aeruginosa*. *Antimicrob. Agents Chemother.* 39, 1948–1953.

Li, X. Z., Poole, K., and Nikaido, H. (2003). Contributions of MexAB-OprM and an EmrE homolog to intrinsic resistance of *Pseudomonas aeruginosa* to aminoglycosides and dyes. *Antimicrob. Agents Chemother.* 47, 27–33.

Li, X. Z., and Nikaido, H. (2004). Efflux-mediated drug resistance in bacteria. *Drugs* 64, 159–204.

Li, X. Z., and Nikaido, H. (2009). Efflux-mediated drug resistance in bacteria: an update. *Drugs* 69, 1555–1623.

Lindemann, A., Koch, M., Pessi, G., Muller, A. J., Balsiger, S., Hennecke, H., et al. (2010). Host-specific symbiotic requirement of BdeAB, a RegR-controlled RND-type efflux system in *Bradyrhizobium japonicum*. *FEMS Microbiol. Lett.* 312, 184–191.

Lister, P. D., Wolter, D. J., and Hanson, N. D. (2009). Antibacterial-resistant *Pseudomonas aeruginosa*: clinical impact and complex regulation of chromosomally encoded resistance mechanisms. *Clin. Microbiol. Rev.* 22, 582–610.

Llanes, C., Hocquet, D., Vogne, C., Benali-Baitich, D., Neuwirth, C., and Plesiat, P. (2004). Clinical strains of *Pseudomonas aeruginosa* overproducing MexAB-OprM and MexXY efflux pumps simultaneously. *Antimicrob. Agents Chemother.* 48, 1797–1802.

Llanes, C., Neuwirth, C., El Garch, F., Hocquet, D., and Plesiat, P. (2006). Genetic analysis of a multiresistant strain of *Pseudomonas aeruginosa* producing PER-1 beta-lactamase. *Clin. Microbiol. Infect.* 12, 270–278.

Llanes, C., Kohler, T., Patry, I., Dehecq, B., van Delden, C., and Plesiat, P. (2011). Role of the MexEF-OprN efflux system in low-level resistance of *Pseudomonas aeruginosa* to ciprofloxacin. *Antimicrob. Agents Chemother.* 55, 5676–5684.

Lomovskaya, O., Warren, M. S., Lee, A., Galazzo, J., Fronko, R., Lee, M., et al. (2001). Identification and characterization of inhibitors of multidrug resistance efflux pumps in *Pseudomonas aeruginosa*: novel agents for combination therapy. *Antimicrob. Agents Chemother.* 45, 105–116.

Magnet, S., Courvalin, P., and Lambert, T. (2001). Resistance-nodulation-cell division-type efflux pump involved in aminoglycoside resistance in *Acinetobacter baumannii* strain BM4454. *Antimicrob. Agents Chemother.* 45, 3375–3380.

Maniati, M., Ikonomidis, A., Mantzana, P., Daponte, A., Maniatis, A. N., and Pournaras, S. (2007). A highly carbapenem-resistant *Pseudomonas aeruginosa* isolate with a novel blaVIM-4/blaP1b integron overexpresses two efflux pumps and lacks OprD. *J. Antimicrob. Chemother.* 60, 132–135.

Mao, W., Warren, M. S., Lee, A., Mistry, A., and Lomovskaya, O. (2001). MexXY-OprM efflux pump is required for antagonism of aminoglycosides by divalent cations in *Pseudomonas aeruginosa*. *Antimicrob. Agents Chemother.* 45, 2001–2007.

Marchand, I., Damier-Piolle, L., Courvalin, P., and Lambert, T. (2004). Expression of the RND-type efflux pump AdeABC in *Acinetobacter baumannii* is regulated by the AdeRS two-component system. *Antimicrob. Agents Chemother.* 48, 3298–3304.

Martha, B., Croisier, D., Durand, D., Hocquet, D., Plesiat, P., Piroth, L., et al. (2006). *In-vivo* impact of the MexXY efflux system on aminoglycoside efficacy in an experimental model of *Pseudomonas aeruginosa* pneumonia treated with tobramycin. *Clin. Microbiol. Infect.* 12, 426–432.

Masuda, N., Sakagawa, E., Ohya, S., Gotoh, N., Tsujimoto, H., and Nishino, T. (2000a). Contribution of the MexX-MexY-oprM efflux system to intrinsic resistance in *Pseudomonas aeruginosa*. *Antimicrob. Agents Chemother.* 44, 2242–2246.

Masuda, N., Sakagawa, E., Ohya, S., Gotoh, N., Tsujimoto, H., and Nishino, T. (2000b). Substrate specificities of MexAB-OprM, MexCD-OprJ, and MexXY-oprM efflux pumps in *Pseudomonas aeruginosa*. *Antimicrob. Agents Chemother.* 44, 3322–3327.

Matsumoto, Y., Hayama, K., Sakakihara, S., Nishino, K., Noji, H., Iino, R., et al. (2011). Evaluation of multidrug efflux pump inhibitors by a new method using microfluidic channels. *PLoS ONE* 6, e18547. doi: 10.1371/journal.pone.0018547

Matsuo, T., Hayashi, K., Morita, Y., Koterasawa, M., Ogawa, W., Mizushima, T., et al.i (2007). VmeAB, an RND-type multidrug efflux transporter in *Vibrio parahaemolyticus*. *Microbiology* 153, 4129–4137.

Matsuo, Y., Eda, S., Gotoh, N., Yoshihara, E., and Nakae, T. (2004). MexZ-mediated regulation of mexXY multidrug efflux pump expression in *Pseudomonas aeruginosa* by binding on the mexZ-mexX intergenic DNA. *FEMS Microbiol. Lett.* 238, 23–28.

McLaughlin, H. P., Caly, D. L., McCarthy, Y., Ryan, R. P., and Dow, J. M. (2012). An orphan chemotaxis sensor regulates virulence and antibiotic tolerance in the human pathogen *Pseudomonas aeruginosa*. *PLoS ONE* 7, e42205. doi: 10.1371/journal.pone.0042205

Medeiros, A. A., O'Brien, T. F., Wacker, W. E., and Yulug, N. F. (1971). Effect of salt concentration on the apparent *in-vitro* susceptibility of *Pseudomonas* and other Gram-negative bacilli to gentamicin. *J. Infect. Dis.* 124(Suppl), S59–S64.

Merlin, T. L., Corvo, D. L., Gill, J. H., and Griffith, J. K. (1989a). Enhanced gentamicin killing of *Escherichia coli* by tet gene expression. *Antimicrob. Agents Chemother.* 33, 230–232.

Merlin, T. L., Davis, G. E., Anderson, W. L., Moyzis, R. K., and Griffith, J. K. (1989b). Aminoglycoside uptake increased by tet gene expression. *Antimicrob. Agents Chemother.* 33, 1549–1552.

Mesaros, N., Glupczynski, Y., Avrain, L., Caceres, N. E., Tulkens, P. M., and Van Bambeke, F. (2007). A combined phenotypic and genotypic method for the detection of Mex efflux pumps in *Pseudomonas aeruginosa*. *J. Antimicrob. Chemother.* 59, 378–386.

Mima, T., and Schweizer, H. P. (2010). The BpeAB-OprB efflux pump of *Burkholderia pseudomallei* 1026b does not play a role in quorum sensing, virulence factor production, or extrusion of aminoglycosides but is a broad-spectrum drug efflux system. *Antimicrob. Agents Chemother.* 54, 3113–3120.

Mine, T., Morita, Y., Kataoka, A., Mizushima, T., and Tsuchiya, T. (1998). Evidence for chloramphenicol/H^+ antiport in Cmr (MdfA) system of *Escherichia coli* and properties of the antiporter. *J. Biochem.* 124, 187–193.

Mine, T., Morita, Y., Kataoka, A., Mizushima, T., and Tsuchiya, T. (1999). Expression in *Escherichia coli* of a new multidrug efflux pump, MexXY, from *Pseudomonas aeruginosa*. *Antimicrob. Agents Chemother.* 43, 415–417.

Moore, R. A., DeShazer, D., Reckseidler, S., Weissman, A., and Woods, D. E. (1999). Efflux-mediated aminoglycoside and macrolide resistance in *Burkholderia pseudomallei*. *Antimicrob. Agents Chemother.* 43, 465–470.

Morita, Y., Kodama, K., Shiota, S., Mine, T., Kataoka, A., Mizushima, T., et al. (1998). NorM, a putative multidrug efflux protein, of *Vibrio parahaemolyticus* and its homolog in *Escherichia coli*. *Antimicrob. Agents Chemother.* 42, 1778–1782.

Morita, Y., Kataoka, A., Shiota, S., Mizushima, T., and Tsuchiya, T. (2000). NorM of *Vibrio parahaemolyticus* is an Na(+)-driven multidrug efflux pump. *J. Bacteriol.* 182, 6694–6697.

Morita, Y., Kimura, N., Mima, T., Mizushima, T., and Tsuchiya, T. (2001a). Roles of MexXY- and MexAB-multidrug efflux pumps in intrinsic multidrug resistance of *Pseudomonas aeruginosa* PAO1. *J. Gen. Appl. Microbiol.* 47, 27–32.

Morita, Y., Komori, Y., Mima, T., Kuroda, T., Mizushima, T., and Tsuchiya, T. (2001b). Construction of a series of mutants lacking all of the four major mex operons for multidrug efflux pumps or possessing each one of the operons from *Pseudomonas aeruginosa* PAO1: MexCD-OprJ is an inducible pump. *FEMS Microbiol. Lett.* 202, 139–143.

Morita, Y., Murata, T., Mima, T., Shiota, S., Kuroda, T., Mizushima, T., et al. (2003). Induction of mexCD-oprJ operon for a multidrug efflux pump by disinfectants in wild-type *Pseudomonas aeruginosa* PAO1. *J. Antimicrob. Chemother.* 51, 991–994.

Morita, Y., Sobel, M. L., and Poole, K. (2006). Antibiotic inducibility of the MexXY multidrug efflux system of *Pseudomonas aeruginosa*: involvement of the antibiotic-inducible PA5471 gene product. *J. Bacteriol.* 188, 1847–1855.

Morita, Y., Gilmour, C., Metcalf, D., and Poole, K. (2009). Translational control of the antibiotic inducibility of the PA5471 gene required for mexXY multidrug efflux gene expression in *Pseudomonas aeruginosa*. *J. Bacteriol.* 191, 4966–4975.

Morita, Y., Narita, S., Tomida, J., Tokuda, H., and Kawamura, Y. (2010). Application of an inducible system to engineer unmarked conditional mutants of essential genes of *Pseudomonas aeruginosa*. *J. Microbiol. Methods* 82, 205–213.

Morita, Y., Tomida, J., and Kawamura, Y. (2012). Primary mechanisms mediating aminoglycoside resistance in the multidrug-resistant *Pseudomonas aeruginosa* clinical isolate PA7. *Microbiology* 158, 1071–1083.

Mulet, X., Moya, B., Juan, C., Macia, M. D., Perez, J. L., Blazquez, J., et al. (2011). Antagonistic interactions of *Pseudomonas aeruginosa* antibiotic resistance mechanisms in planktonic but not biofilm growth. *Antimicrob. Agents Chemother.* 55, 4560–4568.

Muller, C., Plesiat, P., and Jeannot, K. (2011). A two-component regulatory system interconnects resistance to polymyxins, aminoglycosides, fluoroquinolones, and beta-lactams in *Pseudomonas aeruginosa. Antimicrob. Agents Chemother.* 55, 1211–1221.

Murakami, S., Nakashima, R., Yamashita, E., and Yamaguchi, A. (2002). Crystal structure of bacterial multidrug efflux transporter AcrB. *Nature* 419, 587–593.

Murata, T., Gotoh, N., and Nishino, T. (2002). Characterization of outer membrane efflux proteins OpmE, OpmD and OpmB of *Pseudomonas aeruginosa*: molecular cloning and development of specific antisera. *FEMS Microbiol. Lett.* 217, 57–63.

Nagano, K., and Nikaido, H. (2009). Kinetic behavior of the major multidrug efflux pump AcrB of *Escherichia coli. Proc. Natl. Acad. Sci. U.S.A.* 106, 5854–5858.

Nakashima, R., Sakurai, K., Yamasaki, S., Nishino, K., and Yamaguchi, A. (2011). Structures of the multidrug exporter AcrB reveal a proximal multisite drug-binding pocket. *Nature* 480, 565–569.

Nemec, A., Maixnerova, M., van der Reijden, T. J., van den Broek, P. J., and Dijkshoorn, L. (2007). Relationship between the AdeABC efflux system gene content, netilmicin susceptibility and multidrug resistance in a genotypically diverse collection of *Acinetobacter baumannii* strains. *J. Antimicrob. Chemother.* 60, 483–489.

Ngeow, Y. F., and Puthucheary, S. D. (1985). Antibiotic susceptibilities of *Achromobacter xylosoxydans. Singapore Med. J.* 26, 519–522.

Nikaido, H. (1994). Prevention of drug access to bacterial targets: permeability barriers and active efflux. *Science* 264, 382–388.

Nikaido, H. (1996). Multidrug efflux pumps of gram-negative bacteria. *J. Bacteriol.* 178, 5853–5859.

Nikaido, H. (2011). Structure and mechanism of RND-type multidrug efflux pumps. *Adv. Enzymol. Relat. Areas Mol. Biol.* 77, 1–60.

Nikaido, H., and Pages, J. M. (2012). Broad-specificity efflux pumps and their role in multidrug resistance of Gram-negative bacteria. *FEMS Microbiol. Rev.* 36, 340–363.

Nishino, K., and Yamaguchi, A. (2001). Analysis of a complete library of putative drug transporter genes in *Escherichia coli. J. Bacteriol.* 183, 5803–5812.

Nishino, K., Yamada, J., Hirakawa, H., Hirata, T., and Yamaguchi, A. (2003). Roles of TolC-dependent multidrug transporters of *Escherichia coli* in resistance to beta-lactams. *Antimicrob. Agents Chemother.* 47, 3030–3033.

Nishino, K., Latifi, T., and Groisman, E. A. (2006). Virulence and drug resistance roles of multidrug efflux systems of *Salmonella enterica* serovar Typhimurium. *Mol. Microbiol.* 59, 126–141.

Nishino, K., Nikaido, E., and Yamaguchi, A. (2009). Regulation and physiological function of multidrug efflux pumps in *Escherichia coli* and *Salmonella. Biochim. Biophys. Acta* 1794, 834–843.

Nishino, K., Yamasaki, S., Hayashi-Nishino, M., and Yamaguchi, A. (2010). Effect of NlpE overproduction on multidrug resistance in *Escherichia coli. Antimicrob. Agents Chemother.* 54, 2239–2243.

Papadopoulos, J. S., and Agarwala, R. (2007). COBALT: constraint-based alignment tool for multiple protein sequences. *Bioinformatics* 23, 1073–1079.

Pasca, M. R., Dalla Valle, C., De Jesus Lopes Ribeiro, A. L., Buroni, S., Papaleo, M. C., Bazzini, S., et al. (2012). Evaluation of fluoroquinolone resistance mechanisms in *Pseudomonas aeruginosa* multidrug resistance clinical isolates. *Microb. Drug Resist.* 18, 23–32.

Pena, C., Suarez, C., Tubau, F., Juan, C., Moya, B., Dominguez, M. A., et al. (2009). Nosocomial outbreak of a non-cefepime-susceptible ceftazidime-susceptible *Pseudomonas aeruginosa* strain overexpressing MexXY-OprM and producing an integron-borne PSE-1 betta-lactamase. *J. Clin. Microbiol.* 47, 2381–2387.

Piddock, L. J. (2006). Clinically relevant chromosomally encoded multidrug resistance efflux pumps in bacteria. *Clin. Microbiol. Rev.* 19, 382–402.

Piel, J. (2011). Approaches to capturing and designing biologically active small molecules produced by uncultured microbes. *Annu. Rev. Microbiol.* 65, 431–453.

Pirnay, J. P., Bilocq, F., Pot, B., Cornelis, P., Zizi, M., Van Eldere, J., et al. (2009). *Pseudomonas aeruginosa* population structure revisited. *PLoS ONE* 4, e7740. doi: 10.1371/journal.pone.0007740

Poole, K., Heinrichs, D. E., and Neshat, S. (1993a). Cloning and sequence analysis of an EnvCD homologue in *Pseudomonas aeruginosa*: regulation by iron and possible involvement in the secretion of the siderophore pyoverdine. *Mol. Microbiol.* 10, 529–544.

Poole, K., Krebes, K., McNally, C., and Neshat, S. (1993b). Multiple antibiotic resistance in *Pseudomonas aeruginosa*: evidence for involvement of an efflux operon. *J. Bacteriol.* 175, 7363–7372.

Poole, K., Gotoh, N., Tsujimoto, H., Zhao, Q., Wada, A., Yamasaki, T., et al. (1996). Overexpression of the mexC-mexD-oprJ efflux operon in nfxB-type multidrug-resistant strains of *Pseudomonas aeruginosa. Mol. Microbiol.* 21, 713–724.

Poole, K. (2004). Efflux-mediated multiresistance in Gram-negative bacteria. *Clin. Microbiol. Infect.* 10, 12–26.

Poole, K. (2011). *Pseudomonas aeruginosa*: resistance to the max. *Front. Microbiol.* 2:65. doi: 10.3389/fmicb.2011.00065

Poole, K. (2012). "Efflux-mediated antimicrobial resistance," in *Antibiotic Discovery and Development*, Vol. 1, eds T. J. Dougherty and M. J. Pucci (New York, NY: Springer), 349–395.

Queenan, A. M., Shang, W., Bush, K., and Flamm, R. K. (2010). Differential selection of single-step AmpC or efflux mutants of *Pseudomonas aeruginosa* by using cefepime, ceftazidime, or ceftobiprole. *Antimicrob. Agents Chemother.* 54, 4092–4097.

Remans, K., Vercammen, K., Bodilis, J., and Cornelis, P. (2010). Genome-wide analysis and literature-based survey of lipoproteins in *Pseudomonas aeruginosa. Microbiology* 156, 2597–2607.

Roca, I., Espinal, P., Marti, S., and Vila, J. (2011). First identification and characterization of an AdeABC-like efflux pump in Acinetobacter genomospecies 13TU. *Antimicrob. Agents Chemother.* 55, 1285–1286.

Rosenberg, E. Y., Ma, D., and Nikaido, H. (2000). AcrD of *Escherichia coli* is an aminoglycoside efflux pump. *J. Bacteriol.* 182, 1754–1756.

Roy, P. H., Tetu, S. G., Larouche, A., Elbourne, L., Tremblay, S., Ren, Q., et al. (2010). Complete genome sequence of the multiresistant taxonomic outlier *Pseudomonas aeruginosa* PA7. *PLoS ONE* 5, e8842. doi: 10.1371/journal.pone.0008842

Ruzin, A., Keeney, D., and Bradford, P. A. (2007). AdeABC multidrug efflux pump is associated with decreased susceptibility to tigecycline in *Acinetobacter calcoaceticus-Acinetobacter baumannii* complex. *J. Antimicrob. Chemother.* 59, 1001–1004.

Segonds, C., Clavel-Batut, P., Thouverez, M., Grenet, D., Le Coustumier, A., Plesiat, P., et al. (2009). Microbiological and epidemiological features of clinical respiratory isolates of *Burkholderia gladioli. J. Clin. Microbiol.* 47, 1510–1516.

Seo, Y. S., Lim, J., Choi, B. S., Kim, H., Goo, E., Lee, B., et al. (2011). Complete genome sequence of *Burkholderia gladioli* BSR3. *J. Bacteriol.* 193, 3149.

Shiota, S., Shimizu, M., Sugiyama, J., Morita, Y., Mizushima, T., and Tsuchiya, T. (2004). Mechanisms of action of corilagin and tellimagrandin I that remarkably potentiate the activity of beta-lactams against methicillin-resistant *Staphylococcus aureus. Microbiol. Immunol.* 48, 67–73.

Sidhu, K., Talbot, M., Mil, K. V., and Verstraete, M. (2012). Treatment with sub-inhibitory kanamycin induces adaptive resistance to aminoglycoside antibiotics via the AcrD multidrug efflux pump in *Escherichia coli* K-12. *J. Exp. Microbiol. Immunol.* 16, 11–16.

Simpson, A. J., White, N. J., and Wuthiekanun, V. (1999). Aminoglycoside and macrolide resistance in *Burkholderia pseudomallei. Antimicrob. Agents Chemother.* 43, 2332.

Smith, E. E., Buckley, D. G., Wu, Z., Saenphimmachak, C., Hoffman, L. R., D'Argenio, D. A., et al. (2006). Genetic adaptation by *Pseudomonas aeruginosa* to the airways of cystic fibrosis patients. *Proc. Natl. Acad. Sci. U.S.A.* 103, 8487–8492.

Sobel, M. L., McKay, G. A., and Poole, K. (2003). Contribution of the MexXY multidrug transporter to aminoglycoside resistance in *Pseudomonas aeruginosa* clinical isolates. *Antimicrob. Agents Chemother.* 47, 3202–3207.

Sobel, M. L., Neshat, S., and Poole, K. (2005). Mutations in PA2491 (mexS) promote MexT-dependent mexEF-oprN expression and multidrug resistance in a clinical strain of *Pseudomonas aeruginosa. J. Bacteriol.* 187, 1246–1253.

Srikumar, R., Li, X. Z., and Poole, K. (1997). Inner membrane efflux components are responsible for beta-lactam specificity of multidrug efflux pumps in *Pseudomonas aeruginosa*. *J. Bacteriol.* 179, 7875–7881.

Stavri, M., Piddock, L. J., and Gibbons, S. (2007). Bacterial efflux pump inhibitors from natural sources. *J. Antimicrob. Chemother.* 59, 1247–1260.

Stover, C. K., Pham, X. Q., Erwin, A. L. Mizoguchi, S, D., Warrener, P., Hickey, M. J., et al. (2000). Complete genome sequence of *Pseudomonas aeruginosa* PAO1, an opportunistic pathogen. *Nature* 406, 959–964.

Sun, J. R., Chan, M. C., Chang, T. Y., Wang, W. Y., and Chiueh, T. S. (2010). Overexpression of the adeB gene in clinical isolates of tigecycline-nonsusceptible *Acinetobacter baumannii* without insertion mutations in adeRS. *Antimicrob. Agents Chemother.* 54, 4934–4938.

Sun, J. R., Perng, C. L., Chan, M. C., Morita, Y., Lin, J. C., Su, C. M., et al. (2012). A truncated AdeS kinase protein generated by ISAba1 insertion correlates with tigecycline resistance in *Acinetobacter baumannii. PLoS ONE* . doi: 10.1371/journal.pone.0049534

Takatsuka, Y., and Nikaido, H. (2006). Threonine-978 in the transmembrane segment of the multidrug efflux pump AcrB of *Escherichia coli* is crucial for drug transport as a probable component of the proton relay network. *J. Bacteriol.* 188, 7284–7289.

Tanaka, N., and Shuman, S. (2011). RtcB is the RNA ligase component of an *Escherichia coli* RNA repair operon. *J. Biol. Chem.* 286, 7727–7731.

Thibault, F. M., Hernandez, E., Vidal, D. R., Girardet, M., and Cavallo, J. D. (2004). Antibiotic susceptibility of 65 isolates of *Burkholderia pseudomallei* and *Burkholderia mallei* to 35 antimicrobial agents. *J. Antimicrob. Chemother.* 54, 1134–1138.

Trunck, L. A., Propst, K. L., Wuthiekanun, V., Tuanyok A., Beckstrom-Sternberg, S. M., Beckstrom-Sternberg, J. S., et al. (2009). Molecular basis of rare aminoglycoside susceptibility and pathogenesis of *Burkholderia pseudomallei* clinical isolates from Thailand. *PLoS Negl. Trop. Dis.* 3, e519. doi: 10.1371/journal.pntd.0000519

Vermis, K., Vandamme, P. A., and Nelis, H. J. (2003). *Burkholderia cepacia* complex genomovars: utilization of carbon sources, susceptibility to antimicrobial agents and growth on selective media. *J. Appl. Microbiol.* 95, 1191–1199.

Vettoretti, L., Floret, N., Hocquet, D., Dehecq, B., Plesiat, P., Talon, D., et al. (2009a). Emergence of extensive-drug-resistant *Pseudomonas aeruginosa* in a French university hospital. *Eur. J. Clin. Microbiol. Infect. Dis.* 28, 1217–1222.

Vettoretti, L., Plesiat, P., Muller, C., El Garch, F., Phan, G., Attree, I., et al. (2009b). Efflux unbalance in *Pseudomonas aeruginosa* isolates from cystic fibrosis patients. *Antimicrob. Agents Chemother.* 53, 1987–1997.

Vogne, C., Aires, J. R., Bailly, C., Hocquet, D., and Plesiat, P. (2004). Role of the multidrug efflux system MexXY in the emergence of moderate resistance to aminoglycosides among *Pseudomonas aeruginosa* isolates from patients with cystic fibrosis. *Antimicrob. Agents Chemother.* 48, 1676–1680.

Westbrock-Wadman, S., Sherman, D. R., Hickey, M. J., Coulter, S. N., Zhu, Y. Q., Warrener, P., et al. (1999). Characterization of a *Pseudomonas aeruginosa* efflux pump contributing to aminoglycoside impermeability. *Antimicrob. Agents Chemother.* 43, 2975–2983.

Winsor, G. L., Lam, D. K., Fleming, L., Lo, R., Whiteside, M. D., Yu, N. Y., et al. (2011). *Pseudomonas* Genome Database: improved comparative analysis and population genomics capability for Pseudomonas genomes. *Nucleic Acids Res.* 39, D596-600.

Wolter, D. J., Smith-Moland, E., Goering, R. V., Hanson, N. D., and Lister, P. D. (2004). Multidrug resistance associated with mexXY expression in clinical isolates of *Pseudomonas aeruginosa* from a Texas hospital. *Diagn. Microbiol. Infect. Dis.* 50, 43–50.

Wyka, M. A., and St John, A. C. (1990). Effects of production of abnormal proteins on the rate of killing of *Escherichia coli* by streptomycin. *Antimicrob. Agents Chemother.* 34, 534–538.

Xavier, D. E., Picao, R. C., Girardello, R., Fehlberg, L. C., and Gales, A. C. (2010). Efflux pumps expression and its association with porin down-regulation and beta-lactamase production among *Pseudomonas aeruginosa* causing bloodstream infections in Brazil. *BMC Microbiol.* 10, 217. doi: 10.1186/1471-2180-10-217

Yamamoto, M., Ueda, A., Kudo, M., Matsuo, Y., Fukushima, J., Nakae, T., et al. (2009). Role of MexZ and PA5471 in transcriptional regulation of mexXY in *Pseudomonas aeruginosa. Microbiology* 155, 3312–3321.

Yamasaki, S., Nagasawa, S., Hayashi-Nishino, M., Yamaguchi, A., and Nishino, K. (2011). AcrA dependency of the AcrD efflux pump in *Salmonella enterica* serovar Typhimurium. *J. Antibiot. (Tokyo)* 64, 433–437.

Yerushalmi, H., Lebendiker, M., and Schuldiner, S. (1995). EmrE, an *Escherichia coli* 12-kDa multidrug transporter, exchanges toxic cations and H+ and is soluble in organic solvents. *J. Biol. Chem.* 270, 6856–6863.

Yu, E. W., Aires, J. R., and Nikaido, H. (2003). AcrB multidrug efflux pump of *Escherichia coli*: composite substrate-binding cavity of exceptional flexibility generates its extremely wide substrate specificity. *J. Bacteriol.* 185, 5657–5664.

Zgurskaya, H. I., and Nikaido, H. (1999). Bypassing the periplasm: reconstitution of the AcrAB multidrug efflux pump of *Escherichia coli*. *Proc. Natl. Acad. Sci. U.S.A.* 96, 7190–7195.

Zhao, Q., Li, X. Z., Srikumar, R., and Poole, K. (1998). Contribution of outer membrane efflux protein OprM to antibiotic resistance in *Pseudomonas aeruginosa* independent of MexAB. *Antimicrob. Agents Chemother.* 42, 1682–1688.

4

Comparison of multi-drug resistant environmental methicillin-resistant *Staphylococcus aureus* isolated from recreational beaches and high touch surfaces in built environments

Marilyn C. Roberts[1]*, Olusegun O. Soge[2] and David No[1]

[1] Department of Environmental and Occupational Health Sciences, University of Washington, Seattle, WA, USA
[2] Department of Global Health, University of Washington, Seattle, WA, USA

Edited by:
Marcelo Tolmasky, California State University Fullerton, USA

Reviewed by:
David Dryden, University of Edinburgh, UK
Charles W. Knapp, University of Strathclyde, UK

***Correspondence:**
Marilyn C. Roberts, Department of Environmental and Occupational Health Sciences, School of Public Health, University of Washington, Box 357234, Seattle, WA 98195-7234, USA.
e-mail: marilynr@u.washington.edu

Over the last decade community-acquired methicillin-resistant *Staphylococcus aureus* (MRSA) has emerged as a major cause of disease in the general population with no health care exposure or known classical risk factors for MRSA infections. The potential community reservoirs have not been well defined though certain strains such as ST398 and USA300 have been well studied in some settings. MRSA has been isolated from recreational beaches, high-touch surfaces in homes, universities, and other community environmental surfaces. However, in most cases the strains were not characterized to determine if they are related to community-acquired or hospital-acquired clinical strains. We compared 55 environmental MRSA from 805 samples including sand, fresh, and marine water samples from local marine and fresh water recreational beaches ($n = 296$), high touch surfaces on the University of Washington campus ($n = 294$), surfaces in UW undergraduate housing ($n = 85$), and the local community ($n = 130$). Eleven USA300, representing 20% of the isolates, were found on the UW campus surfaces, student housing surfaces, and on the community surfaces but not in the recreational beach samples from the Northwest USA. Similarly, the predominant animal ST133 was found in the recreational beach samples but not in the high touch surface samples. All USA300 isolates were multi-drug resistant carrying two to six different antibiotic resistance genes coding for kanamycin, macrolides and/or macrolides-lincosamides-streptogramin B, and tetracycline, with the majority (72%) carrying four to six different antibiotic resistance genes. A surprising 98% of the 55 MRSA isolates were resistant to other classes of antibiotics and most likely represent reservoirs for these genes in the environment.

Keywords: MRSA, environmental, recreational beaches, high touch surfaces, USA300

INTRODUCTION

Staphylococcus aureus is part of the normal flora and can be found in the anterior nares as well as on the skin, axilla, perineum, and pharynx. It has been estimated that 25–35% of healthy humans in the general community have *S. aureus* in their anterior nares (Grundmann et al., 2006). However the range varies depending on the population examined and when the study was done. It is now thought that ~20% of population almost always carries *S. aureus*, another 20% rarely carries *S. aureus*, and the remaining 60% of the population is intermittently colonized (Kluytmans et al., 1997).

Methicillin-resistant *S. aureus* (MRSA) was first identified over 50 years ago and has become a major nosocomial and community pathogen. MRSA strains are *S. aureus* that have a *mecA* gene which codes for a unique penicillin-binding protein that has decreased affinity for β-lactams. This protein allows for cell growth in the presence of penicillins and other β-lactam antibiotics, which are the antibiotics of choice for staphylococcal skin and soft tissue infections (Eady and Cove, 2003; Grundmann et al., 2006). Over the last decade community-acquired MRSA (CA-MRSA) causing primarily skin and soft tissue infections has emerged as a major cause of disease in the general population with no health care exposure or known classical risk factors for MRSA infections around the world (King et al., 2006). In 2005 there were ~19,000 deaths due to MRSA in hospitalized USA patients. More importantly three fourth of the US MRSA infections were in people that had not been previously hospitalized, had no contact with hospitals, and were part of the general community (Klevens et al., 2007). CA-MRSA morbidity and mortality per 100,000 people have been estimated at 4.6 and 0.5, respectively (Klevens et al., 2007). CA-MRSA strains initially from community patients are now entering the hospital environments to become the predominant nosocomial MRSA isolates (Popovich et al., 2008). In North America, most CA-MRSA disease is due to a single strain, USA300, which produces a number of toxins and has the ability to cause skin and soft tissue infections in otherwise healthy individuals and appears to be more robust on fomites (Desai et al., 2011). In other geographical locations, CA-MRSA can be a variety of different strains (Nimmo and Coombs, 2008; Bartels et al., 2009). Originally CA-MRSA causing disease was less likely to be resistant to other antimicrobial agents than MRSA strains isolated from the high-antibiotic selection pressure of the hospital environment (Eady and Cove, 2003).

Staphylococcus aureus and MRSA can be transmitted from people-to-people, from fomites-to-people, and from air-to-people (Huang et al., 2006; Zuckerman et al., 2009). People colonized or infected with *S. aureus* or MRSA shed into their environments contaminating surfaces and fomites at concentrations sufficient for survival for extended periods of time in the environment which should allow for transfer to skin, clothing, and other fomites (Boyce et al., 1997; Otter et al., 2011).

Environmental reservoirs associated with healthcare settings and closed communities such as daycares, schools, prisons, and sport teams have been examined (Centers for Disease Control and Prevention, 2001; Eady and Cove, 2003; Nguyen et al., 2005; Roberts et al., 2011a,b,c). *S. aureus* and MRSA contamination in the marine environment have been examined including shedding from recreational bathers, untreated wastewater, and urban runoff (Selvakumar and Borst, 2006; Elmir et al., 2007; Börjesson et al., 2009; Plano et al., 2011). Over the past several years, *S. aureus* and MRSA have been isolated from marine water, stream water, and intertidal sand samples from beaches in California (Goodwin and Pobuda, 2009), Florida (Abdelzaher et al., 2010), Hawaii (Tice et al., 2010; Viau et al., 2011), and the Pacific Northwest (Soge et al., 2009). MRSA spatial distribution or strain characterization was not addressed in the studies by Goodwin and Pobuda (2009) in California and Tice et al. (2010) in Hawaii. A more recent study sampled fresh water streams draining into coastal beaches on O'ahu Hawaii found *S. aureus* (Viau et al., 2011). Temporal and spatial distribution of pathogenic microorganisms including *S. aureus* was examined in a Florida study (Abdelzaher et al., 2010), however none of the presumptive *S. aureus* isolates were biochemically confirmed as *S. aureus.* The study by Soge et al. (2009) identified MRSA and/or *S. aureus* isolated in 2008, from 6 of 10 marine beaches from the Pacific Northwest, however the number of samples taken was limited. That study found that the MRSA isolates were related to strains previously associated with hospital-acquired MRSA (five SSC*mec* type I, and one non-typeable and ST types 30, 45, 59, 1405), and the *S. aureus* isolates (ST15, ST30, ST59) suggested that they are related to hospital-acquired MRSA. ST5, ST30, ST45, ST59 were all major clonal complexes found in the United States (Schwalm et al., 2011).

In this current paper we compare 55 environmental MRSA isolates, including 11 USA300, collected from 805 samples taken from fresh and marine beaches, high touch surfaces within the community and the University of Washington. This represents the first comparison of characterized MRSA isolates from different natural and built environments.

MATERIALS AND METHODS

BACTERIAL ISOLATES

All samples from recreational marine or fresh water beaches, and swabs from the environmental surfaces were enriched in Bacto® m *Staphylococcus* broth (1.5×) (Difco Laboratories, Sparks, MD, USA) supplemented with a final concentration of 75 μg/L polymyxin B and 0.1% potassium tellurite (Sigma Co., St. Louis, MO, USA) and 50 ml of media was used for wash clothes used for sampling the washing machines as previously described (Roberts et al., 2011c; Levin-Edens et al., 2012). All samples were incubated in 5% CO_2 at 36.5°C until turbid and black. Positive samples were diluted and plated onto Bacto® *Staphylococcus* Medium 110 (Difco) supplemented with 10 μg/ml methicillin and 0.01% potassium tellurite and Bacto® Mannitol Salts Agar (Difco), and the resulting strains were biochemically verified as *S. aureus* and confirmed as *mecA* positive by PCR assay as previously described (Roberts et al., 2011c; Levin-Edens et al., 2012). Twenty-two MRSA isolated from fresh water draining into recreational marine or fresh water beaches, seven MRSA isolates collected from sand, and two MRSA isolates collected from marine water identified from sand, fresh, and marine water samples from local marine and fresh water recreational beaches ($n = 296$) in 2010 (Levin-Edens et al., 2012) were included in the study. An additional 24 MRSA isolates from frequently touched 509 non-hospital environmental surfaces taken at a large university ($n = 294$), student homes ($n = 85$), and local community sites ($n = 130$) collected 2009–2010 (Roberts et al., 2011c) were included in the comparison (**Table 1**).

CHARACTERIZATION OF MRSA STRAINS

The SCC*mec* typing was done by multiplex PCR assay for types I–V using positive controls. SCC*mec* typing classifies the SCC*mec* elements based on their structural differences and has been used to discriminate MRSA strains and define MRSA clones[1]. Those that were not SCC*mec* type I–V were labeled as non-typeable (NT) (Soge et al., 2009). The MLST was previously determined by PCR and sequencing of the PCR products for the seven housekeeping genes (Soge et al., 2009). Alleles were assigned by a comparison of their sequences with the corresponding loci in the *S. aureus* MLST database and combined into an allelic profile with unique sequence type (ST)[2]. Drug resistance genes including kanamycin resistance gene, *aadD*, macrolide-lincosamide-streptogramin B resistance genes *erm*(A), *erm*(B), *erm*(C), and macrolide-streptogramin B resistant *msr*(A) gene, and tetracycline resistance genes *tet*(M) and *tet*(K) were previously determined by PCR assays (Soge et al., 2009). These specific antibiotic resistance genes were selected because they have previously been identified in MRSA isolates or have been associated with SCC*mec* elements (Soge et al., 2009; McDougal et al., 2010; Roberts et al., 2011a,b,c; Levin-Edens et al., 2012). Pulsed-field gel electrophoresis (PFGE) analysis was previously done and isolates were compared to four clinical MRSA USA300 strains used as positive controls to determine whether the environmental isolates were related to USA300 clone (McDougal et al., 2010).

RESULTS AND DISCUSSION

DISTRIBUTION OF MRSA ISOLATES

Methicillin-resistant *Staphylococcus aureus* was isolated from 10/85 (11.8%) university student homes surfaces and five (63%) of the eight undergraduate student homes had MRSA positive samples. The percentage of MRSA positive samples, which include only samples that yielded MRSA isolates and was a portion of the

[1] http://www.staphylococcus.net/

[2] http://saureus.mlst.net/

samples which were contaminated with *S. aureus*, in our university study was 10-fold higher than the 1.1% MRSA positive found from 1,320 surface samples taken from 35 homes in the Boston area (Scott et al., 2009). Our study had higher number of MRSA positive homes compared to the 9/35 (25.7%) of the homes that were contaminated with MRSA in the Boston study. In the university study, eight (9.4%) methicillin-susceptible *S. aureus* (MSSA) isolates from 3 (37.5%) homes versus the Boston study which found MSSA contaminated surfaces in 34 (97.1%) of 35 Boston homes. However, the demographics of the household members did vary between the current and previous study as did the number of samples per home and the number of homes tested (Scott et al., 2009). Thirty-one (10.5%) of the 296 recreational beach samples were positive for MRSA with 22 isolates (71%) coming from fresh water streams running into the marine and freshwater beaches. Fourteen (4.7%) of the recreational beach samples were *S. aureus* positive with 12 (85.7%) of the isolates coming from the fresh water stream samples draining into the marine beaches. A recent study in Hawaii found *S. aureus* in 19 (86.4%) of 22 fresh water streams with 42 (48.8%) of the 86 samples positive for *S. aureus* and one (5.2%) sample positive for MRSA (Viau et al., 2011). The source of the isolates was not identified nor was potential environmental sources examined or isolates further characterized in the Viau et al. (2011) study. Ten (3.4%) out of 294 university surface samples were MRSA positive, while nine (3.1%) were MSSA. This compares to an earlier study which found no MRSA from 70 high touch surfaces in a large urban US university, though samples from keyboards, telephone mouthpieces, and an elevator button were positive for *S. aureus* (Brooke et al., 2009). Four (3.1%) out of 130 community samples were MRSA positive, and one (0.8%) sample was MSSA positive. The closest community studies for comparison have been from public transport system. A London study found 9 (8%) of the 112 samples taken from hand-touch surfaces in the public transport system and in public areas of a hospital were positive for *S. aureus* but no MRSA was isolated (Otter and French, 2009). A recent study from Japan where environmental samples were collected from 2008 to 2010 found 8 (2.3%) of the 349 trains examined were positive for MRSA (Iwao et al., 2012).

Eleven (20%) of the 55 isolates had PFGE patterns that indicated that they were USA300 strains, the most prevalent community-acquired MRSA in the United States (Tenover and Goering, 2009). However in other parts of the world other strains of CA-MRSA have been identified (Nimmo and Coombs, 2008; Bartels et al., 2009). The USA300 isolates were not evenly distributed in all the environments sampled since all 11 came from samples in built environmental high touch surfaces (student housing 6/10; university 4/10; and community 1/4). Three different MLST types were associated with the USA300 PFGE pattern including ST5, ST8, and ST30 (**Table 1**).

DRUG RESISTANCE CHARACTERIZATION

Originally, CA-MRSA isolates were less likely to be resistant to other classes of antibiotics, however over the last decade USA300 isolates have become increasingly resistant to fluoroquinolones with 54% resistant by 2006 (Eady and Cove, 2003; McDougal et al., 2010). An early collection of 187 MRSA strains identified 30 USA300 isolates that were multiple-drug resistant and carried macrolide [*msr*(A) gene], and/or macrolide, lincosamide-streptogramin B [*erm*(A), *erm*(C) genes], and/or tetracycline resistance gene [*tet*(K)], and/or levofloxacin resistance due to gyrase mutations (Tenover et al., 2006). While a more recent study of 823 USA300 clinical isolates from the Centers for Disease Control and Prevention (CDC) collection found that 43% of the isolates were resistant to erythromycin and carried the *msr*(A) gene and 43% were resistant to erythromycin due to the presence of the *msr*(A) gene plus levofloxacin resistance due to gyrase mutations, and 8.4% were resistant to tetracycline due to presence of the *tet*(K) gene of which some also carried the *msr*(A) gene and/or the gyrase mutations, leaving just 5.6% susceptible to other classes of antibiotics examined (McDougal et al., 2010). However few groups have characterized the antibiotic resistance patterns of MRSA isolates found in the environment besides the study of Soge et al. (2009). In that study, five MRSA SCC*mec* type I isolates were resistant to one to four classes of antibiotics and all five carried the *erm*(A) gene, one carried both *tet*(K) and *tet*(M) genes, and one carried the *tet*(K) and the other carried the *tet*(M) tetracycline resistance genes. One of the MRSA isolates was able to transfer the *tet*(M) and *erm*(A) genes in mating experiment suggesting that MRSA strains could be environmental reservoirs for antibiotic resistance genes. In addition, 17/21 (81%) of the methicillin-resistant coagulase negative *Staphylococcus* spp. (MRCoNS) were resistant to one to five other classes of antibiotics and carried combinations of *erm*(B), *erm*(C), *msr*(A), *tet*(K), and/or *tet*(M) genes suggesting that MRCoNS strains could also be environmental reservoirs for mobile antibiotic resistance genes. In contrast, none of the environmental MSSA isolates carried any of the resistance genes examined.

Fifty-two (95%) isolates in the current study carried a variety of other antibiotic resistance genes and were multi-drug resistant, including all 11 USA300 isolates. Only three (5.5%) of the 55 MRSA isolates were negative by PCR for all seven antibiotic resistance genes examined and represented three different MLST types (**Table 1**). The most commonly found gene *aadD* was identified in 45 (82%) isolates, 42 (76%) isolates were positive for *msr*(A), 46 (84%) isolates positive for either *tet*(K) and/or *tet*(M), 27 (49%) isolates positive for *erm*(C), and 7 (13%) isolates positive for *erm*(A). None of the MRSA isolates carried the *erm*(B) gene. Iwao et al. (2012) examined susceptibilities of eight MRSA isolates from the public trains to nine other non-β-lactam antimicrobial agents and all were resistant to two to seven of the agents tested though specific resistance genes present were not determined. Seven (87.5%) of the eight strains resistant to kanamycin likely carried the *aadD* gene, which is similar to the 82% found in the current study, while 4 (50%) were macrolide resistant and 3 (37.5%) were clindamycin resistant. Three (75%) of the four Japanese isolates identified as ST8 CA-MRSA were resistant to gentamicin and kanamycin.

Nineteen (35%) of the MRSA isolates were positive for one to three different antibiotic resistance genes, and included 8 (57%) of the 13 MLST types from all the different environments and five of the USA300 strains. While 33 (60%) of the MRSA isolates carried four to six of the genes analyzed and included isolates from all the different environments with all the 13 MLST types and 6 of the 11 USA300 included in this group (**Table 1**).

Table 1 | Genotypic characteristics of MRSA isolates from recreational beaches and built environmental high touch surfaces.

Isolate	Source	SCC*mec* type[a]	MLST[b]	PFGE type	USA300	Antibiotic resistance genes[c]
***n* = 31**	**Recreational beaches 2010**					
401	Fresh water	IV	5	L		*tet*(M), *tet*(K), *erm*(C), *msr*(A), *aadD*
PC3	Fresh water	NT	6			*tet*(M), *tet*(K), *msr*(A), *aadD*
1012	Fresh water	NT	6			*tet*(M), *tet*(K), *msr*(A), *aadD*
111	Sand	IV	8	K		*erm*(C), *msr*(A), *aadD*
3mid	Sand	IV	15	G		*tet*(M), *tet*(K), *msr*(A), *aadD*
118	Fresh water	IV	15			*tet*(M), *tet*(K), *erm*(C), *msr*(A), *aadD*
603	Sand	IV	30	H		*tet*(M), *tet*(K), *erm*(C), *msr*(A), *aadD*
1112 (2)	Fresh water	II	45	M		*erm*(A), *aadD*
Seep1	Marine sand	IV	88			*tet*(M), *tet*(K), *msr*(A), *aadD*
257	Marine sand	IV	97	N		*tet*(K), *erm*(C), *msr*(A), *aadD*
302	Marine water	IV	109	F		*tet*(M), *tet*(K), *erm*(A), *msr*(A), *aadD*
308	Marine water	IV	109	F		*tet*(M), *erm*(A), *erm*(C), *msr*(A), *aadD*
361	Sand	IV	109	F		*tet*(M), *erm*(A), *erm*(C), *msr*(A), *aadD*
1112	Fresh water	I	133	B		None
244	Fresh water	IV	133	A		*erm*(C), *msr*(A), *aadD*
248	Fresh water	IV	133	A		*tet*(K), *msr*(A), *aadD*
252	Fresh water	IV	133	B		*tet*(K), *erm*(C), *msr*(A), *aadD*
125	Fresh water	IV	133	C		*tet*(K), *erm*(C), *msr*(A), *aadD*
909	Fresh water	IV	133	D		*tet*(K), *erm*(C), *msr*(A), *aadD*
910	Sand	IV	133	D		*tet*(K), *erm*(C), *msr*(A), *aadD*
512	Fresh water	IV	133	E		*tet*(K), *erm*(C), *msr*(A), *aadD*
824	Fresh water	NT	133			*tet*(K), *erm*(C), *msr*(A), *aadD*
515	Fresh water	IV	1875			*tet*(K), *erm*(C), *msr*(A), *aadD*
526	Fresh water	IV	1875			*tet*(M), *tet*(K), *msr*(A), *aadD*
813	Fresh water	IV	1875			*tet*(M), *tet*(K), *erm*(C), *msr*(A), *aadD*
823	Fresh water	NT	1875			*tet*(M), *tet*(K), *erm*(C), *msr*(A), *aadD*
1113	Fresh water	I	1956	J		None
1124	Fresh water	I	1956			*aadD*
827	Fresh water	IV	1956	I		*tet*(K), *erm*(C), *msr*(A), *aadD*
1017	Fresh water	NT	2049			*erm*(C), *aadD*
1019	Fresh water	NT	2049			*tet*(K), *erm*(C), *msr*(A), *aadD*
***n* = 10**	**Student homes 2010**					
S3–23	TV remote	IV	5	3	Yes	*tet*(M), *tet*(K), *msr*(A), *aadD*
S9–18	Bathroom floor	IV	5	3	Yes	*tet*(M), *msr*(A), *aadD*
S5–28	Bathroom light switch	IV	5	3	Yes	*tet*(M), *tet*(K), *aadD*
T4–38	Washing machine	IV	5	5		*tet*(M), *tet*(K), *msr*(A), *aadD*
J-5	Dorm water fountain	NT	8	1		None
R501	Couch	IV	8	4	Yes	*tet*(M), *msr*(A), *aadD*
R502	Toilet flush handle	IV	8 (931)[d]	4	Yes	*tet*(M), *tet*(K), *msr*(A), *aadD*
R509	Bathroom door knob	IV	8 (931)[d]	4	Yes	*tet*(M), *tet*(K), *msr*(A), *aadD*
A3–6	Microwave touchpad	IV	45	2		*tet*(M), *msr*(A), *aadD*
A4–3	Couch	IV	45	2		*tet*(M), *msr*(A), *aadD*
***n* = 10**	**University campus 2010**					
3–36	Bathroom	IV	5	3	Yes	*erm*(C), *msr*(A)
20	ATM	IV	5	3	Yes	*tet*(M), *tet*(K), *erm*(A), *erm*(C), *msr*(A), *aadD*
3–22	Bathroom	NT	5	12		*tet*(M)
3–2	Elevator button	I	8	9		*tet*(M), *erm*(C), *msr*(A)
8–509	Locker handle	IV	8	8	Yes	*tet*(M), *tet*(K), *msr*(A), *aadD*
26	ATM	IV	30	6	Yes	*tet*(M), *tet*(K), *erm*(A), *erm*(C), *msr*(A), *aadD*
36	ATM	I	45	7		*tet*(M), *tet*(K), *erm*(A), *erm*(C), *aadD*

(Continued)

Table 1 | Continued

Isolate	Source	SCC*mec* type[a]	MLST[b]	PFGE type	USA300	Antibiotic resistance genes[c]
3–6	Bathroom floor	NT	97	11		*tet*(M)
3–8	Elevator button	NT	97	10		*tet*(M)
3–10	Study lounge floor	NT	97	10		*tet*(M), *erm*(C)
***n* = 4**	**Community 2009–2010**					
40	ATM	NT	5	3	Yes	*tet*(M), *msr*(A)
55	ATM	IV	8	13		*tet*(M), *erm*(C), *msr*(A), *aadD*
5–3	Library computer touch screen	NT	30	14		*tet*(K), *aadD*
5–4	Library computer touch screen	IV	30	14		*tet*(M), *tet*(K), *msr*(A), *aadD*

[a]*SCCmec I–V was tested. If not one of these types, listed as non-typeable (NT);* [b]*MLST typing using seven housekeeping genes;* [c]*Kanamycin resistance gene, aadD; macrolide, lincosamide-streptogramin B resistance genes erm(A), erm(B), erm(C), and msr(A) gene and tetracycline resistance genes tet(M) and tet(K) were tested;* [d]*ST931 has recently been reassigned as ST8 due to revision of the gmk locus (Larsen et al., 2012).*

Twenty-two (40%) isolates carried four different antibiotic resistance genes and were isolated from the recreational beaches ($n = 15$), student homes ($n = 4$), university sites ($n = 1$), and community sites ($n = 2$). Ten of the isolates carried *aadD*, *erm*(C), *msr*(A), and *tet*(K) genes and included ST97 ($n = 1$), ST133 ($n = 6$), ST1875 ($n = 1$), ST1956 ($n = 1$), and ST2049 ($n = 1$), and eight were SCC*mec* IV and two NT. Eleven isolates carried *aadD*, *msr*(A), *tet*(K), and *tet*(M) genes and included ST5 ($n = 2$), ST6 ($n = 2$), ST8 ($n = 3$), ST15 ($n = 1$), ST30 ($n = 1$), ST88 ($n = 1$), and ST1875 ($n = 1$). Four (36%) of the 11 MRSA were USA300 strains by PFGE analysis.

The highest number of resistance genes was found in two USA300 isolates, from the University of Washington sites. They were positive for 6 genes [*aadD*, *erm*(A), *erm*(C), *msr*(A), *tet*(K), and *tet*(M)], included ST5 and ST30, and both isolates carried the SCC*mec* IV element. Nine (16%) isolates which carried five different antibiotic resistance genes were isolated from the recreational beaches $n = 8$, and university sites $n = 1$. Five isolates were positive for *aadD*, *erm*(C), *msr*(A), *tet*(K), and *tet*(M) genes, included ST5 ($n = 1$), ST15 ($n = 1$), ST30 ($n = 1$), ST1875 ($n = 2$), and four of the five isolates carried the SCC*mec* IV element. Two SCC*mec* IV, ST109 MRSA isolates from the recreational beaches were positive for *aadD*, *erm*(A), *erm*(C), *msr*(A), and *tet*(M) genes. One other SCC*mec* IV, ST109 isolate from the beach was positive for *aadD*, *erm*(A), *msr*(A), *tet*(K), and *tet*(M) genes (**Table 1**). One SCC*mec* I, ST45 isolate from the university site was positive for *aadD*, *erm*(A), *erm*(C), *tet*(K), and *tet*(M) genes (**Table 1**).

COMPARISON OF SCC*mec* TYPING AND MLST OF ISOLATES ACROSS DIFFERENT WA ENVIRONMENTS

Of the 55 MRSA isolates, 35 (63.6%) carried the SCC*mec* IV, while 14 (25.5%) were non-typeable which meant they did not carry SCC*mec* I–V, five (9.1%) carried the SCC*mec* I and one (1.8%) carried the SCC*mec* II (**Table 1**). In the much smaller Japanese study (Iwao et al., 2012), the SCC*mec* IV was also the most common [4/8 (50%)] with three (37.5%) isolates carrying the SCC*mec* II and one (12.5%) the SCC*mec* I elements. Few other studies of environmental MRSA have SCC*mec* typed their isolates.

There were 13 different MLST types identified from the WA isolates. Nine (69%) of these MLST types have commonly been isolated from humans (see text footnote 2). All 13 of the MLST types were found in MRSA isolated from the WA recreational beaches, five MLST types were found in MRSA isolated from the university, three MLST types (ST5, ST8, and ST45) were found in MRSA isolated from student home surfaces, and three MLST types (ST5, ST8, and ST30) were found in MRSA from the community surfaces. Two new MLST types ST1875 ($n = 4$), three SCC*mec* IV and one NT, and ST2049 ($n = 2$) both NT, were identified in recreational beach samples. The ST2049 is closely related to ST1962 which has previously been identified in squirrels as has ST1956 (see text footnote 2), both of which were found in the recreational beach samples. Interestingly, two of the three ST1956 isolates carried SCC*mec* I, more commonly associated with hospital-acquired MRSA. ST1875 (SCC*mec* IV, $n = 3$; NT, $n = 1$) is closely related to recently identified human ST1176 (CC5) from Brazil (Carmo et al., 2011) and a hospital-acquired ST1176 MRSA strain 2929B reported from Boston, MA, USA and thus could be of human origin (see text footnote 2).

Twenty-six (47%) of the MRSA belonged to three of the 13 MLST types and included nine isolates of ST133 (CC133), nine isolates of ST5 (CC5), and eight isolates of ST8 (CC8). ST5 and ST8 were found in all four environments (**Table 1**). All nine ST133 isolates were from both the marine and fresh recreational beaches and surrounding fresh water streams draining into the recreational beaches at multiple time points (Levin-Edens et al., 2012). Based on difference in PFGE patterns the nine isolates represented at least five different strains (**Table 1**). Seven of the MRSA strains representing all five different PFGE patterns carried the SCC*mec* IV element, one carried SCC*mec* I element, and one carried an element that was different than the I–V. Smyth et al. (2009) stated that *S. aureus* ST133 is an ungulate-animal-specific genotype with no association with humans reported in the literature. The ST133 was the most common lineage reported in *S. aureus* isolates collected from Danish small ruminants (65% of 179 sheep and 55% of 17 goats) (Eriksson et al., 2013). ST133 has been isolated from German wild boars (Meemken et al., 2013), and Japanese cats and dogs (Sasaki et al., 2012). More recently a single MRSA ST133 has been identified from 66 MRSA isolates with seven major clonal complexes from nasal swabs collected from patients upon admission to intensive care units at Pennsylvania State University (Schwalm et al., 2011). Thus it is likely that MRSA ST133 is only rarely associated with humans, which correlates with its absence from human built environment surfaces. It is possible that ST133 is associated with common wild and/or pet animals found in urban areas such as Seattle in addition to ungulates and thus explains the wide distribution among the recreational beach areas at multiple time points within the city but its absence from surfaces in built environments in the same geographical area.

The nine ST5 isolates were found at the beaches ($n = 1$), and on the high touch surfaces in the student homes ($n = 4$), university campus ($n = 3$), and community sites ($n = 1$) (**Table 1**), represented four different PFGE patterns, seven were SCC*mec* IV and two were NT. ST5 has been associated with humans, chickens, turkey, and pork (see text footnote 2). USA100 a common hospital MRSA is ST5 and is part of the major clonal complex which is widely distributed (Schwalm et al., 2011; Iwao et al., 2012; Verghese et al., 2012; Kawaguchiya et al., 2013). ST5 was found in all four WA environments studied (**Table 1**).

There were eight ST8 isolates and like ST5 found in all environments sampled (recreational $n = 1$; students homes $n = 4$; university $n = 2$; community $n = 1$). Six of the ST8 were SCC*mec* IV isolated at the beaches, student homes, university campus, and community, while ST8 SCC*mec* I was isolated on a university surface and the ST8 NT isolated from student dorm. ST8 has been associated with USA300 clonal type which is now being found in hospital setting (Kawaguchiya et al., 2013) and four of the isolates had PFGE patterns that indicated that they were USA300 strains. ST8 MRSA has also been isolated from chickens, cows, horses, turkey, beef, and pork samples (see text footnote 2). One of the eight isolates was the only MRSA (strain 8-509) in the study to be Panton-Valentine Leukocidin (PVL) positive while the remaining MRSA were all PVL-negative in the WA samples as compared to four of eight MRSA isolates PVL+ in the Japanese study (Iwao et al., 2012).

Other ST types found in humans ST109 ($n = 3$), humans and animals ST15 ($n = 2$), ST45 ($n = 4$), ST88 ($n = 1$), ST97 ($n = 4$), or humans and meat products ST6 ($n = 2$), ST30 ($n = 4$), and ST40 ($n = 4$). ST97 is rarely found in humans and ~90% of the submissions to the MLST website lists cow milk, bovine mastitis, or pigs (see text footnote 2). ST30 and ST45 belong to major clonal complexes CC30 and CC45 respectively and are often associated with human disease (Simor et al., 2002; Moore et al., 2010; Isobe et al., 2012). The MRSA ST30 clone, found in three of the WA environments, has been predominantly identified in Japanese hospitalized patients since the 1980s (Isobe et al., 2012) and have also been reported in MRSA infections from other parts of the world (Hetem et al., 2012). MRSA ST45, also found in three of the WA environments, is associated with USA600 which has been reported as an epidemic strain in Central European and Canadian hospitals (Witte et al., 1997; Simor et al., 2002) and been implicated in outbreaks of bloodstream infections in Detroit, MI, USA (Abdel-Haq et al., 2009; Moore et al., 2010).

CONCLUSION

Unlike recent studies of clinical USA300, all the environmental USA300 isolates in the current study were multi-drug resistant carrying two to six different antibiotic resistance genes. The majority (72%) carried four to six different antibiotic resistance genes and ~95% of all the other MRSA isolates were multi-drug resistant. Similar results were found in the Japanese study of MRSA isolates from 2008 to 2010 (Iwao et al., 2012). Why there was such a high level of antibiotic resistance in environmental MRSA isolates is certainly not clear but does correlate with our previous small study (Soge et al., 2009). It is unlikely that the level of resistance found in the environmental MRSA isolates is unique to the Seattle, WA area or to the selected environmental surfaces examined. It will also be of interest to know if the environmental MRSA isolates are acquiring their antibiotic resistance genes from other members of the environmental bacterial community or if some of these genes have originated from bacteria in the hospital setting. The data suggests that the environmental MRSA isolates collected in the current study are potential antibiotic resistance gene reservoirs and should be able to act as donors to the microbes and the environmental antibiotic resistance gene pool and potentially contribute to the human microbiome antibiotic resistance gene pool.

A major difference between MRSA isolates isolated from WA recreational beaches and freshwater streams versus other WA environments is that we found no isolates related to USA300 by PFGE, though MLST type associated with USA300 and SCC*mec* IV were present. In contrast, in the built environments, USA300 MRSA isolates comprised 25–60% of the total number of MRSA isolates recovered (**Table 1**). Another major difference was that ST133 which has until recently thought to be exclusively an animal clone was one of the most commonly isolated ST type from recreational beaches 9/31 (29%) but was absent from the built environmental sites.

From all environmental sites, SCC*mec* IV was the most common 36/55 (66%) which is comparable with what is occurring in the health care setting with SCC*mec* IV replacing other SCC*mec* types (Healy et al., 2004; D'Agata et al., 2009). The most diversity of MLST types were found in the recreational beaches but this could be due to the larger number of different MRSA isolates included. There are a limited number of studies that have characterized environmental MRSA. The recreational beach study of Seifried et al. (2007) identified 18 USA300 isolates from recreational seawater in Hawaii. These isolates represented eight different *spa* types, at least three different SCC*mec* types and a variety of PFGE types. We did not find USA300 in our recreational samples but did find significant diversity of the MRSA strains as was found in Hawaii. Another study in California suggested that beachgoers could be a possible source of MRSA and *S. aureus* isolated in sand and seawater (Goodwin et al., 2012) though the isolates were not characterized to verify this hypothesis. Thus the differences we have found between MRSA strains isolated at the three recreational beaches in the Seattle and the built environmental surfaces may vary geographically with less differences between recreational beaches isolates taken from California, Hawaii or where the water is warmer and many more people swim. However it is clear that more studies characterizing the MRSA isolated in environmental setting need to be done to allow better understanding of the potential risk involved with environmental contact with MRSA and/or *S. aureus* contaminated community high touch surfaces and recreational beaches.

REFERENCES

Abdel-Haq, N., Al-Tatari, H., Chearskul, P., Salimnia, H., Asmar, B., Fairfax, M., et al. (2009). Methicillin-resistant *Staphylococcus aureus* (MRSA) in hospitalized children: correlation of molecular analysis with clinical presentation and antibiotic susceptibility testing (ABST) results. *Eur. J. Clin. Microbiol. Infect. Dis.* 28, 547–551.

Abdelzaher, A. M., Wright, M. E., Ortega, C., Solo-Gabriele, H. M., Miller, G., Elmir, S., et al. (2010). Presence of pathogens and indicator microbes at a non-point source subtropical recreational marine beach. *Appl. Environ. Microbiol.* 76, 724–732.

Bartels, M. D., Kristoffersen, K., Boye, K., and Westh, H. (2009). Rise and subsequent decline of community-associated methicillin-resistant *Staphylococcus aureus* ST30-IVc in Copenhagen. *Clin. Microbiol. Infect.* 16, 78–83.

Börjesson, S., Matussek, A., Melin, S., Löfgren, S., and Lindgren, P. E. (2009). Methicillin-resistant *Staphylococcus aureus* (MRSA) in municipal wastewater: an uncharted threat? *J. Appl. Microbiol.* 108, 1244–1251.

Boyce, J. M., Potter-Bynoe, G., Chenevert, C., and King, T. (1997). Environmental contamination due to methicillin-resistant *Staphylococcus aureus*: possible infection control implications. *Infect. Control Hosp. Epidemiol.* 18, 622–627.

Brooke, J. S., Annand, J. W., Hammer, A., Dembkowski, K., and Shulman, S. T. (2009). Investigation of bacterial pathogens on 70 frequently used environmental surfaces in a large urban US. university. *J. Environ. Health* 71, 17–22.

Carmo, M. S., Inoue, F., Andrade, S. S., Paschoal, L., Silva, F. M., Olieira, V. G. S., et al. (2011). New multilocus sequence typing of MRSA in Sao Paulo. *Braz. J. Med. Biolog. Res.* 44, 1013–1017.

Centers for Disease Control and Prevention. (2001). Methicillin-resistant *Staphylococcus aureus* skin or soft tissue infections in a state prison-Mississippi, 2001. *MMWR Morb. Mortal. Wkly. Rep.* 50, 919–922.

D'Agata, E. M.,Webb, G. F., Horn, M. A., Moellering, R. C. Jr., and Ruan, S. (2009) Modeling the invasion of community-acquired methicillin-resistant *Staphylococcus aureus* into hospitals. *Clin. Infect. Dis.* 48, 274–284.

Desai, R., Pannaraj, P. S., Agopian, J., Sugar, C. A., Liu, G. Y., and Miller, L. G. (2011). Survival and transmission of community-associated methicillin-resistant *Staphylococcus aureus* from fomites. *Am. J. Infect Control* 39, 219–225.

Eady, E. A., and Cove, J. H. (2003). Staphylococcal resistance revisited: community-acquired methicillin resistant *Staphylococcus aureus*-an emerging problem for the management of skin and soft tissue infections. *Curr. Opin. Infect. Dis.* 16, 103–124.

Elmir, S. M., Wright, M. E., Abdelzaher, A., Solo-Gabriele, H. M., Fleming, L. E., Miller, G., et al. (2007). Quantitative evaluation of bacteria released by bathers in marine water. *Water Res.* 41, 3–10.

Eriksson, J., Espinosa-Gongora, C., Stamphøj, I., Larsen, A. R., and Guardabassi, L. (2013). Carriage frequency, diversity and methicillin resistance of *Staphylococcus aureus* in Danish small ruminants. *Vet. Microbiol.* 163, 110–115.

Goodwin, K. D., McNay, M., Cao, Y., Ebentier, D., Madison, M., and Griffity, J. F. (2012). A multi-beach study of *Staphylococcus aureus*, MRSA, and enterococci in seawater and beach sand. *Water Res.* 46, 4195–4207.

Goodwin, K. D., and Pobuda, M. (2009). Performance of CHROMagar Staph aureus and CHROMagar MRSA for detection of *Staphylococcus aureus* in seawater and beach sand – comparison of culture, agglutination, and molecular analysis. *Water Res.* 43, 4802–4811.

Grundmann, H., Aires-de-Sousa, M., Boyce, J., and Tiemersma, E. (2006). Emergence and resurgence of methicillin-resistant *Staphylococcus aureus* as a public-health threat. *Lancet* 368, 874–885.

Healy, C. M., Hulten, K. G., Palazzi, D. L., Campbell, J. R., and Baker, C. J. (2004). Emergence of new strains of methicillin-resistant *Staphylococcus aureus* in a neonatal intensive care unit. *Clin. Infect. Dis.* 39, 1460–1466.

Hetem, D. J., Westh, H., Boye, K., Jarløv, J. O., Bonten, M. J., and Bootsma, M. C. (2012). Nosocomial transmission of community-associated methicillin-resistant *Staphylococcus aureus* in Danish Hospitals. *J. Antimicrob. Chemother.* 67, 1775–1780.

Huang, R., Mehta, S., Weed, D., and Price, C. S. (2006). Methicillin-resistance *Staphylococcus aureus* survival on hospital fomites. *Infect. Control Hosp. Epidemiol.* 27, 1267–1269.

Isobe, H., Takano, T., Nishiyama, A., Hung, W. C., Kuniyuki, S., Shibuya, Y., et al. (2012). Evolution and virulence of Panton-Valentine leukocidin-positive ST30 methicillin-resistant *Staphylococcus aureus* in the past 30 years in Japan. *Biomed. Res.* 33, 97–109.

Iwao, Y., Yabe, S., Takano, T., Higuchi, W., Nishiyama, A., and Yamamoto, T. (2012). Isolation and molecular characterization of methicillin-resistance *Staphylococcus aureus* from public transport. *Microbiol. Immunol.* 56, 76–82.

Kawaguchiya, M., Urushibara, N., Yamanoto, D., Yamsahita, T., Shinagawa, M., Watanabe, N., et al. (2013). Characterization of PVL/ACME-positive methicillin-resistance *Staphylococcus aureus* (genotypes ST8-MRSA-IV and ST5-MRSA-II) isolated from a university hospital in Japan. *Microb. Drug Resist.* 19, 48–56.

King, M. D., Humphrey, B. J., Wang, Y. F., Kourbatova, E. V., Ray, S. M., and Blumberg, H. M. (2006). Emergence of community-acquired methicillin-resistant *Staphylococcus aureus* USA 300 clone as the predominant cause of skin and soft-tissue infections. *Ann. Intern. Med.* 144, 309–317.

Klevens, R. M., Morrison, M. A., Nadle, J., Petit, S., Gersham, K., Ray, S., et al. (2007). Invasive methicillin-resistant *Staphylococcus aureus* infections in the United States. *JAMA* 298, 1763–1771.

Kluytmans, J., van Belkum, A., and Verbrugh, H. (1997). Nasal carriage of *Staphylococcus aureus*: epidemiology, underlying mechanism, and associated risks. *Clin. Microbiol. Rev.* 10, 505–520.

Larsen, J., Enright, M. C., Godoy, D., Spratt, B. G., Larsen, A. R., and Skov, R. L. (2012). Multilocus sequence typing scheme for *Staphylococcus aureus*: revision of the *gmk* locus. *J. Clin. Microbiol.* 50, 2538–2539.

Levin-Edens, E., Soge, O. O., No, D. B., Stiffarm, A., Meschke, J. S., and Roberts, M. C. (2012). Methicillin-resistant *Staphylococcus aureus* from Northwest marine and fresh water recreational beaches. *FEMS Microbiol. Ecol.* 79, 412–420.

McDougal, L. K., Fosheim, G. E., Nicholson, A., Bulens, S. N., Limbago, B. M., Shearer, J. E. S., et al. (2010). Emergence of resistance among USA300 methicillin-resistant *Staphylococcus aureus* isolates causing invasive disease in the Unite States. *Antimicrob. Agents Chemother* 54, 3804–3811.

Meemken, D., Blaha, T., Hotzel, H., Strommenger, B., Klein, G., Ehricht, R., et al. (2013). Genotypic and phenotypic characterization of *Staphylococcus aureus* from wild boars. *Appl. Environ. Microbiol.* 79, 1739–1742.

Moore, C. L., Osaki-Kiyan, P., Perri, M., Donabedian, S., Haque, N. Z., Chen, A., et al. (2010). USA600 (ST45) methicillin-resistant *Staphylococcus aureus* bloodstream infections in urban Detroit. *J. Clin. Microbiol.* 48, 2307–2310.

Nguyen, D. M., Mascola, L., and Brancoft, E. (2005). Recurring methicillin-resistant *Staphylococcus aureus* infections in a football team. *Emerg. Infect. Dis.* 11, 526–532.

Nimmo, G. R., and Coombs, G. W. (2008). Community-associated methicillin-resistant *Staphylococcus aureus* (MRSA) in Australia. *Int. J. Antimicob. Agents* 31, 401–410.

Otter, J. A., and French, G. L. (2009). Bacterial contamination on touch surfaces in the public transport system and in public areas of a hospital in London. *Lett. App. Microbiol.* 49, 803–805.

Otter, J. A., Yezli, S., and French, G. L. (2011). The role played by contaminated surfaces in the transmission of nosocomial pathogens. *Infect. Control Hosp. Epidemiol.* 32, 687–699.

Plano, L. R. W., Garza, A. C., Shibata, T., Elmir, S. M., Kish, J., Sinigalliano, C. D., et al. (2011). Shedding of *Staphylococcus aureus* and methicillin-resistant *Staphylococcus aureus* from adult and pediatric bathers in marine waters. *BMC Microbiol.* 11:5. doi:10.1186/1471-2180-11-5

Popovich, K. J., Weinstein, R. A., and Hota, B. (2008). Are community-associated methicillin-resistant *Staphylococcus aureus* (MRSA) strains replacing traditional nosocomial MRSA strains? *Clin. Infect. Dis.* 46, 787–794.

Roberts, M. C., Soge, O. O., Horst, J. A., Ly, K. A., and Milgrom, P. (2011a). MRSA from dental school surfaces and students. *Am. J. Infect. Control.* 39, 628–632.

Roberts, M. C., Soge, O. O., No, D. B., Beck, N., and Meschke, J. S. (2011b). Isolation and characterization of methicillin-resistant *Staphylococcus aureus* (MRSA) from fire stations in two Northwest fire districts. *Am. J. Infect. Control* 39, 382–389.

Roberts, M. C., Soge, O. O., No, D. B., Helgeson, S. E., and Meschke,

J. S. (2011c). Characterization of methicillin-resistant *Staphylococcus aureus* isolated from public surfaces on a University campus, student homes and local community. *J. Appl. Microbiol.* 110, 1531–1537.

Sasaki, T., Tsubakishita, S., Tanaka, Y., Ohtsuka, M., Hongo, I., Fukata, T., et al. (2012). Population genetic structures of *Staphylococcus aureus* isolates from cats and dogs in Japan. *J. Clin. Microbiol.* 50, 2152–2155.

Schwalm, N. D. III., Verghese, B., and Knabel, S. J. (2011). A novel multiplex PCR method for detecting the major clonal complexes of MRSA in nasal isolates form a Pennsylvania hospital. *J. Microbiol. Methods* 86, 379–382.

Scott, E., Duty, S., and McCue, K. (2009). A critical evaluation of methicillin-resistant *Staphylococcus aureus* and other bacteria of medical interest on commonly touched household surfaces in relation to household demographics. *Am. J. Infect. Control.* 37, 447–453.

Seifried, S. E., Tice, A. D., and Eischen, M. (2007). Diversity of community-associated strains of methicillin-resistant *Staphylococcus aureus* in Hawaii. *J. Infect. Dis.* 195, 305.

Selvakumar, A., and Borst, M. (2006). Variation of microorganism concentration sin urban stormwater runoff with land use and seasons. *J. Water Health* 4, 109–124.

Simor, A. E., Ofner-Agostini, M., Bryce, E., McGeer, A., Paton, S., and Mulvey, M. R. (2002). Laboratory characterization of methicillin-resistant *Staphylococcus aureus* in Canadian hospitals: results of 5 years of national surveillance, 1995–1999. *J. Infect. Dis.* 186, 652–660.

Smyth, D. S., Feil, E. J., Meaney, W. J., Hartigan, P. J., Tollersrud, T., Fitzgerald, J. R., et al. (2009). Molecular genetic typing reveals further insights into the diversity of animal-associated *Staphylococcus aureus. J. Med. Microbiol.* 58, 1343–1353.

Soge, O. O., Meschke, J. S., No, D. B., and Roberts, M. C. (2009). Characterization of methicillin-resistant *Staphylococcus aureus* (MRSA) and methicillin-resistant coagulase-negative *Staphylococcus* spp. (MRCoNS) isolated from West Coast public marine beaches. *J. Antimicrob. Chemother.* 64, 1148–1155.

Tenover, F. C., McDougal, L. K., Goering, R. V., Killgove, G., Porhan, S. J., Patel, J. B., and Dunmann, P. M. (2006). Characterization of a strain of community-associated Methicillin-resistant *Staphylococcus aureus* widely disseminated in the United States. *J. Clin. Microbiol.* 44, 108–118.

Tenover, F. C., and Goering, R. V. (2009). Methicillin-resistant *Staphylococcus aureus* strain USA300: origin and epidemiology. *J. Antimicrob. Chemother.* 64, 441–446.

Tice, A. D., Pombo, D., Hui, J., Kurano, M., Bankowski, M. J., and Seifried, S. E. (2010). Quantification of *Staphylococcus aureus* in seawater using CHROMagar SA. *Hawaii Med. J.* 69, 8–12.

Verghese, B., Schwalm, N. D. III., Gudley, E. G., and Knabel, S. J. (2012). A combined multi-virulence-locus sequence typing and Staphylococcal cassette chromosome *mec* typing scheme possesses enhanced discriminatory power for genotyping MRSA. *Infect. Genet. Evol.* 12, 1816–1821.

Viau, E. J., Goodwin, K. D., Yamahara, K. M., Layton, B. A., Sassoubre, L. M., Burns, S. L., et al. (2011). Bacterial pathogens in Hawaiian coastal streams – associations with fecal indicators, land cover, and water quality. *Water Res.* 45, 3279–3290.

Witte, W., Kresken, M., Braulke, C., and Cuny, C. (1997). Increasing incidence and widespread dissemination of methicillin-resistant *Staphylococcus aureus* (MRSA) in hospitals in central Europe, with special reference to German hospitals. *Clin. Microbiol. Infect.* 3, 414–422.

Zuckerman, J. B., Zuaro, D. E., Prato, B. S., Ruoff, K. L., Sawicki, R. W., Quinton, H. B., et al. (2009). Bacterial contamination of cystic fibrosis clinics. *J. Cystic Fibros* 8, 186–192.

5

Antibiotic resistance shaping multi-level population biology of bacteria

Fernando Baquero[1,2,3]*, Ana P. Tedim[1,2] and Teresa M. Coque[1,2,3]

[1] Department of Microbiology, Hospital Universitario Ramón y Cajal, Instituto Ramón y Cajal de Investigación Sanitaria, Madrid, Spain
[2] Centros de Investigación Biomédica en Red de Epidemiología y Salud Pública, Madrid, Spain
[3] Unidad de Resistencia a Antibióticos y Virulencia Bacteriana asociada al Consejo Superior de Investigaciones Científicas, Madrid, Spain

Edited by:
Fiona Walsh, Agroscope Changins Wädenswil, Switzerland

Reviewed by:
Jose L. Martinez, Centro Nacional de Biotecnología, Spain
Andres Moya, University of Valencia, Spain

***Correspondence:**
Fernando Baquero, Department of Microbiology, Hospital Universitario Ramón y Cajal, Instituto Ramón y Cajal de Investigación Sanitaria, Carretera de Colmenar Viejo, km. 9.100, 28034 Madrid, Spain.
e-mail: baquero@bitmailer.net

Antibiotics have natural functions, mostly involving cell-to-cell signaling networks. The anthropogenic production of antibiotics, and its release in the microbiosphere results in a disturbance of these networks, antibiotic resistance tending to preserve its integrity. The cost of such adaptation is the emergence and dissemination of antibiotic resistance genes, and of all genetic and cellular vehicles in which these genes are located. Selection of the combinations of the different evolutionary units (genes, integrons, transposons, plasmids, cells, communities and microbiomes, hosts) is highly asymmetrical. Each unit of selection is a self-interested entity, exploiting the higher hierarchical unit for its own benefit, but in doing so the higher hierarchical unit might acquire critical traits for its spread because of the exploitation of the lower hierarchical unit. This interactive trade-off shapes the population biology of antibiotic resistance, a composed-complex array of the independent "population biologies." Antibiotics modify the abundance and the interactive field of each of these units. Antibiotics increase the number and evolvability of "clinical" antibiotic resistance genes, but probably also many other genes with different primary functions but with a resistance phenotype present in the environmental resistome. Antibiotics influence the abundance, modularity, and spread of integrons, transposons, and plasmids, mostly acting on structures present before the antibiotic era. Antibiotics enrich particular bacterial lineages and clones and contribute to local clonalization processes. Antibiotics amplify particular genetic exchange communities sharing antibiotic resistance genes and platforms within microbiomes. In particular human or animal hosts, the microbiomic composition might facilitate the interactions between evolutionary units involved in antibiotic resistance. The understanding of antibiotic resistance implies expanding our knowledge on multi-level population biology of bacteria.

Keywords: antibiotics, resistance, population biology, multi-level selection, evolution, evolvability, resistome, microbiome

Antibiotics produced by natural organisms play a role in their interactions shaping the lifestyle and homeostasis of bacterial populations and communities (Waksman, 1961; Davies, 2006; Fajardo and Martínez, 2008; Aminov, 2009). Such interactions might be of antagonistic nature as the production of antibiotics serves to inhibit other bacterial populations. Inhibition does not necessarily intend to kill competitive bacterial organisms, but rather prevent undesirable local overgrowth of partners in shared ecosystems. The diffusion of antibiotics in the environment assures an "exclusive zone" at a certain distance from the producer population. At the borders of such a zone, the potentially competing organisms are confronted with very low antibiotic concentrations, probably sufficient to decrease their growth rate, but not to kill the competing neighbor. In this sense, it is highly possible that the production of antagonistic (allelopathic) substances by microorganisms has more a defensive than offensive nature (Chao and Levin, 1981). In addition, mutual inhibition is frequently desirable for the maintenance of healthy species diversity in a particular ecosystem (Czárán et al., 2002; Becker et al., 2012; Cordero et al., 2012). It is of note that natural antibiotic production, decreasing the growth rate of the competing population, not only restricts its local predominance, but also assures that this population is preserved, as antibiotic-promoted cessation of growth is a highly effective system to avoid antibiotic killing.

However, the production of natural antibiotics might only have functions unrelated with inter-bacterial antagonisms. Antagonism might arise in particular contexts as a side-effect of cell-to-cell signaling effects resulting in self-regulation of growth, virulence, sporulation, motility, mutagenesis, SOS stress response, phage induction, transformation, lateral gene transfer, intra-chromosomal recombination, or biofilm formation (Goh et al., 2002; Ubeda et al., 2005; Linares et al., 2006; Yim et al., 2007; Martínez, 2008; Couce and Blázquez, 2009; Kohanski et al., 2010; Allen et al., 2011; Baharoglu and Mazel, 2011; Pedró et al., 2011; Looft and Allen, 2012; Looft et al., 2012).

Natural antibiotic resistance modulates the effect of the natural production of antibiotics, so antibiotic production and antibiotic resistance act as two complementary sides of the same process assuring the homeostasis of microbial populations and communities. In fact, communities with a cohesive habitat association might act as units in terms of antibiotic production and resistance. In these clusters, antibiotics are frequently produced by few bacterial organisms, whereas other members of the club are resistant (Cordero et al., 2012).

As in the case of natural antibiotic production, natural antibiotic resistance might not only focus on "defense against antibiotics" or "self-protection" in antibiotic producers. In fact, this "defense" is frequently a side-effect of other functions of the "natural resistance mechanisms," including nutrition, metabolism, detoxification of noxious substances, and catabolic processes (Dantas et al., 2008; Martínez, 2008; Alvarez-Ortega et al., 2011; Martínez and Rojo, 2011; Qu and Spain, 2011).

The so-called "intrinsic resistome," the ensemble of non-acquired genes and functions normally present in bacterial cells which influence the susceptibility to antibiotics, might account for 3% of the bacterial genome (Fajardo et al., 2008). Obviously, such a huge number of "defensive" genes reflects the unspecific nature of their functions in which antibiotic resistance is concerned (Fajardo et al., 2008; Alvarez-Ortega et al., 2011). That does not mean that these genes were not submitted to horizontal gene transfer before the crisis provoked by the industrial antibiotics pollution, illustrating that besides direct selection by clinical antibiotics other factors contribute to dissemination and maintenance of antibiotic resistance genes in bacterial populations (Biel and Hartl, 1983; Aminov and Mackie, 2007; Mindlin et al., 2008; Allen et al., 2009; D'Costa et al., 2011). In any case, it has been recently suggested that the close identity of resistance genes (and resistance platforms) from clinical strains and environmental strains might indicate recent exchange events (Forsberg et al., 2012). From this perspective, natural antibiotics and antibiotic "resistance" mechanisms have a natural regulatory role in shaping both population biology and evolutionary biology of bacterial organisms. However, the amount of active antibiotic determining this physiological natural "antibiotic environment" is extremely low (Halling-Sørensen et al., 1998). Of course antibiotic-producer organisms are endowed with "mechanisms for self-protection," which have been considered as the origin of modern functions involved in clinical antibiotic resistance (Benveniste and Davies, 1973). However, phylogenetic studies suggest that current clinical resistance genes are not found in antibiotic producers, and its emergence in clinical strains cannot be explained by recent horizontal gene transfer from these organisms. Nevertheless, they might have been historically submitted to duplications and frequent horizontal gene transfer, so that "modern" resistance genes might have evolved along complex evolutionary processes pre-existing the industrial release of antibiotics. In fact many identical "resistance genes" are found in environmental and clinical organisms (Cantón et al., 1999; Forsberg et al., 2012). In any case, what we denominate "antibiotic resistance" for clinical microorganisms is extremely rare in nature; other kinds of "resistance" genes, those of the "intrinsic resistome," able to protect cells from tiny concentrations of natural antibiotics, dominate in the wild environments.

The main problem that we are examining in this manuscript derives from the huge escalation of the amount of antibiotics released into the microbial environments as an effect of anthropogenic action, greatly exceeding the amount of natural antibiotics signaling and controlling the homeostasis of the bacterial world. Moreover, the amount of antimicrobials of anthropogenic origin entering into the environment assures the presence of every possible antibiotic concentration in contact with bacteria. The consequences of such an extensive release of inhibitory and regulatory molecules have an important impact on the population biology and evolutionary biology of bacteria.

POPULATION BIOLOGY OF THE UNITS OF SELECTION

The units of selection define the evolutionary individuals (Lewontin, 1970; Brandon, 1987; Mayr, 1997; Okasha, 2004; Dupré and O'Malley, 2007; Lloyd, 2008; Doolittle and Zhaxybayeva, 2010; Baquero, 2011; Rodriguez-Valera and Ussery, 2012). But what is selected in the case of antibiotic resistance? Possible units of selection in antibiotic resistance are discrete genetic sequences, genes, operons, functional genetic modules, mobile genetic elements (MGEs) as integrons, transposons, integrative–conjugative elements (ICEs), plasmids, or at the cellular and supra-cellular levels, genomes and cells (organisms), clones, clonal complexes, species, communities, and ecosystems. Note that all these possible units belong to different hierarchical levels, ranging from the relatively simple to the complex, as resistance genes are part of integrons, integrons part of transposons, transposons part of plasmids, plasmids part of cells, cells part of clones, clones part of species, and so on. Each unit is a "vessel" for the other(s), affecting not only its potential dissemination but also its rate of introgressive descent and evolution (Doolittle and Zhaxybayeva, 2010; Baquero, 2011; Bapteste et al., 2012; Cordero et al., 2012). The investigation of such a trans-hierarchical landscape clearly requires a multi-level population genetic approach (Baquero and Coque, 2011; Day et al., 2011; Cordero et al., 2012).

What we propose in this work is essentially a mental heuristic exercise. Let us imagine that we are aware of a kind of replicators called genes but we still ignore the existence of cells. We could observe changes in the frequency and variety of genes, and we might consider populations of genes, submitted to evolutionary dynamics and natural selection. If we were only conscious of the existence of transposons, we would establish population biology of transposons. If we considered plasmids, we would refer to the pan-plasmidome, the plasmid population harbored by a particular microbiome or a particular bacterial group (Fondi and Fani, 2010; Mizrahi, 2012). This would apply for every unit of selection. We would of course be able to observe changes in the abundance and variety of each unit involving a resistance trait as a consequence of the presence of antibiotics in the environment. Each unit of selection is a self-interested entity (Rankin et al., 2011b) exploiting the higher hierarchical unit for its own benefit (resistance plasmids exploit successful bacterial clones), but the higher unit might acquire critical traits for its spread because of the exploitation of the lower hierarchy unit (bacterial clones, bacterial communities, or microbiomes might be successful because of resistance plasmids, ICEs, or elements within those; Castillo et al., 2005; Mizrahi, 2012; Novais et al., 2012b). This trade-off of interactions shapes the global population biology of antibiotic resistance. In a certain sense, this multi-level perspective represents a "second line of complexity" in the classic view of antibiotics-driven natural selection processes, from the selection of a resistant cell to multi-level selections. Such processes should increase the absolute density (number) of all pieces involved in antibiotic resistance, and consequently might favor their interactions and emergence of novel combinatorial patterns (Baquero, 2004). Prediction of which pieces and patterns will evolve is a crucial issue for the management of multiantibiotic resistance, and might be possible if we have the right data (Martínez et al., 2007; Baquero, 2011; Partridge, 2011).

ANTIBIOTICS AND POPULATIONS OF RESISTANCE GENES

Have antibiotics increased the abundance of highly effective resistance genes in the bacterial world? Confronted with antibiotics, bacterial populations might adapt by selecting "more effective" mutants of wild genes endowed with other functions, but providing low level of resistance. Such process is favored by gene duplication, so that wild genes having a "small effect" on resistance could increase in number to increase protection. It is of note that this process might be much more frequent than mutation (Näsvall et al., 2012). A high number of gene-copies might in fact transitorily accumulate during selection, producing a full resistance phenotype. The question is if such gene duplications might contribute to the emergence of novel resistance genes. Once the permanence of a functional copy of a given gene is guaranteed, the second (or *n*-) copy has the evolutionary freedom (liberation from purifying selection) to be modified, eventually leading to a variant or novel gene (Kondrashov et al., 2002; Näsvall et al., 2012). It is of note that not all genes have equal chances of duplication, and certainly there are adaptive genes with a higher potential variability, containing highly variable regions interspersed among well-conserved, "segmentally variable genes," as ABC transporters involved in multidrug resistance (Zheng et al., 2004). Mutational changes in genes, leading to novel resistance genes, are facilitated under circumstances of enhanced mutagenesis in the host strain. Hyper-mutable bacteria ("mutators") are enriched in allelic variants of resistance genes, eventually providing wider resistance spectrum, as in the case of beta-lactamases (Baquero et al., 2005). Indeed organisms with enhanced mutation rates (frequently involving failures in the mismatch repair system) see their possibility of survival increased, and inside these strains, other genes could be modified to provide antibiotic resistance. Note that hyper-mutation and gene variation at large, might result from the effects of the antibiotic themselves (Blázquez et al., 2012).

Indeed, intra- and inter-bacterial gene movement and recombinational events between genetic platforms contribute to the total amount of resistance genes. In fact, the "biological success" of a resistance gene is dependent on its wider genetic context (Walsh, 2006; Wozniak and Waldor, 2010; Bertels and Rainey, 2011). Moreover, hybrid resistance genes resulting from recombinational events are not infrequent in nature (Goffin and Ghuysen, 1998; Maiden, 1998; Novais et al., 2012b). Under antibiotic exposure, bacterial pathogens in humans and animals (and commensals) might fix and further refine acquired resistance genes originated in areas less exposed to antimicrobials, as in the soil (including the rhizosphere!), or water bodies (including sewage!) (Aminov, 2009; Lupo et al., 2012).

If antibiotics have polluted the entire globe, including wild environments, specialized antibiotic resistance genes, identical to those found in hospitals, can be found everywhere else, including the most remote and wild regions (Gilliver et al., 1999; Osterblad et al., 2001; Sjölund et al., 2008; Allen et al., 2009; Quinteira et al., 2011; Stalder et al., 2012). However, the variety of natural bacterial genes that can provide antibiotic resistance in a heterologous host is much larger than that actually found in human pathogens (Dantas et al., 2008). Why only a very small fraction of "resistance genes" present in the "global resistome" have entered in human pathogens is a poorly addressed question. Of course genes from phylogenetically remote organisms should have functional connectivity and concert with the host systems, and that certainly constitutes an important bottleneck for their acceptance (Halary et al., 2010; Martínez, 2011). However, relatively "independent" functionally connected gene clusters (Zheng et al., 2005) determining resistance might be better tolerated and eventually fixed (Popa et al., 2011). In any case, as stated recently (Skippington and Ragan, 2011), the network and evolutionary dynamics that allow the stoichiometric participation of horizontally transferred genes in cellular networks remains poorly addressed, even though new bioinformatic advances have recently been made available (Cohen et al., 2012).

Considering potential sets of "acceptable" resistance genes able to evolve in bacterial populations, eventually only the "fittest genes" resulting from competition among genes might finally reach high densities. Competition is expected to occur mostly among orthologs or paralogs (for instance resulting from recent duplications) occupying the same functional niches (Kondrashov et al., 2002; Francino, 2012). Antibiotics could have enriched the more efficient adaptive genes among competing genes (for instance the more detoxifying ones; Novais et al., 2010b). However, the "fittest genes" are not necessarily those with the best intrinsic activity in terms of providing antibiotic resistance. Different resistance genes impose different biological costs for the host strain. As it was stated above, successful novel resistance genes should be fit in a particular genetic context, that is, the epigenetic compatibility of a new gene with the host genome is critical in the acquisition of resistance (Sánchez and Martínez, 2012). Such fitness bottleneck will select, in combination with the detoxifying efficiency, the novel successful genes.

Alternatively, the quantitative success of a particular gene (as bla_{TEM-1} in *Escherichia coli*, or *blaZ* in *Staphylococcus aureus*) might result only from a "founder effect" (Livermore, 2000; Martinez et al., 2009), that is, the first gene that by chance conferred a selective advantage in particular conditions was fixed and that resulted in a successful wide spread. This founder effect in human and animal pathogens might have occurred because of multiple selective events in environmental organisms exposed to dynamic landscapes. In fact, founder effects are expected to occur in a continuous and cumulative way (Aguilée et al., 2009). In turn, such emergent events might have been facilitated by changes in environmental conditions (as animal crowding in farms) resulting in local fluctuations in the size of particular bacterial populations, thus favoring acquisition by lateral genetic transfer of adaptive traits from environmental bacteria (Balloux, 2010). Similarly, the changes in the environment, the landscape dynamics, influence the probability of founders fixation, as well as the possibilities for extinction and re-emergence (Aguilée et al., 2011). It is not impossible that many resistance genes, even those rarely found or never found in the clinical environment, could have also been enriched by environmental antibiotic exposure (Martinez et al., 2009; Sommer et al., 2009).

How can we explain that the same resistance gene of plausible environmental origin (as bla_{CTX-Ms} or bla_{CMYs}) appears to have been captured in separate events by different gene-capturing elements as IS*Ecp*, IS*CR1*, or IS*26*? (Barlow and Hall, 2002; Toleman et al., 2006; Valverde et al., 2009; Partridge, 2011). There is a contemporary enrichment in organisms as Enterobacteriaceae of captured gene(s) with apparently the same function, and a bloom of a diversity of new genes coding for resistance to beta-lactams (Cantón and Coque, 2006; Coque et al., 2008; Poirel et al., 2012). This might be due to a dense interactive field resulting from an in the number of environmental species (donors) where it originated from, as well as an environmental increase in population density of a variety of "good recipients" as *E. coli* or *Klebsiella pneumoniae*. Recipients increase could result from both the augmentation of the total number of Enterobacteriaceae in the gut microbiota of mammals, probably due to antibiotic exposure, and the massive release of human-and animal sewage to the environment (see later).

Other less-successful resistance or pre-resistance genes might not be relevant in the clinical setting, but constitute an increasing reservoir of unpredictable consequences, and undoubtedly might influence the population ecology of bacteria. On the other hand, the selection of variant genes might occur at very low antibiotic concentrations (Henderson-Begg et al., 2006; Gullberg et al., 2011) particularly among natural concentration gradients (Baquero and Negri, 1997; Negri et al., 2000; Hermsen et al., 2012). It can be suggested that the overall increase in the amount of resistance genes on Earth also has a positive effect in maintaining the desirable homeostasis of bacterial populations in a heavily antibiotic-polluted environment.

An interesting point in gene population biology is the question of why a number of resistance genes maintain their full sequence integrity through myriads of replications in spite of an apparently insufficient level of antibiotic selection. Even considering that they are co-selected with genes under active selection (for instance being part of the collection of gene cassettes of an integron), their functionality seems to be better preserved than could be expected. This might suggest that the current function of a number of classic "resistance genes" is something other than antibiotic resistance (exaptation; Alonso and Gready, 2006; Petrova et al., 2011; Sánchez and Martínez, 2012).

Resistance genes tend to be collected in particular clones and clustered in common genetic platforms (Partridge and Hall, 2004; Ktari et al., 2006; Partridge, 2011; Potron et al., 2013), probably following the "genetic capitalism principle," that is, the more resistant clones and the most fit resistance-providing platforms are selected, and then their ability to acquire novel adaptive traits is favored (Lawrence, 1997; Baquero, 2004). As we will see along this review, the extensive antibiotic-promoted selection of resistant bacterial organisms is a selection of the "vehicles" where antibiotic resistance genes are located, and the selection of "vehicles" assures the selection of the genes that they contain. Consequently, the total amount of resistance genes should increase under selection. Interestingly, some "vehicles" (as MGEs are more frequently associated with resistance genes than others. As complementary explanations, we can recall here the founder effect (advantages for the first gene-capturing MGEs), the influence of genes and platforms on the overall fitness of the recipient cells, or the higher prevalence of particular MGEs in the organisms more exposed to antibiotics, heavy metals, biocides, or other ecological stressors (Stokes and Gillings, 2011).

ANTIBIOTICS AND POPULATIONS OF RESISTANCE INTEGRONS

Have antibiotics increased the abundance, in the microbial world, of integrons able to capture resistance genes? Integrons possess a site-specific recombination system able to integrate, rearrange, and express adaptive genes, including antibiotic resistance genes (Mazel, 2006; Partridge, 2011; Stokes and Gillings, 2011; Moura et al., 2012). These genetic platforms are ancient structures (several hundred million years old) that were already involved in the initial outbreaks of antibiotic resistance in the 1950s (Liebert et al., 1999; Mazel, 2006; Revilla et al., 2008). The same type of integrons, now carrying a diversity of antibiotic resistance genes, are preserved in the current bacterial world, and have installed themselves in natural environments along extended periods of time (Petrova et al., 2011; Stokes and Gillings, 2011; Stalder et al., 2012). Integrons evolution often results in the local array of resistance genes, and other genes of adaptive nature (Labbate et al., 2009; Moura et al., 2012; Stalder et al., 2012), which increases the possibilities of their selective multiplication.

In other words, exposure to antibiotics, biocides, or heavy metals and a high multiplicity of other different environmental factors results in an increase of cells containing integrons (Gaze et al., 2005, 2011; Wright et al., 2008; Stalder et al., 2012). Moreover, exposure to different antibiotics (aminoglycosides, beta-lactams, fluoroquinolones, trimethoprim, metronidazole) facilitates extensive gene cassette recombination; occasionally involving the SOS-triggered IntI1 integrase over-expression (Guerin et al., 2009; Hocquet et al., 2012). Other recombinational events (often mediated by ISs) influence shuffling of resistance genes contained in different integrons, giving rise to multi-resistance regions (Partridge, 2011) and further facilitating the evolution and selection of the upper-level host vehicles (Domingues et al., 2012). In fact, integrons are not mobile, but are frequently associated with transposons and/or plasmids and therefore should increase in abundance as a result of conjugation or transposition events mediated by Tn*21*-like and IS*26*-like elements. For instance class 1 integrons located in Tn*402*, which are often part of Tn*501*-like transposons on conjugative plasmids, have greatly contributed to the spread of integrons among γ and β-proteobacteria (Tato et al., 2010; Partridge, 2011).

The frequent association of integrons with a variety of specialized DNA recombination systems enhances both transferability and genetic diversification. For instance, insertion sequences (IS) of the IS*110*/IS*492* family as IS*4321* and IS*5075* (members of IS*1111* subgroup) target the terminal inverted repeats of Tn*21* family transposons (Partridge and Hall, 2003; Novais et al., 2010a). The outcome is the initiation of a non-standard transposition resulting in only a single copy appearing in the transposed product (Cain et al., 2010; Martinez et al., 2012). Such mobilization of integrons by specialized transposition is a powerful mechanism for integrons spread in both environmental competent and non-competent bacteria (Domingues et al., 2012; Stokes et al., 2012). Also, IS-mediated mobilization of relevant antibiotic resistance genes contained in the integron contributes to enhance gene expression and mosaic genetic diversity, which should be reflected in higher possibilities of dissemination. That is the case for insertion sequences targeting the pseudo-palindromes of integron *attC* sites, as the IS*1111-attC* group elements of the IS*110*/IS*492* family (Tetu and Holmes, 2008), or IS*4*-like elements as IS*1999* (Aubert et al., 2006; Post and Hall, 2009; Poirel et al., 2010). Note that the antibiotic-mediated selection of strains, plasmids, or transposons containing integrons necessarily implies selection of IS sequences, and therefore the capture of resistance genes and the combinatorial evolution of resistance platforms. In fact, ISs mobilizing adjacent sequences by rolling-circle (RC) transposition as, IS*Ecp1* and the insertion sequence common regions (IS*CRs*), favor the capture and mobilization of a full series of antibiotic resistance genes leading to complex multi-resistance class 1 integrons (del Pilar Garcillán-Barcia et al., 2001; Garcillán-Barcia and de la Cruz, 2002; Aubert et al., 2006; Toleman et al., 2006; Poirel et al., 2010).

ANTIBIOTICS AND POPULATIONS OF RESISTANCE TRANSPOSABLE ELEMENTS

Have antibiotics increased the abundance of resistance transposable elements in the microbiosphere? Transposable elements encode an enzyme, transposase, which is required for excising and inserting the mobile element. Transposases (revised in Hickman et al., 2010 and references herein) seem to be the most abundant genes in known sequenced genomes and environmental metagenomes (Aziz et al., 2010).

Among transposases, class II dsDNA transposases constitute the most common group, followed by serine and tyrosine recombinases and RC transposases which are linked to different MGEs (IS, composite transposons, class II transposons, bacteriophages, and genetic islands). The wide spread and maintenance of different classes of transposable elements in bacterial populations has been obviously favored by antibiotic selection because of their association with antibiotic resistance genes. However, most of the contemporary antibiotic resistance transposable elements belong to a few families that have been detected in ancient isolates, often linked to alternative functional roles, thus suggesting antibiotic resistance might have overshadowed previous selection forces.

For instance, some transposable elements, as IS or composite transposons, as Tn*5* or Tn*10*, confer growth rate advantages under different conditions of nutrient availability, enabling populations to rapidly adapt to different physiological conditions (Biel and Hartl, 1983; Hartl et al., 1983; Blot et al., 1994). Also, the highly specialized targeting system of Tn*7* able to selectively direct transposition into both mobile and stationary DNA pools (see later), avoids the occurrence of deleterious insertions and allows the host population or community to recruit genes through a variety of mobile DNAs, thus favoring the adaptation of diverse groups of bacteria to survive or adapt to different conditions (Parks and Peters, 2009; Parks et al., 2009). Selection by different ecological conditions and stressors (including antibiotics) multiplies the chances for expansion, recombination, and diversification (Partridge and Iredell, 2012; Seputiene et al., 2012).

The main group within dsDNA transposases corresponds to DDE transposases (designation given due to the presence of a highly conserved catalytic triad of two aspartate (D) and one glutamate (E) residue), originally identified in the retrovirus integrase and having a role during the transfer of the DNA strand. Most IS families use this catalytic reaction for transposition with the exception of IS*1*/IS*110* and the RCR IS*91*-like elements. IS-DDE transposases have been detected in more than 70 bacterial genera, more than one third being iso-elements (>95% of identity at protein level, >90% at DNA level). They are frequently located on plasmids associated with composite transposons containing antibiotic resistance genes (Merlin et al., 2000).

Tn*7* poses an unique fine-tuned regulated transposition array (TnsABCDE) involved in the regulation of transposition (the core machinery coding for TnsA, TnsB, TnsC) and the mobilization of the element (TnsE, TnsD; Parks and Peters, 2009, Parks et al., 2009). Such regulation allows Tn*7* to use two target-site selection pathways and move to different hosts. Tn*7* belongs to a family of MGE that encodes a transposase and an ATP-utilizing protein (TnsC) that controls the activity of such transposase and often its target site selection. Members of the ATP-subunit superfamily comprise widespread AbR transposons that differ in the transposase (also a DDE enzyme) and the number of proteins in the transposition module (for revision see Craig, 2002). Some examples are Tn*1825*/Tn*1826*, Tn*552*-IS*21*, and Tn*402*–Tn*5053* (Craig, 2002). All are widely distributed and they are related with trimethoprim and heavy metals resistance (Kholodii et al., 2003; Partridge, 2011). Please note that in this case trimethoprim resistance is the currently recognizable phenotype, but the genes might have been selected before trimethoprim exposure for other reasons (Alonso and Gready, 2006).

Members of the Tn*3* family are mainly derivatives of transposon subfamilies Tn*3* (Tn*3*, Tn*5393*, Tn*5403*) or Tn*501* (Tn*21*, Tn*501*, Tn*1721*) and all of them were already detectable in ancient bacteria from permafrost (Tolmasky, 1990; Graidy, 2002; Kholodii et al., 2003; Mindlin et al., 2008). Members of the Tn*501* subfamily of Tn*3* transposons could have been enriched by mercury exposure, as they carry mercury-detoxifying genes. These genes probably originated in hydrothermal environments, where geochemically derived mercury is at high concentrations (Boyd and Barkay, 2012). Mercury-transposons provide target sites for Tn*501*-type transposons, and include a diversity of Tn*21*, Tn*1696*, and Tn*501* related elements carrying class 1 integrons. Enrichment of Tn*3*-type transposons by environmental pollutants, as heavy metals, might have contributed to increase the connectivity with organisms and genetic platforms harboring resistance genes, eventually included in integrons (most frequently of class 1), and have converted this family in the "flagship" of floating resistance genes (Liebert et al., 1999; Partridge and Hall, 2004; Partridge and Iredell, 2012).

Beside classic antibiotic resistance gene cassettes, emerging beta-lactamase genes as bla_{VIM}, bla_{IMP} bla_{VEB}, or bla_{GES} are located in integrons on different Tn*501* derivatives (Partridge, 2011). Other widespread "new" beta-lactamase genes have been directly recruited by host-specific Tn*3*-like transposons as Tn*1440* carrying bla_{KPC} (a Tn*5403*-like transposon from *Klebsiella* which belongs to the Tn*3* subfamily; (Naas et al., 2008).

Such process of gene capture contributes to further increase the number of these transposons, which in turn will facilitate its diversification and eventually novel resistance gene recruitments. Indeed the capture of bla_{TEM1a} by Tn*2* led to, in a landscape of high consumption of aminopenicillins in the 60s and 70s of the past century, a huge amplification of this transposon, now widespread in all environments. Other transposons were less-successful, as Tn*1* (with bla_{TEM-2}), and Tn*3* (carrying bla_{TEM-1a}; Novais et al., 2010a; Bailey et al., 2011), probably because of the reduced numbers and connectivities (influencing success) of the vehicles in which they were located (plasmids, clones; Cain et al., 2010; Novais et al., 2010a; Partridge, 2011).

Transposable elements also increase in number by inserting extra copies in the host genomes. Of course this might cause an "intergenomic conflict," as such insertions might affect chromosomal balance and produce mutations, being so, transposons might be a "bitter–sweet" pill for host bacteria (Toleman and Walsh, 2011). This is why genomes have evolved suppressors limiting transposon spread (Pomiankowski, 1999). Eventually, equilibrium is reached by diminishing the transposition frequency. Successful transposons as Tn*3* have this kind of "transposition immunity" to ensure a maximum of two copies per replicon.

On the other hand, transposition might compete with the host genome replication. Some transposases as that of Tn*7* (and possibly Tn*917*) can bind to "processivity factors" involved DNA replication; competition for this interaction could limit their proliferation. However, a benefit for the transposons appear to be derived from the fact that the interaction of transposases with processivity factors favors "target site selection," so that activation of transposition with Tn*7* (transposon excision and insertion) does not occur until an appropriate target has been identified, most frequently mobile plasmids, providing Tn*7* with a means of spreading to a new host (Parks et al., 2009).

As in the case of integrons, transposable elements are very ancient on Earth, but the very same molecular structures are found in modern resistance-bearing transposons (Bisercić and Ochman, 1993; Mindlin et al., 2005; Vishnivetskaya and Kathariou, 2005; Petrova et al., 2009; Aziz et al., 2010). The acquisition of resistance genes seems to have occurred preferentially by particular transposable elements that were afterward amplified by antibiotics. Interestingly, a number of transposons carrying resistance genes have been recovered from ancient permafrost and seem to have been selected before the antibiotic era (Mindlin et al., 2008). Widespread transposons in our days, as those belonging to Tn*7* or Tn*3* superfamilies, certainly have a very ancient origin. Most probably they were selected by pre-antibiotic forces, increasing their absolute amount, followed by their spread and diversification in different plasmids and organisms. Exposure to early chemotherapeutic agents has reinforced these evolutionary events.

ANTIBIOTICS AND POPULATIONS OF RESISTANCE MOBILE GENETIC ELEMENTS (PLASMIDS, ICEs)

Have antibiotics increased the abundance of plasmids and ICEs carrying resistance genes in bacterial populations and communities? Conjugative plasmids and ICEs are quite similar genomic objects, in fact they appear to be short-term variants of identical backbone elements (Guglielmini et al., 2011); the main difference is that the replication of ICEs occurs only by integration in the host's chromosome (Wozniak and Waldor, 2010). For instance a close relationship resulting from a common phylogeny can be found between IncA/C plasmids and SXT/R391 ICEs (Wozniak and Waldor, 2010; Toleman and Walsh, 2011). Note that the traditional association of highly transmissible elements with plasmids is not necessarily true.

Plasmids are abundant in nature and consistently isolated from microbial communities of different habitats with and without anthropogenic exposure (Coombs, 2009; Sobecky and Hazen, 2009). In fact, contemporary resistance plasmids are based on plasmid backgrounds existing in the pre-antibiotic era (Datta and Hughes, 1983; Hughes and Datta, 1983). Maintenance of plasmids and ICEs in bacterial populations results from both the selfish features that promote acquisition and persistence within bacterial populations ("the parasitic hypothesis") and the beneficial effects they confer to individual bacterial hosts and communities ("the evolvability hypothesis"; Werren, 2011). MGEs are increasingly being considered within this multi-hierarchical model, as clonal-, species-, or community-specific mobile elements (Carattoli, 2009; Garcillán-Barcia et al., 2009; Lim et al., 2010; Shearer et al., 2011; Heuer et al., 2012; Williams et al., 2012; Clewell et al., 2013; Guglielmini et al., 2013). Between and also within these hierarchical levels, plasmids may eventually evolve toward mutualism (Rankin et al., 2011b). Plasmids might assure their permanent linkage with a particular host, bacterial lineage, or multi-specific community by post-segregation killer strategies that cause the death of non-carrying bacterial offspring. This is caused by toxin–antitoxin (TA), restriction-modification (R-M), or clustered regularly interspaced short palindromic repeats (CRISPR) systems, and also probably by "plasmid domestication," which is produced by changes either in the plasmid and host genome that lead to a more stable coexistence (Bouma and Lenski, 1988; Jones, 2010; Marraffini and Sontheimer, 2010; García-Quintanilla and Casadesús, 2011).

The diversity of bacterial communities, the relative population densities of their components, the spatial separation, and nutrient availability greatly influence plasmid host-range, content, and transferability (Coombs, 2009). It is interesting to suggest that the selective processes exerted by antibiotics will modify bacterial diversity and population densities, forcing the coexistence of plasmids and particular hosts, favoring recombination and other processes that lead to plasmid domestication (Boyd et al., 1996). The robustness of interactions between particular plasmids and particular clones is shaped by epistatic processes (Silva et al., 2011; San Millán et al., 2012) mediated by nucleoid-associated transcriptional regulators (Doyle et al., 2007; Yun et al., 2010; Fernández-Alarcón et al., 2011; Humphrey et al., 2012) and the clonal interferences that might result from these interactions (Hughes et al., 2012). A robust interaction is reflected in a non-cost or even negative-cost coexistence, and will tie the fate of plasmid density to the abundance of their specific bacterial hosts, resulting in a necessary "in-host" plasmid evolution linked to "with plasmid" host evolution (Dionisio et al., 2005; Halary et al., 2010).

A major topic in plasmid population biology is the consideration of advantages and inconveniences of plasmid or ICE broad-host-range. It is of note that host-range does not necessarily mean transfer ability to a particular host or long-term maintenance in bacterial populations, but stable replication in a new host (De Gelder et al., 2007; Suzuki et al., 2010). Certainly, broad-host-range conjugative plasmids favor the penetration of adaptive traits as "new" antibiotic resistance genes (Fernández-Alarcón et al., 2011; Sen et al., 2011; Hamprecht et al., 2012; Heuer and Smalla, 2012) and, in turn, antibiotics can favor the abundance of these plasmids promoting transfer and by selection of plasmid containing bacteria (Lang et al., 2012). The frequent observation of different systems of replication (recognizing host primases) in the same plasmid suggests adaptive ways of increasing host-range (Del Solar et al., 1996; Clewell et al., 2013). Globally spread plasmids identified in hospitals, soils, agriculture, and marine habitats have a complex mosaic structure that reflects inter-genomic historical adaptations to phylogenetically distant bacterial hosts (Schlüter et al., 2007; Norberg et al., 2011; Heuer et al., 2012; Partridge and Iredell, 2012). In addition, broad-host-range plasmids lacking transfer systems can be transferred to phylogenetically close or distantly related bacteria by helper conjugation systems located in narrow-host-range plasmids containing a conjugation system (Smorawinska et al., 2012).

Long-term maintenance and dispersion of broad-host-range plasmids in bacterial populations and communities seems to be related with the local availability of hosts (De Gelder et al., 2007), but also with the "social interactions between plasmids" eventually leading to unbearable costs for their hosts (Smith, 2012). Eventually, exclusion mechanisms between plasmids (one plasmid excludes the incoming one) might be softened by inter-plasmid recombination that might result in hybrids able to evade exclusion. CRISPR is a genetic interference system by which bacteria with CRISPR regions carrying DNA copies of previously encountered plasmids can abort the replication of plasmids with these sequences. Hypothetically that might favor plasmid dispersal among different strains, providing a weak selective advantage for the host cell (Levin, 2010), although an increased benefit could be predicted for host coalitions, as genetic exchange communities (GECs; see later). This system also controls phages, but the possible populational interactions (competition–cooperation) between phages and plasmids have scarcely been investigated.

Antibiotic exposure might have increased the absolute number of plasmids with resistance determinants in bacterial populations due to the selection of clones harboring them. The possibility that broad-host conjugative plasmids have been submitted to a more effective enrichment than narrow-host plasmids (because of selection in multiple hosts and environmental compartments) poses an interesting question. Eventually, the biological cost of resistance plasmids for the host could be compensated by higher transmission (Garcillán-Barcia et al., 2011). As Stokes and Gillings pointed out, an increase in the general *tempo* of resistance genes dissemination is highly probable, due to selection of cells with inherently higher rates of lateral transfer (Stokes and Gillings, 2011).

Finally, we can consider bacteriophages as mobile mediators of inter-bacterial transfer of resistance genes. Also in this case antibiotics might modulate phage–bacteria population dynamics by processes as "phage-antibiotic synergy," a non-SOS mechanism of virulent phage induction caused by exposure to sub-inhibitory concentrations of beta-lactams (Comeau et al., 2007; Allen et al., 2011; Looft et al., 2012). Antibiotics promote the number of phages and pro-phages linked to antibiotic resistance platforms, favoring dissemination of these platforms, and consequently amplifying the dissemination of resistance and virulence genes (Allen et al., 2011).

ANTIBIOTICS AND POPULATIONS OF BACTERIAL CLONES AND SPECIES

Bacterial clones are constituted by isolates that have a close common phylogenetic origin. High-risk clones are defined as clones with an enhanced ability to colonize, spread, and persist in a variety of niches, which acquire adaptive traits that increase pathogenicity or antibiotic resistance (Baquero and Coque, 2011). They constitute the main vehicles dispersing antibiotic resistance at a global scale (Willems et al., 2011; Woodford et al., 2011). Examples of these high-risk clones are *E. coli* ST131 (phylogroup B2), ST155 and ST393 (phylogroup B1), or ST69, ST405, and ST648 (phylogroup D); *K. pneumoniae* ST258, ST14 or ST37; *Enterococcus faecium*, ST18, ST17, ST78; *Enterococcus faecalis* ST6; *S. aureus*, ST45, ST5, ST8, ST30, or ST22. A number of these clones were ancient lineages, well-adapted to colonization and transmission between particular hosts, that acquired antibiotic resistance and consequently enhanced capabilities of dispersal (McBride et al., 2007; Brisse et al., 2009; Chambers and Deleo, 2009; Willems et al., 2012). Multiplication and spread of highly successful clones implies multiplication and spread of all the antibiotic resistance genes and platforms they contain, increasing their absolute numbers. In fact, it is not unusual that a single successful clone might contribute to the spread of different plasmids, genetic platforms, and resistance genes, both in Gram-positives (Chambers and Deleo, 2009) and in Gram-negatives (Carattoli, 2009; Andrade et al., 2011; Woodford et al., 2011; Novais et al., 2012a; Partridge and Iredell, 2012). Such multi-lateral collaboration probably contributes to the local ecological success of variants arising in these clones, leading to a clonal diversification (clonalization) which assures a long-term permanence in complex adaptive landscapes, following the "never put all the eggs in the same basket" principle (Wiedenbeck and Cohan, 2011; de Regt et al., 2012; Freitas et al., 2013). Focusing only on mutational evolution, it has been suggested that there is an acceleration of emergence of bacterial antibiotic resistance in connected microenvironments (Zhang et al., 2011; Hallatschek, 2012) but this might also occur in the case of gene flow.

Local clonalization might result in a restricted gene flow among resulting subpopulations (Willems et al., 2012). However, recombinational events might spare those regions required for adaptation to local microniches, assuring divergence, and be maintained for other regions (ecological speciation with-gene-flow; Via, 2012). The increased recovery of isolates belonging to high-risk clonal complexes of important human pathogens as *E. coli*, *S. aureus*, *E. faecalis*, or *E. faecium*, that cause both human infections and mucosal colonization, and even the expansion of these clones to novel hosts is most probably related with the acquisition of antibiotic resistance genes (Hidron et al., 2008; Baquero, 2012; Novais et al., 2012a, 2013)

An interesting question is if the selection of particular clones because of antibiotic resistance might decrease the overall clonal diversity as might be inferred from recent studies (Ghosh et al., 2011). Actually, that might be compensated by clonal diversification, in a "*ex pluribus unum/ex unibus plurum*" evolutionary dynamics (Baquero, 2011). It is easy to conclude that any outbreak produced by antibiotic resistant bacteria will locally enrich the involved evolutionary units, facilitating further events of antibiotic resistance development and possibly transmission (Chambers and Deleo, 2009; Freitas et al., 2013).

ANTIBIOTICS AND POPULATIONS OF BACTERIAL COMMUNITIES

Imbedded into the high complexity of the microbiomes, of humans and animals, in the soil or in the water sediments, it is possible to recognize "clubs" of bacterial clones and species where genes and genetic platforms circulate via lateral transfer, the GECs. In a very restrictive manner, Skippington and Ragan (2011) have recently defined a GEC as a group of organisms (entities) in which each entity has over time both donated genetic material to, and received genetic material from every other entity in that GEC, via a path of lateral gene transfer. What do the members of such clubs have in common? Network modeling and co-occurrence statistical approaches indicate that lifestyle and shared environments, functional complementarities, and most probably, continued physical clustering (granularity) determine the size and connectivity of GECs (Freilich et al., 2010; Smillie et al., 2011; Faust and Raes, 2012; Faust et al., 2012). In many cases, this also means a closed shared phylogeny (Skippington and Ragan, 2012). In fact, GECs members are linked not only by genetic exchanges, but also by metabolic and functional cooperation, providing a certain ecological compartmentalization inside particular microbial megasystems (as intestinal microbiota; Faust and Raes, 2012; Faust et al., 2012). We can consider here some kind of cooperative "niche construction" (Laland et al., 1999; Kylafis and Loreau, 2011). Genetic transfer, particularly considering mixed-granular "surface-associated populations" with a kind of "lattice reciprocity" (Zhong et al., 2010, 2012) might assure a "collective" adaptation of such functional GEC units, increasing relatedness among members and fixing common evolutionary boundaries (Nogueira et al., 2009; Rankin et al., 2011a,b). The development of more studies on the "physics" of genetic transfer, is certainly advisable, for instance, to investigate to what extent genetic transfer can be influenced by mixing movements or the viscosity or fluidity of the surrounding medium, as in the intestinal content (particularly during enteric diseases) or in water bodies, influencing cell-to-cell contacts and therefore GECs integrities (Zhong et al., 2010; Jeffery et al., 2012).

An important topic is the possibility of "multiclonal GECs" as a form of organization of the lifestyle of a particular species or closely phylogenetically related coalitions in changing environments (Skippington and Ragan, 2012), where different sub-specific ecotypes exploiting neighbor nano-niches (Wiedenbeck and Cohan, 2011) and taking advantage of a common "public good" are frequently encoded by conjugative elements (Norman et al., 2009; Rankin et al., 2011b). The distribution among GECs members of such plasmid-mediated "public goods" is favored by common characteristics in the consortium, as nearly identical immune phenotypes mediated by CRISPR, or common DNA uptake mechanisms or quorum sensing responses. Plasmid-mediated common benefits will probably lead to GEC-plasmid coevolution (Skippington and Ragan, 2012). Along the same line, addiction-type TA complexes can spread on plasmids, favoring coexistence and/or competition in spatially structured environments (Rankin et al., 2012) highlighting the role of kin effects in GECs selection (taking "kin" in a wider sense than just intra-specific ties). It is of note, however, that possibly most organisms and environments might act as conduits for resistance gene flow (Stokes and Gillings, 2011), acting as "sources" from where resistance genes are directed to GECs, acting as "sinks," according to the Perron et al. (2007) metaphor. The possibility of "go-between" organisms traveling from GECs of different microbiotic systems (humans, animals, rhizosphere, and water sediments) should be taken into consideration, as they might contribute to the inter-environmental globalization of antibiotic resistance genes. The existence of "ubiquitous" organisms or species able to transit in different environments has been suggested (Fondi and Fani, 2010; Freilich et al., 2010; Tamames et al., 2010). Candidates for efficient "go-between" organisms are groups of the same bacterial species but specialized in particular environments, as the case of human or animal-adapted versus environmental *E. coli* clades, where probably only ecological barriers prevent gene flow (Freilich et al., 2010; Luo et al., 2011). Mixing of human or animal derived water effluents into the environment, a practice that is surprisingly perpetuated even in modern societies will facilitate conduits for resistance gene flow (Baquero et al., 2008; Czekalski et al., 2012; Lupo et al., 2012). Such flow occurs because of the confluence of human microbiota from different human hosts, different animals and the indigenous environmental microbiota.

Among these GECs, the most relevant for the transmission of antibiotic resistance are those including species from Gammaproteobacteria (as *E. coli*) and Firmicutes (as *Enterococcus*; Antonopoulos et al., 2009; Freilich et al., 2010; Skippington and Ragan, 2011; Faust et al., 2012). These groups of organisms are enriched in the microbiota during antibiotic exposure (Antonopoulos et al., 2009; Sommer et al., 2009). Antibiotic-mediated reduction in number or loss of some species, favors bacterial species able to explore and temporarily exploit empty niches due to short generation times (Allen et al., 2011; Looft and Allen, 2012). Antibiotic exposure will increase the absolute number (overgrowth) of GECs-associated organisms, for instance, by antibiotic exposure of the infant gut (Fouhy et al., 2012; Looft and Allen, 2012). Probably the same might occur in environmental GECs submitted either to antibiotic pollution or sanitation procedures (Baquero et al., 2008). For instance, metagenomic analysis indicates that drinking water chlorination could concentrate populations containing insertion sequences, integrons, and antibiotic resistance plasmids (Shi et al., 2013). These effects will contribute to the dissemination of resistance genes and the genetic platforms in which they are located.

The identification of GECs among members of the "microbial guilds" in the three identified major microbiome "enterotypes" (Arumugam et al., 2011) needs to be investigated. These major enterotypes (clusters of species) should probably be tightly maintained into host populations, and therefore the local spread of antibiotic resistance genes could serve to maintain their integrity in an antibiotic-polluted environment. At the same time, low-abundance enterotype-species, but providing critical functions, could have low possibilities of getting resistance genes in the absence of GECs. Consequently, a deep and permanent contamination by antibiotic resistance genes of the normal microbiota of humans and animals is a reasonable possibility. Complex microbiota of humans and animals are reproducible systems, not only along time in the same individual, but also across individuals. These systems are frequently based in a microbiotic "core" composed by organisms belonging to a relatively small number of phylogroups, and probably metabolically linked with the host (Dethlefsen et al., 2006; Ley et al., 2006; Marchesi, 2011). Newborns have a sterile gut, but the human microbiota is "reproduced" with a relatively low number of variations on each of them (Baquero and Nombela, 2012; Vallès et al., 2012). Possibly there is also an "epidemiology of bacterial consortia" even in hospitals, which remains to be investigated. Exposure to antimicrobial agents might affect the frequency and absolute number of GECs; in a number of cases, antibiotic resistance might contribute to the temporal stability and resilience of microbiomes in an antibiotic-polluted environment (Allison and Martiny, 2008; Antonopoulos et al., 2009). Of course that occurs at the expenses of maintenance and spread of the full range of antibiotic resistance evolutionary units.

Finally, we cannot discard individual variations in the microbiotic communities caused by diet, host genetics, particular illnesses, inflammation, or infectious agents including viruses and parasites which might lead to microbial communities more prone to capture and propagate antibiotic resistance (Marchesi, 2010; Claesson et al., 2012; Looft and Allen, 2012). For instance, a high-fat diet determines the composition of the murine gut microbiome independently of obesity, with an increase of Proteobacteria and Firmicutes, heavily involved in resistance gene mobilization (Hildebrandt et al., 2009; Tagliabue and Elli, 2012). In several microbiota communities studied in the elderly, the proportion of phylum Proteobacteria, very active in the mobilization of antibiotic resistance genes and vehicles, was ten times higher than average (20 versus 2%; Claesson et al., 2011). *E. coli* numbers are higher in the microbiota of women with excessive weight gain than in women with normal weight gain during pregnancy (Santacruz et al., 2010).

A number of surgical interventions (as surgery for morbid obesity) increases Proteobacteria even in a higher proportion (50 times increase; Li et al., 2011; Graessler et al., 2012). Unfortunately, these populational microbiotic shifts favoring the active populations and communities contributing to the emergence, dispersal and maintenance of antibiotic resistance might also occur as a consequence of undernutrition (10 times increase in Proteobacteria, 46 versus 5% in healthy children in Bangladesh; Monira et al., 2011). Possibly the deleterious effect of antibiotics in promoting antibiotic resistance will be significantly increased. Finally, it could be considered, under certain circumstances, as during the colonization of the neonatal intestinal tract, that rapidly growing populations might be more prone to the dissemination of antibiotic resistance. Also the unexpected possibility of resistance gene exchange between Actinobacteria (*Bifidobacterium* belongs to this group!) and Gammaproteobacteria has been recently shown under the same conditions (Tamminen et al., 2012).

ANTIBIOTICS IN THE ANTHROPOCENE: EFFECTS ON GLOBAL ECOLOGY AND EVOLUTION

Evolution is a natural trend of complex systems, and might be accelerated by changing and stressful conditions. The Anthropocene is the current human-dominated geological epoch where nature is changed and stressed by the action of humans (Zalasiewicz et al., 2011; Biermann et al., 2012). Industrial antibiotics are a paradigmatic example of substances exerting a powerful effect of anthropogenic origin on the bacterial communities of the microbiosphere. Not only most of these substances are unspecifically killing bacterial organisms, and selecting for resistance, but directly influence the mechanisms of genetic variation (mutation, recombination, transposition, modularization, gene transfer; Baquero, 2009; Gillings and Stokes, 2012).

Such effects on microorganisms will be further enhanced by a diversity of other anthropogenic effects as the release of biopharmaceuticals, biocides, heavy metals, industrial and agricultural residues, and plastic materials or changes in the environmental conditions. The mixing of bacterial populations (human organisms with other human, animal, or environmental organisms), that makes the emergence and spread of resistance possible is also favored by poor sanitation, facilitating contact of human or animal sewage with the soil. Some of these effects might escalate with other anthropogenic effects as destruction of diversity in food animals (Baquero, 2012) or even global warming (Baquero et al., 2008; Baquero, 2009; Balbus et al., 2013). The fight against antibiotic resistance should focus not only on acting on its appropriate usage in human and veterinary medicine, but by considering possible initiatives at ecological and evolutionary levels, as eco-evo drugs and strategies (Baquero et al., 2011) in accordance with the environmental distribution of bacterial organisms (Tamames et al., 2010), in the scope of progressing toward a protective and restorative planet medicine (Baquero, 2009).

ACKNOWLEDGMENTS

The authors' work was sponsored by grants from the European Union (PAR-241476 and EvoTAR-282004), the Instituto de Salud Carlos III – Ministry of Economy and Competitiveness of Spain (FIS-PS09-02381; FIS-PI10-02588, PI12-01581), and the Regional Government of Madrid in Spain (PROMPT- S2010/BMD2414). The authors are also grateful to the Spanish Network for the Study of Plasmids and Extrachromosomal Elements (REDEEX) for encouraging and funding cooperation among Spanish microbiologists working on the biology of mobile genetic elements (grant BFU 2012-0079-E/BMC; Spanish Ministry of Science and Innovation).

REFERENCES

Aguilée, R., Claessen, D., and Lambert, A. (2009). Allele fixation in a dynamic metapopulation: founder effects vs refuge effects. *Theor. Popul. Biol.* 76, 105–117.

Aguilée, R., Lambert, A., and Claessen, D. (2011). Ecological speciation in dynamic landscapes. *J. Evol. Biol.* 24, 2663–2677.

Allen, H. K., Looft, T., Bayles, D. O., Humphrey, S., Levine, U. Y., Alt, D., et al. (2011). Antibiotics in feed induce prophages in swine fecal microbiomes. *MBio* 2, e00260–e00211.

Allen, H. K., Moe, L. A., Rodbumrer, J., Gaarder, A., and Handelsman, J. (2009). Functional metagenomics reveals diverse beta-lactamases in a remote Alaskan soil. *ISME J.* 3, 243–251.

Allison, S. D., and Martiny, J. B. H. (2008). Colloquium paper: resistance, resilience, and redundancy in microbial communities. *Proc. Natl. Acad. Sci. U.S.A.* 105, 11512–11519.

Alonso, H., and Gready, J. E. (2006). Integron-sequestered dihydrofolate reductase: a recently redeployed enzyme. *Trends Microbiol.* 14, 236–242.

Alvarez-Ortega, C., Wiegand, I., Olivares, J., Hancock, R. E. W., and Martínez, J. L. (2011). The intrinsic resistome of *Pseudomonas aeruginosa* to β-lactams. *Virulence* 2, 144–146.

Aminov, R. I. (2009). The role of antibiotics and antibiotic resistance in nature. *Environ. Microbiol.* 11, 2970–2988.

Aminov, R. I., and Mackie, R. I. (2007). Evolution and ecology of antibiotic resistance genes. *FEMS Microbiol. Lett.* 271, 147–161.

Andrade, L. N., Curiao, T., Ferreira, J. C., Longo, J. M., Clímaco, E. C., Martinez, R., et al. (2011). Dissemination of bla_{KPC-2} by the spread of *Klebsiella pneumoniae* clonal complex 258 clones (ST258, ST11, ST437) and plasmids (IncFII, IncN, IncL/M) among Enterobacteriaceae species in Brazil. *Antimicrob. Agents Chemother.* 55, 3579–3583.

Antonopoulos, D. A., Huse, S. M., Morrison, H. G., Schmidt, T. M., Sogin, M. L., and Young, V. B. (2009). Reproducible community dynamics of the gastrointestinal microbiota following antibiotic perturbation. *Infect. Immun.* 77, 2367–2375.

Arumugam, M., Raes, J., Pelletier, E., Le Paslier, D., Yamada, T., Mende, D. R., et al. (2011). Enterotypes of the human gut microbiome. *Nature* 473, 174–180.

Aubert, D., Naas, T., Héritier, C., Poirel, L., and Nordmann, P. (2006). Functional characterization of IS1999, an IS4 family element involved in mobilization and expression of beta-lactam resistance genes. *J. Bacteriol.* 188, 6506–6514.

Aziz, R. K., Breitbart, M., and Edwards, R. A. (2010). Transposases are the most abundant, most ubiquitous genes in nature. *Nucleic Acids Res.* 38, 4207–4217.

Baharoglu, Z., and Mazel, D. (2011). *Vibrio cholerae* triggers SOS and mutagenesis in response to a wide range of antibiotics: a route towards multiresistance. *Antimicrob. Agents Chemother.* 55, 2438–2441.

Bailey, J. K., Pinyon, J. L., Anantham, S., and Hall, R. M. (2011). Distribution of the blaTEM gene and blaTEM-containing transposons in commensal *Escherichia coli. J. Antimicrob. Chemother.* 66, 745–751.

Balbus, J. M., Boxall, A. B. A., Fenske, R. A., McKone, T. E., and Zeise, L. (2013). Implications of global climate change for the assessment and management of human health risks of chemicals in the natural environment. *Environ. Toxicol. Chem.* 32, 62–78.

Balloux, F. (2010). "Demographic influences on bacterial population structure," in *Bacterial Population Genetics in Infectious Disease*, eds D. A. Robinson, D. Falush, and E. J. Feil (Hoboken: John Wiley & Sons, Inc.), 103–120.

Bapteste, E., Lopez, P., Bouchard, F., Baquero, F., McInerney, J. O., and Burian, R. M. (2012). Evolutionary analyses of non-genealogical bonds produced by introgressive descent. *Proc. Natl. Acad. Sci. U.S.A.* 109, 18266–18272.

Baquero, F. (2009). Environmental stress and evolvability in microbial systems. *Clin. Microbiol. Infect.* 15, 5–10.

Baquero, F. (2004). From pieces to patterns: evolutionary engineering in bacterial pathogens. *Nat. Rev. Microbiol.* 2, 510–518.

Baquero, F. (2012). On the shifting balance: the case of *Staphylococcus aureus* CC398. *MBio* 3, e00078–12.

Baquero, F. (2011). The 2010 Garrod Lecture: the dimensions of evolution in antibiotic resistance: ex unibus plurum et ex pluribus unum. *J. Antimicrob. Chemother.* 66, 1659–1672.

Baquero, F., and Coque, T. M. (2011). Multilevel population genetics in antibiotic resistance. *FEMS Microbiol. Rev.* 35, 705–706.

Baquero, F., Coque, T. M., and de la Cruz, F. (2011). Ecology and evolution as targets: the need for novel eco-evo drugs and strategies to fight antibiotic resistance. *Antimicrob. Agents Chemother.* 55, 3649–3660.

Baquero, F., Martínez, J.-L., and Cantón, R. (2008). Antibiotics and antibiotic resistance in water environments. *Curr. Opin. Biotechnol.* 19, 260–265.

Baquero, F., and Negri, M. C. (1997). Selective compartments for resistant microorganisms in antibiotic gradients. *Bioessays* 19, 731–736.

Baquero, F., and Nombela, C. (2012). The microbiome as a human organ. *Clin. Microbiol. Infect.* 18, 2–4.

Baquero, M.-R., Galán, J. C., Del Carmen Turrientes, M., Cantón, R., Coque, T. M., Martínez, J. L., et al. (2005). Increased mutation frequencies in *Escherichia coli* isolates harboring extended-spectrum beta-lactamases. *Antimicrob. Agents Chemother.* 49, 4754–4756.

Barlow, M., and Hall, B. G. (2002). Origin and evolution of the AmpC beta-lactamases of *Citrobacter freundii. Antimicrob. Agents Chemother.* 46, 1190–1198. .

Becker, J., Eisenhauer, N., Scheu, S., and Jousset, A. (2012). Increasing antagonistic interactions cause bacterial communities to collapse at high diversity. *Ecol. Lett.* 15, 468–474.

Benveniste, R., and Davies, J. (1973). Aminoglycoside antibiotic-inactivating enzymes in actinomycetes similar to those present in clinical isolates of antibiotic-resistant bacteria. *Proc. Natl. Acad. Sci. U.S.A.* 70, 2276–2280.

Bertels, F., and Rainey, P. B. (2011). Within-genome evolution of REPINs: a new family of miniature mobile DNA in bacteria. *PLoS Genet.* 7:e1002132. doi: 10.1371/journal.pgen.1002132

Biel, S. W., and Hartl, D. L. (1983). Evolution of transposons: natural selection for Tn5 in *Escherichia coli* K12. *Genetics* 103, 581–592.

Biermann, F., Abbott, K., Andresen, S., Bäckstrand, K., Bernstein, S., Betsill, M. M., et al. (2012). Science and government. Navigating the anthropocene: improving Earth system governance. *Science* 335, 1306–1307.

Bisercić, M., and Ochman, H. (1993). Natural populations of *Escherichia coli* and *Salmonella typhimurium* harbor the same classes of insertion sequences. *Genetics* 133, 449–454.

Blázquez, J., Couce, A., Rodríguez-Beltrán, J., and Rodríguez-Rojas, A. (2012). Antimicrobials as promoters of genetic variation. *Curr. Opin. Microbiol.* 15, 561–569.

Blot, M., Hauer, B., and Monnet, G. (1994). The Tn5 bleomycin resistance gene confers improved survival and growth advantage on *Escherichia coli. Mol. Gen. Genet.* 242, 595–601.

Bouma, J. E., and Lenski, R. E. (1988). Evolution of a bacteria/plasmid association. *Nature* 335, 351–352.

Boyd, E. F., Hill, C. W., Rich, S. M., and Hartl, D. L. (1996). Mosaic structure of plasmids from natural populations of *Escherichia coli. Genetics* 143, 1091–1100.

Boyd, E. S., and Barkay, T. (2012). The mercury resistance operon: from an origin in a geothermal environment to an efficient detoxification machine. *Front. Microbiol.* 3:349. doi: 10.3389/fmicb.2012.00349

Brandon, R. (1987). The levels of selection: a hierarchy of interactors," in *The Role of Behavior in Evolution*, ed. H. Plotkin (Cambridge: MIT Press), 124–146.

Brisse, S., Fevre, C., Passet, V., Issenhuth-Jeanjean, S., Tournebize, R., Diancourt, L., et al. (2009). Virulent clones of *Klebsiella pneumoniae*: identification and evolutionary scenario based on genomic and phenotypic characterization. *PloS ONE* 4:e4982. doi: 10.1371/journal.pone.0004982

Cain, A. K., Liu, X., Djordjevic, S. P., and Hall, R. M. (2010). Transposons related to Tn1696 in IncHI2 plasmids in multiply antibiotic resistant *Salmonella enterica* serovar Typhimurium from Australian animals. *Microb. Drug Resist.* 16, 197–202.

Cantón, R., and Coque, T. M. (2006). The CTX-M beta-lactamase pandemic. *Curr. Opin. Microbiol.* 9, 466–475.

Cantón, R., Mir, N., Sánchez, M., and Baquero, F. (1999). MIC distribution and inoculum effect of LY333328: a study of vancomycin-susceptible and VanA-type and VanC-type enterococci obtained from intensive care unit patient surveillance cultures. *Clin. Microbiol. Infect.* 5, 554–559.

Carattoli, A. (2009). Resistance plasmid families in Enterobacteriaceae. *Antimicrob. Agents Chemother.* 53, 2227–2238. .

Castillo, A., Eguiarte, L. E., and Souza, V. (2005). A genomic population genetics analysis of the pathogenic enterocyte effacement island in *Escherichia coli*: the search for the unit of selection. *Proc. Natl. Acad. Sci. U.S.A.* 102, 1542–1547.

Chambers, H. F., and Deleo, F. R. (2009). Waves of resistance: *Staphylococcus aureus* in the antibiotic era. *Nat. Rev. Microbiol.* 7, 629–641.

Chao, L., and Levin, B. R. (1981). Structured habitats and the evolution of anticompetitor toxins in bacteria. *Proc. Natl. Acad. Sci. U.S.A.* 78, 6324–6328.

Claesson, M. J., Cusack, S., O'Sullivan, O., Greene-Diniz, R., De Weerd, H., Flannery, E., et al. (2011). Composition, variability, and temporal stability of the intestinal microbiota of the elderly. *Proc. Natl. Acad. Sci.* U.S.A. 108, 4586–4591.

Claesson, M. J., Jeffery, I. B., Conde, S., Power, S. E., O'Connor, E. M., Cusack, S., et al. (2012). Gut microbiota composition correlates with diet and health in the elderly. *Nature* 488, 178–184.

Clewell, D. B., Weaver, K. E., Dunny, G. M., Coque, T. M., Francia, M. V., and Hayes, F. (2013). "Extrachromosomal and mobile elements," in *Enterococci. Transmission, Maintenance, and Epidemiology*, ed. M. S. Gilmore (in press).

Cohen, O., Ashkenazy, H., Burstein, D., and Pupko, T. (2012). Uncovering the co-evolutionary network among prokaryotic genes. *Bioinformatics* 28, i389–i394.

Comeau, A. M., Tétart, F., Trojet, S. N., Prère, M.-F., and Krisch, H. M. (2007). Phage-Antibiotic Synergy (PAS): beta-lactam and quinolone antibiotics stimulate virulent phage growth. *PloS ONE* 2:e799. doi: 10.1371/journal.pone.0000799

Coombs, J. M. (2009). Potential for horizontal gene transfer in microbial communities of the terrestrial subsurface. *Methods Mol. Biol.* 532, 413–433.

Coque, T. M., Baquero, F., and Canton, R. (2008). Increasing prevalence of ESBL-producing Enterobacteriaceae in Europe. *Euro Surveill.* 13, 19044.

Cordero, O. X., Wildschutte, H., Kirkup, B., Proehl, S., Ngo, L., Hussain, F., et al. (2012). Ecological populations of bacteria act as socially cohesive units of antibiotic production and resistance. *Science* 337, 1228–1231.

Couce, A., and Blázquez, J. (2009). Side effects of antibiotics on genetic variability. *FEMS Microbiol. Rev.* 33, 531–538.

Craig, N. L. (2002). "Tn7," in *Mobile DNA II*, eds. N. Craig, R. Craigie, M. Gellet, and A. M. Lambowitz (Washington: ASM Press), 432–456.

Czekalski, N., Berthold, T., Caucci, S., Egli, A., and Bürgmann, H. (2012). Increased levels of multiresistant bacteria and resistance genes after wastewater treatment and their dissemination into lake geneva, Switzerland. *Front. Microbiol.* 3:106. doi: 10.3389/fmicb.2012.00106

Czárán, T. L., Hoekstra, R. F., and Pagie, L. (2002). Chemical warfare between microbes promotes biodiversity. *Proc. Natl. Acad. Sci. U.S.A.* 99, 786–790.

Dantas, G., Sommer, M. O. A., Oluwasegun, R. D., and Church, G. M. (2008). Bacteria subsisting on antibiotics. *Science* 320, 100–103.

Datta, N., and Hughes, V. M. (1983). Plasmids of the same Inc groups in Enterobacteria before and after the medical use of antibiotics. *Nature* 306, 616–617.

Davies, J. (2006). Are antibiotics naturally antibiotics? *J. Ind. Microbiol. Biotechnol.* 33, 496–499.

Day, M. D., Beck, D., and Foster, J. A. (2011). Microbial communities as experimental units. *Bioscience* 61, 398–406.

D'Costa, V. M., King, C. E., Kalan, L., Morar, M., Sung, W. W. L., Schwarz, C., et al. (2011). Antibiotic resistance is ancient. *Nature* 477, 457–461.

De Gelder, L., Ponciano, J. M., Joyce, P., and Top, E. M. (2007). Stability of a promiscuous plasmid in different hosts: no guarantee for a long-term relationship. *Microbiology* 153, 452–463.

del Pilar Garcillán-Barcia, M., Bernales, I., Mendiola, M. V., and De la Cruz, F. (2001). Single-stranded DNA intermediates in IS91 rolling-circle transposition. *Mol. Microbiol.* 39, 494–501.

Del Solar, G., Alonso, J. C., Espinosa, M., and Díaz-Orejas, R. (1996). Broad-host-range plasmid replication: an open question. *Mol. Microbiol.* 21, 661–666.

de Regt, M. J. A., Van Schaik, W., Van Luit-Asbroek, M., Dekker, H. A. T., Van Duijkeren, E., Koning, C. J. M., et al. (2012). Hospital and community ampicillin-resistant *Enterococcus faecium* are evolutionarily closely linked but have diversified through niche adaptation. *PloS ONE* 7:e30319. doi: 10.1371/journal.pone.0030319

Dethlefsen, L., Eckburg, P. B., Bik, E. M., and Relman, D. A. (2006). Assembly of the human intestinal microbiota. *Trends Ecol. Evol.* 21, 517–523.

Dionisio, F., Conceição, I. C., Marques, A. C. R., Fernandes, L., and Gordo, I. (2005). The evolution of a conjugative plasmid and its ability to increase bacterial fitness. *Biol. Lett.* 1, 250–252.

Domingues, S., Harms, K., Fricke, W. F., Johnsen, P. J., Da Silva, G. J., and Nielsen, K. M. (2012). Natural transformation facilitates transfer of transposons, integrons and gene cassettes between bacterial species. *PLoS Pathog.* 8:e1002837. doi: 10.1371/journal.ppat.1002837

Doolittle, W. F., and Zhaxybayeva, O. (2010). Metagenomics and the units of biological organization. *BioScience* 60, 102–112.

Doyle, M., Fookes, M., Ivens, A., Mangan, M. W., Wain, J., and Dorman, C. J. (2007). An H-NS-like stealth protein aids horizontal DNA transmission in bacteria. *Science* 315, 251–252.

Dupré, J., and O'Malley, M. A. (2007). Metagenomics and biological ontology. *Stud. Hist. Philos. Biol. Biomed. Sci.* 38, 834–846.

Fajardo, A., and Martínez, J. L. (2008). Antibiotics as signals that trigger specific bacterial responses. *Curr. Opin. Microbiol.* 11, 161–167.

Fajardo, A., Martínez-Martín, N., Mercadillo, M., Galán, J. C., Ghysels, B., Matthijs, S., et al. (2008). The neglected intrinsic resistome of bacterial pathogens. *PloS ONE* 3:e1619. doi: 10.1371/journal.pone.0001619

Faust, K., and Raes, J. (2012). Microbial interactions: from networks to models. *Nat. Rev. Microbiol.* 10, 538–550.

Faust, K., Sathirapongsasuti, J. F., Izard, J., Segata, N., Gevers, D., Raes, J., et al. (2012). Microbial co-occurrence relationships in the human microbiome. *PLoS Comput. Biol.* 8:e1002606. doi: 10.1371/journal.pcbi.1002606

Fernández-Alarcón, C., Singer, R. S., and Johnson, T. J. (2011). Comparative genomics of multidrug resistance-encoding IncA/C plasmids from commensal and pathogenic *Escherichia coli* from multiple animal sources. *PloS One* 6:e23415. doi: 10.1371/journal.pone.0023415

Fondi, M., and Fani, R. (2010). The horizontal flow of the plasmid resistome: clues from inter-generic similarity networks. *Environ. Microbiol.* 12: 3228–3242.

Forsberg, K. J., Reyes, A., Wang, B., Selleck, E. M., Sommer, M. O. A., and Dantas, G. (2012). The shared antibiotic resistome of soil bacteria and human pathogens. *Science* 337, 1107–1111.

Fouhy, F., Guinane, C. M., Hussey, S., Wall, R., Ryan, C. A., Dempsey, E. M., et al. (2012). High-throughput sequencing reveals the incomplete, short-term recovery of infant gut microbiota following parenteral antibiotic treatment with ampicillin and gentamicin. *Antimicrob. Agents Chemother.* 56, 5811–5820.

Francino, M. P. (2012). The ecology of bacterial genes and the survival of the new. *Int. J. Evol. Biol.* 2012, 394026.

Freilich, S., Kreimer, A., Meilijson, I., Gophna, U., Sharan, R., and Ruppin, E. (2010). The large-scale organization of the bacterial network of ecological co-occurrence interactions. *Nucleic Acids Res.* 38, 3857–3868.

Freitas, A. R., Novais, C., Tedim, A. P., Francia, M. V., Baquero, F., and Coque, T. M. (2013). Microevolutionary events involving narrow host plasmid influences local fixation of vancomycin-resistance in *Enterococcus. PloS ONE* (in press).

Garcillán-Barcia, M. P., Alvarado, A., and De la Cruz, F. (2011). Identification of bacterial plasmids based on mobility and plasmid population biology. *FEMS Microbiol. Rev.* 35, 936–956.

Garcillán-Barcia, M. P., Francia, M. V., and De la Cruz, F. (2009). The diversity of conjugative relaxases and its application in plasmid classification. *FEMS Microbiol. Rev.* 33, 657–687.

Garcillán-Barcia, M. P., and de la Cruz, F. (2002). Distribution of IS91 family insertion sequences in bacterial genomes: evolutionary implications. *FEMS Microbiol. Ecol.* 42, 303–313.

García-Quintanilla, M., and Casadesús, J. (2011). Virulence plasmid interchange between strains ATCC 14028, LT2, and SL1344 of *Salmonella enterica* serovar Typhimurium. *Plasmid* 65, 169–175.

Gaze, W. H., Abdouslam, N., Hawkey, P. M., and Wellington, E. M. H. (2005). Incidence of class 1 integrons in a quaternary ammonium compound-polluted environment. *Antimicrob. Agents Chemother.* 49, 1802–1807.

Gaze, W. H., Zhang, L., Abdouslam, N. A., Hawkey, P. M., Calvo-Bado, L., Royle, J., et al. (2011). Impacts of anthropogenic activity on the ecology of class 1 integrons and integron-associated genes in the environment. *ISME J.* 5, 1253–1261.

Ghosh, A., Dowd, S. E., and Zurek, L. (2011). Dogs leaving the ICU carry a very large multi-drug resistant enterococcal population with capacity for biofilm formation and horizontal gene transfer. *PloS ONE* 6:e22451. doi: 10.1371/journal.pone.0022451

Gillings, M. R., and Stokes, H. W. (2012). Are humans increasing bacterial evolvability? *Trends Ecol. Evol.* 27, 346–352.

Gilliver, M. A., Bennett, M., Begon, M., Hazel, S. M., and Hart, C. A. (1999). Antibiotic resistance found in wild rodents. *Nature* 401, 233–234.

Goffin, C., and Ghuysen, J. M. (1998). Multimodular penicillin-binding proteins: an enigmatic family of orthologs and paralogs. *Microbiol. Mol. Biol. Rev.* 62, 1079–1093.

Goh, E.-B., Yim, G., Tsui, W., McClure, J., Surette, M. G., and Davies, J. (2002). Transcriptional modulation of bacterial gene expression by subinhibitory concentrations of antibiotics. *Proc. Natl. Acad. Sci. U.S.A.* 99, 17025–17030.

Graessler, J., Qin, Y., Zhong, H., Zhang, J., Licinio, J., Wong, M.-L., et al. (2012). Metagenomic sequencing of the human gut microbiome before and after bariatric surgery in obese patients with type 2 diabetes: correlation with inflammatory and metabolic parameters. *Pharmacogenomics J.* doi: 10.1038/tpj.2012.43 [Epub ahead of print].

Graidy, N. G. (2002). "The movement of Tn3-like elements. Transposase and cointegrate resolution," in *Mobile DNA II*, eds. N. L. Craig, R. Craigie, M. Gellet, and A. M. Lambowitz (Washington: ASM Press), 272–304.

Guerin, E., Cambray, G., Sanchez-Alberola, N., Campoy, S., Erill, I., Da Re, S., et al. (2009). The SOS response controls integron recombination. *Science* 324, 1034.

Guglielmini, J., De la Cruz, F., and Rocha, E. P. C. (2013). Evolution of conjugation and type IV secretion systems. *Mol. Biol. Evol.* 30, 315–331.

Guglielmini, J., Quintais, L., Garcillán-Barcia, M. P., De la Cruz, F., and Rocha, E. P. C. (2011). The repertoire of ICE in prokaryotes underscores the unity, diversity, and ubiquity of conjugation. *PLoS Genet.* 7:e1002222. doi: 10.1371/journal.pgen.1002222

Gullberg, E., Cao, S., Berg, O. G., Ilbäck, C., Sandegren, L., Hughes, D., et al. (2011). Selection of resistant bacteria at very low antibiotic concentrations. *PLoS Pathog.* 7:e1002158. doi:10.1371/journal.ppat.1002158

Halary, S., Leigh, J. W., Cheaib, B., Lopez, P., and Bapteste, E. (2010). Network analyses structure genetic diversity in independent genetic worlds. *Proc. Natl. Acad. Sci. U.S.A.* 107, 127–132.

Hallatschek, O. (2012). Bacteria evolve to go against the grain. *Physics* 5, 93.

Halling-Sørensen, B., Nors Nielsen, S., Lanzky, P. F., Ingerslev, F., Holten Lützhøft, H. C., and Jørgensen, S. E. (1998). Occurrence, fate and effects of pharmaceutical substances in the environment–a review. *Chemosphere* 36, 357–393.

Hamprecht, A., Poirel, L., Göttig, S., Seifert, H., Kaase, M., and Nordmann, P. (2012). Detection of the carbapenemase GIM-1 in *Enterobacter cloacae* in Germany. *J. Antimicrob. Chemother.* doi: 10.1093/jac/dks447 [Epub ahead of print].

Hartl, D. L., Dykhuizen, D. E., Miller, R. D., Green, L., and De Framond, J. (1983). Transposable element IS*50* improves growth rate of *E. coli* cells without transposition. *Cell* 35, 503–510.

Henderson-Begg, S. K., Livermore, D. M., and Hall, L. M. C. (2006). Effect of subinhibitory concentrations of antibiotics on mutation frequency in *Streptococcus pneumoniae*. *J. Antimicrob. Chemother.* 57, 849–854.

Hermsen, R., Deris, J. B., and Hwa, T. (2012). On the rapidity of antibiotic resistance evolution facilitated by a concentration gradient. *Proc. Natl. Acad. Sci. U.S.A.* 109, 10775–10780.

Heuer, H., Binh, C. T. T., Jechalke, S., Kopmann, C., Zimmerling, U., Krögerrecklenfort, E., et al. (2012). IncP-1ε plasmids are important vectors of antibiotic resistance genes in agricultural systems: diversification driven by class 1 integron gene cassettes. *Front. Microbiol.* 3:2. doi: 10.3389/fmicb.2012.00002

Heuer, H., and Smalla, K. (2012). Plasmids foster diversification and adaptation of bacterial populations in soil. *FEMS Microbiol. Rev.* 36, 1083–1104.

Hickman, A. B., Chandler, M., and Dyda, F. (2010). Integrating prokaryotes and eukaryotes: DNA transposases in light of structure. *Crit. Rev. Biochem. Mol. Biol.* 45, 50–69.

Hidron, A. I., Edwards, J. R., Patel, J., Horan, T. C., Sievert, D. M., Pollock, D. A., et al. (2008). NHSN annual update: antimicrobial-resistant pathogens associated with healthcare-associated infections: annual summary of data reported to the National Healthcare Safety Network at the Centers for Disease Control and Prevention, 2006-2007. *Infect. Control Hosp. Epidemiol.* 29, 996–1011.

Hildebrandt, M. A., Hoffmann, C., Sherrill-Mix, S. A., Keilbaugh, S. A., Hamady, M., Chen, Y.-Y., et al. (2009). High-fat diet determines the composition of the murine gut microbiome independently of obesity. *Gastroenterology* 137, 1716–1724.

Hocquet, D., Llanes, C., Thouverez, M., Kulasekara, H. D., Bertrand, X., Plésiat, P., et al. (2012). Evidence for induction of integron-based antibiotic resistance by the SOS response in a clinical setting. *PLoS Pathog.* 8:e1002778. doi: 10.1371/journal.ppat.1002778

Hughes, J. M., Lohman, B. K., Deckert, G. E., Nichols, E. P., Settles, M., Abdo, Z., et al. (2012). The role of clonal interference in the evolutionary dynamics of plasmid-host adaptation. *MBio* 3, e00077-12.

Hughes, V. M., and Datta, N. (1983). Conjugative plasmids in bacteria of the "pre-antibiotic" era. *Nature* 302, 725–726.

Humphrey, B., Thomson, N. R., Thomas, C. M., Brooks, K., Sanders, M., Delsol, A. A., et al. (2012). Fitness of *Escherichia coli* strains carrying expressed and partially silent IncN and IncP1 plasmids. *BMC Microbiol.* 12:53. doi: 10.1186/1471-2180-12-53

Jeffery, I. B., Claesson, M. J., O'Toole, P. W., and Shanahan, F. (2012). Categorization of the gut microbiota: enterotypes or gradients? *Nat. Rev. Microbiol.* 10, 591–592.

Jones, B. V. (2010). The human gut mobile metagenome: a metazoan perspective. *Gut Microbes* 1, 415–431.

Kholodii, G., Mindlin, S., Petrova, M., and Minakhina, S. (2003). Tn*5060* from the Siberian permafrost is most closely related to the ancestor of Tn*21* prior to integron acquisition. *FEMS Microbiol. Lett.* 226, 251–255.

Kohanski, M. A., DePristo, M. A., and Collins, J. J. (2010). Sublethal antibiotic treatment leads to multidrug resistance via radical-induced mutagenesis. *Mol. Cell* 37, 311–320.

Kondrashov, F. A., Rogozin, I. B., Wolf, Y. I., and Koonin, E. V. (2002). Selection in the evolution of gene duplications. *Genome Biol.* 3, research0008.1–research0008.9.

Ktari, S., Arlet, G., Mnif, B., Gautier, V., Mahjoubi, F., Ben Jmeaa, M., et al. (2006). Emergence of multidrug-resistant *Klebsiella pneumoniae* isolates producing VIM-4 metallo-beta-lactamase, CTX-M-15 extended-spectrum beta-lactamase, and CMY-4 AmpC beta-lactamase in a Tunisian university hospital. *Antimicrob. Agents Chemother.* 50, 4198–4201.

Kylafis, G., and Loreau, M. (2011). Niche construction in the light of niche theory. *Ecol. Lett.* 14, 82–90.

Labbate, M., Case, R. J., and Stokes, H. W. (2009). The integron/gene cassette system: an active player in bacterial adaptation. *Methods Mol. Biol.* 532, 103–125.

Laland, K. N., Odling-Smee, F. J., and Feldman, M. W. (1999). Evolutionary consequences of niche construction and their implications for ecology. *Proc. Natl. Acad. Sci. U.S.A.* 96, 10242–10247.

Lang, K. S., Danzeisen, J. L., Xu, W., and Johnson, T. J. (2012). Transcriptome mapping of pAR060302, a blaCMY-2-positive broad-host-range IncA/C plasmid. *Appl. Environ. Microbiol.* 78, 3379–3386.

Lawrence, J. G. (1997). Selfish operons and speciation by gene transfer. *Trends Microbiol.* 5, 355–359.

Levin, B. R. (2010). Nasty viruses, costly plasmids, population dynamics, and the conditions for establishing and maintaining CRISPR-mediated adaptive immunity in bacteria. *PLoS Genet.* 6:e1001171. doi: 10.1371/journal.pgen.1001171

Lewontin, R. C. (1970). The units of selection. *Annu. Rev. Ecol. Syst.* 1, 1–18.

Ley, R. E., Turnbaugh, P. J., Klein, S., and Gordon, J. I. (2006). Microbial ecology: human gut microbes associated with obesity. *Nature* 444, 1022–1023.

Li, J. V., Ashrafian, H., Bueter, M., Kinross, J., Sands, C., Le Roux, C. W., et al. (2011). Metabolic surgery profoundly influences gut microbial-host metabolic cross-talk. *Gut* 60, 1214–1223.

Liebert, C. A., Hall, R. M., and Summers, A. O. (1999). Transposon Tn*21*, flagship of the floating genome. *Microbiol. Mol. Biol. Rev.* 63, 507–522.

Lim, J. Y., Yoon, J., and Hovde, C. J. (2010). A brief overview of *Escherichia coli* O157:H7 and its plasmid O157. *J. Microbiol. Biotechnol.* 20, 5–14.

Linares, J. F., Gustafsson, I., Baquero, F., and Martinez, J. L. (2006). Antibiotics as intermicrobial signaling agents instead of weapons. *Proc. Natl. Acad. Sci. U.S.A.* 103, 19484–19489.

Livermore, D. M. (2000). Antibiotic resistance in staphylococci. *Int. J. Antimicrob. Agents* 16, S3–S10.

Lloyd, E. (2008). "Units and levels of selection," in *The Stanford Encyclopedia of Philosophy*, ed. E. N. Zalta.

Looft, T., and Allen, H. K. (2012). Collateral effects of antibiotics on mammalian gut microbiomes. *Gut Microbes* 3, 463–467.

Looft, T., Johnson, T. A., Allen, H. K., Bayles, D. O., Alt, D. P., Stedtfeld, R. D., et al. (2012). In-feed antibiotic effects on the swine intestinal microbiome. *Proc. Natl. Acad. Sci. U.S.A.* 109, 1691–1696.

Luo, C., Walk, S. T., Gordon, D. M., Feldgarden, M., Tiedje, J. M., and Konstantinidis, K. T. (2011). Genome sequencing of environmental *Escherichia coli* expands understanding of the ecology and speciation of the model bacterial species. *Proc. Natl. Acad. Sci. U.S.A.* 108, 7200–7205.

Lupo, A., Coyne, S., and Berendonk, T. U. (2012). Origin and evolution of antibiotic resistance: the common mechanisms of emergence and spread in water bodies. *Front. Microbiol.* 3:18. doi: 10.3389/fmicb.2012.00018

Maiden, M. C. (1998). Horizontal genetic exchange, evolution, and spread of antibiotic resistance in bacteria. *Clin. Infect. Dis.* 27, S12–S20.

Marchesi, J. R. (2010). Prokaryotic and eukaryotic diversity of the human gut. *Adv. Appl. Microbiol.* 72, 43–62.

Marchesi, J. R. (2011). Shifting from a gene-centric to metabolite-centric strategy to determine the core gut microbiome. *Bioeng. Bugs* 2, 309–314.

Marraffini, L. A., and Sontheimer, E. J. (2010). CRISPR interference: RNA-directed adaptive immunity in bacteria and archaea. *Nat. Rev. Genet.* 11, 181–190.

Martinez, E., Marquez, C., Ingold, A., Merlino, J., Djordjevic, S. P., Stokes, H. W., et al. (2012). Diverse mobilized class 1 integrons are common in the chromosomes of pathogenic *Pseudomonas aeruginosa* clinical isolates. *Antimicrob. Agents Chemother.* 56, 2169–2172.

Martinez, J. L., Fajardo, A., Garmendia, L., Hernandez, A., Linares, J. F., Martínez-Solano, L., et al. (2009). A global view of antibiotic resistance. *FEMS Microbiol. Rev.* 33, 44–65.

Martínez, J. L. (2008). Antibiotics and antibiotic resistance genes in natural environments. *Science* 321, 365–367.

Martínez, J. L. (2011). Bottlenecks in the transferability of antibiotic resistance from natural ecosystems to human bacterial pathogens. *Front. Microbiol.* 2:265. doi: 10.3389/fmicb.2011.00265

Martínez, J. L., Baquero, F., and Andersson, D. I. (2007). Predicting antibiotic resistance. *Nat. Rev. Microbiol.* 5, 958–965.

Martínez, J. L., and Rojo, F. (2011). Metabolic regulation of antibiotic resistance. *FEMS Microbiol. Rev.* 35, 768–789.

Mayr, E. (1997). The objects of selection. *Proc. Natl. Acad. Sci. U.S.A.* 94, 2091–2094.

Mazel, D. (2006). Integrons: agents of bacterial evolution. *Nat. Rev. Microbiol.* 4, 608–620.

McBride, S. M., Fischetti, V. A., Leblanc, D. J., Moellering, R. C., and Gilmore, M. S. (2007). Genetic diversity among *Enterococcus faecalis*. *PloS ONE* 2:e582. doi: 10.1371/journal.pone.0000582

Merlin, C., Mahillon, J., Nesvera, J., and Toussaint, A. (2000). "Gene recruiters and transporters: the modular structure of bacterial mobile elements," in *The Horizontal Gene Pool. Bacterial Plasmids and Gene Spread*, ed. C. M. Thomas (Harwood Academic Press), 363–409.

Mindlin, S., Minakhin, L., Petrova, M., Kholodii, G., Minakhina, S., Gorlenko, Z., et al. (2005). Present-day mercury resistance transposons are common in bacteria preserved in permafrost grounds since the Upper Pleistocene. *Res. Microbiol.* 156, 994–1004.

Mindlin, S. Z., Soina, V. S., Petrova, M. A., and Gorlenko, Z. M. (2008). Isolation of antibiotic resistance bacterial strains from Eastern Siberia permafrost sediments. *Russ. J. Genet.* 44, 27–34.

Mizrahi, I. (2012). The rumen plasmidome: a genetic communication hub for the rumen microbiome. *Mob. Genet. Elements* 2, 152–153.

Monira, S., Nakamura, S., Gotoh, K., Izutsu, K., Watanabe, H., Alam, N. H., et al. (2011). Gut microbiota of healthy and malnourished children in bangladesh. *Front. Microbiol.* 2:228. doi: 10.3389/fmicb.2011.00228

Moura, A., Pereira, C., Henriques, I., and Correia, A. (2012). Novel gene cassettes and integrons in antibiotic-resistant bacteria isolated from urban wastewaters. *Res. Microbiol.* 163, 92–100.

Naas, T., Cuzon, G., Villegas, M.-V., Lartigue, M.-F., Quinn, J. P., and Nordmann, P. (2008). Genetic structures at the origin of acquisition of the beta-lactamase bla KPC gene. *Antimicrob. Agents Chemother.* 52, 1257–1263.

Negri, M.-C., Lipsitch, M., Blazquez, J., Levin, B. R., and Baquero, F. (2000). Concentration-dependent selection of small phenotypic differences in TEM beta-lactamase-mediated antibiotic resistance. *Antimicrob. Agents Chemother.* 44, 2485–2491.

Nogueira, T., Rankin, D. J., Touchon, M., Taddei, F., Brown, S. P., and Rocha, E. P. C. (2009). Horizontal gene transfer of the secretome drives the evolution of bacterial cooperation and virulence. *Curr. Biol.* 19, 1683–1691.

Norberg, P., Bergström, M., Jethava, V., Dubhashi, D., and Hermansson, M. (2011). The IncP-1 plasmid backbone adapts to different host bacterial species and evolves through homologous recombination. *Nat. Commun.* 2, 268.

Norman, A., Hansen, L. H., and Sørensen, S. J. (2009). Conjugative plasmids: vessels of the communal gene pool. *Philos. Trans. R. Soc. Lond. B Biol. Sci.* 364, 2275–2289.

Novais, A., Baquero, F., Machado, E., Cantón, R., Peixe, L., and Coque, T. M. (2010a). International spread and persistence of TEM-24 is caused by the confluence of highly penetrating enterobacteriaceae clones and an IncA/C2 plasmid containing Tn1696::Tn1 and IS5075-Tn21. *Antimicrob. Agents Chemother.* 54, 825–834.

Novais, A., Comas, I., Baquero, F., Cantón, R., Coque, T. M., Moya, A., et al. (2010b). Evolutionary trajectories of beta-lactamase CTX-M-1 cluster enzymes: predicting antibiotic resistance. *PLoS Pathog.* 6:e1000735. doi: 10.1371/journal.ppat.1000735

Novais, A., Pires, J., Ferreira, H., Costa, L., Montenegro, C., Vuotto, C., et al. (2012a). Characterization of globally spread *Escherichia coli* ST131 isolates (1991 to 2010). *Antimicrob. Agents Chemother.* 56, 3973–3976.

Novais, C., Freitas, A. R., Silveira, E., Baquero, F., Peixe, L., Roberts, A. P., et al. (2012b). A tet(S/M) hybrid from CTn6000 and CTn916 recombination. *Microbiology* 158, 2710–2711.

Novais, A., Vuotto, C., Pires, J., Montenegro, C., Donelli, G., Coque, T. M., et al. (2013). Diversity and biofilm-production ability among isolates of epidemic clonal groups (ST69, ST393 and ST405) of *Escherichia coli* phylogroup D. *Antimicrob. Agents Chemother.* (in press).

Näsvall, J., Sun, L., Roth, J. R., and Andersson, D. I. (2012). Real-time evolution of new genes by innovation, amplification, and divergence. *Science* 338, 384–387.

Okasha, S. (2004). Multilevel selection and the partitioning of covariance: a comparison of three approaches. *Evolution* 58, 486–494.

Osterblad, M., Norrdahl, K., Korpimäki, E., and Huovinen, P. (2001). Antibiotic resistance. How wild are wild mammals? *Nature* 409, 37–38.

Parks, A. R., Li, Z., Shi, Q., Owens, R. M., Jin, M. M., and Peters, J. E. (2009). Transposition into replicating DNA occurs through interaction with the processivity factor. *Cell* 138, 685–695.

Parks, A. R., and Peters, J. E. (2009). Tn7 elements: engendering diversity from chromosomes to episomes. *Plasmid* 61, 1–14.

Partridge, S. R. (2011). Analysis of antibiotic resistance regions in Gram-negative bacteria. *FEMS Microbiol. Rev.* 35, 820–855.

Partridge, S. R., and Hall, R. M. (2004). Complex multiple antibiotic and mercury resistance region derived from the r-det of NR1 (R100). *Antimicrob. Agents Chemother.* 48, 4250–4255.

Partridge, S. R., and Hall, R. M. (2003). The IS*1111* family members IS*4321* and IS*5075* have subterminal inverted repeats and target the terminal inverted repeats of Tn*21* family transposons. *J. Bacteriol.* 185, 6371–6384.

Partridge, S. R., and Iredell, J. R. (2012). Genetic Contexts of blaNDM-1. *Antimicrob. Agents Chemother.* 56, 6065–6067.

Pedró, L., Baños, R. C., Aznar, S., Madrid, C., Balsalobre, C., and Juárez, A. (2011). Antibiotics shaping bacterial genome: deletion of an IS91 flanked virulence determinant upon exposure to subinhibitory antibiotic concentrations. *PloS ONE* 6:e27606. doi: 10.1371/journal.pone.0027606

Perron, G. G., Gonzalez, A., and Buckling, A. (2007). Source-sink dynamics shape the evolution of antibiotic resistance and its pleiotropic fitness cost. *Proc. Biol. Sci.* 274, 2351–2356.

Petrova, M., Gorlenko, Z., and Mindlin, S. (2009). Molecular structure and translocation of a multiple antibiotic resistance region of a Psychrobacter psychrophilus permafrost strain. *FEMS Microbiol. Lett.* 296, 190–197.

Petrova, M., Gorlenko, Z., and Mindlin, S. (2011). Tn5045, a novel integron-containing antibiotic and chromate resistance transposon isolated from a permafrost bacterium. *Res. Microbiol.* 162, 337–345.

Poirel, L., Bonnin, R. A., and Nordmann, P. (2012). Genetic support and diversity of acquired extended-spectrum β-lactamases in Gram-negative rods. *Infect. Genet. Evol.* 12, 883–893.

Poirel, L., Rodríguez-Martínez, J.-M., Al Naiemi, N., Debets-Ossenkopp, Y. J., and Nordmann, P. (2010). Characterization of DIM-1, an integron-encoded metallo-beta-lactamase from a *Pseudomonas stutzeri* clinical isolate in the Netherlands. *Antimicrob. Agents Chemother.* 54, 2420–2424.

Pomiankowski, A. (1999). "Intragenomic conflict," in *Levels of Selection in Evolution*, ed. L. Keller (Princeton University Press), 121–152.

Popa, O., Hazkani-Covo, E., Landan, G., Martin, W., and Dagan, T. (2011). Directed networks reveal genomic barriers and DNA repair bypasses to lateral gene transfer among prokaryotes. *Genome Res.* 21, 599–609.

Post, V., and Hall, R. M. (2009). Insertion sequences in the IS*1111* family that target the *attC* recombination sites of integron-associated gene cassettes. *FEMS Microbiol. Lett.* 290, 182–187.

Potron, A., Nordmann, P., Rondinaud, E., Jaureguy, F., and Poirel, L. (2013). A mosaic transposon encoding OXA-48 and CTX-M-15: towards pan-resistance. *J. Antimicrob. Chemother.* 68, 476–477.

Qu, Y., and Spain, J. C. (2011). Catabolic pathway for 2-nitroimidazole involves a novel nitrohydrolase that also confers drug resistance. *Environ. Microbiol.* 13, 1010–1017.

Quinteira, S., Novais, C., Antunes, P., Campos, J., Freitas, A. R., Abdukadir, A., et al. (2011). Tracking antibiotic resistance along the Silk Road. *Clin. Microbiol. Infect.* 17, s58–s59.

Rankin, D. J., Ginty, S. E. M., Nogueira, T., Touchon, M., Taddei, F., Rocha, E. P. C., et al. (2011a). Bacterial cooperation controlled by mobile elements: kin selection and infectivity are part of the same process. *Heredity* 107, 279–281.

Rankin, D. J., Rocha, E. P. C., and Brown, S. P. (2011b). What traits are carried on mobile genetic elements, and why? *Heredity* 106, 1–10.

Rankin, D. J., Turner, L. A., Heinemann, J. A., and Brown, S. P. (2012). The coevolution of toxin and antitoxin genes drives the dynamics of bacterial addiction complexes and intragenomic conflict. *Proc. Biol. Sci.* 279, 3706–3715.

Revilla, C., Garcillán-Barcia, M. P., Fernández-López, R., Thomson, N. R., Sanders, M., Cheung, M., et al. (2008). Different pathways to acquiring resistance genes illustrated by the recent evolution of IncW plasmids. *Antimicrob. Agents Chemother.* 52, 1472–1480.

Rodriguez-Valera, F., and Ussery, D. W. (2012). Is the pan-genome also a pan-selectome? *F1000 Res.* 1:16.

San Millán, A., Heilbron, K., and MacLean, R. C. (2012). Positive epistasis between co-infecting plasmids promotes plasmid stability and maintenance of multidrug resistance. in IPBC (Santander).

Santacruz, A., Collado, M. C., García-Valdés, L., Segura, M. T., Martín-Lagos, J. A., Anjos, T., et al. (2010). Gut microbiota composition is associated with body weight, weight gain and biochemical parameters in pregnant women. *Br. J. Nutr.* 104, 83–92.

Schlüter, A., Szczepanowski, R., Pühler, A., and Top, E. M. (2007). Genomics of IncP-1 antibiotic resistance plasmids isolated from wastewater treatment plants provides evidence for a widely accessible drug resistance gene pool. *FEMS Microbiol. Rev.* 31, 449–477.

Sen, D., Van der Auwera, G. A., Rogers, L. M., Thomas, C. M., Brown, C. J., and Top, E. M. (2011). Broad-host-range plasmids from agricultural soils have IncP-1 backbones with diverse accessory genes. *Appl. Environ. Microbiol.* 77, 7975–7983.

Seputiene, V., Povilonis, J., and Suziedeliene, E. (2012). Novel variants of AbaR resistance islands with a common backbone in *Acinetobacter baumannii* isolates of European clone II. *Antimicrob. Agents Chemother.* 56, 1969–1973.

Shearer, J. E. S., Wireman, J., Hostetler, J., Forberger, H., Borman, J., Gill, J., et al. (2011). Major families of multiresistant plasmids from geographically and epidemiologically diverse *staphylococci. G3* 1, 581–591.

Shi, P., Jia, S., Zhang, X.-X., Zhang, T., Cheng, S., and Li, A. (2013). Metagenomic insights into chlorination effects on microbial antibiotic resistance in drinking water. *Water Res.* 47, 111–120.

Silva, R. F., Mendonça, S. C. M., Carvalho, L. M., Reis, A. M., Gordo, I., Trindade, S., et al. (2011). Pervasive sign epistasis between conjugative plasmids and drug-resistance chromosomal mutations. *PLoS Genet.* 7:e1002181. doi: 10.1371/journal.pgen.1002181

Sjölund, M., Bonnedahl, J., Hernandez, J., Bengtsson, S., Cederbrant, G., Pinhassi, J., et al. (2008). Dissemination of multidrug-resistant bacteria into the Arctic. *Emerg. Infect. Dis.* 14, 70–72.

Skippington, E., and Ragan, M. A. (2011). Lateral genetic transfer and the construction of genetic exchange communities. *FEMS Microbiol. Rev.* 35, 707–735.

Skippington, E., and Ragan, M. A. (2012). Phylogeny rather than ecology or lifestyle biases the construction of *Escherichia coli-Shigella* genetic exchange communities. *Open Biol.* 2, 120112.

Smillie, C. S., Smith, M. B., Friedman, J., Cordero, O. X., David, L. A., and Alm, E. J. (2011). Ecology drives a global network of gene exchange connecting the human microbiome. *Nature* 480, 241–244.

Smith, J. (2012). Tragedy of the commons among antibiotic resistance plasmids. *Evolution* 66, 1269–1274.

Smorawinska, M., Szuplewska, M., Zaleski, P., Wawrzyniak, P., Maj, A., Plucienniczak, A., et al. (2012). Mobilizable narrow host range plasmids as natural suicide vectors enabling horizontal gene transfer among distantly related bacterial species. *FEMS Microbiol. Lett.* 326, 76–82.

Sobecky, P. A., and Hazen, T. H. (2009). Horizontal gene transfer and mobile genetic elements in marine systems. *Methods Mol. Biol.* 532, 435–453.

Sommer, M. O. A., Dantas, G., and Church, G. M. (2009). Functional characterization of the antibiotic resistance reservoir in the human microflora. *Science* 325, 1128–1131.

Stalder, T., Barraud, O., Casellas, M., Dagot, C., and Ploy, M.-C. (2012). Integron involvement in environmental spread of antibiotic resistance. *Front. Microbiol.* 3:119. doi: 10.3389/fmicb.2012.00119

Stokes, H. W., and Gillings, M. R. (2011). Gene flow, mobile genetic elements and the recruitment of antibiotic resistance genes into Gram-negative pathogens. *FEMS Microbiol. Rev.* 35, 790–819.

Stokes, H. W., Martinez, E., Roy Chowdhury, P., and Djordjevic, S. (2012). Class 1 integron-associated spread of resistance regions in *Pseudomonas aeruginosa*: plasmid or chromosomal platforms? *J. Antimicrob. Chemother.* 67, 1799–1800.

Suzuki, H., Yano, H., Brown, C. J., and Top, E. M. (2010). Predicting plasmid promiscuity based on genomic signature. *J. Bacteriol.* 192, 6045–6055.

Sánchez, M. B., and Martínez, J. L. (2012). Differential epigenetic compatibility of qnr antibiotic resistance determinants with the chromosome of *Escherichia coli. PloS ONE* 7:e35149. doi: 10.1371/journal.pone.0035149

Tagliabue, A., and Elli, M. (2012). The role of gut microbiota in human obesity: Recent findings and future perspectives. *Nutr. Metab. Cardiovasc. Dis.* (in press).

Tamames, J., Abellán, J. J., Pignatelli, M., Camacho, A., and Moya, A. (2010). Environmental distribution of prokaryotic taxa. *BMC Microbiol.* 10:85. doi: 10.1186/1471-2180-10-85

Tamminen, M., Virta, M., Fani, R., and Fondi, M. (2012). Large-scale analysis of plasmid relationships through gene-sharing networks. *Mol. Biol. Evol.* 29, 1225–1240.

Tato, M., Coque, T. M., Baquero, F., and Cantón, R. (2010). Dispersal of carbapenemase *bla*$_{VIM-1}$ gene associated with different Tn*402* variants, mercury transposons, and conjugative plasmids in Enterobacteriaceae and *Pseudomonas aeruginosa. Antimicrob. Agents Chemother.* 54, 320–327.

Tetu, S. G., and Holmes, A. J. (2008). A family of insertion sequences that impacts integrons by specific targeting of gene cassette recombination sites, the IS*1111-attC* Group. *J. Bacteriol.* 190, 4959–4970.

Toleman, M. A., Bennett, P. M., and Walsh, T. R. (2006). ISCR elements: novel gene-capturing systems of the 21st century? *Microbiol. Mol. Biol. Rev.* 70, 296–316.

Toleman, M. A., and Walsh, T. R. (2011). Combinatorial events of insertion sequences and ICE in Gram-negative bacteria. *FEMS Microbiol. Rev.* 35, 912–935.

Tolmasky, M. E. (1990). Sequencing and expression of aadA, bla, and tnpR from the multiresistance transposon Tn1331. *Plasmid* 24, 218–226.

Ubeda, C., Maiques, E., Knecht, E., Lasa, I., Novick, R. P., and Penadés, J. R. (2005). Antibiotic-induced SOS response promotes horizontal dissemination of pathogenicity island-encoded virulence factors in staphylococci. *Mol. Microbiol.* 56, 836–844.

Vallès, Y., Gosalbes, M. J., De Vries, L. E., Abellán, J. J., and Francino, M. P. (2012). Metagenomics and development of the gut microbiota in infants. *Clin. Microbiol. Infect.* 18, 21–26.

Valverde, A., Cantón, R., Garcillán-Barcia, M. P., Novais, A., Galán, J. C., Alvarado, A., et al. (2009). Spread of bla(CTX-M-14) is driven mainly by IncK plasmids disseminated among *Escherichia coli* phylogroups A, B1, and D in Spain. *Antimicrob. Agents Chemother.* 53, 5204–5212.

Via, S. (2012). Divergence hitchhiking and the spread of genomic isolation during ecological speciation-with-gene-flow. *Philos. Trans. R. Soc. Lond. B Biol. Sci.* 367, 451–460.

Vishnivetskaya, T. A., and Kathariou, S. (2005). Putative transposases conserved in Exiguobacterium isolates from ancient Siberian permafrost and from contemporary surface habitats. *Appl. Environ. Microbiol.* 71, 6954–6962.

Waksman, S. A. (1961). "The role of antibiotics in nature," in *Perspectives in Biology and Medicine*, Vol. 4 (Chicago: University of Chicago Press), 271–287.

Walsh, T. R. (2006). Combinatorial genetic evolution of multiresistance. *Curr. Opin. Microbiol.* 9, 476–482.

Werren, J. H. (2011). Selfish genetic elements, genetic conflict, and evolutionary innovation. *Proc. Natl. Acad. Sci. U.S.A.* 108, 10863–10870.

Wiedenbeck, J., and Cohan, F. M. (2011). Origins of bacterial diversity through horizontal genetic transfer and adaptation to new ecological niches. *FEMS Microbiol. Rev.* 35, 957–976.

Willems, R. J. L., Hanage, W. P., Bessen, D. E., and Feil, E. J. (2011). Population biology of Gram-positive pathogens: high-risk clones for dissemination of antibiotic resistance. *FEMS Microbiol. Rev.* 35, 872–900.

Willems, R. J. L., Top, J., Van Schaik, W., Leavis, H., Bonten, M., Sirén, J., et al. (2012). Restricted gene flow among hospital subpopulations of *Enterococcus faecium*. *MBio* 3, e00151-12.

Williams, L. E., Wireman, J., Hilliard, V. C., and Summers, A. O. (2012). Large plasmids of *Escherichia coli* and *Salmonella* encode highly diverse arrays of accessory genes on common replicon families. *Plasmid* 69, 36–48.

Woodford, N., Turton, J. F., and Livermore, D. M. (2011). Multiresistant Gram-negative bacteria: the role of high-risk clones in the dissemination of antibiotic resistance. *FEMS Microbiol. Rev.* 35, 736–755.

Wozniak, R. A. F., and Waldor, M. K. (2010). Integrative and conjugative elements: mosaic mobile genetic elements enabling dynamic lateral gene flow. *Nat. Rev. Microbiol.* 8, 552–563.

Wright, M. S., Baker-Austin, C., Lindell, A. H., Stepanauskas, R., Stokes, H. W., and McArthur, J. V. (2008). Influence of industrial contamination on mobile genetic elements: class 1 integron abundance and gene cassette structure in aquatic bacterial communities. *ISME J.* 2, 417–428.

Yim, G., Wang, H. H., and Davies, J. (2007). Antibiotics as signalling molecules. *Philos. Trans. R. Soc. Lond. B. Biol. Sci.* 362, 1195–1200.

Yun, C.-S., Suzuki, C., Naito, K., Takeda, T., Takahashi, Y., Sai, F., et al. (2010). Pmr, a histone-like protein H1 (H-NS) family protein encoded by the IncP-7 plasmid pCAR1, is a key global regulator that alters host function. *J. Bacteriol.* 192, 4720–4731.

Zalasiewicz, J., Williams, M., Haywood, A., and Ellis, M. (2011). The Anthropocene: a new epoch of geological time? *Philos. Transact. A Math. Phys. Eng. Sci.* 369, 835–841.

Zhang, Q., Lambert, G., Liao, D., Kim, H., Robin, K., Tung, C., et al. (2011). Acceleration of emergence of bacterial antibiotic resistance in connected microenvironments. *Science* 333, 1764–1767.

Zheng, Y., Anton, B. P., Roberts, R. J., and Kasif, S. (2005). Phylogenetic detection of conserved gene clusters in microbial genomes. *BMC Bioinformatics* 6:243. doi:10.1186/1471-2105-6-243

Zheng, Y., Roberts, R. J., and Kasif, S. (2004). Segmentally variable genes: a new perspective on adaptation. *PLoS Biol.* 2:E81. doi: 10.1371/journal.pbio.0020081

Zhong, X., Droesch, J., Fox, R., Top, E. M., and Krone, S. M. (2012). On the meaning and estimation of plasmid transfer rates for surface-associated and well-mixed bacterial populations. *J. Theor. Biol.* 294, 144–152.

Zhong, X., Krol, J. E., Top, E. M., and Krone, S. M. (2010). Accounting for mating pair formation in plasmid population dynamics. *J. Theor. Biol.* 262, 711–719.

6

Design of a large-scale femtoliter droplet array for single-cell analysis of drug-tolerant and drug-resistant bacteria

Ryota Iino[1,2]*, Yoshimi Matsumoto[3], Kunihiko Nishino[3], Akihito Yamaguchi[4,5] and Hiroyuki Noji[1,2]

[1] *Department of Applied Chemistry, Graduate School of Engineering, The University of Tokyo, Tokyo, Japan*
[2] *Core Research for Evolutional Science and Technology, Japan Science and Technology Agency, Tokyo, Japan*
[3] *Laboratory of Microbiology and Infectious Diseases, Institute of Scientific and Industrial Research, Osaka University, Osaka, Japan*
[4] *Department of Cell Membrane Biology, Institute of Scientific and Industrial Research, Osaka University, Osaka, Japan*
[5] *Graduate School of Pharmaceutical Sciences, Osaka University, Osaka, Japan*

Edited by:
Jun Lin, The University of Tennessee, USA

Reviewed by:
Shigetoshi Eda, University of Tennessee, USA
Ahmad S. Khalil, Boston University, USA
Aldo Jesorka, Chalmers University of Technology, Sweden

*Correspondence:
Ryota Iino, Department of Applied Chemistry, Graduate School of Engineering, The University of Tokyo, 7-3-1 Hongo, Bunkyo-ku, Tokyo, Japan
e-mail: iino@appchem.t.u-tokyo.ac.jp

Single-cell analysis is a powerful method to assess the heterogeneity among individual cells, enabling the identification of very rare cells with properties that differ from those of the majority. In this Methods Article, we describe the use of a large-scale femtoliter droplet array to enclose, isolate, and analyze individual bacterial cells. As a first example, we describe the single-cell detection of drug-tolerant persisters of *Pseudomonas aeruginosa* treated with the antibiotic carbenicillin. As a second example, this method was applied to the single-cell evaluation of drug efflux activity, which causes acquired antibiotic resistance of bacteria. The activity of the MexAB-OprM multidrug efflux pump system from *Pseudomonas aeruginosa* was expressed in *Escherichia coli* and the effect of an inhibitor D13-9001 were assessed at the single cell level.

Keywords: single-cell analysis, microdevice, drug tolerance, persister, drug resistance, drug efflux, transporter

INTRODUCTION

Opportunistic infection with bacteria resistant to multiple antibiotics is a continuing clinical challenge (Taubes, 2008). The antibiotic resistance of bacteria can be classified into two categories, natural resistance (tolerance) and acquired resistance. In natural resistance, a very small proportion of the bacterial population is resistant to multiple antibiotics despite having the same genotype as the sensitive majority. These bacteria are often referred to as "persisters" (Lewis, 2010). However, the nature of these persisters is not fully understood because they occur at a very low frequency in a bacterial population (typically less than 1%), which makes systematic studies difficult (Allison et al., 2011; Balaban, 2011, Gerdes and Maisonneuve, 2012; Kint et al., 2012). In the first section of this review article, we describe a microdroplet-based method to identify and culture individual bacterial cells for efficient detection of persisters. In contrast, acquired antibiotic resistance is caused by a change in the genotype of the sensitive strain. The four main mechanisms of acquired resistance are suppression of drug influx into the cell due to decreased expression of membrane channel proteins, inactivation of drugs by intracellular and extracellular enzymes, mutations in the target proteins of drugs, and active efflux of the drugs from the cell due to increased expression of efflux pumps (Fischbach and Walsh, 2009; Nikaido, 2009). Here we focused on the active efflux of drugs from the cell. In the second section, we introduce a microdroplet-based method for assessing the drug efflux activity of single bacterial cells.

ADVANTAGES OF SINGLE-CELL ANALYSIS USING A MICRODEVICE

Single-cell analysis is a powerful approach for detecting variations among the cells in a population, such as differences in the expression of proteins, the copy number of genes, and the concentration of metabolites (Li and Xie, 2011; Trouillon et al., 2013). Single-cell analysis can overcome the limitations associated with ensemble-averaged data from multiple cells, and enable the identification of very rare cells with properties that differ from those of the majority. Microfabricated devices have contributed greatly to the development of massively parallel and high-throughput single-cell analyses.

However, in most microdevices, the target cells are eukaryotic, such as mammalian cells and yeasts (Sims and Allbritton, 2007; Gupta et al., 2010, Lindstrom and Andersson-Svahn, 2010), because their size, a few millimeters to tens of micrometers, allows for easy handling compared to bacteria, which are much smaller in size. Thus far, only a few studies have used microdevices for single bacterial cell analysis (Balaban et al., 2004; Cai et al., 2006, Ottesen et al., 2006; Weibel et al., 2007, Boedicker et al., 2009; Teng et al., 2013, Wakamoto et al., 2013). In addition, in many microdevices that are based on microfluidic channels and valves or droplets generated in a microfluidic channel, the closed nature of the system makes the collection of cells from the device and their subsequent use difficult. Therefore, the development of microdevices from which individual bacterial cells can be recovered has been highly anticipated.

LARGE-SCALE FEMTOLITER DROPLET ARRAY FOR SINGLE BACTERIAL CELL ANALYSIS

We recently developed a micron-sized femtoliter droplet array fixed on a hydrophilic-in-hydrophobic micropatterned surface (Sakakihara et al., 2010). In our new microdevice, a large number of dome-shaped femtoliter droplets can be prepared that enclose individual bacterial cells (Iino et al., 2012a). One prominent feature of this array is that the individual droplets containing the enclosed cells can be accessed and collected with a micropipette. The array can also be used for mass culture and gene and protein analyses.

We prepared the hydrophilic-in-hydrophobic micropatterned surface through conventional microfabrication (**Figure 1A**). A hydrophobic polymer of carbon-fluorine (CYTOP; Asahi Glass, Japan) was deposited on a SiO_2 cover glass, and photolithography was performed using a high-viscosity photoresist. The resist-patterned substrate surface was dry-etched with O_2 plasma by using a reactive ion-etching system to produce circular micropatterns on a hydrophilic SiO_2 glass surface. The diameter of the exposed hydrophilic SiO_2 surfaces was 10–30 μm, and they were surrounded by a hydrophobic polymer layer with a height of 1 μm. A fabricated micropatterned cover glass was attached to the bottom of a perforated petri dish (**Figure 1B**). The circular micropatterns were grouped into islands and were numbered to identify the individual droplets and the cells enclosed in each droplet.

To form a droplet array containing bacteria, we covered the micropatterned cover glass with medium containing a bacterial suspension (**Figure 1C**, left). Then, fluorinated oil (Fluorinert FC-40; Sigma Aldrich, USA), which has a higher density than water, was flowed over the medium near the surface. The hydrophilic SiO_2 glass surfaces retained the medium and the bacteria, whereas the hydrophobic surface was replaced with oil. As a result, many droplets containing one or more bacteria were formed (**Figure 1C**, right). More than 3×10^5 droplets could be simultaneously prepared in a 1-cm^2 area in a single device. Enclosure of the cells in the droplets was stochastic and was dependent on the cell density of the bacterial suspension. At an optical density (turbidity) at 600 nm (OD_{600}) of 0.6, approximately 20–30% of the droplets contained single cells. Increasing the diameter of the hydrophilic surfaces to 20 or 30 μm increased the fraction of droplets containing multiple cells; however, the fraction of droplets containing single cells did not increase significantly (**Figure 1D**). In contrast, the number of droplets formed increased significantly when we used a device with hydrophilic surfaces of a smaller diameter. Therefore, to increase the total number of droplets containing single cells, we used a microdevice containing hydrophilic surfaces with a diameter of 10 μm.

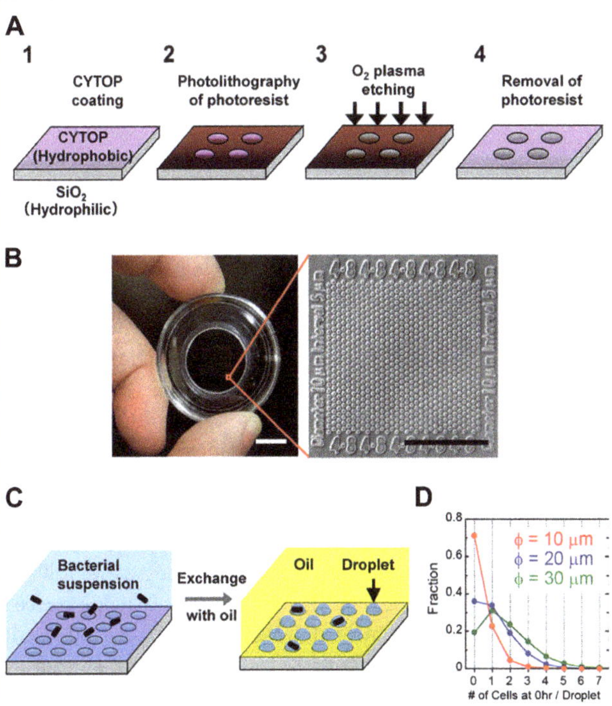

FIGURE 1 | Formation of a femtoliter droplet array containing bacteria. **(A)** Schematic of the fabrication procedure for preparation of a hydrophilic-in-hydrophobic micropatterned surface. **(B)** Image of the assembled device (left). Scale bar, 10 mm. Microscopic image of the hydrophilic-in-hydrophobic micropatterned surface (right). Scale bar, 200 μm. **(C)** Procedure for bacterial enclosure into the femtoliter droplet array. **(D)** The number of bacterial cells in each droplet in microdevices with different hydrophilic surface diameters just after enclosure.

DETECTION OF PERSISTER BACTERIA IN A FEMTOLITER DROPLET ARRAY

We generated a femtoliter droplet array of *Pseudomonas aeruginosa* PAO1 using our microdevice to detect persisters under an optical microscope. In the control experiment without antibiotic treatment, most cells underwent multiple cell divisions after incubation overnight at 37°C (**Figures 2A,B**). The divided cells showed active flagellar motion, indicative of high metabolic activity. To detect persisters, an antibiotic, carbenicillin (at final concentration of 5 mg/mL, which is ~100 times higher than the minimal inhibitory concentration), was added to the bacterial suspension that was grown to late exponential phase (OD_{600} ~1.0) in trypticase soy broth. The suspension was further incubated at 37°C for 3 h, and then the cells were collected, washed, resuspended in fresh medium (OD_{600} ~0.2). This suspension was enclosed in a droplet array. After enclosure, the whole device was placed in an incubator at 37°C, and the cells were cultured overnight. The persisters were easily identified under an optical microscope the overnight culture (**Figure 3A**). The divided cells were not cells that acquired resistance, but were actually persisters. This was confirmed by collecting the cells with a micropipette with an aperture diameter of 10–15 μm (**Figures 3B,C**), inoculating a culture in test tubes, and antibiotic susceptibility testing.

Bacterial cells that divided multiple times were counted, and the frequency of persisters was calculated. The frequency of persisters in the femtoliter droplet array (1.5 ± 0.72%, $N = 4$; **Figure 3D**) was quite unexpectedly much higher than that estimated by conventional agar plate assays (0.10 ± 0.03%, $N = 4$). In the plate assays, the carbenicillin-treated preculture sample was prepared as described above along with an untreated culture sample, and then the samples were serially diluted and cultured overnight at 37°C on agar plates. The number of colonies on the plates

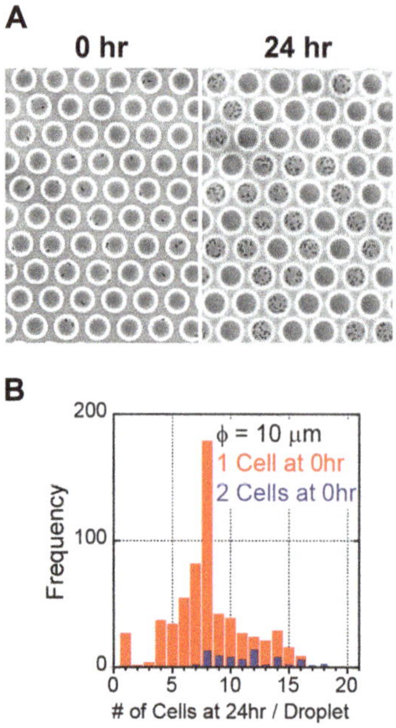

FIGURE 2 | Enclosure and culture of bacteria in a femtoliter droplet array. (A) Images of *P. aeruginosa* PAO1 after 0 h (left) and 24 h (right) of culture in the femtoliter droplet array. **(B)** Distribution of the number of cells after 24 h of culture.

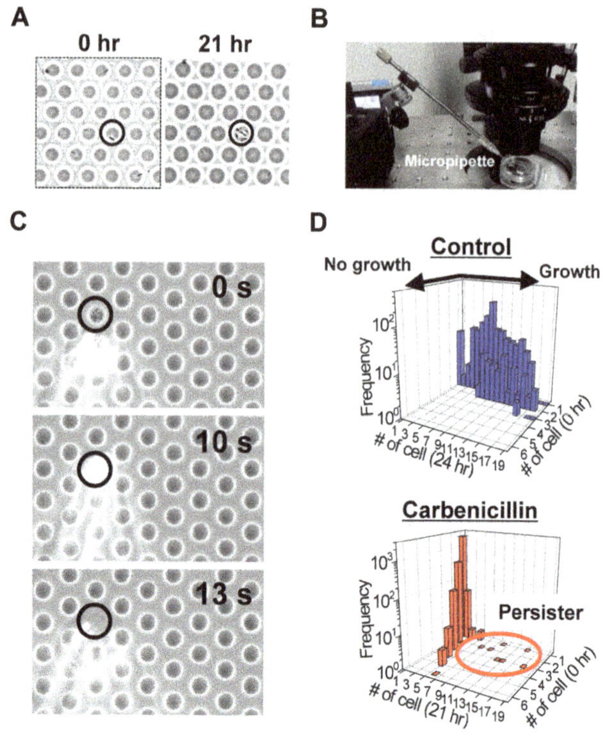

FIGURE 3 | Detection of the persisters in the femtoliter droplet array. (A) Images of *P. aeruginosa* PAO1 persisters (indicated by circle) after 0 h (left) and 21 h (right) of culture in the femtoliter droplet array. **(B)** Image of the micropipette used for droplet collection. **(C)** Sequential images of droplet collection. **(D)** Distribution of the number of cells in each droplet before and after overnight culture. Top, control cells without carbenicillin treatment. Bottom, carbenicillin-treated cells.

from carbenicillin-treated and untreated preculture samples were counted and compared. It has been recently reported that quorum sensing autoinducer increased the frequency of persister appearance (Moker et al., 2010; Leung and Levesque, 2012, Vega et al., 2012), and that inhibiting the quorum signal restored antibiotic susceptibility (Pan et al., 2012, 2013). Furthermore, the quorum-sensing signal could be transduced even in single isolated cells when PAO1 was enclosed in picoliter-volume droplets (Boedicker et al., 2009). Therefore, enclosure of a single cell in a femtoliter droplet may enhance the quorum sensing signal and increase persister frequency. The effect of the quorum sensing signal on the frequency of persister appearance in the femtoliter droplet array can be more clearly confirmed by treating the cells with antibiotic after enclosure in the droplets by adding the antibiotic with a micropipette (Sakakihara et al., 2010).

A SINGLE-CELL DRUG EFFLUX ASSAY IN A FEMTOLITER DROPLET ARRAY

The AcrAB-TolC multicomponent efflux pump system recognizes and expels a wide variety of compounds, including antibiotics, dyes, and detergents. In this system, AcrA is the membrane fusion protein that stabilizes the complex (Zgurskaya and Nikaido, 1999), AcrB is the inner membrane transporter protein that belongs to the resistance-nodulation-division (RND) family (Murakami et al., 2006; Nakashima et al., 2011, 2013), and TolC is the outer membrane channel protein (Koronakis et al., 2000). The AcrAB-TolC efflux system is responsible for both intrinsic and acquired drug resistance of Gram-negative bacteria such as *Escherichia coli* and *Salmonella enterica* (Nishino and Yamaguchi, 2008; Nikaido and Takatsuka, 2009). Two systems *P. aeruginosa* that are homologous to the AcrAB-TolC system, MexAB-OprM and MexXY-OprM, lead to multidrug resistance in clinical isolates (Morita et al., 2001; Livermore, 2002; Hocquet et al., 2006, 2007; Henrichfreise et al., 2007).

We have recently developed a single-cell drug efflux assay using the femtoliter droplet array (**Figure 4**; Iino et al., 2012a). In this assay, *E. coli* cultured in test tubes was mixed with a fluorogenic substrate, fluorescein-di-β-D-galactopyranoside (FDG), enclosed in a droplet array, and then cultured for 15–20 min at room temperature. Upon entering the cytoplasm of *E. coli*, FDG is hydrolyzed into the fluorescent dye fluorescein by β-galactosidase. Both FDG and fluorescein are substrates for the AcrAB-TolC system (Matsumoto et al., 2011; Iino et al., 2012b). In wild-type cells, FDG was effectively pumped out before hydrolysis, and no fluorescence was detected (**Figure 4A**, left, and **Figure 4B**, top). In contrast, when FDG was imported into Δ*acrB* (ΔB) and Δ*tolC* (ΔC) strains it was hydrolyzed to fluorescein. In ΔB cells, not only the cells, but also the droplets themselves fluoresced (**Figure 4A**, center, and **Figure 4B**, middle) because the remaining minor RND efflux pumps slowly pumped out the fluorescein. Although only a small amount of the dye was pumped out, it could be easily detected because it was confined to the femtoliter droplet (Rondelez et al., 2005; Sakakihara et al., 2010, Kim et al., 2012). In ΔC cells, fluorescein accumulated in the cell (**Figure 4A**, right, and

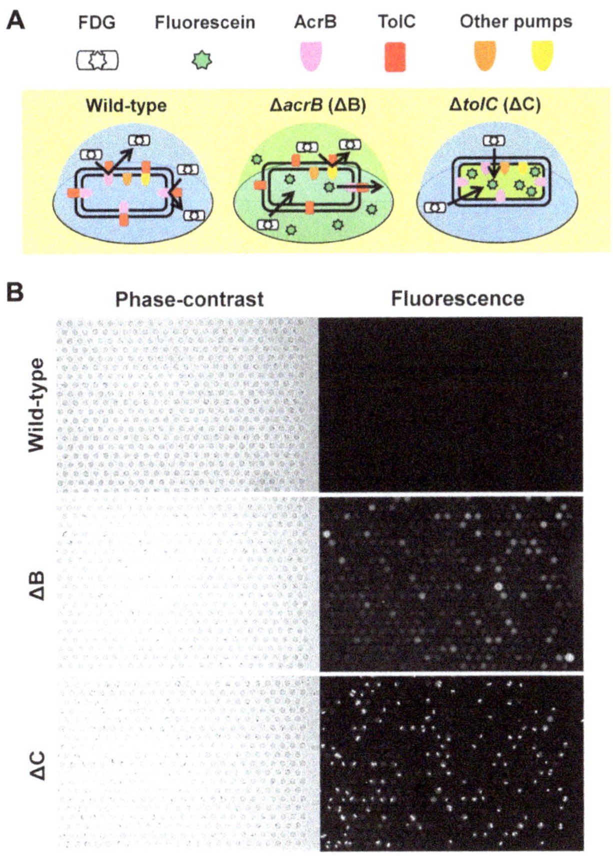

FIGURE 4 | Single-cell drug efflux assay. (A) Schematic of the principle of the single-cell drug efflux assay. **(B)** A representative assay. Phase-contrast (left) and fluorescence (right) images of the same field are shown.

Figure 4B, bottom) because TolC is a channel protein common to both the major and minor RND efflux pumps in *E. coli*.

With this method, the inhibitory effect of chemical compounds against the efflux pump can be easily assessed. The effect of an efflux pump inhibitor, D13-9001 (Yoshida et al., 2007), is shown in **Figure 5**. D13-9001 has been reported to enhance the antibacterial activities of several antibiotics by binding tightly to the drug binding pockets of AcrB and MexB (Nakashima et al., 2013). A ΔBΔC double-knockout *E. coli* strain that stably expresses MexAB-OprM from *P. aeruginosa* was used for the experiment. This strain did not fluoresce in our assay, indicating that the exogenously expressed MexAB-OprM worked well in *E. coli*, and that the cells recovered drug efflux activity (**Figure 5**, top). Addition of D13-9001 increased the number of fluorescent cells (**Figure 5**, bottom). The fluorescence intensity of the cells increased as the concentration of D13-9001 increased, indicating a concentration-dependent inhibitory effect. D13-9001 is a specific inhibitor of MexB, a major efflux pump in *P. aeruginosa*. However, it does not inhibit MexY, which is another major efflux pump in *P. aeruginosa* (Yoshida et al., 2007). Our simple and rapid approach would be useful to screen for new inhibitors that are also effective against MexY and other efflux pumps.

FIGURE 5 | Effect of the pump inhibitor D13-9001 on the efflux activity of MexAB-OprM expressed in the ΔBΔC *E. coli* strain. Phase-contrast (left) and fluorescence (right) images of untreated control cells (top) or cells treated with 16 μg/mL D13-9001 (bottom).

PHENOTYPIC CHANGE AFTER GENETIC TRANSFORMATION

As a demonstration of the rapid phenotypic change after genetic transformation, we introduced the *S. enterica tolC* gene into *E. coli* ΔC cells. After electroporation with the expression vector, the cells were incubated for different time durations in the presence of the selection marker kanamycin and drug efflux activity was assessed. The efflux-active phenotype was observed after 3 h (**Figure 6**, top), whereas no phenotypic change was observed in the control experiment (**Figure 6**, bottom).

A prominent feature of the femtoliter droplet array is the ability to access individual droplets. Using a micropipette, not only droplets but also the cells within the droplets can be collected (**Figures 3B,C**). Collected single cells divide multiple times after

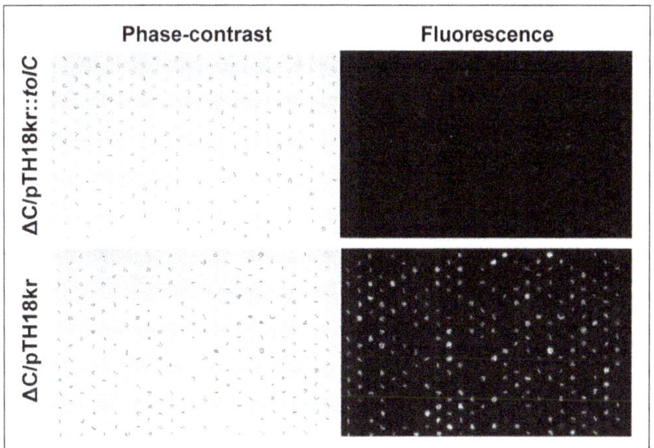

FIGURE 6 | Phenotypic change after genetic transformation. Phase-contrast (left) and fluorescence (right) images of *E. coli* ΔC cells transformed with a vector expressing *tolC* from *Salmonella enterica* (pTH18kr::tolC; top) or a control vector pTH18kr (bottom).

transfer to growth medium in a test tube. The plasmid in the divided cells can be extracted and used for subsequent gene analysis (Iino et al., 2012a). Culturing after cell collection can be omitted by amplifying the DNA by single-cell PCR (Ottesen et al., 2006). Considering the rapid detection (3 h) of the phenotypic change after genetic transformation, single-cell gene analysis would enable high-throughput screening.

PERSPECTIVE

As described above, the femtoliter droplet array is useful for single-bacterial cell analysis. Single-cell analysis of persister bacteria could help elucidate the mechanism of persister appearance and the reversible switching dynamics between persister and sensitive cells. This single-cell drug efflux assay can be used to screen for pump inhibitors, which requires the testing of numerous compounds. Our method is a direct evaluation of efflux activity, it takes only 20-30 min, and its advantage over the conventional method, based on the shift in the minimal inhibitory concentration is evident. Furthermore, with the advantage of individual droplet accessibility, single persister cells and cells exhibiting the efflux-active phenotype can be easily collected and used for subsequent analysis. It should be possible to screen for genes encoding functional efflux pump systems with a plasmid library of cloned genomic fragments. We believe that our approach will aid in addressing the challenge of infectious diseases caused by bacteria that are multidrug tolerant and resistant.

REFERENCES

Allison, K. R., Brynildsen, M. P., and Collins, J. J. (2011). Heterogeneous bacterial persisters and engineering approaches to eliminate them. *Curr. Opin. Microbiol.* 14, 593–598. doi: 10.1016/j.mib.2011.09.002

Balaban, N. Q. (2011). Persistence: mechanisms for triggering and enhancing phenotypic variability. *Curr. Opin. Genet. Dev.* 21, 768–775. doi: 10.1016/j.gde.2011.10.001

Balaban, N. Q., Merrin, J., Chait, R., Kowalik, L., and Leibler, S. (2004). Bacterial persistence as a phenotypic switch. *Science* 305, 1622–1625. doi: 10.1126/science.1099390

Boedicker, J. Q., Vincent, M. E., and Ismagilov, R. F. (2009). Microfluidic confinement of single cells of bacteria in small volumes initiates high-density behavior of quorum sensing and growth and reveals its variability. *Angew. Chem. Int. Ed. Engl.* 48, 5908–5911. doi: 10.1002/anie.200901550

Cai, L., Friedman, N., and Xie, X. S. (2006). Stochastic protein expression in individual cells at the single molecule level. *Nature* 440, 358–362. doi: 10.1038/nature04599

Fischbach, M. A., and Walsh, C. T. (2009). Antibiotics for emerging pathogens. *Science* 325, 1089–1093. doi: 10.1126/science.1176667

Gerdes, K., and Maisonneuve, E. (2012). Bacterial persistence and toxin-antitoxin loci. *Annu. Rev. Microbiol.* 66, 103–123. doi: 10.1146/annurev-micro-092611-150159

Gupta, K., Kim, D. H., Ellison, D., Smith, C., Kundu, A., Tuan, J., et al. (2010). Lab-on-a-chip devices as an emerging platform for stem cell biology. *Lab Chip* 10, 2019–2031. doi: 10.1039/c004689b

Henrichfreise, B., Wiegand, I., Pfister, W., and Wiedemann, B. (2007). Resistance mechanisms of multiresistant *pseudomonas aeruginosa* strains from Germany and correlation with Hypermutation del. *Antimicrob. Agents Chemother.* 51, 4062–4070. doi: 10.1128/aac.0014s-07

Hocquet, D., Nordmann, P., El Garch, F., Cabanne, L., and Plesiat, P. (2006). Involvement of the MexXY-OprM efflux system in emergence of cefepime resistance in clinical strains of *Pseudomonas aeruginosa. Antimicrob. Agents Chemother.* 50, 1347–1351. doi: 10.1128/AAC.50.4.1347-1351.2006

Hocquet, D., Roussel-Delvallez, M., Cavallo, J. D., and Plesiat, P. (2007). MexAB-OprM- and MexXY-overproducing mutants are very prevalent among clinical strains of *Pseudomonas aeruginosa* with reduced susceptibility to ticarcillin. *Antimicrob. Agents Chemother.* 51, 1582–1583. doi: 10.1128/AAC.01334-06

Iino, R., Hayama, K., Amezawa, H., Sakakihara, S., Kim, S. H., Matsumono, Y., et al. (2012a). A single-cell drug efflux assay in bacteria by using a directly accessible femtoliter droplet array. *Lab Chip* 12, 3923–3929. doi: 10.1039/c2lc40394c

Iino, R., Nishino, K., Noji, H., Yamaguchi, A., and Matsumoto, Y. (2012b). A microfluidic device for simple and rapid evaluation of multidrug efflux pump inhibitors. *Front. Microbiol.* 3:40. doi: 10.3389/fmicb.2012.00040

Kim, S. H., Iwai, S., Araki, S., Sakakihara, S., Iino, R., and Noji, H. (2012). Large-scale femtoliter droplet array for digital counting of single biomolecules. *Lab Chip* 12, 4986–4991. doi: 10.1039/c2lc40632b

Kint, C. I., Verstraeten, N., Fauvart, M., and Michiels, J. (2012). New-found fundamentals of bacterial persistence. *Trends Microbiol.* 20, 577–585. doi: 10.1016/j.tim.2012.08.009

Koronakis, V., Sharff, A., Koronakis, E., Luisi, B., and Hughes, C. (2000). Crystal structure of the bacterial membrane protein TolC central to multidrug efflux and protein export. *Nature* 405, 914–919. doi: 10.1038/35016007

Leung, V., and Levesque, C. M. (2012). A stress-inducible quorum-sensing peptide mediates the formation of persister cells with noninherited multidrug tolerance. *J. Bacteriol.* 194, 2265–2674. doi: 10.1128/JB.06707-11

Lewis, K. (2010). Persister cells. *Annu. Rev. Microbiol.* 64, 357–372. doi: 10.1146/annurev.micro.112408.134306

Li, G. W., and Xie, X. S. (2011). Central dogma at the single-molecule level in living cells. *Nature* 475, 308–315. doi: 10.1038/nature10315

Lindstrom, S., and Andersson-Svahn, H. (2010). Overview of single-cell analyses: microdevices and applications. *Lab Chip* 10, 3363–3372. doi: 10.1039/c0lc00150c

Livermore, D. M. (2002). Multiple mechanisms of antimicrobial resistance in *Pseudomonas aeruginosa*: our worst nightmare? *Clin. Infect. Dis.* 34, 634–640.

Matsumoto, Y., Hayama, K., Sakakihara, S., Nishino, K., Noji, H., Iino, R., et al. (2011). Evaluation of multidrug efflux pump inhibitors by a new method using microfluidic channels. *PLoS ONE* 6:e18547. doi: 10.1371/journal.pone.0018547

Moker, N., Dean, C. R., and Tao, J. (2010). *Pseudomonas aeruginosa* increases formation of multidrug-tolerant persister cells in response to quorum-sensing signaling molecules. *J. Bacteriol.* 192, 1946–1955. doi: 10.1128/JB.01231-09

Morita, Y., Kimura, N., Mima, T., Mizushima, T., and Tsuchiya, T. (2001). Roles of MexXY- and MexAB-multidrug efflux pumps in intrinsic multidrug resistance of *Pseudomonas aeruginosa* PAO1. *J. Gen. Appl. Microbiol.* 47, 27–32.

Murakami, S., Nakashima, R., Yamashita, E., Matsumoto, T., and Yamaguchi, A. (2006). Crystal structures of a multidrug transporter reveal a functionally rotating mechanism. *Nature* 443, 173–179. doi: 10.1038/nature05076

Nakashima, R., Sakurai, K., Yamasaki, S., Hayashi, K., Nagata, C., Hoshino, K., et al. (2013). Structural basis for the inhibition of bacterial multidrug exporters. *Nature* 500, 102–106. doi: 10.1038/nature12300

Nakashima, R., Sakurai, K., Yamasaki, S., Nishino, K., and Yamaguchi, A. (2011). Structures of the multidrug exporter AcrB reveal a proximal multisite drug-binding pocket. *Nature* 480, 565–569. doi: 10.1038/nature10641

Nikaido, H. (2009). Multidrug resistance in bacteria. *Annu. Rev. Biochem.* 78, 119–146. doi: 10.1146/annurev.biochem.78.082907.145923

Nikaido, H., and Takatsuka, Y. (2009). Mechanisms of RND multidrug efflux pumps. *Biochim. Biophys. Acta* 1794, 769–781. doi: 10.1016/j.bbapap.2008.10.004

Nishino, K., and Yamaguchi, A. (2008). Role of xenobiotic transporters in bacterial drug resistance and virulence. *IUBMB Life* 60, 569–574. doi: 10.1002/iub.90

Ottesen, E. A., Hong, J. W., Quake, S. R., and Leadbetter, J. R. (2006). Microfluidic digital PCR enables multigene analysis of individual environmental bacteria. *Science* 314, 1464–1467. doi: 10.1126/science.1131370

Pan, J., Bahar, A. A., Syed, H., and Ren, D. (2012). Reverting antibiotic tolerance of *Pseudomonas aeruginosa* PAO1 persister cells by (Z)-4-bromo-5-(bromomethylene)-3-methylfuran-2(5H)-one. *PLoS ONE* 7:e45778. doi: 10.1371/journal.pone.0045778

Pan, J., Song, F., and Ren, D. (2013). Controlling persister cells of *Pseudomonas aeruginosa* PDO300 by (Z)-4-bromo-5-(bromomethylene)-

3-methylfuran-2(5H)-one. *Bioorg. Med. Chem. Lett.* 23, 4648–4651. doi: 10.1016/j.bmcl.2013.06.011

Rondelez, Y., Tresset, G., Tabata, K. V., Arata, H., Fujita, H., Takeuchi, S., et al. (2005). Microfabricated arrays of femtoliter chambers allow single molecule enzymology. *Nat. Biotechnol.* 23, 361–365. doi: 10.1038/nbt1072

Sakakihara, S., Araki, S., Iino, R., and Noji, H. (2010). A single-molecule enzymatic assay in a directly accessible femtoliter droplet array. *Lab Chip* 10, 3355–3362. doi: 10.1039/c0lc00062k

Sims, C. E., and Allbritton, N. L. (2007). Analysis of single mammalian cells on-chip. *Lab Chip* 7, 423–440. doi: 10.1039/b615235j

Taubes, G. (2008). The bacteria fight back. *Science* 321, 356–361. doi: 10.1126/science.321.5887.356

Teng, S. W., Mukherji, S., Moffitt, J. R., de Buyl, S., and O'Shea, E. K. (2013). Robust circadian oscillations in growing cyanobacteria require transcriptional feedback. *Science* 340, 737–740. doi: 10.1126/science.1230996

Trouillon, R., Passarelli, M. K., Wang, J., Kurczy, M. E., and Ewing, A. G. (2013). Chemical analysis of single cells. *Anal. Chem.* 85, 522–542. doi: 10.1021/ac303290s

Vega, N. M., Allison, K. R., Khalil, A. S., and Collins, J. J. (2012). Signaling-mediated bacterial persister formation. *Nat. Chem. Biol.* 8, 431–433. doi: 10.1038/nchembio.915

Wakamoto, Y., Dhar, N., Chait, R., Schneider, K., Signorino-Gelo, F., Leibler, S., et al. (2013). Dynamic persistence of antibiotic-stressed mycobacteria. *Science* 339, 91–95. doi: 10.1126/science.1229858

Weibel, D. B., Diluzio, W. R., and Whitesides, G. M. (2007). Microfabrication meets microbiology. *Nat. Rev. Microbiol.* 5, 209–218. doi: 10.1038/nrmicro1616

Yoshida, K., Nakayama, K., Ohtsuka, M., Kuru, N., Yokomizo, Y., Sakamoto, A., et al. (2007). MexAB-OprM specific efflux pump inhibitors in *Pseudomonas aeruginosa.* Part 7: highly soluble and in vivo active quaternary ammonium analogue D13-9001, a potential preclinical candidate. *Bioorg. Med. Chem.* 15, 7087–7097.

Zgurskaya, H. I., and Nikaido, H. (1999). AcrA is a highly asymmetric protein capable of spanning the periplasm. *J. Mol. Biol.* 285, 409–420. doi: 10.1006/jmbi.1998.2313

7

Sterol C-22 desaturase ERG5 mediates the sensitivity to antifungal azoles in *Neurospora crassa* and *Fusarium verticillioides*

Xianyun Sun[1], Wenzhao Wang[1], Kangji Wang[1], Xinxu Yu[2], Jie Liu[3], Fucai Zhou[3], Baogui Xie[2] and Shaojie Li[1]*

[1] *State Key Laboratory of Mycology, Institute of Microbiology, Chinese Academy of Sciences, Beijing, China*
[2] *Mycological Research Center, College of Life Sciences, Fujian Agriculture and Forestry University, Fuzhou, China*
[3] *College of Bioscience and Biotechnology, Yangzhou University, Yangzhou, China*

Edited by:
Lixin Zhang, Chinese Academy of Sciences, China

Reviewed by:
Christopher Morton Thomas, University of Birmingham, UK
Dmitri Debabov, NovaBay Pharmaceuticals, USA

***Correspondence:**
Shaojie Li, Institute of Microbiology, Chinese Academy of Sciences, No. 8 Beiertiao, Zhongguancun, Beijing 100080, China.
e-mail: shaojieli@gmail.com

Antifungal azoles inhibit ergosterol biosynthesis by interfering with lanosterol 14α-demethylase. In this study, seven upregulated and four downregulated ergosterol biosynthesis genes in response to ketoconazole treatment were identified in *Neurospora crassa*. Azole sensitivity test of knockout mutants for six ketoconazole-upregulated genes in ergosterol biosynthesis revealed that deletion of only sterol C-22 desaturase ERG5 altered sensitivity to azoles: the *erg5* mutant was hypersensitive to azoles but had no obvious defects in growth and development. The *erg5* mutant accumulated higher levels of ergosta 5,7-dienol relative to the wild type but its levels of 14α-methylated sterols were similar to the wild type. ERG5 homologs are highly conserved in fungal kingdom. Deletion of *Fusarium verticillioides erg5* also increased ketoconazole sensitivity, suggesting that the roles of ERG5 homologs in azole resistance are highly conserved among different fungal species, and inhibition of ERG5 could reduce the usage of azoles and thus provide a new target for drug design.

Keywords: resistance to antifungal agents, ergosterol biosynthesis, azole, *Neurospora crassa*, *Fusarium verticillioides*

INTRODUCTION

Antifungal azoles are the most commonly used drugs for controlling fungal infections. Azoles inhibit ergosterol biosynthesis by disrupting essential P450 superfamily protein lanosterol 14α-demethylase CYP51 (syn. ERG11) (Bossche et al., 1984; Kelly et al., 1993). In addition, the inhibition of lanosterol 14α-demethylase also results in the accumulation of the toxic 14-α methylated sterols, like 14α-methyl-ergosta-8,24(28)-dien-3β,6α-diol (Kelly et al., 1995). Incorporation of such compounds into fungal membranes reduces their rigidity (Abe et al., 2009).

Biological processes of sterol biosynthesis are highly conserved in fungal kingdom (Ferreira et al., 2005). In response to azole treatments, significant transcriptional increases in several genes involved in ergosterol biosynthesis, such as *ERG2* (C-8 sterol isomerase), *ERG3* (C-5 sterol desaturase), *ERG5* (C-22 sterol desaturase), *ERG6* (C-24 sterol methyltransferase), *ERG25* (C-4 methyl sterol oxidase), and *ERG11*, are consistently observed in many fungal species such as *Saccharomyces cerevisiae* (Bammert and Fostel, 2000; Agarwal et al., 2003), *Candida albicans* (De Backer et al., 2001; Liu et al., 2005), *Aspergillus fumigatus* (da Silva Ferreira et al., 2006), *Trichophyton rubrum* (Yu et al., 2007), *Cryptococcus neoformans* (Florio et al., 2011), and *Fusarium graminearum* (Liu et al., 2010; Becher et al., 2011). Many reports have shown that increased expression of *ERG11* could reduce azole susceptibility (Hamamoto et al., 2000; Schnabel and Jones, 2001; Du et al., 2004; Ma et al., 2006). In addition to *ERG11*, *ERG3*, and *ERG5* have also been shown to be related to drug susceptibility. Many *ERG3* mutants of *S. cerevisiae* or *C. albicans* with defects in C5-6 desaturase showed increased resistance to azoles (Watson et al., 1989; Martel et al., 2010a; Morio et al., 2012; Vale-Silva et al., 2012). A clinical isolate of *C. albicans* with mutations in both *ERG11* and *ERG5* is cross resistance to azoles and amphotericin B (Martel et al., 2010b). However, due to lack of systemic analysis, except *ERG11*, contributions of most of these azole-responsive genes to azole resistance were not fully understood.

Since the non-pathogenic *Neurospora crassa* has less redundant genes in ergosterol biosynthesis relative to other filamentous pathogenic fungi and has knockout mutants available for most of ergosterol synthesis genes, it can be an excellent model for systemic analysis of the contributions of these azole-responsive genes to azole resistance. In this study, we demonstrate that ERG5 mediates the sensitivity to antifungal azoles in both *N. crassa* and *Fusarium verticillioides*.

MATERIALS AND METHODS

STRAINS AND CULTURE CONDITIONS

Neurospora crassa strains used in this study are listed in **Table 1**. All of them were obtained from the Fungal Genetics Stock Center[1] (University of Kansas Medical Center). Vogel's minimum medium (Vogel, 1956), supplemented with 2% (w/v) sucrose for slants or 2% glucose for plates and the liquid medium, was used for

[1]www.fgsc.net

Table 1 | *Neurospora* strains used in this study.

Strain	Genotype
FGSC#4200	Wild type, a
FGSC#18507	*erg2* (NCU04156), a, hetero
FGSC#13802	*erg5* (NCU05278), a
FGSC#13803	*erg5* (NCU05278), A
FGSC#12752	*erg6* (NCU03006), a
FGSC#12753	*erg6* (NCU03006), A
FGSC#18506	*erg24* (NCU08762), a, hetero
FGSC#17674	*erg25* (NCU06402), a

culturing strains. All cultures were grown at 28°C in the light. Antifungal compounds were added as needed.

DRUG SUSCEPTIBILITY TEST

Ketoconazole, fluconazole, and itraconazole were dissolved in dimethyl sulfoxide (DMSO) and then aseptically added to the autoclaved medium before making agar plates. The final concentrations of ketoconazole, fluconazole, and itraconazole in the agar plates were 2, 25, and 10 μg/ml, respectively. The final DMSO concentration was below 0.25% (v/v). Two microliters of conidial suspension were inoculated on plates ($\Phi = 9$ cm) with or without antifungal drugs and incubated at 28°C for 66 h.

MIC DETERMINATION OF KETOCONAZOLE, ITRACONAZOLE, AND FLUCONAZOLE

The MICs of three azoles for each strain were determined in 96-well microtiter plate according to National Committee for Clinical Laboratory Standards (CLSI, 2008). Briefly, 100 μl of 2× azole solution and 100 μl of conidial suspension were added into each well. The final conidial concentration was approximately 1×10^6 conidia/ml. The plates were incubated at 28°C for 24 h. The MIC was determined as the lowest drug concentration without growth.

RNA EXTRACTION AND DIGITAL GENE EXPRESSION PROFILING ANALYSIS

The transcriptional responses of ergosterol biosynthesis genes to ketoconazole treatment in the wild-type strain were detected by digital gene expression (DGE) profiling (Nielsen et al., 2006). Briefly, conidia of the wild-type strain was inoculated into 20-ml liquid medium in a plate ($\Phi = 9$ cm) and incubated for 24 h at 28°C in darkness to form mycelial mat on the surface of the liquid medium. Mycelial mat then was cut into small pieces ($\Phi = 10$ mm) and transferred to the liquid medium (2 pieces/100 ml). Cultures were incubated at 28°C with shaking at 180 rpm for 12 h. Ketoconazole was then added into the medium to reach a final concentration of 2.5 μg/ml. After 24 h of incubation, mycelia were harvested and total RNA was extracted and subjected to DGE analysis as described by Sun et al. (2011).

STEROL EXTRACTION AND ANALYSIS

Sterols of dried mycelium (0.3 g) was extracted into 1.5-ml chloroform under ultrasonication for 12 h. The extracts were dried and subsequently dissolved into 150 μl methanol under ultrasonication for 1 h. After filtration with a Millipore filter, the extracts were subjected to HPLC-MS analysis following the method reported by Cañabate-Díaz et al. (2007) with some modifications.

Liquid chromatography separation was performed on an Agilent Zorbax Extend-C18 1.8 μm 2.1 mm × 50 mm column using an Agilent 1200 Series system (Agilent, USA). Total flow rate was 0.4 ml min^{-1}; mobile phase A consisted of water with 0.01% acetic acid and mobile phase B consisted of acetonitrile. Total elution program was 27 min. Gradient began with 70% mobile phase B, changed to 100% B over 2 min, maintained a constant level from 2 to 18 min at 100% B and then decreased to 70% B over 1 min prior to re-stabilization over 8 min before the next injection. The column temperature was maintained at 40°C. The injection volume was 10 μl.

Mass spectra were acquired with an Agilent Accurate-Mass-Q-TOF MS 6520 system. Analytes were detected in the positive ionization mode with an APCI probe. For Q-TOF/MS conditions, fragmentor and capillary voltages were kept at 130 and 3500 V, respectively. Nitrogen was supplied as the nebulizing and drying gas. Temperature of the drying gas and vaporizer were both set at 350°C. The corona was set to 4 μA. The flow rate of the drying gas and the pressure of the nebulizer were 3 l min^{-1} and 50 psi, respectively. Full-scan spectra were acquired over a scan range of m/z 80–1000 at 1.03 spectra s^{-1}. The derived sterols were identified with reference molecular weight and fragmentation spectra for known standards.

PHYLOGENETIC ANALYSIS

Protein sequences were aligned with the Clustal X 2.1 software (Larkin et al., 2007). Then, the neighbor-joining (NJ) tree was constructed using MEGA 5 software (Tamura et al., 2011). To assess the confidence of phylogenetic relationships, the bootstrap tests were conducted with 1000 resamplings.

KNOCKOUT OF *erg5* HOMOLOG GENE IN *FUSARIUM VERTICILLIOIDES*

In order to knockout *erg5* homologous genes (*erg5A*: FVEG_07284; *erg5B*: FVEG_08786) in *F. verticillioides*, the upstream and downstream flanking sequences of the FVEG_07284 and FVEG_08786 were amplified. The primer pairs were shown in **Table 2**.

The resulting PCR products were cloned into the plasmid pCX62 (Zhao et al., 2004) and results in knockout construct pCX62-ΔFv07284 and pCX62-ΔFv08786, in which the PCR products were ligated with the hygromycin phosphotransferase (*hph*) gene. Then, the deletion cassette was transformed into *F. verticillioides* 7600 and resulted in deletion mutants. Fungal transformation followed the protocol reported by Miller et al. (1985), with minor modification as described by Li et al. (2006).

RESULTS

TRANSCRIPTIONAL RESPONSES TO KETOCONAZOLE STRESS BY GENES INVOLVED IN ERGOSTEROL BIOSYNTHESIS

Genome-wide transcriptional responses to ketoconazole treatment from two independent experiments were analyzed by DGE method. For genes involved in ergosterol biosynthesis, seven were

Table 2 | Primer pairs used for knockout of *erg5* homolog gene in *F. verticillioides*.

Primers	Sequence (5′ → 3′)	Product size (bp)	Amplified region
Fv07284(p)F-*Xho*I	CCGCTCGAGCACCCGATGAACTCGCCAATA	1859	FVEG_07284 5′ flanking region
Fv07284(p)R-*Eco*RI	CGGAATTCATCATACGCAACGCAAAGAGC		
Fv07284(3)F-*Bam*HI	CGGGATCCATGATGGGAAAGCGAGTTGA	1717	FVEG_07284 3′ flanking region
Fv07284(3)R-*Xba*I	GCTCTAGAGCTGACAGCGACCAGTAGGA		
Fv08786(p)F-*Kpn*I	GCGGTACCCGAGGATGATTGCTTGGTGAG	1455	FVEG_08786 5′ flanking region
Fv08786(p)R-*Eco*RI	CGGAATTCCATGCTGGGTCTAGTTGAGGG		
Fv08786(3)F-*Xba*I	GCTCTAGAGGGGCAAGGTGTTTGTGAATA	1797	FVEG_08786 3′ flanking region
Fv08786(3)R-*Xba*I	GCTCTAGAAATGCCACTGAGTTCGGATG		

Table 3 | Transcriptional response to ketoconazole stress by genes involved in ergosterol biosynthesis in *N. crassa* wild type.

Locus	Gene	Function	TPM-wt1	TPM-wt(k)1	Fold [wt(k)1/wt1]	TPM-wt2	TPM-wt(k)2	Fold [wt(k)2/wt2]
NCU08280	*erg1*	Squalene epoxidase	78.1	34.6	0.44	16.1	27.4	1.70
NCU04156	*erg2*	Sterol biosynthesis	107.1	327.7	3.06	26.8	296.4	11.07
NCU06207	*erg3*	C-5 sterol desaturase	1000.3	767.0	0.77	639.5	999.0	1.56
NCU01333	*erg4*	C-24 reductase	1.4	0.6	0.42	1.4	2.0	1.36
NCU05278	*erg5*	C-22 sterol desaturase	67.4	308.9	4.58	83.5	174.6	2.09
NCU03006	*erg6*	C-24 sterol methyltransferase	23.8	791.5	33.20	19.3	174.6	9.06
NCU01119	*erg7*	Oxidosqualene:lanosterol cyclase/lanosterol synthase	34.0	11.3	0.33	23.0	4.5	0.19
NCU08671	*erg8*	Phosphomevalonate kinase	24.7	8.7	0.35	26.5	10.6	0.40
NCU06054	*erg9*	Squalene synthetase	21.1	14.7	0.70	10.1	14.6	1.44
NCU02571	*erg10*	Acetoacetyl-CoA thiolase	181.6	178.8	0.98	323.8	103.8	0.32
NCU02624	*erg11*	Cytochrome P450 lanosterol 14α-Demethylase	110.1	812.0	7.37	69.1	676.7	9.80
NCU03633	*erg12*	Mevalonate kinase	70.1	90.6	1.29	21.6	77.5	3.59
NCU03922	*erg13*	Hydroxymethylglutaryl-coenzyme A synthase	117.0	47.3	0.40	227.4	35.0	0.15
NCU11381	*erg19*	Mevalonate pyrophosphate decarboxylase	38.6	21.1	0.55	49.5	18.2	0.37
NCU01175	*erg20*	Polyprenyl synthetase	188.5	81.1	0.43	116.0	50.9	0.44
NCU08762	*erg24*	Sterol C-14 reductase	7.1	11.8	1.66	9.2	34.7	3.77
NCU06402	*erg25*	C-4 methyl sterol oxidase	2512.8	5111.7	2.03	2894.3	5348.9	1.85
NCU02693	*erg26*	C-3 sterol dehydrogenase	57.0	63.2	1.11	81.5	48.4	0.59
NCU05991	*erg27*	3-Keto sterol reductase	3.0	4.6	1.53	0.6	1.7	2.90
NCU04461	*erg28*	Endoplasmic reticulum membrane protein	67.7	28.9	0.43	30.2	33.3	1.10
NCU04144	*are2*	Acyl-CoA:sterol acyltransferase	1.4	1.4	1.05	0.6	0.1	0.17
NCU00712	*hmg1/hmg2*	Hydroxymethylglutaryl-coenzyme A reductase	14.8	8.1	0.55	9.8	10.1	1.03
NCU07719	*idi1*	Isopentenyl diphosphate isomerase	59.2	15.6	0.26	39.4	37.5	0.95
NCU08139	*mvd1*	Diphosphomevalonate decarboxylase	0	0	–	0	0	–

wt1 and wt(k)1 represent the first batch samples, wt2 and wt(k)2 represent the second batch samples; wt: wild type; wt(k): wild type treated with ketoconazole.

consistently upregulated while four consistently downregulated upon ketoconazole treatment in two independent experiments (**Table 3**). The most dramatically upregulated genes were *erg11* (NCU2624), *erg6* (NCU03006), *erg2* (NCU04156), and *erg5* (NCU05278), which were consistently increased upon ketoconazole treatment by at least three folds in two independent experiments. The consistently downregulated genes include *erg7* (NCU01119), *erg8* (NCU08671), *erg13* (NCU03922), and *erg20* (NCU11381). However, the transcriptional changes in these downregulated genes were less dramatic than those in *erg11*, *erg6*, *erg2*, and *erg5*. None of them had a transcriptional change higher than three folds.

DELETION OF *erg5* INCREASES AZOLE SUSCEPTIBILITY IN *N. CRASSA*

Six ketoconazole-responsive genes involved in ergosterol synthesis have the knockout mutants available in Fungal Genetics Stock Center. All these genes are ketoconazole-upregulated genes, including *erg2*, *erg3*, *erg5*, *erg6*, *erg24*, and *erg25*. On the solid medium without antifungal drugs, all deletion mutants had the growth rates similar to the wild-type strain and no obvious defect was observed in their asexual and sexual reproduction (the data not shown)[2]. Drug sensitivity test showed that the deletion of only

[2] http://www.broadinstitute.org/annotation/genome/neurospora/Phenotypes.html

erg5 altered the sensitivity to azoles. On agar plates, all three tested azoles, including ketoconazole, itraconazole, and fluconazole, had greater inhibition to the *erg5* mutants than the wild-type strain (**Figure 1**). MIC analysis in the liquid medium showed that MIC values of the *ERG5* mutants for ketoconazole, itraconazole, and fluconazole were only 60, 50, and 40% of that of the wild-type strain, respectively (**Table 4**).

DELETION OF *erg5* DOES NOT CAUSE ACCUMULATION OF 14α-METHYLATED STEROLS DURING KETOCONAZOLE STRESS IN *N. CRASSA*

ERG5 catalyzes the biosynthesis of ergosta 5,7,22,24(28)-trienol, a direct precursor for ergosterol biosynthesis. ERG5 mutations caused accumulation of ergosta 5,7,24(28)-trienol and ergosta 5,7-dienol in *S. cerevisiae ERG5* deletion mutant (Barton et al., 1974; Skaggs et al., 1996). Thus, it is possible that the *erg5* mutant might accumulate more toxic 14α-methylated sterols than the wild-type strain. To test this possibility, a comparative analysis of sterol profiles between the *erg5* mutant and the wild type was performed by HPLC-MS. Our results showed that, in the normal liquid medium without ketoconazole, the *erg5* mutant produced more ergosta 5,7-dienol than the wild-type strain. As expected, ergosterol in the *erg5* mutant was almost undetectable (**Figure 2**). When treated with ketoconazole, 4,4-dimethyl-ergosta 8,14,24(28)-trienol, the direct product catalyzed by ERG11 (lanosterol 14α-methylase), was reduced in the wild-type strain and the *erg5* mutant at the similar level. Ketoconazole treatment greatly increased levels of 14α-methylated sterols, such as eburicol and 14α-methyl-ergosta-8,24(28)-dien-3β, 6α-diol, in both the wild-type strain and the *erg5* mutant (**Figure 2**). However, the levels of these compounds were similar between the wild-type strain and the *erg5* mutant, suggesting that the azole-hypersensitive phenotype in the *erg5* mutant is not due to over-accumulation of 14α-methylated sterols.

ERG5 HOMOLOGS ARE HIGHLY CONSERVED IN FUNGAL KINGDOM

To gain an insight into the sequence conservation and phylogenic relationship of ERG5 homologs in fungi, Blast and phylogenetic analysis were conducted. Blast analysis revealed that ERG5 homologs are high conserved in amino acid sequences. Phylogenetic analysis with amino acid sequences of 27 ERG5 homologs (*E* value = 0; Alignment coverage >90%; sequence similarity >76%) from 3 yeast fungal species (*C. albicans, S. cerevisiae, Schizosaccharomyces pombe*) and 16 filamentous fungal species showed that all ERG5 homologs were clustered into 2 big clades (**Figure 3**). The ERG5 homologs from yeast fungal species were distributed in the first clade (clade I), which represents the most ancestral group, while those from filamentous fungal species were located in the second clade (clade II).

As shown in **Figure 3**, ERG5 in filamentous fungi can be further categorized into two classes based on their phylogenic relationship, namely Type IIA and Type IIB, respectively. *N. crassa, N. fischeri, A. niger, A. nidulans, T. reesei, M. grisea*, and *V. albo-atrum* have only one *erg5* gene, all in Type IIA. *A. fumigatus, A. oryzae*, and *A. clavatus* and all examined *Fusarium* species have two *erg5* genes, one in Type IIA and the other in Type IIB. *A. terreus* is the only species that has three *erg5* genes, two in Type IIA and one in Type IIB. Similar to ERG5, multiple ERG3 and ERG11 homologs were also found in *Aspergillus* and *Fusarium* species (Ferreira et al., 2005; Liu et al., 2010; Becher et al., 2011).

DELETION OF *erg5* INCREASES AZOLE SUSCEPTIBILITY IN *F. VERTICILLIOIDES*

To see if ERG5 in other filamentous fungi also mediate azole sensitivity, gene knockout mutants for Type IIA *erg5* gene *erg5A* (FVEG_07284) and for Type IIB *erg5* gene *erg5B* (FVEG_08786), in the pathogenic fungus *F. verticillioides* were generated. As shown in **Figure 4**, on the medium without drug, the growth rates of the *erg5* deletion mutants were similar to that of the wild-type strain and no defect in conidiation was observed in the mutants. When inoculated on the medium with 0.5 μg/ml ketoconazole, both *erg5A* and *erg5B* mutant displayed greater growth inhibition than the wild-type strain, indicating the ERG5 homologs have similar roles in azole resistance among different fungal species.

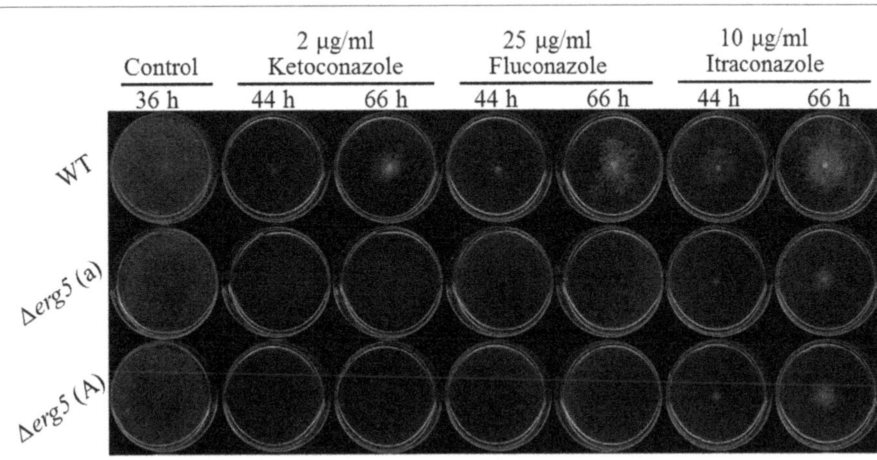

FIGURE 1 | Drug susceptibility analysis of the *erg5* knockout mutant of *N. crassa*. Two microliters of conidial suspension (1 × 104) conidia/ml were inoculated on the center of plates (Φ = 9 cm) with or without antifungal drugs, then incubated at 28°C for 66 h. Each test had three replicates and the experiment was independently repeated twice.

DISCUSSION

Although transcriptional responses by genes of sterol biosynthesis to azole stress have been observed in many fungal species (Bammert and Fostel, 2000; De Backer et al., 2001; Agarwal et al., 2003; Liu et al., 2005, 2010; da Silva Ferreira et al., 2006; Yu et al., 2007; Becher et al., 2011; Florio et al., 2011), it is still mysterious about the biological significance of transcriptional activation for most of these genes. Taking advantage of the availability of knockout mutants of *N. crassa*, we analyzed the contributions of six ketoconazole-responsive genes in ergosterol biosynthesis, including *erg2*, *erg3*, *erg5*, *erg6*, *erg24*, and *erg25*, to azole resistance, and demonstrated that deletion of *erg5*, but not other ergosterol genes, could make *N. crassa* more susceptible to antifungal azoles. Since the deletion of *erg5* should result in an effect opposite to its overexpression, transcriptional increase of *erg5* upon azole stress might positively contribute to the azole resistance. As *erg5* deletion consistently resulted in azole hypersensitivity in both *N. crassa* and *F. verticillioides*, strategies that either silencing the expression of *erg5* or disrupting C-22 sterol desaturase (ERG5) activity can make fungal pathogens more susceptible to antifungal azoles. ERG5, thus, can be a promising target for antifungal drug design or fungal disease management in crops. Although no alteration in azole sensitivity was observed in the mutants for the rest of ergosterol biosynthesis genes, their transcriptional increases during azole treatment suggest that these genes are involved in the adaptation to azole stress. Their contributions to azole resistance might be able to be detected by combined mutation of multiple genes. Nevertheless, *erg5* is the most important contributor to azole resistance among these azole-responsive genes.

Table 4 | MIC of the *erg5* mutant and wild type for azoles.

	MIC for ketoconazole (μg/ml)	MIC for fluconazole (μg/ml)	MIC for itraconazole (μg/ml)
WT	2.5 ± 0	31.25 ± 0	5.0 ± 0
Δ*erg5 (a)*	1.5 ± 0	12.5 ± 0	2.5 ± 0
Δ*erg5 (A)*	1.5 ± 0	12.5 ± 0	2.5 ± 0

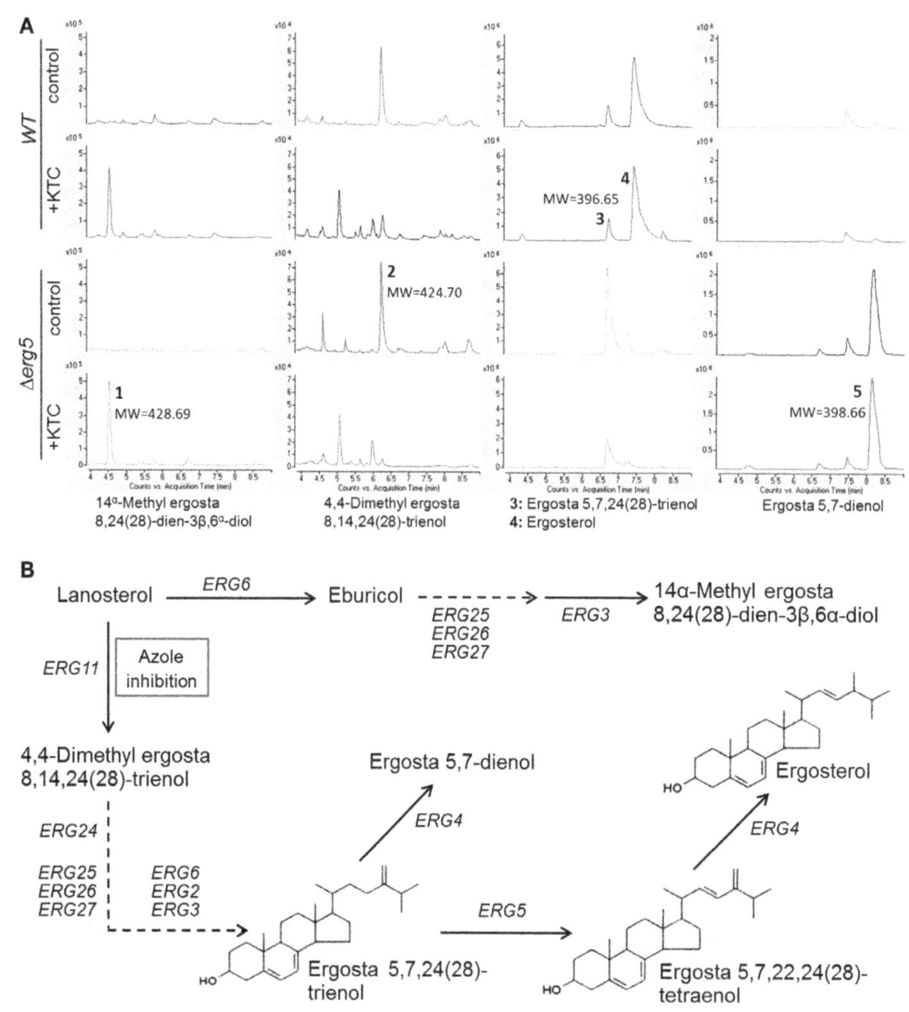

FIGURE 2 | HPLC-MS chromatogram of sterol extracts (A) and schematic representation of the ergosterol biosynthetic pathway (B) in *N. crassa*.

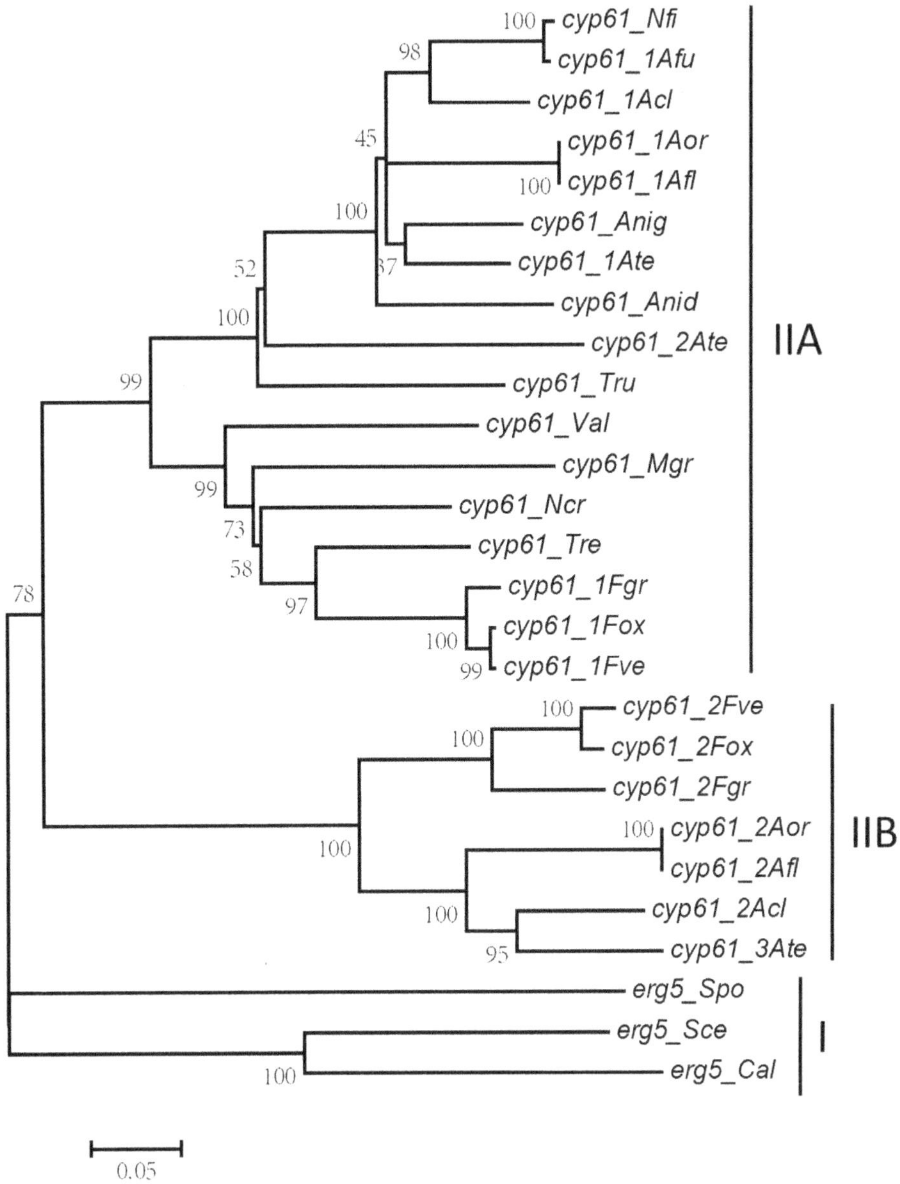

FIGURE 3 | Phylogenic analysis of fungal ERG5 homologs. Predicted REG5 proteins from 19 fungal species were aligned and a condensed neighbor-joining (NJ) tree was constructed with cut-off bootstrap values of 50% obtained from 1000 replicates using MEGA 5 software (Tamura et al., 2011). (*Cal, C. albicans*; *Sce, S. cerevisiae*; *Spo, S. pombe*; *Ncr, N. crassa*; *Afu, A. fumigatus*; *Afl, A. flavus*; *Anid, A. nidulans*; *Anig, A. niger*; *Acl, A. clavatus*; *Ate, A. terreus*; *Aor, A. oryzae*; *Nfi, N. fischeri*; *Fve, F. verticillioides*; *Fox, F. oxysporum*; *Fgr, F. graminearum*; *Tru, T. rubrum*; *Val, V. albo-atrum*; *Tre, T. reesei*; *Mag, M. grisea*).

Membrane sterols regulate membrane fluidity, permeability, the activity of membrane-bound enzymes and growth rate (Skaggs et al., 1996). In *S. cerevisiae*, genes involved in early steps of ergosterol biosynthesis, such as *ERG9* (squalene synthase), *ERG1* (squalene epoxidase), *ERG7* (lanosterol synthase), *ERG11* (lanosterol 14α demethylase), and *ERG24* (C-14 reductase), are essential, while genes participating the late steps of ergosterol biosynthesis, such as *ERG2*, *ERG3*, *ERG6*, *ERG5*, *ERG25*, and *ERG4*, are not essential (Fryberg et al., 1973; Lees et al., 1995). In *N. crassa*, viable homokaryotic mutants for only these non-essential genes were generated. Thus, the end-product ergosterol is not necessary for fungal survival. When ergosterol is absent, other sterol intermediates might function as substitutes of ergosterol. Similar to previous observation in *S. cerevisiae* (Kelly et al., 1995), our data showed that disruption of lanosterol 14α-demethylase by ketoconazole reduced 4,4-dimethyl-ergosta 8,14,24(28)-trienol biosynthesis and accumulated 14α methylated sterols such as 14α-methyl-ergosta-8,24(28)-dien-3,6-diol. ERG5 catalyzes the chemical reaction downstream to 4,4-dimethyl-ergosta 8,14,24(28)-trienol biosynthesis. As shown in **Figure 2**, deletion of *erg5*

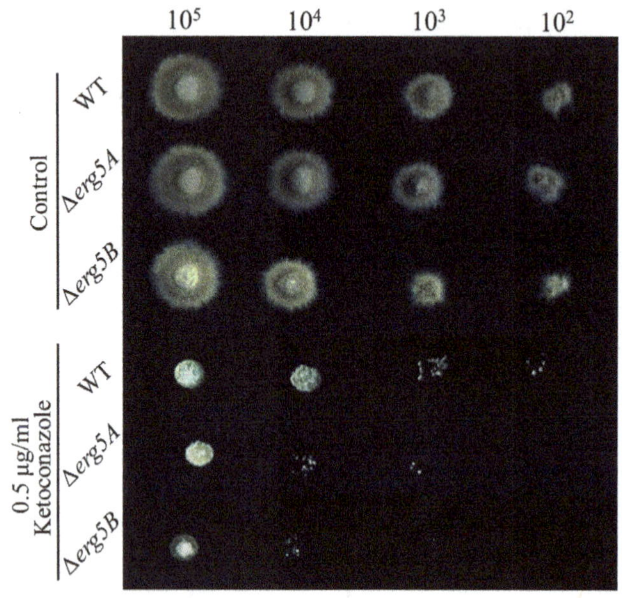

FIGURE 4 | Drug susceptibility analysis of the *erg5A* (FVEG_07284) and *erg5B* (FVEG_08786) knockout mutants of *F. verticillioides*. Two microliters of conidial suspensions with different concentration (1 × 105, 1 × 104, 1 × 103, or 1 × 102 conidia/ml, respectively) were inoculated on the plates (Φ = 9 cm) with or without antifungal drugs, and incubated at 28°C for 72 h. Each test had three replicates and the experiment was independently repeated twice.

is not likely to reduce the biosynthesis of 4,4-dimethyl-ergosta 8,14,24(28)-trienol under ketoconazole stress. Therefore, the azole-hypersensitive phenotype in *erg5* mutants is not related to the biosynthesis of 4,4-dimethyl-ergosta 8,14,24(28)-trienol. In addition, deletion of *erg5* did not lead an increase in accumulation of 14α-methylated sterols upon ketoconazole stress. Thus, over-accumulation of 14α-methylated sterols is also not a possible cause to the azole-hypersensitive phenotype in *erg5* mutants. An *in vitro* experiment has shown that ketoconazole can bind to ERG5 (CYP61) of *S. cerevisiae* with an affinity similar to that of ERG11 (Kelly et al., 1997). Binding of azole to ERG5 might reduce the concentration of azoles attacking ERG11, providing a protective buffer to ERG11. If it is true, removal of *erg5* will increase azole sensitivity. In addition, when ergosterol is absent, localization of some membrane proteins, such as azole pumps, might be affected and make cells accumulate more azoles. The real mechanism requires further investigation.

In summary, this study reported azole sensitivities of knockout mutants for 6 azole-responsive genes involved in ergosterol biosynthesis and demonstrated that deletion of *erg5* increase azole sensitivity in both *N. crassa* and *F. verticillioides*. Our findings provide a new insight into in the mechanism of azole resistance.

ACKNOWLEDGMENTS

This project is supported by grants 31170087 (to Shaojie Li) and 31000551 (to Xianyun Sun) from National Natural Science Foundation of China and a "100 Talent Program" grant from Chinese Academy of Sciences (to Shaojie Li).

REFERENCES

Abe, F., Usui, K., and Hiraki, T. (2009). Fluconazole modulates membrane rigidity, heterogeneity, and water penetration into the plasma membrane in *Saccharomyces cerevisiae*. *Biochemistry* 48, 8494–8504.

Agarwal, A. K., Rogers, P. D., Baerson, S. R., Jacob, M. R., Barker, K. S., Cleary, J. D., et al. (2003). Genome-wide expression profiling of the response to polyene, pyrimidine, azole, and echinocandin antifungal agents in *Saccharomyces cerevisiae*. *J. Biol. Chem.* 278, 34998–35015.

Bammert, G. F., and Fostel, J. M. (2000). Genome-wide expression patterns in *Saccharomyces cerevisiae*: comparison of drug treatments and genetic alterations affecting biosynthesis of ergosterol. *Antimicrob. Agents Chemother.* 44, 1255–1265.

Barton, D. H. R., Corrie, J. E. T., Widdowson, D. A., Bard, M., and Woods, R. A. (1974). Biosynthesis of terpenes and steroids. IX. The sterols of some mutant yeasts and their relationship to the biosynthesis of ergosterol. *J. Chem. Soc. Perkin Trans. I* 1, 1326–1333.

Becher, R., Weihmann, F., Deising, H., and Wirsel, S. (2011). Development of a novel multiplex DNA microarray for *Fusarium graminearum* and analysis of azole fungicide responses. *BMC Genomics* 12:52. doi:10.1186/1471-2164-12-52

Bossche, H. V., Lauwers, W., Willemsens, G., Marichal, P., Cornelissen, F., and Cools, W. (1984). Molecular basis for the antimycotic and antibacterial activity of N-substituted imidazoles and triazoles: the inhibition of isoprenoid biosynthesis. *Pestic. Sci.* 15, 188–198.

Cañabate-Díaz, B., Segura Carretero, A., Fernández-Gutiérrez, A., Belmonte Vega, A., Garrido Frenich, A., Martínez Vidal, J. L., et al. (2007). Separation and determination of sterols in olive oil by HPLC-MS. *Food Chem.* 102, 593–598.

Ferreira, M. E., Colombo, A. L., Paulsen, I., Ren, Q., Wortman, J., Huang, J., et al. (2005). The ergosterol biosynthesis pathway, transporter genes, and azole resistance in *Aspergillus fumigatus*. *Med. Mycol.* 43, 313–319.

De Backer, M. D., Ilyina, T., Ma, X.-J., Vandoninck, S., Luyten, W. H. M. L., and Vanden Bossche, H. (2001). Genomic profiling of the response of *Candida albicans* to itraconazole treatment using a DNA microarray. *Antimicrob. Agents Chemother.* 45, 1660–1670.

Du, W., Coaker, M., Sobel, J., and Akins, R. (2004). Shuttle vectors for *Candida albicans*: control of plasmid copy number and elevated expression of cloned genes. *Curr. Genet.* 45, 390–398.

da Silva Ferreira, M., Malavazi, I., Savoldi, M., Brakhage, A., Goldman, M., Kim, H. S., et al. (2006). Transcriptome analysis of *Aspergillus fumigatus* exposed to voriconazole. *Curr. Genet.* 50, 32–44.

Florio, A., Ferrari, S., De Carolis, E., Torelli, R., Fadda, G., Sanguinetti, M., et al. (2011). Genome-wide expression profiling of the response to short-term exposure to fluconazole in *Cryptococcus neoformans* serotype A. *BMC Microbiol.* 11:97. doi:10.1186/1471-2180-11-97

Fryberg, M., Oehlschlager, A. C., and Unrau, A. M. (1973). Biosynthesis of ergosterol in yeast. Evidence for multiple pathways. *J. Am. Chem. Soc.* 95, 5747–5757.

Hamamoto, H., Hasegawa, K., Nakaune, R., Lee, Y. J., Makizumi, Y., Akutsu, K., et al. (2000). Tandem repeat of a transcriptional enhancer upstream of the sterol 14α-demethylase gene (*CYP51*) in *Penicillium digitatum*. *Appl. Environ. Microbiol.* 66, 3421–3426.

Kelly, S. L., Arnoldi, A., and Kelly, D. E. (1993). Molecular genetic analysis of azole antifungal mode of action. *Biochem. Soc. Trans.* 21, 1034–1038.

Kelly, S. L., Lamb, D. C., Baldwin, B. C., Corran, A. J., and Kelly, D. E. (1997). Characterization of *Saccharomyces cerevisiae CYP61*, sterol Δ22-desaturase, and inhibition by azole antifungal agents. . *J. Biol. Chem.* 272, 9986–9988.

Kelly, S. L., Lamb, D. C., Corran, A. J., Baldwin, B. C., and Kelly, D. E. (1995). Mode of action and resistance to azole antifungals associated with the formation of 14α-methylergosta-8,24(28)-dien-3β,6α-diol. *Biochem. Biophys. Res. Commun.* 207, 910–915.

Larkin, M. A., Blackshields, G., Brown, N. P., Chenna, R., McGettigan, P. A., McWilliam, H., et al. (2007). Clustal W and Clustal X version 2.0. *Bioinformatics* 23, 2947–2948.

Lees, N. D., Skaggs, B., Kirsch, D. R., and Bard, M. (1995). Cloning of the late genes in the ergosterol biosynthetic pathway of *Saccharomyces cerevisiae* – a review. *Lipids* 30, 221–226.

Li, S., Myung, K., Guse, D., Donkin, B., Proctor, R. H., Grayburn, W. S., et al. (2006). FvVE1 regulates filamentous growth, the ratio of microconidia to macroconidia and cell wall formation in *Fusarium verticillioides. Mol. Microbiol.* 62, 1418–1432.

Liu, T., Lee, R., Barker, K., Lee, R., Wei, L., Homayouni, R., et al. (2005). Genome-wide expression profiling of the response to azole, polyene, echinocandin, and pyrimidine antifungal agents in *Candida albicans. Antimicrob. Agents Chemother.* 49, 2226–2236.

Liu, X., Jiang, J., Shao, J., Yin, Y., and Ma, Z. (2010). Gene transcription profiling of *Fusarium graminearum* treated with an azole fungicide tebuconazole. *Appl. Microbiol. Biotechnol.* 85, 1105–1114.

Ma, Z., Proffer, T. J., Jacobs, J. L., and Sundin, G. W. (2006). Overexpression of the 14α-demethylase target gene (*CYP51*) mediates fungicide resistance in *Blumeriella jaapii. Appl. Environ. Microbiol.* 72, 2581–2585.

Martel, C. M., Parker, J. E., Bader, O., Weig, M., Gross, U., Warrilow, A. G. S., et al. (2010a). A clinical isolate of *Candida albicans* with mutations in *ERG11* (encoding sterol 14α-demethylase) and *ERG5* (encoding C22 desaturase) is cross resistant to azoles and amphotericin B. *Antimicrob. Agents Chemother.* 54, 3578–3583.

Martel, C. M., Parker, J. E., Bader, O., Weig, M., Gross, U., Warrilow, A. G. S., et al. (2010b). Identification and characterization of four azole-resistant *erg3* mutants of *Candida albicans. Antimicrob. Agents Chemother.* 54, 4527–4533.

Miller, B. L., Miller, K. Y., and Timberlake, W. E. (1985). Direct and indirect gene replacements in *Aspergillus nidulans. Mol. Cell. Biol.* 5, 1714–1721.

Morio, F., Pagniez, F., Lacroix, C., Miegeville, M., and Le Pape, P. (2012). Amino acid substitutions in the *Candida albicans* sterol Δ5,6-desaturase (Erg3p) confer azole resistance: characterization of two novel mutants with impaired virulence. *J. Antimicrob. Chemother.* 67, 2131–2138.

Nielsen, K. L., Høgh, A. L., and Emmersen, J. (2006). DeepSAGE – digital transcriptomics with high sensitivity, simple experimental protocol and multiplexing of samples. *Nucleic Acids Res.* 34, e133.

Schnabel, G., and Jones, A. L. (2001). The 14α-demethylase(*CYP51A1*) gene is overexpressed in *Venturia inaequalis* strains resistant to myclobutanil. *Phytopathology* 91, 102–110.

Skaggs, B. A., Alexander, J. F., Pierson, C. A., Schweitzer, K. S., Chun, K. T., Koegel, C., et al. (1996). Cloning and characterization of the *Saccharomyces cerevisiae* C-22 sterol desaturase gene, encoding a second cytochrome P-450 involved in ergosterol biosynthesis. *Gene* 169, 105–109.

Sun, X., Zhang, H., Zhang, Z., Wang, Y., and Li, S. (2011). Involvement of a helix-loop-helix transcription factor CHC-1 in CO(2)-mediated conidiation suppression in *Neurospora crassa. Fungal Genet. Biol.* 48, 1077–1086.

Tamura, K., Peterson, D., Peterson, N., Stecher, G., Nei, M., and Kumar, S. (2011). MEGA5: molecular evolutionary genetics analysis using maximum likelihood, evolutionary distance, and maximum parsimony methods. *Mol. Biol. Evol.* 28, 2731–2739.

Vale-Silva, L. A., Coste, A. T., Ischer, F., Parker, J. E., Kelly, S. L., Pinto, E., et al. (2012). Azole resistance by loss of function of the sterol Δ5,6-desaturase gene (*ERG3*) in *Candida albicans* does not necessarily decrease virulence. *Antimicrob. Agents Chemother.* 56, 1960–1968.

Vogel, H. J. (1956). A convenient growth medium for *Neurospora* (Medium N). *Microb. Genet. Bull.* 13, 42–43.

Watson, P. F., Rose, M. E., Ellis, S. W., England, H., and Kelly, S. L. (1989). Defective sterol C5-6 desaturation and azole resistance: a new hypothesis for the mode of action of azole antifungals. *Biochem. Biophys. Res. Commun.* 164, 1170–1175.

Yu, L., Zhang, W., Wang, L., Yang, J., Liu, T., Peng, J., et al. (2007). Transcriptional profiles of the response to ketoconazole and amphotericin B in *Trichophyton rubrusm. Antimicrob. Agents Chemother.* 51, 144–153.

Zhao, X., Xue, C., Kim, Y., and Xu, J. (2004). A Ligation-PCR approach for generating gene replacement constructs in *Magnaporthe grisea. Fungal Genet. Newsl.* 51, 17–18.

8

Novel resistance functions uncovered using functional metagenomic investigations of resistance reservoirs

Erica C. Pehrsson*[1]*, Kevin J. Forsberg*[1]*, Molly K. Gibson*[1]*, Sara Ahmadi*[1,2] *and Gautam Dantas*[1,2,3]**

[1] *Center for Genome Sciences and Systems Biology, Washington University School of Medicine, St. Louis, MO, USA*
[2] *Department of Pathology and Immunology, Washington University School of Medicine, St. Louis, MO, USA*
[3] *Department of Biomedical Engineering, Washington University, St. Louis, MO, USA*

Edited by:
Marilyn C. Roberts, University of Washington, USA

Reviewed by:
Gerry Wright, McMaster University, Canada
George Jacoby, Lahey Clinic, USA

****Correspondence:***
Gautam Dantas, Center for Genome Sciences and Systems Biology, Washington University School of Medicine, 4444 Forest Park Blvd., 6th floor, Campus Box 8510, St. Louis, MO 63108, USA
e-mail: dantas@wustl.edu

Rates of infection with antibiotic-resistant bacteria have increased precipitously over the past several decades, with far-reaching healthcare and societal costs. Recent evidence has established a link between antibiotic resistance genes in human pathogens and those found in non-pathogenic, commensal, and environmental organisms, prompting deeper investigation of natural and human-associated reservoirs of antibiotic resistance. Functional metagenomic selections, in which shotgun-cloned DNA fragments are selected for their ability to confer survival to an indicator host, have been increasingly applied to the characterization of many antibiotic resistance reservoirs. These experiments have demonstrated that antibiotic resistance genes are highly diverse and widely distributed, many times bearing little to no similarity to known sequences. Through unbiased selections for survival to antibiotic exposure, functional metagenomics can improve annotations by reducing the discovery of false-positive resistance and by allowing for the identification of previously unrecognizable resistance genes. In this review, we summarize the novel resistance functions uncovered using functional metagenomic investigations of natural and human-impacted resistance reservoirs. Examples of novel antibiotic resistance genes include those highly divergent from known sequences, those for which sequence is entirely unable to predict resistance function, bifunctional resistance genes, and those with unconventional, atypical resistance mechanisms. Overcoming antibiotic resistance in the clinic will require a better understanding of existing resistance reservoirs and the dissemination networks that govern horizontal gene exchange, informing best practices to limit the spread of resistance-conferring genes to human pathogens.

Keywords: functional metagenomics, antibiotic resistance, bifunctional resistance gene, environmental resistance, resistance reservoir, transferable resistance

OVERVIEW

It is estimated that infection with antibiotic-resistant pathogens incurs over $25 billion in societal and healthcare costs annually in the United States (CDC, 2011). More than 70% of hospital-acquired bacterial infections are currently resistant to at least one of the major antibiotics used as standard treatment (Stone, 2009), and patient deaths as a result of hospital-acquired infections have increased by over 675% during the past 20 years (NIAID, 2012). As the incidence and spectrum of antibiotic resistance increases (Arias and Murray, 2009), antibiotic development has slowed to a trickle (Spellberg et al., 2008), further hindering the effectiveness of antibiotics to treat infectious disease. The majority of acquired antibiotic resistance genes in bacterial pathogens are obtained via horizontal gene transfer (HGT) (Ochman et al., 2000), likely with environmental origins (Benveniste and Davies, 1973; Wright, 2010; D'Costa et al., 2011). Accordingly, an increasing impetus has been placed on cataloging antibiotic resistance reservoirs (Allen et al., 2009b, 2010), determining how resistance genes are most readily transferred to the clinic (Marshall and Levy, 2011; Smillie et al., 2011), and identifying resistance mechanisms heretofore unseen in clinical settings (Jeon et al., 2011; Tao et al., 2012).

TRADITIONAL MECHANISMS OF ANTIBIOTIC RESISTANCE

An antibiotic-resistant phenotype can be either an acquired trait or intrinsic to the bacterium in question. In the case of intrinsic resistance, antibiotic therapy is rendered ineffective due to a pre-existing physiological trait of the species, such as reduced accessibility to or absence of a drug target (Alekshun and Levy, 2007; Martinez, 2008; Davies and Davies, 2010; Dantas and Sommer, 2012). Examples of intrinsic antibiotic resistance include vancomycin tolerance in Gram-negative bacteria (the outer cell membrane reduces access to the peptidoglycan target) (Arthur and Courvalin, 1993) and biofilm formation in numerous organisms (perhaps providing resistance via reduced drug penetration and/or altered microenvironments) (Stewart and Costerton, 2001). Conversely, acquired antibiotic resistance stems from the expression of a specific resistance gene and is commonly the result of *de novo* mutation or the acquisition of resistance-conferring genes on mobile genetic elements (e.g., plasmids, transposons, integrons) (Walsh, 2003). The antibiotic resistance genes present in a microbial community that are capable of transfer to a new host are collectively referred to as the "transferable resistome." Intrinsic resistance is, by definition, limited to the context of the parent organism, whereas acquired resistance represents a more flexible phenotype, and its prevalence is more immediately responsive to selection pressure (Martinez, 2008). As nearly all infectious bacteria were antibiotic-susceptible prior to the introduction of antibiotic therapy (Houndt and Ochman, 2000; Davies and Davies, 2010), the exceeding majority of resistance in human pathogens is acquired, either through mutation or HGT (Alekshun and Levy, 2007). This resistance represents a diversity of biochemical mechanisms that break down into three general categories (Walsh, 2000, 2003): (1) inactivation of the antibiotic, (2) reducing intracellular antibiotic concentration through efflux or permeability barriers, and (3) altering the cellular target of the antibiotic, reducing their association.

Perhaps the most intuitive of resistance mechanisms, antibiotic inactivation, is sub-categorized into two groups: enzymes that inactivate drugs via degradation (e.g., the β-lactamases) vs. those that function via chemical modification. The β-lactamases are characterized by their ability to cleave the four-membered ring present in all β-lactam antibiotics and are some of the best-studied and widely-distributed antibiotic resistance genes (for review, see Jacoby and Munoz-Price, 2005). These enzymes confer high-level antibiotic resistance and are found associated with mobile DNA elements and integrated into bacterial chromosomes. β-lactamases function via either a serine active site or metal cation cofactor (Jacoby and Munoz-Price, 2005) and can be found across bacterial phyla. Antibiotic-modifying enzymes are also phylogenetically widespread, as well as mechanistically diverse. These enzymes can confer tolerance toward numerous drugs, including the aminoglycoside (Davies and Wright, 1997), tetracycline (Yang et al., 2004), amphenicol (Schwarz et al., 2004), and macrolide-lincosamide-streptogramin (Weisblum, 1998) antibiotics, typically functioning via covalent modification of the drug with some functional moiety (e.g., acetyl, phosphoryl, nucleotidyl, glycosyl, and hydroxyl groups) (Alekshun and Levy, 2007).

The intracellular concentration of any given antibiotic can be reduced by either efflux mechanisms to remove the drug from the cytosol or permeability barriers that limit the drug's uptake. Many antibiotics have poor activity against Gram-negative pathogens due to efflux systems (Levy, 1992), most notably the RND superfamily transporters (Li and Nikaido, 2004, 2009). Other major families of efflux systems include the MFS, SMR, and ABC superfamily transporters, which are present in both Gram-negative and -positive organisms (Li and Nikaido, 2004, 2009). Although commonly chromosomal, many efflux systems are found on plasmids and other mobile elements and can confer drug-specific, class-specific, or multidrug resistance (Poole, 2005). Some permeability barriers, such as the Gram-negative outer membrane (Arthur and Courvalin, 1993), represent intrinsic antibiotic resistance, while in other instances, permeability barriers are acquired. Examples include multidrug-resistance via the altered expression of Gram-negative porin proteins (e.g., OmpF in *Escherichia coli* and OprD in *Pseudomonas*) (Delcour, 2009) and glycopeptide resistance due to thickened Gram-positive cell walls (Cui et al., 2006).

Antibiotic resistance via cellular target modification often occurs via chromosomal mutation and represents a common means by which the fluoroquinolone, sulfonamide, and trimethroprim antibiotics, among others, are tolerated (Alekshun and Levy, 2007). In the case of the fluoroquinolones, mutations to a variety of residues within the quinolone-resistance-determining-region (QRDR) of the DNA gyrase GyrA or topoisomerase IV ParC/GrlA prevent the interaction of the synthetic antibiotic with its target, facilitating resistance (Hooper, 1999). Importantly, resistance to fluoroquinolones via mutation is typically recessive, suppressing the acquisition of a resistant phenotype in the presence of wild-type GyrA or ParC/GrlA and thus preventing widespread horizontal dissemination of resistant gene variants (Wolfson and Hooper, 1989; Soussy et al., 1993). However, a plasmid-borne GyrA protection protein, Qnr, has been discovered that confers low-level fluoroquinolone resistance (Tran and Jacoby, 2002) and can potentiate the incidence of QRDR mutations, which combined provide high levels of resistance (Jacoby, 2005). Both the sulfonamides and trimethroprim competitively inhibit enzymes within the folate biosynthesis pathway: mutations to the dihydropteroate synthase and dihydrofolate reductase (DHFR) enzymes can reduce affinity for sulfonamides and trimethroprim, respectively, and provide tolerance to the antibiotics (Huovinen et al., 1995). In addition to arising *de novo*, both sulfonamide- and trimethroprim-resistant enzymes are present on mobile DNA elements, providing resistance to numerous bacteria via HGT (Alekshun and Levy, 2007). Other highly mobile mechanisms of target-modification include vancomycin resistance via the modification of peptidoglycan precursors (Bugg et al., 1991), aminoglycoside resistance via methylation of the 16S rRNA subunit (Galimand et al., 2003), and macrolide resistance from 23S rRNA methylases (Zhanel et al., 2001).

RESERVOIRS OF TRANSFERABLE ANTIBIOTIC RESISTANCE

Research on antibiotic resistance over the past 70 years has focused on traditionally pathogenic bacteria isolated in a clinical setting and the role of antibiotic resistance genes already present in those species (Sommer et al., 2009; Davies and Davies, 2010). The resistance phenotype, however, is an ancient function of environmental bacteria (D'Costa et al., 2011), despite being largely absent from human pathogens prior to the antibiotic age (Hughes and Datta, 1983; Houndt and Ochman, 2000), with estimates that β-lactamases have existed for over 2 billion years (Hall and Barlow, 2004; Hall et al., 2004). Moreover, diverse mechanisms of antibiotic resistance have been discovered in nearly all environments (D'Costa et al., 2006; Allen et al., 2010; Davies and Davies, 2010; Wright, 2010); seemingly each new metagenomic study uncovers numerous examples of resistance genes previously unreported in public databases (Allen et al., 2009b; Sommer et al., 2009; Donato et al., 2010; Forsberg et al., 2012). In short, the diversity and abundance of antibiotic resistance in commensal microbiota and environmental settings dwarfs that which is seen in the context of human pathogens.

Importantly, environmental antibiotic resistance is not only widespread, but also represents the likely origins of the resistance seen in human pathogens. It has been known for 40 years that environmental bacteria share the same resistance mechanisms as those seen in pathogens (Benveniste and Davies, 1973), with documented examples of environmental resistance genes moving from natural settings into human pathogens (Poirel et al., 2002, 2005). It is becoming increasingly evident that human pathogens and environmental organisms share antibiotic resistance genes; a recent study described seven resistance genes from non-pathogenic soil organisms, conferring tolerance to five antibiotic classes, with perfect identity to genes from phylogenetically and geographically diverse pathogens (Forsberg et al., 2012). Given the staggering diversity of environmental resistance, high adaptability of bacteria, and strong selection pressure for antibiotic resistance, the question of antibiotic resistance is "not a matter of if but only a matter of when" (Walsh, 2000).

To understand *when* novel resistance will appear in human pathogens and perhaps diminish its impact, one must understand *how* new resistance genes are most frequently acquired by pathogenic bacteria. Since the answer is, most commonly, *via HGT* (Hughes and Datta, 1983; Ochman et al., 2000; Alekshun and Levy, 2007), understanding the complement of resistance genes most likely to be transferred to pathogens is crucial to predicting resistance acquisition. Although cataloging the repertoire of resistance genes on Earth remains a prohibitively large undertaking, techniques for interrogating the resistance properties of complex microbial communities exist and are being applied toward the identification of diverse and novel resistance from numerous settings. Importantly, these studies are focused not only on environmental locales, but also on the resistomes associated with human and animal microbiota (Shoemaker et al., 2001; Sommer et al., 2010b; Sommer and Dantas, 2011). Although antibiotic resistance may have its origins in the environment (Benveniste and Davies, 1973; Wright, 2010; D'Costa et al., 2011), the commensal resistome shares many resistance genes with both pathogens (Sommer et al., 2010b) and environmental organisms (Forsberg et al., 2012) and represents a likely route through which these populations exchange resistance genes (Smillie et al., 2011; Sommer and Dantas, 2011). Focused efforts to understand how pathogens acquire antibiotic resistance will require a greater appreciation for the diversity of resistance genes and in which environments and under what conditions these resistance genes are most accessible to human pathogens.

INTERROGATING ANTIBIOTIC RESISTANCE PROPERTIES IN COMPLEX MICROBIAL COMMUNITIES

Traditionally, either culture-based (D'Costa et al., 2006) or PCR-based approaches (Perez-Perez and Hanson, 2002) have been used to study antibiotic resistance properties from microbial communities. While both techniques have led to major discoveries (Galan et al., 2013), both have inherent limitations that have contributed to an under-sampling of resistance genes from diverse microbial habitats. The majority of bacteria remain recalcitrant to culturing (Daniel, 2005) and are therefore not interrogated when culture-dependent techniques are employed. Additionally, linking a resistance phenotype to a causal genotype is a time-consuming process, often necessitating experimental scope to be limited to a small number of organisms, rather than whole communities. PCR screens are an effective means to identify or quantify resistance genes of known sequence, circumventing the need for culture (Knapp et al., 2010), but are only able to detect previously described genes and often require expression cloning and subsequent experimentation to verify function. In addition, annotation of antibiotic resistance genes in shotgun-sequenced microbial communities has proven challenging, as homology-based functional gene comparisons often fail due to low sequence similarity to previously discovered resistance genes, and *in silico* analyses are unable to confirm resistance function.

In contrast with standard techniques, *functional metagenomics* is a culture- and sequence-independent means of identifying transferrable antibiotic resistance in complex metagenomes. This method (**Figure 1**) involves shotgun-cloning total community DNA into an expression vector and transforming the library into an indicator host (commonly the model organism *E. coli*). The resulting transformants are then selected for the desired function (e.g., antibiotic resistance), and metagenomic DNA fragments are sequenced and annotated to identify causal survival-conferring genes (Allen et al., 2009b; Sommer et al., 2009). Functional metagenomics offers three classical advantages for the unbiased interrogation of complex resistomes (Daniel, 2005; Sommer and Dantas, 2011): (1) no need to culture organisms, (2) no required knowledge of resistance gene sequence, and (3) direct association between a genotype and a demonstrated resistance phenotype. Additionally, functional metagenomic selections specifically identify those genes within a metagenome capable of conferring antibiotic tolerance to the indicator host when expressed exogenously (i.e., they distinguish transferrable resistance from intrinsic resistance) (Dantas and Sommer, 2012). Recent improvements to the throughput of functional metagenomics (Forsberg et al., 2012) unlock the potential for the experiments of scale needed identify the specific sequences, and environments, most readily able to confer resistance to human pathogens, frequently represented by the opportunistic pathogen *E. coli.*

NOVEL RESISTANCE MECHANISMS UNCOVERED BY FUNCTIONAL METAGENOMIC SELECTIONS

The following sections review novel resistance mechanisms and genes uncovered by functional metagenomic selections; these studies are summarized in **Table 1**.

GENES HIGHLY DIVERGENT FROM KNOWN RESISTANCE GENES

PCR-based screens for known resistance genes are able to detect novel variants with minor sequence differences, but due to the requirement for conserved primer binding sites, they are often unable to detect genes that have diverged significantly from the canonical example. In comparison, functional metagenomic selections for antibiotic resistance frequently identify genes that are less than 65% identical at the amino acid level to known resistance genes. In this way, functional metagenomics expands our knowledge of what sequence variants are tolerated in a resistance gene while preserving the resistance mechanism, as well as what mutations lead to expanded specificity profiles.

β-lactamases are one of the largest and best studied classes of resistance determinants, and yet, novel β-lactamases are regularly uncovered with sequence-independent techniques (Allen et al., 2009b; Sommer et al., 2009; Donato et al., 2010; Cheng

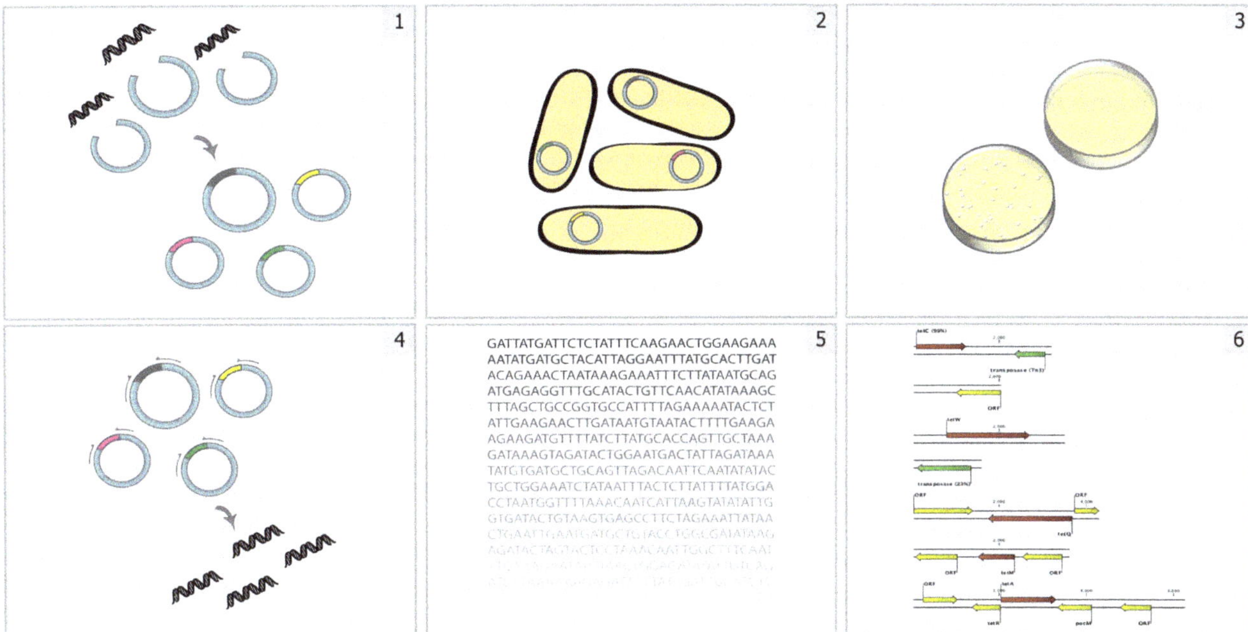

FIGURE 1 | Overview of functional metagenomic selections. Total metagenomic DNA is extracted from a microbial community sample, sheared, and ligated into an expression vector (Step 1) and is subsequently transformed into a suitable library host (Step 2) to create a metagenomic library. The library is then plated on media containing antibiotics inhibitory to the wild-type host (Step 3) to select for metagenomic fragments conferring antibiotic resistance. Metagenomic fragments present in colonies growing on antibiotic selection media are then PCR-amplified (Step 4) and sequenced using either traditional Sanger sequencing or next-generation sequencing methods (Step 5). Finally, reads are assembled and annotated in order to identify the causative antibiotic resistance genes (Step 6).

et al., 2012; Forsberg et al., 2012). In the first functional metagenomic selection for antibiotic resistance in the human gut microbiome, Sommer et al. identified ten novel β-lactamase families whose eleven members were only 35–61% identical to known genes (Sommer et al., 2009). Based on phylogenetic analysis with PhyloPythia, (McHardy et al., 2007) these genes originated primarily from the Firmicutes and Bacteroidetes phyla, which comprise the majority of the human gut microbiota but have been undersampled because they are less readily culturable in aerobic environments than Proteobacteria. Functional selection for β-lactam resistance in metagenomic libraries constructed from remote Alaskan soil revealed 13 novel β-lactamases of all four Ambler classes that were ≤67% identical to any known, functionally characterized gene (Allen et al., 2009b). In the case of the class B β-lactamases, several genes appear to be more closely related to the ancestral gene of that class than to clinically isolated genes, providing context for the evolution of clinical isolates. The study also confirmed that overall sequence similarity does not necessarily confer similar drug susceptibility profiles, supporting discovery techniques that confirm the function of identified genes.

Functional metagenomic selections also enable the detection of highly diverse classes of resistance genes, defined by substrate specificity more than shared sequence identity. For instance, aminoglycoside 6′-N-acetyltransferases [AAC(6′)s] are difficult to identify via PCR because of their high sequence diversity (Riesenfeld et al., 2004). Sommer et al. identified six AAC(6′)s with less than 48% amino acid identity to known genes and a methyltransferase conferring resistance to sisomycin with only 26.3% shared identity. Riesenfeld et al. and other studies have identified many aminoglycoside resistance genes less than 70% identical to previously reported sequences (Riesenfeld et al., 2004; Donato et al., 2010; Torres-Cortes et al., 2011; Cheng et al., 2012; McGarvey et al., 2012). Similarly, two novel bleomycin resistance genes were isolated from an activated sludge metagenomic library (Mori et al., 2008). Bleomycin resistance proteins act primarily by sequestering the antibiotic through electrostatic interactions, so their sequences tolerate an extreme amount of divergence while still maintaining the resistance function. Nevertheless, the study confirmed that all known bleomycin resistance proteins contain a proline near the N-terminus and have an acidic pI of <5, improving computational annotation of this class. Finally, McGarvey et al. identified an ADP-ribosyltransferase that was much longer any previously characterized using functional metagenomic selections (McGarvey et al., 2012). This full-length gene may not have been identified by PCR-based screens, but its discovery, enabled by functional metagenomics, expands our knowledge of the sequence diversity tolerated within this resistance class.

RESISTANCE GENES THAT WOULD NOT HAVE BEEN PREDICTED BY SEQUENCE

A major limitation of sequence-based metagenomics is its restriction to antibiotic resistance genes that are recognizable as members of a previously characterized class. BLAST, the most

Table 1 | Functional metagenomic investigations of antibiotic resistance reservoirs.

Resistance reservoir	Date	Novel resistance function identified	Total DNA queried*	References
FUNCTIONAL METAGENOMIC INVESTIGATIONS OF ENVIRONMENTAL RESERVOIRS				
Soil (remnant oak savannah)	2004	First use of functional metagenomic selections to investigate environmental antibiotic resistance; Nine novel aminoglycoside-resistance genes	5.4 GB	Riesenfeld et al., 2004
Activated sludge	2008	Two novel bleomycin-resistance genes	3.2 GB	Mori et al., 2008
Remote Alaskan soil	2009	13 novel β-lactamases; First discovery of bifunctional β-lactamase	12.4 GB	Allen et al., 2009b
Gypsy moth larvae midgut isolates	2009	*ramA* (AraC transcriptional regulator)	0.3 GB	Allen et al., 2009a
Remote Alaskan soil	2010	*pexA* (novel chloramphenicol transporter)	13.2 GB	Lang et al., 2010
Activated sludge	2010	Six novel chloramphenicol-modifying resistance genes; Novel aminoglycoside-resistance gene	1.9 GB	Parsley et al., 2010
Soil (apple orchard)	2010	Nine novel β-lactamases; Three novel aminoglycoside-resistance genes; A novel tetracycline efflux pump	13.4 GB	Donato et al., 2010
Alluvial soil	2011	Est136, chloramphenicol acetate esterase	1.6 GB	Tao, 2011; Tao et al., 2012
Soil (agricultural, nature reserve)	2011	*Tm8-3* (novel dihydrofolate reductase)	3.6 GB	Torres-Cortes et al., 2011
Wetland soil	2011	EstU1, family VIII carboxylesterase	0.3 GB	Kim et al., 2008; Jeon et al., 2011
Gull gut microbiome	2011	31 β-lactam resistance genes of undetermined mechanism	20.5 GB	Martiny et al., 2011
Urban soil	2012	Novel MFS and ABC transporters; Five novel aminoglycoside-resistance genes; ADP-ribosyltransferase longer than any previously discovered	2.8 GB	McGarvey et al., 2012
Multidrug-resistant soil isolates	2012	Novel β-lactamases; D-cycloserine efflux pump	2.6 GB	Forsberg et al., 2012
FUNCTIONAL METAGENOMIC INVESTIGATIONS OF HUMAN-ASSOCIATED RESERVOIRS				
Human oral microbiome	2003	Tetracycline-inactivating protein *tet(37)*	0.4–1.4 MB	Diaz-Torres et al., 2003
Human oral microbiome	2006	Tetracycline-resistance genes of undetermined mechanism	27.8 MB	Diaz-Torres et al., 2006
Human gut and oral microbiome	2009	10 new β-lactamase classes; Seven novel aminoglycoside-resistance genes	9.3 GB	Sommer et al., 2009
Pig gut microbiome	2009	Tetracycline-resistance genes *galE1* and *galE2* of undetermined mechanism	0.1 GB	Kazimierczak et al., 2009
Human gut microbiome	2012	Confirmed bifunctional aminoglycoside-resistance gene; Novel β-lactamase; Novel aminoglycoside-resistance gene	12.5 GB	Cheng et al., 2012

**For comparison, the genome size of E. coli K-12 substrain MG1655 is 4.64 MB.*

commonly used annotation tool, requires a threshold of shared sequence identity for a gene to be considered a member of an established gene class. Therefore, by definition, this method limits the ability to identify novel resistance genes. In addition, while profile hidden Markov model (HMM)-based annotation provides a sensitive, statistically sound analysis method capable of identifying remote homologs, these models still rely on underlying multiple sequences alignments of previously characterized proteins. In addition, current profile HMM databases provide high-level classification of antibiotic resistance genes (e.g., "Beta-Lactamase," rather than "TEM Beta-Lactamase"), providing little functional information about the gene and its potential resistance profile. Therefore, while these techniques have the potential to identify genes that have low sequence identity to known resistance genes, in the absence of additional functional confirmation, they cannot identify novel resistance mechanisms or verify that sequence variants are functional.

Functional metagenomics identifies resistance-conferring elements without prior knowledge of the sequence, circumventing this limitation. For instance, in a selection for tetracycline resistance encoded by the human oral metagenome, Diaz-Torres et al. discovered a novel tetracycline resistance gene, *tet(37)* (Diaz-Torres et al., 2003). *In vitro* analysis indicated that *tet(37)* inactivates tetracycline, making it one of only three tetracycline resistance proteins to utilize this mechanism (Thaker et al., 2010). *tet(37)* resembles flavoproteins, oxidoreductases, and NAD(P)-requiring enzymes in sequence and conserved motifs, but has no identity to *tet(X)*, the first tetracycline-inactivating gene identified. It is therefore unlikely that computational annotation would have identified it as a resistance gene (Diaz-Torres et al., 2003).

Similarly, a study of soil microbiota identified a dihydrofolate-reducing gene, *Tm8-3*, that resembles 3-oxoacyl-(acyl-carrier-protein) reductases but not *dhfr*, the target of trimethoprim (Torres-Cortes et al., 2011). A screen of an activated sludge metagenome also identified six resistance genes that appear to inactivate chloramphenicol through enzymatic modification, but which share no significant identity with known chloramphenicol acetyltransferases (Parsley et al., 2010). Although these genes may become important for clinical resistance in the future, their existence would likely have been overlooked without high-throughput functional selections independent of previous sequence knowledge.

Drug efflux is a widespread resistance mechanism common to many antibiotic classes, but individual transporters identified through computational annotation methods cannot be assigned antibiotic efflux properties without functional validation. Small changes in protein structure can change the drug specificity profile of an efflux pump and confer or eliminate resistance. Therefore, functional metagenomic selections are an attractive alternative for high-throughput characterization of transporters with tentative resistance annotations (Torres-Cortes et al., 2011). For instance, in their study of soil isolate metagenomes, Forsberg et al. identified a novel gene with only low identity to a drug/metabolite transporter. Were it not for functional selection of D-cycloserine resistance, this putative transporter would never have been identified as an antibiotic resistance gene (Forsberg et al., 2012). McGarvey et al. identified five novel MFS transporters and two ABC transporters from an urban soil that conferred resistance to tetracycline, chloramphenicol, or trimethoprim (McGarvey et al., 2012). Lang et al. successfully identified *pexA*, a novel amphenicol MFS transporter, despite its low identity (33%) to other drug resistance transporters, including any known chloramphenicol exporters (Lang et al., 2010).

BIFUNCTIONAL ENZYMES

Broad-spectrum resistance as a result of bifunctional resistance genes, the fusion of two complementary enzymatic functions into a single gene, is recognized as an increasing occurrence in many pathogens (Kim et al., 2006; Perez et al., 2007; Chandrakanth et al., 2008). Functional metagenomics provides an opportunity to identify fusion genes that are functionally active against multiple classes of antibiotic agents from natural resistance reservoirs and commensal organisms, and which have the potential to appear in clinically relevant bacteria.

Recently, functional metagenomic selections of a remote Alaskan soil revealed a novel bifunctional β-lactamase (Allen et al., 2009b). The 609-amino-acid protein is nearly double the length of a typical β-lactamase and is a natural fusion of genes for two different β-lactamase subclasses. The C-terminal domain (356 residues) aligns with class C β-lactamases, while the N-terminal domain (253 residues) aligns with class D β-lactamases, each contributing to the resistance profile of the full-length gene. The class C homologue confers resistance to cephalexin, while the class D homologue is responsible for resistance to amoxicillin, ampicillin, and carbenicillin. The bifunctional fusion gene therefore expands the resistance profile of the full-length gene beyond what either domain is responsible for alone (Allen et al., 2009b).

While this was the first bifunctional β-lactamase to be discovered, bifunctional resistance has been documented in the past, particularly against the aminoglycoside antibiotics (Daigle et al., 1999; Centrón and Roy, 2002; Dubois et al., 2002; Mendes et al., 2004; Robicsek et al., 2006). The most common mechanism of aminoglycoside resistance is deactivation of the molecule through modification by cytoplasmic enzymes: aminoglycoside acetyltransferases (AACs), aminoglycoside phosphotransferases (APHs), or aminoglycoside nucleotidyltransferases (ANTs). Four bifunctional enzymes, combining two complementary aminoglycoside-modifying enzymes as separate domains into a single open reading frame, significantly broadening the resistance profile, are known. Ferretti et al. reported the first bifunctional enzyme, AAC(6′)/APH(2″), demonstrating that it is capable of both acetylation (ACC activity found in N-terminal domain) and phosphorylation (APH activity found in C-terminal domain) of aminoglycosides (Ferretti et al., 1986). This bifunctional enzyme was also discovered in a functional metagenomics study of the human gut microbiota (Cheng et al., 2012). The ability to doubly modify aminoglycosides enables this enzyme to confer resistance to nearly all clinically relevant aminoglycosides except streptomycin and spectinomycin (Daigle et al., 1999). Similarly, the bifunctional resistance enzymes characterized as an AAC(3)-Ib/AAC(6′)-Ib′ (Dubois et al., 2002), an ANT(3″)-Ii/AAC(6′)-IId (Centrón and Roy, 2002), and an AAC(6′)-30/AAC(6′)-Ib′ (Mendes et al., 2004) all exhibit an expanded resistance profile by combining two different aminoglycoside-modifying enzymes into a single gene.

AAC(6′)-Ib-cr is the only bifunctional resistance enzyme identified capable of conferring resistance to two different structural classes of antibiotics, aminoglycosides and fluoroquinolones (Vetting et al., 2008). A variant of a common aminoglycoside acetyltransferase AAC(6′)-Ib, AAC(6′)-Ib-cr is also capable of N-acetylation of fluoroquinolones. Only two codon changes in the original enzyme are responsible for the fluoroquinolone-resistance phenotype (Vetting et al., 2008).

The merger of two genes with complementary enzymatic activities represents a novel mechanism for overcoming the increasing challenge by antibiotics, resulting in extremely broad resistance to entire antibiotic structural classes. It is likely that more examples of bifunctional resistance exist in the environment, and functional metagenomics provides a powerful technique for the discovery of functionally active bifunctional enzymes that may have great clinical implications.

UNUSUAL MECHANISMS OF RESISTANCE

Functional metagenomic selections have the potential to identify another important class of resistance genes, those that have a primary role in the cell other than antibiotic resistance. This includes housekeeping genes whose overexpression provides resistance, general stress response transcription factors, and enzymes with promiscuous activity.

Selections for trimethoprim resistance, for example, frequently identify genes encoding DHFR, the cellular target of trimethoprim (Torres-Cortes et al., 2011; McGarvey et al., 2012). Cloning a *dhfr* homolog into a high copy-number plasmid results in overexpression of DHFR, which sequesters the antibiotic (Flensburg and Skold, 1987). McGarvey et al. identified 19 highly divergent DHFRs from a soil metagenome. The proteins shared only 7–44% amino acid identity in pairwise alignments, but a subset selected for further investigation conferred similar levels of trimethoprim resistance on the host when cloned into the same position of a high-copy number vector (McGarvey et al., 2012). Although clinical isolates of *E. coli* that massively overproduce DHFR as a result of promoter mutations and intrinsically resistant *dhfr* homologs have been identified (Flensburg and Skold, 1987), in most instances, resistance conferred by overexpression of a heterologous gene is likely independent of its ability to replace the host homolog. Rather, the introduced gene may sequester enough of the antibiotic to allow the native homolog to continue functioning. Selections for D-cycloserine resistance that identify D-alanine-D-alanine ligase, the target of the antibiotic, likely fall under the same class (Cheng et al., 2012). Creating and screening libraries in low-copy number vectors is essential in these instances to identify genes that are naturally resistant to the antibiotic, rather than simply selecting for overexpression.

In contrast, antibiotic resistance conferred by transcriptional regulators represents the successful interaction of a heterologous gene with existing host cellular pathways. The AraC transcriptional stress response regulators *marA*, *soxS*, and *rob* share a highly overlapping regulon and mediate low-level antibiotic resistance in *E. coli* and its close relative *E. fergusonii* (Alekshun and Levy, 1997; Martin and Rosner, 2002). As might be expected, these genes are often identified in functional metagenomic selections against chloramphenicol, tetracyclines, and other antibiotics when *E. coli* is the indicator host. A homolog of the AraC transcriptional regulator *ramA*, from Enterobacter sp., was also identified from a gypsy moth larvae gut isolate metagenomic library as conferring resistance to *E. coli* against multiple antibiotics of different classes when overexpressed (Allen et al., 2009a). These results provide valuable information about the ability of horizontally acquired genes from closely related phyla to incorporate into a cell at the regulatory level, a mechanism of antibiotic resistance that has been previously under-considered.

Certain genes identified by functional metagenomic selections are surprising in that they more closely resemble protein families that perform unrelated functions in the cell than previously identified resistance genes. They may represent instances of expanded substrate specificity, where mutation to a gene with an unrelated function confers resistance. By first screening a soil metagenomic library for esterase activity, Jeon et al. identified a family VIII carboxylesterase that hydrolyzes both esters and the amide bond of β-lactams, apparently utilizing the same catalytic site residues for both reactions (Jeon et al., 2011). The protein changes that enable it to also hydrolyze β-lactams are currently unidentified. A novel chloramphenicol acetate esterase, EstDL136, isolated from a soil metagenome, hydrolyzes the amide linkage of both chloramphenicol and its synthetic derivative florfenicol (Tao, 2011; Tao et al., 2012). Many of the surrounding genes in the metagenomic fragment are most closely related to Sphingomonadaceae, which are frequently considered for bioremediation for their ability to degrade many compounds (Stolz, 2009). EstDL136 may have originally evolved to detoxify another compound, later expanding its substrate specificity to chloramphenicol.

FUTURE DIRECTIONS AND CHALLENGES

Functional metagenomic selections have proven to be an excellent technique for the discovery of novel antibiotic resistance mechanisms and genes encoded by varied environmental and human-associated microbial communities. As library sizes continue to increase, diverse indicator hosts are established, and techniques for improved functional selection and mechanistic determination are developed, functional metagenomics will only become better powered to explore the transferable resistome of complex microbial communities.

All of the metagenomic libraries discussed above were constructed in *E. coli*. The commercial availability of competent *E. coli* with extremely high transformation efficiencies has made this organism the preferred host for library construction, and these studies show that *E. coli* permits the heterologous expression of genes from many phyla. However, there are many clinically important classes of antibiotics that are intrinsically inactive against this Gram-negative species (e.g., glycopeptides, macrolides, oxazolidinones), prohibiting functional metagenomic selections in this host from identifying antibiotic resistance genes active against these classes. Development of a Gram-positive indicator host will represent a major step forward for the field (Riesenfeld et al., 2004; Sommer et al., 2009). This host must also exhibit a high transformation efficiency to enable the creation of metagenomic libraries large enough to permit the discovery of novel resistance genes and should lack restriction-modification systems or other host defenses that would prevent the expression of foreign DNA. *E. coli* mutants that mimic Gram-positive species through the alteration of cell membrane and wall structure are another possible alternative (Tamae et al., 2008).

The taxa from which antibiotic resistance genes can be expressed in *E. coli* are also limited by the ability of the host to recognize gene promoters and ribosome binding sites and translate them into functional proteins. Engineering *E. coli* to produce tRNA that recognize rare codons and alternative sigma factors will expand the range of taxa interrogated (Riesenfeld et al., 2004; Sommer et al., 2009, 2010a).

Finally, genes of unknown function should be further investigated to determine their mechanisms of resistance. Functional metagenomic selections that uncover a multitude of confirmed resistance genes in a high-throughput manner often require complementary biochemical experimentation to understand novel mechanisms of antibiotic resistance. Many metagenomic functional selections have identified resistance-conferring inserts whose mechanisms remain obscure because they cannot be determined based on sequence alone (Riesenfeld et al., 2004; Diaz-Torres et al., 2006; Kazimierczak et al., 2009; Martiny et al., 2011; McGarvey et al., 2012). These genes are excellent candidates for future functional characterization.

ALTERNATIVE STRATEGIES TO COMBAT ANTIBIOTIC RESISTANCE

The depth and diversity of antibiotic resistance genes uncovered by functional metagenomic selections, many of which are associated with mobile genetic elements, brings to light the need for novel strategies to combat antibiotic-resistant pathogens. Alternative approaches that modulate the host immune response (e.g., immunomodulatory peptides, vaccination, therapeutic antibodies) or target the pathogen (e.g., anti-virulence initiatives, phage therapy, antibiotic potentiators) have been explored with some success (Planson et al., 2011; Pieren and Tigges, 2012).

For instance, recent studies have suggested engineered bacteriophage as an adjuvant to enhance the bactericidal activity of antibiotics and avoid evolution of resistance to either (Lu and Collins, 2009; Parracho et al., 2012). In this case, bacteriophage is engineered to repress non-essential genes (e.g., the SOS system) not directly targeted by antibiotics, weakening the cell and potentiating antibiotic activity. Other adjuvant compounds that inhibit intrinsic repair pathways or cell tolerance mechanisms are being explored (Fischbach, 2011).

Several permeabilizing products capable of disturbing the cell membrane have been identified, thus allowing antibiotics to penetrate the cells more efficiently. One such product is the low molecular-weight oligosaccharide nanomedicine OligoG, which is able to disturb multidrug-resistant bacteria (Khan et al., 2012).

Drug efflux pumps, both specific and multidrug-resistant, may be inhibited through a variety of strategies. These include interfering with the expression of a functional transporter at different stages between transcription and final assembly, interfering with the assembly of channel proteins, designing inhibitors that compete with the antibiotic for efflux, disrupting the energy source, and blocking the efflux channel (Pages and Amaral, 2009). Deletion of genes involved in expression of porins has been shown to increase antibiotic resistance (Rodrigues et al., 2011). Therefore, strategies combining overexpression of porins used by the antibiotic to penetrate the cell with downregulation of efflux pumps may allow the antibiotic to overcome existing resistance mechanisms.

CONCLUSION

Functional metagenomic selections are a powerful technique for high-throughput characterization of the transferable resistome encoded by environmental and human-associated microbial communities, which have the potential to provide human pathogens with resistance genes through HGT. The advantages of this technique over traditional culture- and sequence-based screens are underlined when considering novel resistance mechanisms. Because resistance genes are selected on the basis of function regardless of sequence, the functional metagenomic selections reviewed above identified numerous genes with sequences highly divergent from other members of their class, as well as novel resistance mechanisms that would not have been recognized as resistance genes based on sequence alone. Conversely, they confirm antibiotic resistance function in putative drug transporters, which are frequently annotated as such regardless of true resistance ability, and permit the accurate annotation of resistance genes typically associated with other cellular functions. They have also led to the discovery of confirmed bifunctional enzymes, with broad resistance spectrums resulting from the fusion of two resistance genes. By providing a broader understanding of the resistance mechanisms currently in existence, functional metagenomic selections will aid the production of new antibiotics less susceptible to existing resistance mechanisms, as well as alternative strategies for combating antibiotic resistance.

ACKNOWLEDGMENTS

This work was supported in part by The Children's Discovery Institute of Washington University and St. Louis Children's Hospital (grant MD-II-2011-117 to Gautam Dantas), The March of Dimes Foundation (grant 6-FY12-394 to Gautam Dantas), the Kenneth Rainin Foundation (grant 12H1 to Gautam Dantas), and the National Institutes of Health (grants DP2-DK098089 and R01-GM099538 to Gautam Dantas). Erica C. Pehrsson is supported by the Department of Defense (DoD) through the National Defense Science & Engineering Graduate Fellowship (NDSEG) Program, Kevin J. Forsberg is a National Science Foundation graduate research fellow (award DGE-1143954), and Molly K. Gibson is a National Science Foundation graduate research fellow (award DGE-1143954).

REFERENCES

Alekshun, M. N., and Levy, S. B. (1997). Regulation of chromosomally mediated multiple antibiotic resistance: the mar regulon. *Antimicrob. Agents Chemother* 41, 2067–2075.

Alekshun, M. N., and Levy, S. B. (2007). Molecular mechanisms of antibacterial multidrug resistance. *Cell* 128, 1037–1050. doi: 10.1016/j.cell.2007.03.004

Allen, H. K., Cloud-Hansen, K. A., Wolinski, J. M., Guan, C., Greene, S., Lu, S., et al. (2009a). Resident microbiota of the gypsy moth midgut harbors antibiotic resistance determinants. *DNA Cell Biol.* 28, 109–117. doi: 10.1089/dna.2008.0812

Allen, H. K., Moe, L. A., Rodbumrer, J., Gaarder, A., and Handelsman, J. (2009b). Functional metagenomics reveals diverse beta-lactamases in a remote Alaskan soil. *ISME J.* 3, 243–251. doi: 10.1038/ismej.2008.86

Allen, H. K., Donato, J., Wang, H. H., Cloud-Hansen, K. A., Davies, J., and Handelsman, J. (2010). Call of the wild: antibiotic resistance genes in natural environments. *Nat. Rev. Microbiol.* 8, 251–259. doi: 10.1038/nrmicro2312

Arias, C. A., and Murray, B. E. (2009). Antibiotic-resistant bugs in the 21st century—a clinical superchallenge. *N. Engl. J. Med.* 360, 439–443. doi: 10.1056/NEJMp0804651

Arthur, M., and Courvalin, P. (1993). Genetics and mechanisms of glycopeptide resistance in enterococci. *Antimicrob. Agents Chemother.* 37, 1563–1571.

Benveniste, R., and Davies, J. (1973). Aminoglycoside antibiotic-inactivating enzymes in actinomycetes similar to those present in clinical isolates of antibiotic-resistant bacteria. *Proc. Natl. Acad. Sci. U.S.A.* 70, 2276–2280.

Bugg, T. D., Wright, G. D., Dutka-Malen, S., Arthur, M., Courvalin, P., and Walsh, C. T. (1991). Molecular basis for vancomycin resistance in *Enterococcus faecium* BM4147: biosynthesis of a depsipeptide peptidoglycan precursor by vancomycin resistance proteins VanH and VanA. *Biochemistry* 30, 10408–10415. doi: 10.1021/bi00107a007

CDC. (2011). *Antimicrobial Resistance Posing Growing Health Threat.* Available online at: http://www.cdc.gov/media/releases/2011/p0407_antimicrobialresistance.html [Accessed]. Press Release: April 7, 2011.

Centrón, D., and Roy, P. H. (2002). Presence of a group II intron in a multiresistant *Serratia marcescens* strain that harbors three integrons and a novel gene fusion. *Antimicrob. Agents Chemother.* 46, 1402–1409.

Chandrakanth, R. K., Raju, S., and Patil, S. A. (2008). Aminoglycoside-resistance mechanisms in multidrug-resistant *Staphylococcus aureus* clinical isolates. *Curr. Microbiol.* 56, 558–562. doi: 10.1007/s00284-008-9123-y

Cheng, G., Hu, Y., Yin, Y., Yang, X., Xiang, C., Wang, B., et al. (2012). Functional screening of antibiotic resistance genes from human gut microbiota reveals a novel gene fusion. *FEMS Microbiol. Lett.* 336, 11–16. doi: 10.1111/j.1574-6968.2012.02647.x

Cui, L., Iwamoto, A., Lian, J. Q., Neoh, H. M., Maruyama, T., Horikawa, Y., et al. (2006). Novel mechanism of antibiotic resistance originating in vancomycin-intermediate *Staphylococcus aureus. Antimicrob. Agents Chemother.* 50, 428–438. doi: 10.1128/AAC.50.2.428-438.2006

D'Costa, V. M., King, C. E., Kalan, L., Morar, M., Sung, W. W. L., Schwarz, C., et al. (2011). Antibiotic resistance is ancient. *Nature* 477, 457–461. doi: 10.1038/nature10388

D'Costa, V. M., McGrann, K. M., Hughes, D. W., and Wright, G. D. (2006). Sampling the antibiotic resistome. *Science* 311, 374–377. doi: 10.1126/science.1120800

Daigle, D. M., Hughes, D. W., and Wright, G. D. (1999). Prodigious substrate specificity of AAC(6′)-APH(2″), an aminoglycoside antibiotic resistance determinant in enterococci and staphylococci. *Chem. Biol.* 6, 99–110. doi: 10.1016/S1074-5521(99)80006-4

Daniel, R. (2005). The metagenomics of soil. *Nat. Rev. Microbiol.* 3, 470–478. doi: 10.1038/nrmicro1160

Dantas, G., and Sommer, M. O. (2012). Context matters - the complex interplay between resistome genotypes and resistance phenotypes. *Curr. Opin. Microbiol.* 15, 577–582. doi: 10.1016/j.mib.2012.07.004

Davies, J., and Davies, D. (2010). Origins and evolution of antibiotic resistance. *Microbiol. Mol. Biol. Rev.* 74, 417–433. doi: 10.1128/MMBR.00016-10

Davies, J., and Wright, G. D. (1997). Bacterial resistance to aminoglycoside antibiotics. *Trends Microbiol.* 5, 234–240. doi: 10.1016/S0966-842X(97)01033-0

Delcour, A. H. (2009). Outer membrane permeability and antibiotic resistance. *Biochim. Biophys. Acta* 1794, 808–816. doi: 10.1016/j.bbapap.2008.11.005

Diaz-Torres, M. L., McNab, R., Spratt, D. A., Villedieu, A., Hunt, N., Wilson, M., et al. (2003). Novel tetracycline resistance determinant from the oral metagenome. *Antimicrob. Agents Chemother.* 47, 1430–1432.

Diaz-Torres, M. L., Villedieu, A., Hunt, N., McNab, R., Spratt, D. A., Allan, E., et al. (2006). Determining the antibiotic resistance potential of the indigenous oral microbiota of humans using a metagenomic approach. *FEMS Microbiol. Lett.* 258, 257–262. doi: 10.1111/j.1574-6968.2006.00221.x

Donato, J. J., Moe, L. A., Converse, B. J., Smart, K. D., Berklein, F. C., McManus, P. S., et al. (2010). Metagenomic analysis of apple orchard soil reveals antibiotic resistance genes encoding predicted bifunctional proteins. *Appl. Environ. Microbiol.* 76, 4396–4401. doi: 10.1128/AEM.01763-09

Dubois, V., Poirel, L., Marie, C., Arpin, C., Nordmann, P., and Quentin, C. (2002). Molecular characterization of a novel class 1 integron containing bla(GES-1) and a fused product of aac3-Ib/aac6′-Ib′ gene cassettes in *Pseudomonas aeruginosa. Antimicrob. Agents Chemother.* 46, 638–645.

Ferretti, J. J., Gilmore, K. S., and Courvalin, P. (1986). Nucleotide sequence analysis of the gene specifying the bifunctional 6′-aminoglycoside acetyltransferase 2″-aminoglycoside phosphotransferase enzyme in Streptococcus faecalis and identification and cloning of gene regions specifying the two activities. *J. Bacteriol.* 167, 631–638.

Fischbach, M. A. (2011). Combination therapies for combating antimicrobial resistance. *Curr. Opin. Microbiol.* 14, 519–523. doi: 10.1016/j.mib.2011.08.003

Flensburg, J., and Skold, O. (1987). Massive overproduction of dihydrofolate reductase in bacteria as a response to the use of trimethoprim. *Eur. J. Biochem.* 162, 473–476. doi: 10.1111/j.1432-1033.1987.tb10664.x

Forsberg, K. J., Reyes, A., Wang, B., Selleck, E. M., Sommer, M. O., and Dantas, G. (2012). The shared antibiotic resistome of soil bacteria and human pathogens. *Science* 337, 1107–1111. doi: 10.1126/science.1220761

Galan, J. C., Gonzalez-Candelas, F., Rolain, J. M., and Canton, R. (2013). Antibiotics as selectors and accelerators of diversity in the mechanisms of resistance: from the resistome to genetic plasticity in the beta-lactamases world. *Front. Microbiol.* 4:9. doi:10.3389/fmicb.2013.00009

Galimand, M., Courvalin, P., and Lambert, T. (2003). Plasmid-mediated high-level resistance to aminoglycosides in Enterobacteriaceae due to 16S rRNA methylation. *Antimicrob. Agents Chemother.* 47, 2565–2571.

Hall, B. G., and Barlow, M. (2004). Evolution of the serine beta-lactamases: past, present and future. *Drug Resist. Updat.* 7, 111–123. doi: 10.1016/j.drup.2004.02.003

Hall, B. G., Salipante, S. J., and Barlow, M. (2004). Independent origins of subgroup Bl + B2 and subgroup B3 metallo-beta-lactamases. *J. Mol. Evol.* 59, 133–141. doi: 10.1007/s00239-003-2572-9

Hooper, D. C. (1999). Mechanisms of fluoroquinolone resistance. *Drug Resist. Updat.* 2, 38–55. doi: 10.1054/drup.1998.0068

Houndt, T., and Ochman, H. (2000). Long-term shifts in patterns of antibiotic resistance in enteric bacteria. *Appl. Environ. Microbiol.* 66, 5406–5409. doi: 10.1128/AEM.66.12.5406-5409.2000

Hughes, V. M., and Datta, N. (1983). Conjugative plasmids in bacteria of the 'pre-antibiotic' era. *Nature* 302, 725–726. doi: 10.1038/302725a0

Huovinen, P., Sundstrom, L., Swedberg, G., and Skold, O. (1995). Trimethoprim and sulfonamide resistance. *Antimicrob. Agents Chemother.* 39, 279–289. doi: 10.1128/AAC.39.2.279

Jacoby, G. A. (2005). Mechanisms of resistance to quinolones. *Clin. Infect. Dis.* 41(Suppl. 2), S120–S126. doi: 10.1086/428052

Jacoby, G. A., and Munoz-Price, L. S. (2005). The new beta-lactamases. *N. Engl. J. Med.* 352, 380–391. doi: 10.1056/NEJMra041359

Jeon, J. H., Kim, S. J., Lee, H. S., Cha, S. S., Lee, J. H., Yoon, S. H., et al. (2011). Novel metagenome-derived carboxylesterase that hydrolyzes beta-lactam antibiotics. *Appl. Environ. Microbiol.* 77, 7830–7836. doi: 10.1128/AEM.05363-11

Kazimierczak, K. A., Scott, K. P., Kelly, D., and Aminov, R. I. (2009). Tetracycline resistome of the organic pig gut. *Appl. Environ. Microbiol.* 75, 1717–1722. doi: 10.1128/AEM.02206-08

Khan, S., Tondervik, A., Sletta, H., Klinkenberg, G., Emanuel, C., Onsoyen, E., et al. (2012). Overcoming drug resistance with alginate oligosaccharides able to potentiate the action of selected antibiotics. *Antimicrob. Agents Chemother.* 56, 5134–5141. doi: 10.1128/AAC.00525-12

Kim, C., Hesek, D., Zajícek, J., Vakulenko, S. B., and Mobashery, S. (2006). Characterization of the Bifunctional Aminoglycoside-Modifying Enzyme ANT(3″)-Ii/AAC(6′)-IId from *Serratia marcescens. Biochemistry* 45, 8368–8377. doi: 10.1021/bi060723g

Kim, S. J., Lee, C. M., Han, B. R., Kim, M. Y., Yeo, Y. S., Yoon, S. H., et al. (2008). Characterization of a gene encoding cellulase from uncultured soil bacteria. *FEMS Microbiol. Lett.* 282, 44–51. doi: 10.1111/j.1574-6968.2008.01097.x

Knapp, C. W., Dolfing, J., Ehlert, P. A., and Graham, D. W. (2010). Evidence of increasing antibiotic resistance gene abundances in archived soils since 1940. *Environ. Sci. Technol.* 44, 580–587. doi: 10.1021/es901221x

Lang, K. S., Anderson, J. M., Schwarz, S., Williamson, L., Handelsman, J., and Singer, R. S. (2010). Novel florfenicol and chloramphenicol resistance gene discovered in Alaskan soil by using functional metagenomics. *Appl. Environ. Microbiol.* 76, 5321–5326. doi: 10.1128/AEM.00323-10

Levy, S. B. (1992). Active efflux mechanisms for antimicrobial resistance. *Antimicrob. Agents Chemother.* 36, 695–703. doi: 10.1128/AAC.36.4.695

Li, X. Z., and Nikaido, H. (2004). Efflux-mediated drug resistance in bacteria. *Drugs* 64, 159–204.

Li, X. Z., and Nikaido, H. (2009). Efflux-mediated drug resistance in bacteria: an update. *Drugs* 69, 1555–1623. doi: 10.2165/11317030-000000000-00000

Lu, T. K., and Collins, J. J. (2009). Engineered bacteriophage targeting gene networks as adjuvants for antibiotic therapy. *Proc. Natl. Acad. Sci. U.S.A.* 106, 4629–4634. doi: 10.1073/pnas.0800442106

Marshall, B. M., and Levy, S. B. (2011). Food animals and antimicrobials: impacts on human health. *Clin. Microbiol. Rev.* 24, 718–733. doi: 10.1128/CMR.00002-11

Martin, R. G., and Rosner, J. L. (2002). Genomics of the marA/soxS/rob regulon of *Escherichia coli*: identification of directly activated promoters by application of molecular genetics and informatics to microarray data. *Mol. Microbiol.* 44, 1611–1624. doi: 10.3410/f.1008106.102720

Martinez, J. L. (2008). Antibiotics and antibiotic resistance genes in natural environments. *Science* 321, 365–367. doi: 10.1126/science.1159483

Martiny, A. C., Martiny, J. B., Weihe, C., Field, A., and Ellis, J. C. (2011). Functional metagenomics reveals previously unrecognized diversity of antibiotic resistance genes in gulls. *Front. Microbiol.* 2:238. doi: 10.3389/fmicb.2011.00238

McGarvey, K. M., Queitsch, K., and Fields, S. (2012). Wide variation in antibiotic resistance proteins identified by functional metagenomic screening of a soil DNA library. *Appl. Environ. Microbiol.* 78, 1708–1714. doi: 10.1128/AEM.06759-11

McHardy, A. C., Martin, H. G., Tsirigos, A., Hugenholtz, P., and Rigoutsos, I. (2007). Accurate phylogenetic classification of variable-length DNA fragments. *Nat. Methods* 4, 63–72. doi: 10.1038/NMETH976

Mendes, R. E., Toleman, M. A., Ribeiro, J., Sader, H. S., Jones, R. N., and Walsh, T. R. (2004). Integron carrying a novel metallo-beta-lactamase gene, blaIMP-16, and a fused form of aminoglycoside-resistant gene aac(6′)-30/aac(6′)-Ib′: report from the SENTRY Antimicrobial Surveillance Program. *Antimicrob. Agents Chemother.* 48, 4693–4702. doi: 10.1128/AAC.48.12.4693-4702.2004

Mori, T., Mizuta, S., Suenaga, H., and Miyazaki, K. (2008). Metagenomic screening for bleomycin resistance genes. *Appl. Environ. Microbiol.* 74, 6803–6805. doi: 10.1128/AEM.00873-08

NIAID. (2012). *Antimicrobial (Drug) Resistance: Quick Facts.* Available online at: http://www.niaid.nih.gov/topics/antimicrobialResistance/Understanding/Pages/quickFacts.aspx [Accessed]. Last Updated: January 05, 2012

Ochman, H., Lawrence, J. G., and Groisman, E. A. (2000). Lateral gene transfer and the nature of bacterial innovation. *Nature* 405, 299–304. doi: 10.1038/35012500

Pages, J. M., and Amaral, L. (2009). Mechanisms of drug efflux and strategies to combat them: challenging the efflux pump of Gram-negative bacteria. *Biochim. Biophys. Acta* 1794, 826–833. doi: 10.1016/j.bbapap.2008.12.011

Parracho, H. M., Burrowes, B. H., Enright, M. C., McConville, M. L., and Harper, D. R. (2012). The role of regulated clinical trials in the development of bacteriophage therapeutics. *J. Mol. Genet. Med.* 6, 279–286.

Parsley, L. C., Consuegra, E. J., Kakirde, K. S., Land, A. M., Harper, W. F. Jr., and Liles, M. R. (2010). Identification of diverse antimicrobial resistance determinants carried on bacterial, plasmid, or viral metagenomes from an activated sludge microbial assemblage. *Appl. Environ. Microbiol.* 76, 3753–3757. doi: 10.1128/AEM.03080-09

Perez-Perez, F. J., and Hanson, N. D. (2002). Detection of plasmid-mediated AmpC beta-lactamase genes in clinical isolates by using multiplex PCR. *J. Clin. Microbiol.* 40, 2153–2162. doi: 10.1128/JCM.40.6.2153-2162.2002

Perez, F., Hujer, A. M., Hujer, K. M., Decker, B. K., Rather, P. N., and Bonomo, R. A. (2007). Global challenge of multidrug-resistant *Acinetobacter baumannii*. *Antimicrob. Agents Chemother.* 51, 3471–3484. doi: 10.1128/AAC.01464-06

Pieren, M., and Tigges, M. (2012). Adjuvant strategies for potentiation of antibiotics to overcome antimicrobial resistance. *Curr. Opin. Pharmacol.* 12, 551–555. doi: 10.1016/j.coph.2012.07.005

Planson, A. G., Carbonell, P., Grigoras, I., and Faulon, J. L. (2011). Engineering antibiotic production and overcoming bacterial resistance. *Biotechnol. J.* 6, 812–825. doi: 10.1002/biot.201100085

Poirel, L., Kampfer, P., and Nordmann, P. (2002). Chromosome-encoded Ambler class A beta-lactamase of Kluyvera georgiana, a probable progenitor of a subgroup of CTX-M extended-spectrum beta-lactamases. *Antimicrob. Agents Chemother.* 46, 4038–4040.

Poirel, L., Rodriguez-Martinez, J. M., Mammeri, H., Liard, A., and Nordmann, P. (2005). Origin of plasmid-mediated quinolone resistance determinant QnrA. *Antimicrobi. Agents Chemother.* 49, 3523–3525. doi: 10.1128/AAC.49.8.3523-3525.2005

Poole, K. (2005). Efflux-mediated antimicrobial resistance. *J. Antimicrob. Chemother.* 56, 20–51. doi: 10.1093/jac/dki171

Riesenfeld, C. S., Goodman, R. M., and Handelsman, J. (2004). Uncultured soil bacteria are a reservoir of new antibiotic resistance genes. *Environ. Microbiol.* 6, 981–989. doi: 10.1111/j.1462-2920.2004.00664.x

Robicsek, A., Jacoby, G. A., and Hooper, D. C. (2006). The worldwide emergence of plasmid-mediated quinolone resistance. *Lancet Infect. Dis.* 6, 629–640. doi: 10.1016/S1473-3099(06)70599-0

Rodrigues, L., Ramos, J., Couto, I., Amaral, L., and Viveiros, M. (2011). Ethidium bromide transport across Mycobacterium smegmatis cell-wall: correlation with antibiotic resistance. *BMC Microbiol.* 11:35. doi: 10.1186/1471-2180-11-35

Schwarz, S., Kehrenberg, C., Doublet, B., and Cloeckaert, A. (2004). Molecular basis of bacterial resistance to chloramphenicol and florfenicol. *FEMS Microbiol. Rev.* 28, 519–542. doi: 10.1016/j.femsre.2004.04.001

Shoemaker, N. B., Vlamakis, H., Hayes, K., and Salyers, A. A. (2001). Evidence for extensive resistance gene transfer among Bacteroides spp. and among Bacteroides and other genera in the human colon. *Appl. Environ. Microbiol.* 67, 561–568. doi: 10.1128/AEM.67.2.561-568.2001

Smillie, C. S., Smith, M. B., Friedman, J., Cordero, O. X., David, L. A., and Alm, E. J. (2011). Ecology drives a global network of gene exchange connecting the human microbiome. *Nature* 480, 241–244. doi: 10.1038/nature10571

Sommer, M. O., Church, G. M., and Dantas, G. (2010a). A functional metagenomic approach for expanding the synthetic biology toolbox for biomass conversion. *Mol. Syst. Biol.* 6, 360. doi: 10.1038/msb.2010.16

Sommer, M. O., Church, G. M., and Dantas, G. (2010b). The human microbiome harbors a diverse reservoir of antibiotic resistance genes. *Virulence* 1, 299–303. doi: 10.4161/viru.1.4.12010

Sommer, M. O., and Dantas, G. (2011). Antibiotics and the resistant microbiome. *Curr. Opin. Microbiol.* 14, 556–563. doi: 10.1016/j.mib.2011.07.005

Sommer, M. O., Dantas, G., and Church, G. M. (2009). Functional characterization of the antibiotic resistance reservoir in the human microflora. *Science* 325, 1128–1131. doi: 10.1126/science.1176950

Soussy, C. J., Wolfson, J. S., Ng, E. Y., and Hooper, D. C. (1993). Limitations of plasmid complementation test for determination of quinolone resistance due to changes in the gyrase A protein and identification of conditional quinolone resistance locus. *Antimicrob. Agents Chemother.* 37, 2588–2592. doi: 10.1128/AAC.37.12.2588

Spellberg, B., Guidos, R., Gilbert, D., Bradley, J., Boucher, H. W., Scheld, W. M., et al. (2008). The epidemic of antibiotic-resistant infections: a call to action for the medical community from the Infectious Diseases Society of America. *Clin. Infect. Dis.* 46, 155–164. doi: 10.1086/524891

Stewart, P. S., and Costerton, J. W. (2001). Antibiotic resistance of bacteria in biofilms. *Lancet* 358, 135–138.

Stolz, A. (2009). Molecular characteristics of xenobiotic-degrading sphingomonads. *Appl. Microbiol. Biotechnol.* 81, 793–811. doi: 10.1007/s00253-008-1752-3

Stone, P. W. (2009). Economic burden of healthcare-associated infections: an American perspective. *Exp. Rev. Pharmacoecon Outcomes Res.* 9, 417–422. doi: 10.1586/erp.09.53

Tamae, C., Liu, A., Kim, K., Sitz, D., Hong, J., Becket, E., et al. (2008). Determination of antibiotic hypersensitivity among 4, 000 single-gene-knockout mutants of *Escherichia coli*. *J. Bacteriol.* 190, 5981–5988. doi: 10.1128/JB.01982-07

Tao, W. (2011). Characterization of two metagenome-derived esterases that reactivate chloramphenicol by counteracting chloramphenicol acetyltransferase. *J. Microbiol. Biotechnol.* 21, 1203–1210.

Tao, W., Lee, M. H., Wu, J., Kim, N. H., Kim, J. C., Chung, E., et al. (2012). Inactivation of chloramphenicol and florfenicol by a novel chloramphenicol hydrolase. *Appl. Environ. Microbiol.* 78, 6295–6301. doi: 10.1128/AEM.01154-12

Thaker, M., Spanogiannopoulos, P., and Wright, G. D. (2010). The tetracycline resistome. *Cell. Mol. Life Sci.* 67, 419–431. doi: 10.1007/s00018-009-0172-6

Torres-Cortes, G., Millan, V., Ramirez-Saad, H. C., Nisa-Martinez, R., Toro, N., and Martinez-Abarca, F. (2011). Characterization of novel antibiotic resistance genes identified by functional metagenomics on soil samples. *Environ. Microbiol.* 13, 1101–1114. doi: 10.1111/j.1462-2920.2010.02422.x

Tran, J. H., and Jacoby, G. A. (2002). Mechanism of plasmid-mediated quinolone resistance. *Proc. Natl. Acad. Sci. U.S.A.* 99, 5638–5642. doi: 10.1073/pnas.082092899

Vetting, M. W., Park, C. H., Hegde, S. S., and Jacoby, G. A. (2008). Mechanistic and Structural Analysis of Aminoglycoside N-Acetyltransferase, AAC (6′)-Ib and Its Bifunctional, Fluoroquinolone-Active, AAC (6′)-Ib-cr Variant†‡. *Biochemistry* 47, 9825–9835. doi: 10.1021/bi800664x

Walsh, C. (2000). Molecular mechanisms that confer antibacterial drug resistance. *Nature* 406, 775–781. doi: 10.1038/35021219

Walsh, C. (2003). *Antibiotics: Actions, Origins, Resistance.* Washington, DC: ASM Press.

Weisblum, B. (1998). Macrolide resistance. *Drug Resist. Updat.* 1, 29–41.

Wolfson, J. S., and Hooper, D. C. (1989). Fluoroquinolone antimicrobial agents. *Clin. Microbiol. Rev.* 2, 378–424.

Wright, G. D. (2010). Antibiotic resistance in the environment: a link to the clinic? *Curr. Opin. Microbiol.* 13, 589–594. doi: 10.1016/j.mib.2010.08.005

Yang, W., Moore, I. F., Koteva, K. P., Bareich, D. C., Hughes, D. W., and Wright, G. D. (2004). TetX is a flavin-dependent monooxygenase conferring resistance to tetracycline antibiotics. *J. Biol. Chem.* 279, 52346–52352. doi: 10.1074/jbc.M409573200

Zhanel, G. G., Dueck, M., Hoban, D. J., Vercaigne, L. M., Embil, J. M., Gin, A. S., et al. (2001). Review of macrolides and ketolides: focus on respiratory tract infections. *Drugs* 61, 443–498.

9

Aerobic digestion reduces the quantity of antibiotic resistance genes in residual municipal wastewater solids

Tucker R. Burch*[1], *Michael J. Sadowsky*[2] *and Timothy M. LaPara*[1,2]

[1] *Department of Civil Engineering, University of Minnesota, Minneapolis, MN, USA*
[2] *Biotechnology Institute, University of Minnesota, St. Paul, MN, USA*

Edited by:
Marilyn C. Roberts, University of Washington, USA

Reviewed by:
M. Pilar Francino, Center for Public Health Research, Spain
Peter Pristas, Slovak Academy of Sciences, Slovakia

****Correspondence:***
Timothy M. LaPara, Department of Civil Engineering, University of Minnesota, 500 Pillsbury Drive SE, Minneapolis, MN 55455, USA.
e-mail: lapar001@umn.edu

Numerous initiatives have been undertaken to circumvent the problem of antibiotic resistance, including the development of new antibiotics, the use of narrow spectrum antibiotics, and the reduction of inappropriate antibiotic use. We propose an alternative but complimentary approach to reduce antibiotic resistant bacteria (ARB) by implementing more stringent technologies for treating municipal wastewater, which is known to contain large quantities of ARB and antibiotic resistance genes (ARGs). In this study, we investigated the ability of conventional aerobic digestion to reduce the quantity of ARGs in untreated wastewater solids. A bench-scale aerobic digester was fed untreated wastewater solids collected from a full-scale municipal wastewater treatment facility. The reactor was operated under semi-continuous flow conditions for more than 200 days at a residence time of approximately 40 days. During this time, the quantities of *tet*(A), *tet*(W), and *erm*(B) decreased by more than 90%. In contrast, *intI1* did not decrease, and *tet*(X) increased in quantity by 5-fold. Following operation in semi-continuous flow mode, the aerobic digester was converted to batch mode to determine the first-order decay coefficients, with half-lives ranging from as short as 2.8 days for *tet*(W) to as long as 6.3 days for *intI1*. These results demonstrated that aerobic digestion can be used to reduce the quantity of ARGs in untreated wastewater solids, but that rates can vary substantially depending on the reactor design (i.e., batch vs. continuous-flow) and the specific ARG.

Keywords: antibiotic resistance genes, municipal wastewater treatment, aerobic digestion, class 1 integrons, qPCR

INTRODUCTION

The resistance of pathogenic bacteria to antibiotic chemotherapy is a growing problem with significant consequences for public health. In the United States, methicillin-resistant *Staphylococcus aureus* (MRSA) infections lead to more fatalities than the combination of HIV/AIDs, Parkinson's disease, and homicides (Spellberg et al., 2011). The estimated economic cost of antibiotic resistance ranges from $21 to 34 billion dollars per year (Spellberg et al., 2011). In response, medical practitioners have attempted to reduce the number of inappropriate and unnecessary antibiotic prescriptions. The biomedical research community is also focusing its research efforts to develop new antibiotics as well as alternatives to antibiotic chemotherapy (Kohanski et al., 2010; Jabes, 2011; Edgar et al., 2012). Finally, in Sweden and Switzerland, the use of antibiotics in agriculture for growth promotion and prophylaxis has been banned (Wierup, 2001; Arnold et al., 2004).

Despite these initiatives, a significant body of research suggests that antibiotic resistant bacteria (ARB) are becoming increasingly more prevalent (Palumbi, 2001; Levy and Marshall, 2004; Levy, 2005). An alternative, but complementary, approach to reducing the prevalence of ARB would be to identify pertinent reservoirs of resistance and then to implement appropriate technologies to ameliorate these reservoirs. Consistent with this approach, numerous studies have identified untreated municipal wastewater (raw sewage) as a significant reservoir of ARB and antibiotic resistance genes (ARGs) (Bönemann et al., 2006; da Silva et al., 2006; Auerbach et al., 2007; Schlüter et al., 2007; Szczepanowski et al., 2009; Zhang et al., 2009a; Galvin et al., 2010; Uyaguari et al., 2011; Zhang and Zhang, 2011). Municipal wastewater treatment processes, therefore, should represent an important opportunity to mitigate the quantity of this reservoir of antibiotic resistance.

Although prior research has demonstrated that the treated municipal wastewater also contains substantial concentrations of ARB and ARGs (da Silva et al., 2006; Pruden et al., 2006; Graham et al., 2011; LaPara et al., 2011), a mass balance on wastewater treatment operations suggests that >99% of the ARB and ARGs in untreated municipal wastewater accumulate in the residual wastewater solids. These are subsequently treated by numerous technologies to reduce their nutrient and pathogen content (to varying degrees) prior to their disposal on agricultural land (Tchobanoglous et al., 2003). There have been relatively few investigations on the different technologies used for treating residual wastewater solids and their associated effectiveness at mitigating ARB and ARGs. Diehl and LaPara (2010) observed relatively little removal of ARGs in aerobic digestion processes operated at 22–55°C, but observed increasingly effective removal of ARGs in anaerobic digestion processes at temperature >37°C. In contrast, Ma et al. (2011) observed little benefit of increasing the temperature of anaerobic digestion beyond 37°C.

In the present research, we undertook a detailed investigation of the effectiveness of a bench-scale conventional aerobic digestion process at mitigating the quantity of ARGs in untreated residual wastewater solids. Although our prior research had observed no effect of aerobic digestion on the quantity of ARGs in wastewater solids (Diehl and LaPara, 2010), these previous experiments were performed in relatively small bioreactors with a mean hydraulic residence time of 4 days. Assuming that ARGs decay at a relatively slow rate (i.e., half-lives > 4 days), this experimental design would have been insufficient to observe significant reductions in ARGs. This short time period used in our prior experimental design is also pertinent because the United States Environmental Protection Agency requires that aerobic digestion processes have a mean hydraulic residence time of 40 days (when operated at 20°C) to qualify as a "process to significantly reduce pathogens" (PSRP), which must be achieved before these treated wastewater solids can be applied to agricultural land for their disposal (albeit with some restrictions) (Tchobanoglous et al., 2003). This research is of considerable practical importance because numerous full-scale municipal wastewater treatment facilities currently utilize aerobic digestion processes to treat their wastewater solids, particularly those that treat less than 10 million gallons of wastewater each day (at higher flow rates, other technologies are considered more practical and economical).

MATERIALS AND METHODS

EXPERIMENTAL DESIGN

A 10-L aerobic digester was operated at room temperature with a mean residence time of 40 days and a minimum dissolved oxygen (DO) concentration of 2 mg/L. The digester was inoculated with 10 L of untreated residual municipal wastewater solids from a full-scale municipal wastewater treatment plant. Mixing and aeration were provided by pumping atmospheric air through a stone diffuser located at the bottom of the reactor vessel at a rate sufficient to prevent settling of solids and to maintain the minimum DO concentration. Typical operating variables, including temperature, DO, pH, total solids, volatile solids, and inert solids, were monitored throughout the entire time period the digester was in operation (Clesceri et al., 1999). The total solids concentration represents the quantity of material remaining after drying at 103°C (i.e., the sum of inorganic and organic material dissolved and suspended in the sample). In contrast, the volatile solids concentration represents the fraction of the total solids concentration that is lost upon ignition at 550°C, whereas the IS concentration represents the fraction of the total solids that is not lost upon ignition at 550°C (i.e., the fraction of the total solids that represents that ash-material). Water loss from the digestor due to evaporation was monitored and replaced by adding appropriate volumes of deionized water to the digester.

The digester was operated for more than 175 days while being fed on a weekly basis untreated residual municipal wastewater solids. The digester was considered to have reached steady-state conditions once the residence time for inert solids (i.e., the average amount of time that an "inert solid" would reside in the aerobic digester) had been maintained at 41.1 ± 0.5 days (mean ± standard deviation) for a time period of 35 days. Once steady-state conditions had been established, the operating mode of the digester was shifted to better reflect continuous-flow operating conditions by feeding untreated residual municipal wastewater solids on a daily basis from Day 180 to Day 191. Following this semi-continuous flow phase, the aerobic digester was operated for an additional 27 days while being fed on a weekly basis untreated residual municipal wastewater solids. On Day 218, half of the digester contents (i.e., 5 L) were replaced with untreated residual municipal wastewater solids to allow the determination of decay coefficients in a batch-like reactor.

SAMPLE COLLECTION AND GENOMIC DNA EXTRACTION AND PURIFICATION

Triplicate samples (100 μL) were collected from larger aliquots (50–300 mL) of digester contents to ensure accurate sample collection volumes. Samples were then diluted with 500 μL of lysis buffer (120 mM sodium phosphate buffer, 5% dodecyl sulfate, pH 8.0 ± 0.1) and subjected to three consecutive freeze-thaw cycles followed by incubation at 70°C for 90 min. Genomic DNA was then extracted using a FastDNA Spin Kit (MP Biomedicals LLC, Solon, OH) according to the manufacturer's instructions.

REAL-TIME PCR

Real-time PCR was used to quantify the concentrations of three different genes that encode resistance to tetracycline [*tet*(A), *tet*(W), and *tet*(X)], one gene that encodes resistance to erythromycin [*erm*(B)], one gene that encodes resistance to sulfonamides (*sulI*), and the integrase gene of class 1 integrons (*intI1*). The three tetracycline resistance genes were selected because they represent each of the three known mechanisms of tetracycline resistance (efflux pumps, ribosomal protection proteins, and enzymatic modification) (Levy et al., 1999). The erythromycin gene, *erm*(B), was chosen because it encodes an rRNA methyltransferase that confers resistance to macrolides, lincosamides, and streptogramin B (Roberts et al., 1999). Prior work has demonstrated that all five of these ARGs are present at substantial concentrations in wastewater and/or wastewater solids (Diehl and LaPara, 2010; LaPara et al., 2011; Munir et al., 2011). Class 1 integrons were quantified because of their association with multiple antibiotic resistance. These integrons enable bacteria to collect multiple, exogenous ARGs and modulate their expression (Mazel, 2006). qPCR was also used to determine the concentrations of 16S rRNA genes (a measure of total bacterial biomass), all *Bacteroides* spp. (a measure of total fecal bacteria), and human-specific *Bacteroides* spp. (a measure of human fecal bacteria) (Muyzer et al., 1993; Bernhard and Field, 2000; Layton et al., 2006). Additional information regarding the use of qPCR to quantify these genes can be found in **Table 1**.

Real-time PCR was carried out on an Eppendorf Mastercycler EP Realplex thermal cycler (Eppendorf, Westbury, NY). PCR assays were optimized to reduce or eliminate the formation of primer-dimers and non-specific products. Typical PCR assays began with a 1 min initial denaturation at 95°C. This step was followed by 40 cycles of denaturation at 95°C for 15 s and combined annealing and extension at the primer-specific annealing temperature for 1 min. Typical reaction volumes were 25 μL and consisted of 12.5 μL of BioRad iTaq SYBR Green Supermix with ROX

Table 1 | Gene targets, resistance mechanisms, primer sequences, amplicon sizes, and annealing temperatures for real-time PCR assays.

Gene target	Resistance mechanism	Primer sequence (5′ → 3′)	Size (bp)	Annealing temperature (°C)	References
16S rRNA gene	NA	F: CCT ACG GGA GGC AGC AG R: ATT ACC GCG GCT GCT GG	202	60	Muyzer et al., 1993
Bacteroides spp.	NA	F: GAG AGG AAG GTC CCC CAC R: CGC TAC TTG GCT GGT TCA G	116	60	Layton et al., 2006
Human-specific *Bacteroides*	NA	F: ATC ATG AGT TCA CAT GTC CG R: TAC CCC GCC TAC TAT CTA ATG	82	56	Bernhard and Field, 2000; Seurinck et al., 2005
erm(B)	Ribosomal protection	F: GAT ACC GTT TAC GAA ATT GG R: GAA TCG AGA CTT GAG TGT GC	364	58	Chen et al., 2007
intI1	Class 1 integron	F: CCT CCC GCA CGA TGA TC R: TCC ACG CAT CGT CAG GC	280	60	Goldstein et al., 2001
sul1	Enzymatic modification	F: CCG TTG GCC TTC CTG TAA AG R: TTG CCG ATC GCG TGA AGT	67	60	Heuer and Smalla, 2007
tet(A)	Efflux	F: GCT ACA TCC TGC TTG CCT TC R: CAT AGA TCG CCG TGA AGA GG	210	60	Ng et al., 2001
tet(W)	Ribosomal protection	F: GAG AGC CTG CTA TAT GCC AGC R: GGG CGT ATC CAC AAT GTT AAC	168	60	Aminov et al., 2001
tet(X)	Enzymatic modification	F: AGC CTT ACC AAT GGG TGT AAA R: TTC TTA CCT TGG ACA TCC CG	278	60	Ghosh et al., 2009

(Life Science Research, Hercules, CA), 25 µg of bovine serum albumin, optimized quantities of forward and reverse primers, and approximately 1 ng of template genomic DNA. Each analysis consisted of three replicates. Standards were made from PCR products that targeted specific genes from either well-described bacterial isolates or from municipal wastewater solids. PCR products were ligated into a pGEM-T Easy cloning vector, transformed into JM109 competent cells, and extracted from cell cultures using the alkaline lysis procedure (Sambrook et al., 1989). It was confirmed that all plasmids contained the specified gene by nucleotide sequence analysis of the extracted plasmid. The DNA concentration of plasmid extracts was quantified using a TD-700 fluorometer and Hoechst 33258 dye. Each standard curve consisted of a 10-fold dilution series containing at least 5 standards ($r^2 \geq 0.99$). Amplification efficiencies were 100 ± 10%.

DATA ANALYSIS

All data obtained from groups of triplicate samples were treated as if they had been obtained from a normal distribution (i.e., means and standard deviations were used to describe the data). This assumption of normal distributions was based on results from Shapiro–Wilk normality tests performed in SigmaPlot 12.0 that indicated the complete semi-continuous flow data series for most gene targets could not be distinguished from a normal distribution ($P > 0.05$). Analysis of variance (ANOVA; Microsoft Excel 2010) was used with data from the semi-continuous flow experiment to determine the statistical significance of differences in gene target concentrations between untreated and treated residual solids samples.

Simple linear regression (Arc 1.06) was used with log-transformed data from the batch experiment to determine the goodness of fit of the data to a first-order kinetic model. The first-order kinetic model was chosen based on previous empirical observations that it tends to fit this type of data well. Values of P used to compare the relative statistical significance of different kinetic coefficients (**Table 4**) were determined using Welch's t-test for unequal n and unequal sample variance. The sample variance for each estimated first-order kinetic coefficient was obtained from the estimated standard error for that coefficient as provided by Arc 1.06.

RESULTS

SEMI-CONTINUOUS FLOW OPERATING MODE

With respect to typically monitored operating variables, the lab-scale aerobic digester performed as an appropriate experimental model simulation during the semi-continuous flow experimental period (**Table 2**). The pH was circumneutral, digester temperature was the same as the ambient air temperature, and DO concentrations were well above the target DO concentration of 2 mg/L. The total and volatile solids concentrations for the untreated and treated solids were well within ranges typically encountered in practice (2–5% total solids, 0.6–3% volatile solids) (Tchobanoglous et al., 2003). The fractions of total and volatile solids destroyed were 26 and 41%, respectively, which is also typical for a full-scale aerobic digestion process (Tchobanoglous et al., 2003).

The aerobic digester eliminated a substantial fraction of bacterial biomass and fecal indicator bacteria (FIB) as measured by

Table 2 | Operating variables during operation in semi-continuous flow mode.

Variable	Mean ± SD	n values
pH	7.5 ± 0.2	n = 12
Temperature (°C)	17.0 ± 0.3	n = 12
Dissolved oxygen (mg/L)	5.8 ± 1.5	n = 12
Hydraulic residence time (days)	13.5 ± 0.7	n = 12
Untreated total solids	4.6% ± 0.04%	n = 4
Treated total solids	3.4% ± 0.3%	n = 4
Total solids destruction	26.3% ± 6.0%	n = 4
Total solids residence time (days)	33.1 ± 0.4	n = 12
Untreated volatile solids	3.2% ± 0.05%	n = 4
Treated volatile solids	1.9% ± 0.1%	n = 4
Volatile solids destruction	41.1% ± 4.8%	n = 4
Volatile solids residence time (days)	27.7 ± 0.6	n = 12
Untreated inert solids	1.5% ± 0.02%	n = 4
Treated inert solids	1.5% ± 0.1%	n = 4
Inert solids destruction	−5.7% ± 8.4%	n = 4
Inert solids residence time (days)	41.7 ± 0.1	n = 12

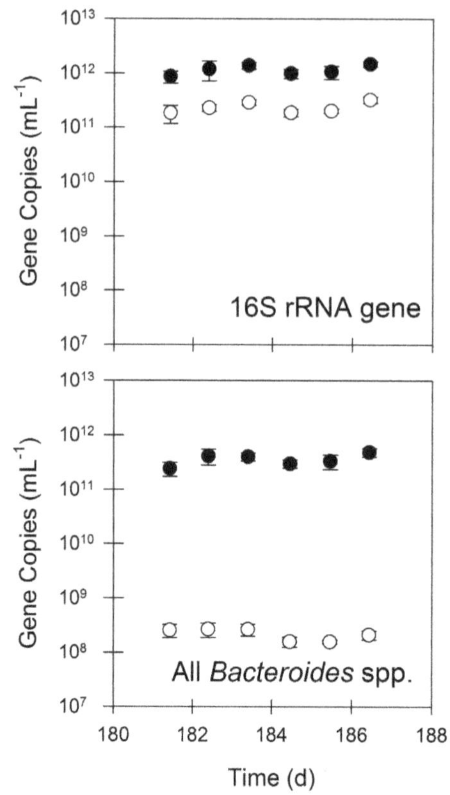

FIGURE 1 | The quantities of 16S rRNA genes and fecal indicator bacteria as measured by 16S rRNA genes of all *Bacteroides* spp. in untreated (closed circles) and treated (open circles) residual solids. Values are the arithmetic mean of triplicate samples; error bars represent one standard deviation. The concentrations of human-specific *Bacteroides* spp. were approximately 5 × 10^8 gene copies mL^{-1} in untreated samples, but were below the detection limit (1 × 10^8 gene copies mL^{-1}) in treated samples.

qPCR targeting the 16S rRNA gene and 16S rRNA genes specific for all *Bacteroides* spp. and for human-specific *Bacteroides* spp. (**Figure 1**). The concentrations of 16S rRNA genes were 77% lower in treated samples compared to the untreated samples. This indicates net destruction of total bacterial biomass in the digester, consistent with the total and volatile solids removal. Significant removal was observed for both types of FIB. The concentrations of all *Bacteroides* spp. were 99.9% lower in treated samples compared to untreated samples. Similarly, the concentrations of human-specific *Bacteroides* spp. were approximately 5 × 10^8 gene copies mL^{-1} in untreated samples, but were below the detection limit (1 × 10^8 gene copies mL^{-1}) in treated samples.

The untreated wastewater solids contained substantial quantities of each of the ARGs investigated in this study. The quantities of *intI1*, *sul1*, and *tet*(W) were similar, present at a concentration of approximately 10^{10} gene copies mL^{-1}. In contrast, the concentration of *erm*(B) was approximately 10^{11} gene copies mL^{-1}, and the concentrations of *tet*(A) and *tet*(X) were approximately 10^9 gene copies mL^{-1}. Given that the concentrations of 16S rRNA genes were approximately 10^{12} gene copies mL^{-1} in the untreated solids, the ratio of the various antibiotic resistance determinants examined in this study to bacterial cells ranged from approximately 0.1% for *tet*(A) and *tet*(X) to 1% for *intI1*, *sul1*, and *tet*(W), and to 10% for *erm*(B).

The bench-scale aerobic digester removed between 85 and 98% of *erm*(B), *sul1*, *tet*(A), and *tet*(W) during the semi-continuous flow experimental period (**Figure 2**), which was substantially greater than that for bacterial biomass (i.e., 16S rRNA genes). In contrast, the quantity of *intI1* was not statistically different ($P = 0.17$) in the untreated and treated solids, suggesting that aerobic digestion operated in semi-continuous flow mode does not eliminate *intI1* (**Figure 3**). Furthermore, the ratio of *intI1* to 16S rRNA genes increased in the treatment process from 0.8 to 3%, indicating that aerobic digestion likely selects for bacterial cells possessing a class 1 integron. Interestingly, the aerobic digestion process also appeared to select for bacterial cells containing *tet*(X), as the quantity of this gene was 5-fold greater in the treated solids than in the untreated solids.

BATCH OPERATING MODE

Following the semi-continuous flow experimental phase, the aerobic digester was shifted to batch mode to determine decay rates for each target gene. As with the previous experimental phase, typically monitored operating variables indicated that the digester operated as an appropriate simulation of a full-scale aerobic digester. The pH rose from a semi-continuous phase value between 7 and 7.5 to just above 8 following the addition of untreated residual solids, but then gradually decreased to between 7 and 7.5. A substantial decrease in DO concentration to less than 1 mg/L was initially observed, but increased to > 4 mg/L within 24 h and remained so for the duration of the batch experiment.

A significant decay rate was observed for 16S rRNA genes and FIB during operation in batch mode (**Figure 4**). The quantities of 16S rRNA genes decayed by 90% during the 20-day batch

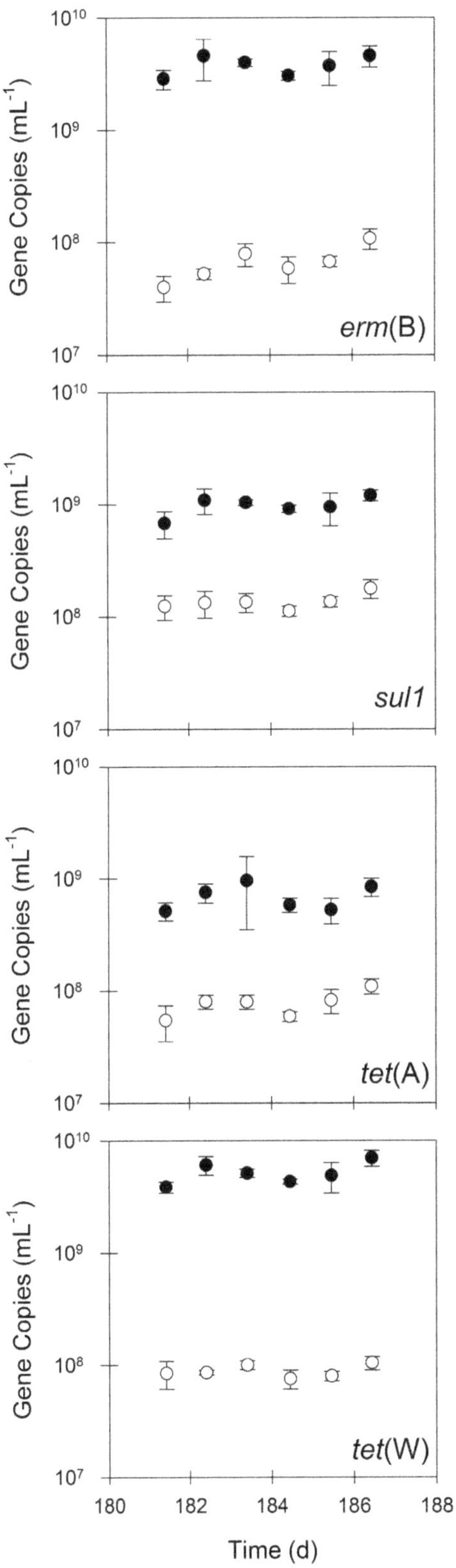

FIGURE 2 | The quantities of *erm*(B), *sul1*, *tet*(A), and *tet*(W) in untreated (closed circles) and treated (open circles) residual solids. Values are the arithmetic mean of triplicate samples; error bars represent one standard deviation.

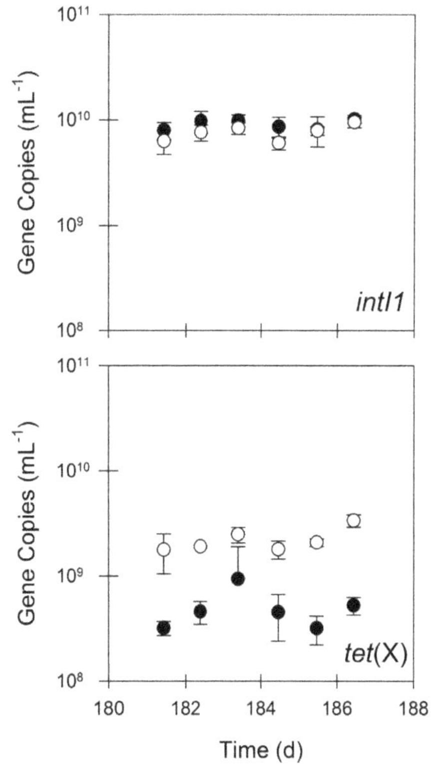

FIGURE 3 | The quantities of *intI1* and *tet*(X) in untreated (closed circles) and treated (open circles) residual solids. Values are the arithmetic mean of triplicate samples; error bars represent one standard deviation.

experiment ($t_{1/2} = 5.5$ d; **Table 3**). In contrast, all *Bacteroides* spp. decayed by nearly four orders of magnitude over 20 days ($t_{1/2} = 1.4$ d; **Table 3**), whereas human-specific *Bacteroides* spp. decayed to below the detection limit within one week of beginning the batch experimental phase ($t_{1/2} = 4.6$ d; **Table 3**).

In contrast to operation in semi-continuous flow mode, the quantities of all of the antibiotic resistance determinants, including *intI1* and *tet*(X), declined in the batch experimental phase (**Figure 5**). The quantities of *erm*(B) and *tet*(W) declined by approximately two orders of magnitude during the 20-day experiment, whereas the quantities of *intI1*, *sul1*, *tet*(A), and *tet*(X) each declined by one order of magnitude during the same time period. Correspondingly, the first-order decay rates varied considerably among individual gene targets. The *intI1* and *tet*(X) genes decayed the most slowly, each with a half-life of approximately 6 days (**Table 3**). These rates of decay were statistically similar to each other as well as to the rate of decay for the 16S rRNA gene (**Table 4**). In contrast, the first-order decay rates were significantly ($P < 0.05$) more rapid for the remaining gene targets, with half-lives ranging from 2.8 to 4.6 days (**Table 3**). These rates of decay were significantly faster than the decay rate for 16S rRNA genes (**Table 4**).

DISCUSSION

The long-term goal of our research is to determine how the numerous technologies used to treat municipal wastewater can

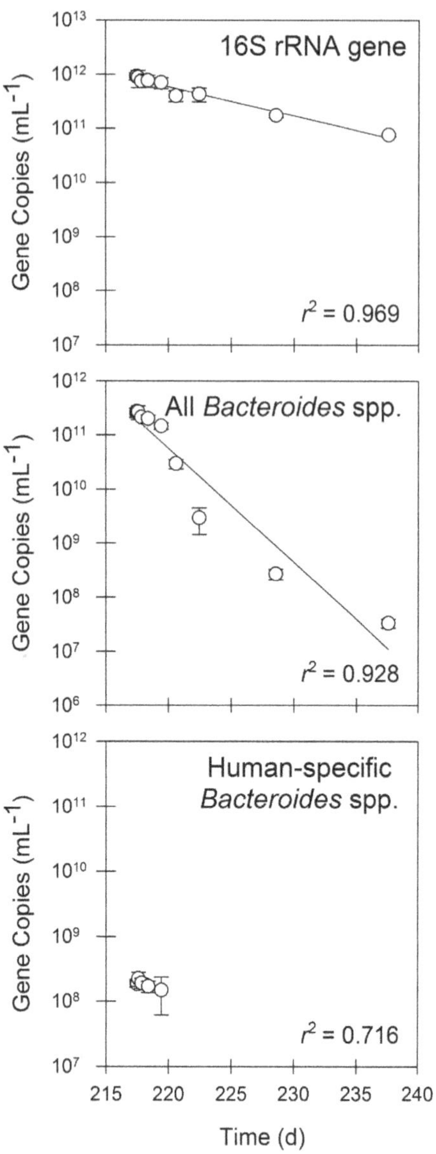

FIGURE 4 | The quantities of 16S rRNA genes, fecal indicator bacteria as measured by 16S rRNA genes of all *Bacteroides* spp., and fecal indicator bacteria as measured by 16S rRNA genes of human-specific *Bacteroides* spp. in residual solids undergoing batch treatment. Values are the arithmetic mean of triplicate samples; error bars represent one standard deviation.

simultaneously be used to eliminate the substantial quantities of ARB and ARGs that are known to exist in untreated sewage. The present study makes an important advance in our knowledge by elucidating the extent and rate by which aerobic digestion can be used to eliminate ARGs. This research is practically important because the overwhelming majority of ARB and ARGs in raw sewage ultimately end up in the residual wastewater solids, and a recent study suggested that more than 2200 municipal wastewater treatment facilities use this technology to produce more than 85,000 dry tons of treated wastewater solids in the United States each year (Beecher et al., 2007).

Table 3 | Summary of first-order degradation kinetic model parameter estimates for the 16S rRNA gene, fecal indicator bacteria as measured by 16S rRNA genes of all *Bacteroides* spp., fecal indicator bacteria as measured by 16S rRNA genes of human-specific *Bacteroides* spp., *erm*(B), *intI1*, *sul1*, *tet*(A), *tet*(W), and *tet*(X) during batch mode operation.

Gene target	k (day^{-1}) ± standard error (day^{-1})	$t_{1/2}$ (days)
16S rRNA gene	0.13 ± 0.008	5.5
Bacteroides spp.	0.49 ± 0.048	1.4
Human-specific *Bacteroides* spp.	0.15 ± 0.047	4.6
erm(B)	0.19 ± 0.025	3.6
intI1	0.11 ± 0.011	6.3
sul1	0.15 ± 0.009	4.6
tet(A)	0.16 ± 0.011	4.4
tet(W)	0.25 ± 0.025	2.8
tet(X)	0.12 ± 0.006	5.7

All rates were regressed from 10 data points (except human-specific Bacteroides spp., $n = 6$) and are statistically significant ($P < 0.05$).

In most cases, the rate of disappearance of different ARGs exceeded that of the total number of bacteria (as measured by 16S rRNA gene copies), suggesting that these ARGs were actively eliminated during the aerobic digestion process. Although there is only very limited data presently available in the published literature, these disappearance rates are generally similar to the rates that were previously observed during anaerobic digestion at 37°C (Diehl and LaPara, 2010). In contrast, the quantities of *tet*(X) and *intI1* decayed at a rate similar to that of all bacteria, suggesting that these genes were passively eliminated, paralleling the decline in the total number of bacteria. This observation is substantially different than our previous study, in which both *tet*(X) and *intI1* rapidly declined in bench-scale anaerobic digestion processes operated at temperatures of 37°C or higher (Diehl and LaPara, 2010). Therefore, the rates by which different ARGs decay in a conventional aerobic digestion process are either similar to or slower than the decay rates observed in anaerobic digestion processes. This apparent inferiority of aerobic digestion is pertinent because anaerobic digestion is also a commonly used technology to treat residual wastewater solids (Tchobanoglous et al., 2003).

This research also demonstrated that reactor design has a major effect on the fate of ARGs during the treatment of residual municipal wastewater solids. The most obvious difference occurred with *tet*(X), which declined under batch experimental conditions but increased substantially in semi-continuous flow conditions. Similarly, the quantity of *intI1* declined under batch conditions but remained static during semi-continuous flow operation. In contrast, model results suggest that the quantities of *erm*(B) and *tet*(W) declined more rapidly in semi-continuous flow operation than would be suggested by the first-order decay coefficient elucidated under batch conditions (analyses not shown). Previous researchers have suggested that reactor design affects the removal of ARGs during wastewater solids digestion (Ma et al., 2011); our results support this

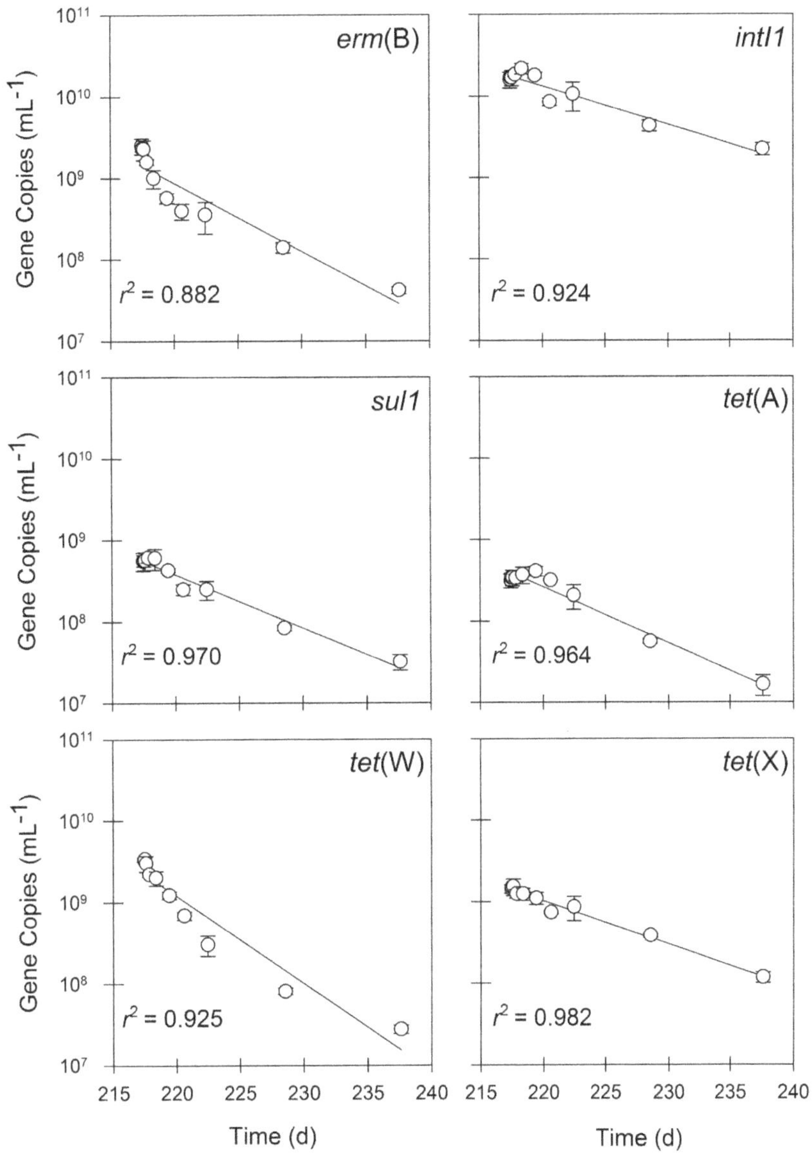

FIGURE 5 | The quantities of *erm*(B), *intI1*, *sul1*, *tet*(A), *tet*(W), and *tet*(X) in residual solids undergoing batch treatment. Values are the arithmetic mean of triplicate samples; error bars represent one standard deviation.

hypothesis. Additional research is needed to clarify the importance of reactor design and the disappearance of ARGs during the digestion of wastewater solids.

A growing body of evidence suggests that class 1 integrons, which are linked to multiple antibiotic resistance, are particularly prominent in wastewater (Ghosh et al., 2009; Zhang et al., 2009b; Ramsden et al., 2010; Ma et al., 2011; Stalder et al., 2012). Our research has shown significant variation in removal efficiencies of *intI1* depending on the specific technology (i.e., anaerobic digestion achieves better and more efficient removal than aerobic digestion) and the specific operating conditions (temperature, flow regime, etc.). Additional research is needed to better understand the fate and gene cassette content of class 1 integrons in residual solids treatment systems.

Prior research has suggested that *sul1* flanks all class 1 integrons (Mazel, 2006). When the aerobic digester was operated in semi-continuous flow mode, however, the quantities of *sul1* genes declined by almost an order of magnitude, whereas the quantities of *intI1* were similar in the treated and in the untreated residual solids. Similarly, the rate by which *sul1* declined in batch operating mode was significantly faster than the rate by which *intI1* declined ($P = 0.01$; **Table 4**). This suggests that the coupling of the *sul1* gene to class 1 integrons is not universal; additional research is needed to better understand the relationship between class 1 integrons and *sul1* genes in the unit operations used to treat wastewater solids.

The most significant limitation of our research is the use of real-time quantitative PCR targeting various ARGs as a surrogate

Table 4 | Values of *P* for comparing the relative statistical significance of different kinetic coefficients determined using Welch's *t*-test for unequal *n* and unequal sample variance.

Gene	16S rRNA gene	*Bacteroides* spp.	Human-specific *Bacteroides* spp.	*erm*(B)	*intI1*	*sul1*	*tet*(A)	*tet*(W)	*tet*(X)
16S rRNA gene	1	3×10^{-5}	0.6	0.02	0.3	0.06	0.03	7×10^{-4}	0.8
Bacteroides spp.		1	2×10^{-4}	1×10^{-4}	2×10^{-5}	5×10^{-5}	6×10^{-5}	6×10^{-4}	3×10^{-5}
Human-specific *Bacteroides* spp.			1	0.4	0.4	1	0.9	0.1	0.6
erm(B)				1	9×10^{-3}	0.1	0.2	0.1	0.02
intI1					1	0.01	5×10^{-3}	2×10^{-4}	0.3
sul1						1	0.6	4×10^{-3}	0.02
tet(A)							1	6×10^{-3}	0.01
tet(W)								1	6×10^{-4}
tet(X)									1

for ARB. The genes quantified here could be present in dead but intact bacteria or in bacteria in which the gene is non-functional. Similarly, the identity of the ARB harboring the ARGs detected in this study, and their clinical significance, remain unknown. Finally, only a select group of ARGs were targeted; even though these genes represent several important classes of antibiotics and all three known molecular mechanisms of resistance to tetracyline, they cover a relatively small cross-section of possible resistance gene targets.

In conclusion, aerobic digestion can be used to eliminate ARGs in untreated wastewater solids, but rates can vary substantially depending on the reactor design and the specific ARG examined. This information represents a critical step toward our long-term goal of applying wastewater treatment technologies to mitigate the spread of antibiotic resistance. This knowledge is particularly useful to wastewater treatment engineers as they compare the relative merits of alternative residual solids treatment technologies and for designing specific unit operations to eliminate ARGs. Specifically, aerobic digestion technology, which is used by numerous full-scale municipal wastewater treatment facilities, appears less effective at eliminating ARGs than both conventional and high temperature anaerobic digestion.

ACKNOWLEDGMENTS

This work was supported, in part, by grant 0967176 from the National Science Foundation.

REFERENCES

Aminov, R. I., Garrigues-Jeanjean, N., and Mackie, R. I. (2001). Molecular ecology of tetracycline resistance: development and validation of primers for detection of tetracycline resistance genes encoding ribosomal protection. *Appl. Environ. Microbiol.* 67, 22–32.

Arnold, S., Gassner, B., Giger, T., and Zwahlen, R. (2004). Banning antimicrobial growth promoters in feedstuffs does not result in increased therapeutic use of antibiotics in medicated feed in pig farming. *Pharmacoepidemiol. Drug Saf.* 13, 323–331.

Auerbach, E. A., Seyfried, E. E., and McMahon, K. D. (2007). Tetracycline resistance genes in activated sludge wastewater treatment plants. *Water Res.* 41, 1143–1151.

Beecher, N., Crawford, K., Goldstein, N., Kester, G., Lono-Batura, M., Dziezyk, E., et al. (2007). *Final Report: A National Biosolids Regulation, Quality, End Use and Disposal Survey.* Tamworth, NH: North East Biosolids and Residuals Association.

Bernhard, A. E., and Field, K. G. (2000). A PCR assay to discriminate human and ruminant feces on the basis of host differences in Bacteroides-Prevotella genes encoding 16S rRNA. *Appl. Environ. Microbiol.* 66, 4571–4574.

Bönemann, G., Stiens, M., Pühler, A., and Schlüter, A. (2006). Mobilizable IncQ-related plasmid carrying a new quinolone resistance gene, qnrS2, isolated from the bacterial community of a wastewater treatment plant. *Antimicrob. Agents Chemother.* 50, 3075–3080.

Chen, J., Yu, Z., Michel, F. C., Wittum, T., and Morrison, M. (2007). Development and application of real-time PCR assays for quantification of erm genes conferring resistance to macrolides-lincosamides-streptogramin B in livestock manure and manure management systems. *Appl. Environ. Microbiol.* 73, 4407–4416.

Clesceri, L. S., Greenberg, A. E., and Eaton, A. D. (eds.). (1999). *Standard Methods for the Examination of Water and Wastewater, 20th Edn.* Washington, DC: American Public Health Association.

da Silva, M. F., Tiago, I., Veríssimo, A., Boaventura, R. A. R., Nunes, O. C., and Manaia, C. M. (2006). Antibiotic resistance of enterococci and related bacteria in an urban wastewater treatment plant. *FEMS Microbiol. Ecol.* 55, 322–329.

Diehl, D. L., and LaPara, T. M. (2010). Effect of temperature on the fate of genes encoding tetracycline resistance and the integrase of Class 1 integrons within anaerobic and aerobic digesters treating municipal wastewater solids. *Environ. Sci. Technol.* 44, 9128–9133.

Edgar, R., Friedman, N., Molshanski-Mor, S., and Qimron, U. (2012). Reversing bacterial resistance to antibiotics by phage-mediated delivery of dominant sensitive genes. *Appl. Environ. Microbiol.* 78, 744–751.

Galvin, S., Boyle, F., Hickey, P., Vellinga, A., Morris, D., and Cormican, M. (2010). Enumeration and characterization of antimicrobial-resistant *Escherichia coli* bacteria in effluent from municipal, hospital, and secondary treatment facility sources. *Appl. Environ. Microbiol.* 76, 4772–4779.

Ghosh, S., Ramsden, S. J., and LaPara, T. M. (2009). The role of anaerobic digestion in controlling the release of tetracycline resistance genes and class 1 integrons from municipal wastewater treatment plants. *Appl. Microbiol. Biotechnol.* 84, 791–796.

Goldstein, C., Lee, M. D., Sanchez, S., Hudson, C., Phillips, B., Register, B., et al. (2001). Incidence of Class 1 and 2 integrases in clinical and commensal bacteria from livestock, companion animals, and exotics. *Antimicrob. Agents Chemother.* 45, 723–726.

Graham, D. W., Olivares-Rieumont, S., Knapp, C. W., Lima, L., Werner, D., and Bowen, E. (2011). Antibiotic resistance gene abundances associated with waste discharges to the Almendares River near Havana, Cuba. *Environ. Sci. Technol.* 45, 418–424.

Heuer, H., and Smalla, K. (2007). Manure and sulfadiazine synergistically increased bacterial antibiotic resistance in soil over at least two months. *Environ. Microbiol.* 9, 657–666.

Jabes, D. (2011). The antibiotic RandD pipeline: an update. *Curr. Opin. Microbiol.* 14, 564–569.

Kohanski, M. A., Dwyer, D. J., and Collins, J. J. (2010). How antibiotics kill bacteria: from targets to networks. *Nat. Rev. Microbiol.* 8, 423–435.

LaPara, T. M., Burch, T. R., McNamara, P. J., Tan, D. T., Yan, M., and Eichmiller, J. J. (2011). Tertiary-treated municipal wastewater is a significant point source of antibiotic resistance genes into Duluth-Superior Harbor. *Environ. Sci. Technol.* 45, 9543–9549.

Layton, A., McKay, L., Williams, D., Garrett, V., Gentry, R., and Sayler, G. (2006). Development of Bacteroides 16S rRNA gene TaqMan-based real-time PCR assays for estimation of total, human, and bovine fecal pollution in water. *Appl. Environ. Microbiol.* 72, 4214–4224.

Levy, S. B. (2005). Antibiotic resistance—the problem intensifies. *Adv. Drug Deliv. Rev.* 57, 1446–1450.

Levy, S. B., and Marshall, B. (2004). Antibacterial resistance worldwide: causes, challenges and responses. *Nat. Med.* 10, 122–129.

Levy, S. B., McMurry, L. M., Barbosa, T. M., Burdett, V., Courvalin, P., Hillen, W., et al. (1999). Nomenclature for new tetracycline resistance determinants. *Antimicrob. Agents Chemother.* 43, 1523–1524.

Ma, Y., Wilson, C. A., Novak, J. T., Riffat, R., Aynur, S., Murthy, S., et al. (2011). Effect of various sludge digestion conditions on sulfonamide, macrolide, and tetracycline resistance genes and class I integrons. *Environ. Sci. Technol.* 45, 7855–7861.

Mazel, D. (2006). Integrons: agents of bacterial evolution. *Nat. Rev. Microbiol.* 4, 608–620.

Munir, M., Wong, K., and Xagoraraki, I. (2011). Release of antibiotic resistant bacteria and genes in the effluent and biosolids of five wastewater utilities in Michigan. *Water Res.* 45, 681–693.

Muyzer, G., de Waal, E. C., and Uitterlinden, A. G. (1993). Profiling of complex microbial populations by denaturing gradient gel electrophoresis analysis of polymerase chain reaction-amplified genes coding for 16S rRNA. *Appl. Environ. Microbiol.* 59, 695–700.

Ng, L.-K., Martin, I., Alfa, M., and Mulvey, M. (2001). Multiplex PCR for the detection of tetracycline resistant genes. *Mol. Cell. Probes* 15, 209–215.

Palumbi, S. R. (2001). Humans as the world's greatest evolutionary force. *Science* 293, 1786–1790.

Pruden, A., Pei, R., Storteboom, H., and Carlson, K. H. (2006). Antibiotic resistance genes as emerging contaminants: studies in northern Colorado. *Environ. Sci. Technol.* 40, 7445–7450.

Ramsden, S. J., Ghosh, S., Bohl, L. J., and LaPara, T. M. (2010). Phenotypic and genotypic analysis of bacteria isolated from three municipal wastewater treatment plants on tetracycline-amended and ciprofloxacin-amended growth media. *J. Appl. Microbiol.* 109, 1609–1618.

Roberts, M. C., Sutcliffe, J., Courvalin, P., Jensen, L. B., Rood, J., and Seppala, H. (1999). Nomenclature for macrolide and macrolide-lincosamide-streptogramin B resistance determinants. *Antimicrob. Agents Chemother.* 43, 2823–2830.

Sambrook, J., Fritsch, E. F., and Maniatis, T. (1989). *Molecular Cloning: A Laboratory Manual.* 2nd Edn. Coldspring Harbor, NY: Coldspring Harbor Laboratory.

Schlüter, A., Szczepanowski, R., Pühler, A., and Top, E. M. (2007). Genomics of IncP-1 antibiotic resistance plasmids isolated from wastewater treatment plants provides evidence for a widely accessible drug resistance gene pool. *FEMS Microbiol. Rev.* 31, 449–477.

Seurinck, S., Defoirdt, T., Verstraete, W., and Siciliano, S. D. (2005). Detection and quantification of the human-specific HF183 Bacteroides 16S rRNA genetic marker with real-time PCR for assessment of human faecal pollution in freshwater. *Environ. Microbiol.* 7, 249–259.

Spellberg, B., Blaser, M., Guidos, R. J., Boucher, H. W., Bradley, J. S., Eisenstein, B. I., et al. (2011). Combating antimicrobial resistance: policy recommendations to save lives. *Clin. Infect. Dis.* 52(Suppl. 5), S397–S428.

Stalder, T., Barraud, O., Casellas, M., Dagot, C., and Ploy, M.-C. (2012). Integron involvement in environmental spread of antibiotic resistance. *Front. Microbiol.* 3:119. doi: 10.3389/fmicb.2012.00119

Szczepanowski, R., Linke, B., Krahn, I., Gartemann, K.-H., Gützkow, T., Eichler, W., et al. (2009). Detection of 140 clinically relevant antibiotic-resistance genes in the plasmid metagenome of wastewater treatment plant bacteria showing reduced susceptibility to selected antibiotics. *Microbiology* 155, 2306–2319.

Tchobanoglous, G., Burton, F. L., and Stensel, H. D. (2003). *Wastewater Engineering: Treatment and Reuse.* 4th Edn. Boston, MA: McGraw-Hill.

Uyaguari, M. I., Fichot, E. B., Scott, G. I., and Norman, R. S. (2011). Characterization and quantitation of a novel {beta}-lactamase gene within a wastewater treatment facility and surrounding coastal ecosystem. *Appl. Environ. Microbiol.* 77, 8226–8233.

Wierup, M. (2001). The Swedish experience of the 1986 year ban of antimicrobial growth promoters, with special reference to animal health, disease prevention, productivity, and usage of antimicrobials. *Microb. Drug Resist.* 7, 183–190.

Zhang, T., Zhang, M., Zhang, X., and Fang, H. H. (2009a). Tetracycline resistance genes and tetracycline resistant Enterobacteriaceae in activated sludge of sewage treatment plants. *Environ. Sci. Technol.* 43, 3455–3460.

Zhang, X.-X., Zhang, T., Zhang, M., Fang, H. H. P., and Cheng, S.-P. (2009b). Characterization and quantification of class 1 integrons and associated gene cassettes in sewage treatment plants. *Appl. Microbiol. Biotechnol.* 82, 1169–1177.

Zhang, X.-X., and Zhang, T. (2011). Occurrence, abundance, and diversity of tetracycline resistance genes in 15 sewage treatment plants across China and other global locations. *Environ. Sci. Technol.* 45, 2598–2604.

10

Chronological change of resistance to β-lactams in *Salmonella enterica* serovar Infantis isolated from broilers in Japan

Takehisa Chuma[1]*, Daisuke Miyasako[1], Hesham Dahshan[1,2], Tomoko Takayama[1], Yuko Nakamoto[1], Francis Shahada[3], Masato Akiba[3] and Karoku Okamoto[1]

[1] Laboratory of Veterinary Public Health, Department of Veterinary Medicine, Joint Faculty of Veterinary Medicine, Kagoshima University, Kagoshima, Japan
[2] Department of Veterinary Public Health, Faculty of Veterinary Medicine, Zagazig University, Zagazig, Egypt
[3] Safety Research Team, National Institute of Animal Health, Tsukuba, Japan

Edited by:
Kunihiko Nishino, Osaka University, Japan

Reviewed by:
Bruno Gonzalez-Zorn, Universidad Complutense de Madrid, Spain
Béla Nagy, Hungarian Academy of Sciences, Hungary

***Correspondence:**
Takehisa Chuma, Laboratory of Veterinary Public Health, Department of Veterinary Medicine, Faculty of Agriculture, Kagoshima University, 1-21-24 Korimoto, Kagoshima 890-0065, Japan.
e-mail: chuma@vet.kagoshima-u.ac.jp

Epidemiologic surveillance study was conducted in southern Japan to determine the antimicrobial resistance phenotypes and characterize the β-lactamase genes and the plasmids harboring these genes in *Salmonella enterica* serovar Infantis (*S.* Infantis) isolates from broilers. Between January, 2007 and December, 2008, a total of 1,472 fecal samples were collected and examined at the Laboratory of Veterinary Public Health, Kagoshima University, Japan. In 93 (6.3%) isolates recovered, 33 (35.5%) isolates showed resistance to cefotaxime, an extended-spectrum cephalosporin (ESC), conferred by TEM-20, TEM-52 and CTX-M-25 extended-spectrum β-lactamases (ESBLs). In addition to ESC-resistance, eight (8.6%) isolates exhibited resistance to cefoxitin mediated by CMY-2 AmpC β-lactamase. Plasmid analysis and polymerase chain reaction replicon typing revealed the bla_{TEM-20} and bla_{CMY-2} genes were associated with IncP plasmids, bla_{TEM-52} was linked with a non-typable plasmid and $bla_{CTX-M-25}$ was carried by an IncA/C plasmid. Non-β-lactam resistance to streptomycin, sulfamethoxazole, and oxytetracycline encoded by the *aadA1*, *sul1*, and *tet*(A) genes, respectively, was found in 86 (92.5%) isolates. Resistance to kanamycin and ofloxacin was exhibited in 12 (12.9%) and 11 (11.8%) isolates, respectively, the former was mediated by *aphA1-lab*. These data indicate that *S.* Infantis isolates producing ESBLs and AmpC β-lactamase have spread among broiler farms in Japan. These data demonstrated that the incidence of ESC-resistant S. Infantis carrying bla_{TEM-52} remarkably increased and *S.* Infantis strains harboring bla_{CMY-2}, bla_{TEM-20}, or $bla_{CTX-M-25}$ genes emerged from broilers in Japan for the first time in 2007 and 2008.

Keywords: antimicrobial resistance, β-lactamase gene, broiler, extended-spectrum cephalosporin, *Salmonella enterica* serovar Infantis, plasmids

INTRODUCTION

Non-typhoidal *Salmonella enterica* serovars (*Salmonella*) are a major cause of bacterial food-borne diseases world-wide (Majowicz et al., 2010). The food poisoning statistics in Japan show that bacterial food poisoning patients during the year 2008 numbered at 10,331 and *Salmonella* were the leading etiological agents accounting for 24.7% of the cases [http://idsc.nih.go.jp/iasr/29/342/graph/t3421.gif]. Poultry products are important vehicles in the transmission, and have been incriminated in several *Salmonella* outbreaks (Kimura et al., 2004; Chittick et al., 2006). Since the late 1990s, *Salmonella enterica* serovar Infantis (*S.* Infantis) has been the commonest serovar of *Salmonella* isolated from both broiler flocks and retail chicken meat in Japan (Asai et al., 2007b; Iwabuchi et al., 2011).

The emergence of multidrug-resistant *Salmonella* has become a serious global health problem because antimicrobial treatment is lifesaving for invasive infections, particularly in neonates of <1 year of age. Preventive antimicrobial treatment is also generally given to patients suffering from immunosuppressive or other predisposing conditions (Hohmann, 2001). The options of first-line therapy for *Salmonella* infection include ampicillin (AMP), sulfamethoxazole-trimethoprim, fluoroquinolones, and extended-spectrum cephalosporins (ESCs). ESCs are among the preferred drugs because of resistance to the other aforementioned drugs is relatively frequent in *Salmonella* isolates (Hohmann, 2001). At present, ESC-resistance in *Salmonella* is mainly attributed to the acquisition of plasmid-mediated extended-spectrum β-lactamases (ESBLs) and AmpC β-lactamases (Bonnet, 2004; Arlet et al., 2006).

Salmonella carrying the bla_{CMY-2} gene were recently recovered from bovine and porcine salmonellosis cases (Dahshan et al., 2010; Sugawara et al., 2011). Besides, *S.* Infantis isolates harboring the bla_{TEM-52} gene were reported from broilers for the first time in the year 2004 (Shahada et al., 2010a). Thus, a major concern has been increased prevalence of resistance to ESCs noted in *S.* Infantis isolates. This study was conducted to determine the antimicrobial resistance phenotypes and characterize the β-lactamase genes and the plasmids harboring these genes in *S.* Infantis isolated from broiler flocks.

MATERIALS AND METHODS

BACTERIAL ISOLATES

Between January, 2007 and December, 2008, a total of 1,472 cecal specimens derived from 92 broiler flocks (ca. 10,000 birds per flock) were collected from a poultry processing plant located in the southern part of Japan. Usually, 16 samples per flock were randomly selected fortnightly. The isolation, identification and serotyping of S. Infantis isolates were performed at the Laboratory of Veterinary Public Health, Kagoshima University, Japan as previously described (Shahada et al., 2008).

DETERMINATION OF MINIMUM INHIBITORY CONCENTRATIONS

Antimicrobial susceptibility testing was assayed by the agar dilution method on Mueller-Hinton (MH) agar (Oxoid Ltd., Basingstoke, Hampshire, England) plates according to the National Committee for Clinical and Laboratory Standards guidelines (National Committee for Clinical Laboratory Standards, 2001). *S.* Infantis isolates were tested for sensitivities to AMP, cefotaxime (CTX), cefoxitin (FOX), chloramphenicol (CHL), streptomycin (STR), sulfamethoxazole (SUL), oxytetracycline (TET), kanamycin (KAN), and ofloxacin (OFX). The MIC range was set at 0.125–512 μg/ml for all tested antimicrobial agents. The MIC breakpoints were interpreted according to the new criteria established by the Clinical and Laboratory Standards Institute (2012). *Escherichia coli* (*E. coli*) ATCC 25922 and *Staphylococcus aureus* ATCC29213 were used as quality control strains.

DOUBLE-DISK SYNERGY ASSAY

The double-disk synergy testing was conducted to screen for ESBLs and AmpC β-lactamases as previously described (Shahada et al., 2010a). This test was performed as a standard Kirby-Bauer disk diffusion assay on MH agar (Oxoid) plates.

DETECTION OF RESISTANCE DETERMINANTS

All DNA templates were prepared using the InstaGene Matrix kit (Bio-Rad Laboratories, Hercules, CA, USA). Detection of resistance genes was performed by polymerase chain reaction (PCR). The amplification reactions were carried out using primers and conditions as previously described (Dahshan et al., 2010; Shahada et al., 2010b). Briefly, the targets were as follows: bla_{TEM}, bla_{OXA}, bla_{PSE}, bla_{SHV}, $bla_{CTX-M-1}$ group, $bla_{CTX-M-2}$ group, $bla_{CTX-M-25}$, and *Toho-1* encoding for penicillinases; bla_{CIT}, bla_{CMY-2}, bla_{DHA}, bla_{FOX}, bla_{MOX}, bla_{ACC}, and bla_{EBC} encoding for cephalosporinases; *tet*(A), *tet*(B), and *tet*(G) mediating tetracycline efflux proteins; *aadA1* and *aadA2* encoding for resistance to STR and spectinomycin; *sul1* conferring resistance to SUL; and *aphA1-Iab* encoding for resistance to KAN.

When β-lactamase-encoding genes were positive following PCR amplification, obtained products were directly sequenced using a BioDye Terminator version 3.1 Ready Reaction sequencing kit and ABI 3100 automated DNA sequencer (Applied Biosystems, Foster City, CA, USA). The DNA alignments and deduced amino acid sequences were examined using the BLAST program (National Center for Biotechnology Information, USA).

PLASMID ANALYSIS

All *S.* Infantis isolates were examined for the carriage of plasmids by employing the alkaline lysis method as previously described (Kado and Liu, 1981). The molecular size of plasmids was determined by using the standard *Salmonella enterica* serovar Choleraesuis ATCC 7001 (50 kbp) and *S.* Typhimurium DT104 strain 300-98 (90 kbp). The plasmid size was estimated by graphing the molecular size of standard strains versus the distance traveled from the wells using logistic graph paper. Conjugation experiments were performed as described previously (Shahada et al., 2010a). In brief, *S.* Infantis donor isolates and rifampicin-resistant *E. coli* DH5α recipient derivatives were used for conjugal mating. Conjugants were selected onto deoxycholate hydrogen sulfide lactose agar containing 128 μg/ml rifampicin and 128 μg/ml AMP, followed by antimicrobial testing and the detection of transferred resistance genes as above. Plasmids were characterized by the PCR-based replicon typing method as described previously (Carattoli et al., 2005) to detect the plasmid types: IncI1, IncA/C, IncHI1, IncHI2, IncN, IncX, IncW, IncY, IncP, IncT, IncFIIs, IncL/M, IncFIA, IncFIB, IncFIC, IncFrepB, IncK/B, and IncB/O.

RESULTS

ANTIMICROBIAL RESISTANCE

S. Infantis isolates were recovered in 54 (58.7%) of 92 flocks surveyed and 93 (6.3%) of 1,472 samples examined. Antimicrobial susceptibility profiles of the isolates are summarized in **Table 1**. Of 93 *S.* Infantis isolates recovered, 34 (36.5%) exhibited resistance to AMP (MIC, 256 to >512 μg/ml), 33 (35.5%) showed resistance to CTX (MIC, 4-256 μg/ml) and eight (8.6%) demonstrated resistance to FOX (MIC, 32–128 μg/ml). From the 93 isolates and with regard to non-β-lactam antibiotics, 86 (92.5%) isolates exhibited resistance to STR (MIC, 16–512 μg/ml, conferred by *aadA1*), SUL (MIC > 512 μg/ml, conferred by *sul1*) and TET (MIC, 64–512 μg/ml, conferred by *tetA*); 12 (12.9%) isolates showed resistance to KAN (MIC, ≥512 μg/ml, conferred by *aphA1*); and 11 (11.8%) isolates demonstrated resistance to OFX (MIC, 2–8 μg/ml). All 93 isolates were fully susceptible to CHL. On the basis of resistance patterns, 11 phenotypes (A to K) were demonstrated as depicted in **Table 2**. The most frequent pattern was STR/SUL/TET (43 isolates) followed by AMP/CTX/STR/SUL/TET (14 isolates).

ESBL AND AMPC CHARACTERIZATION

Double-disk synergy testing revealed 25 ESBL- and eight AmpC β-lactamase-producing *S.* Infantis isolates. TEM-type ESBL was identified in 23 (24.7%) isolates, CTX-M-type ESBL was demonstrated in one isolate and CMY-type AmpC β-lactamase was detected in eight isolates. Nucleotide sequencing of PCR products confirmed that the amplicons were bla_{TEM-52} (22 isolates), bla_{TEM-20} (one isolate), bla_{CTX-25} (one isolate in combination with bla_{TEM-52}), and bla_{CMY-2} (8 isolates). Of 54 S. Infantis-positive flocks, As indicated in **Table 3**, *S.* Infantis isolates harboring bla_{TEM-1} were not detected during the present study; but, they were found during 1998–2003 (one isolate) and 2004–2006 (17 isolates). On the other hand, isolates harboring bla_{TEM-52} were identified during 2004–2006 (11 isolates) and 2007–2008 (22 isolates). Isolates carrying the bla_{TEM-20}, bla_{CTX-25}, and

Table 1 | Antimicrobial susceptibility among 93 *Salmonella* Infantis isolates detected in this study

Antimicrobial agent	MIC breakpoint (μg/m/)	No. of resistant isolates (%)	
		This study	Previous study
		2007–2008	2004–2006[a]
AMP	≥32	34 (36.5)	29 (24.2)
CTX	≥4	33 (35.5)	11 (9.1)
FOX	≥32	8 (8.6)	0 (0)
CHL	≥32	0 (0)	0 (0)
STR	≥16	86 (92.5)	120 (100)
SUL	≥512	86 (92.5)	120 (100)
TET	≥16	86 (92.5)	120 (100)
KAN	≥64	12(12.9)	9 (7.5)
OFX	≥2	11(11.8)	25 (20.8)

CTX, cefotaxime; FOX, cefoxitin; CHL, chloramphenicol; STR, streptomycin; SUL, sulfamethoxazole; TET, oxytetracycline; KAN, kanamycin; OFX, ofloxacin. (a) Cited from the previous study (Shahada et al., 2010b)

bla_{CMY-2} genes were demonstrated during 2007–2008 study period.

PLASMID CHARACTERIZATION

Three plasmid profiles were defined among S. Infantis isolates. Seventy isolates harbored ca. 180-kbp plasmids (profile I), 22 isolates carried two plasmids of ca. 50 and 180 kbp (profile II), and one isolate possessed three plasmids of ca. 50, 125, and 180 kbp (profile III; **Figure 1**). Isolates exhibiting resistance to ESCs displayed diverse profiles: Of 34 ESC-resistant S. Infantis isolates, 22 belonged to profile II, 11 were classified into profile I and one isolate was categorized into profile III (**Table 2**). PCR-based replicon typing revealed three kinds of plasmids. Large-size plasmids (ca.180 kbp) were typed as IncP, intermediate-size plasmid (ca. 125 kbp) was typed as IncA/C and small plasmids (ca. 50 kbp) were non-typable. Large-, intermediate- and small-size plasmids were self-transmissible to *E. coli* recipient strain by conjugation. The bla_{TEM-20} and bla_{CMY-2} genes were associated with large IncP plasmids, $bla_{CTX-M-25}$ was affiliated with intermediate IncA/C plasmid and the bla_{TEM-52} gene was linked to small non-typable plasmids.

DISCUSSION

The results obtained in this study show that resistance to ESCs has increased to 35.5% from the previous 9.2% reported during an earlier investigation (Shahada et al., 2010b). Other new findings include the detection of S. Infantis isolates harboring the bla_{TEM-20}, $bla_{CTX-M-25}$, and bla_{CMY-2} genes. Demonstration of these resistance traits in S. Infantis serovar is a rare phenomenon. This is the first report describing these mechanisms of ESC-resistance exhibited by S. Infantis isolates derived from broilers. Previous reports indicate that β-lactam resistance in broilers was once mediated by bla_{TEM-1}, a narrow-spectrum β-lactamase gene that was demonstrated in one S. Infantis isolate recovered during 1998–2003 (Shahada et al., 2006) and 14.2% of the isolates obtained in 2004–2006 (Shahada et al., 2010a). Besides, during the period of 2004–2006, resistance to ESCs mediated by bla_{TEM-52} was reported for the first time from the broiler industry in Japan (Shahada et al., 2010a).

Table 2 | Distribution of resistance phenotypes, plasmid profiles and β-lactamase phenotypes in *Salmonella* Infantis isolates

Resistance pattern	Resistance phenotype	Plasmid profile	size (ca. kbp)	replicon type	No. of isolates	β-lactamase phenotype
A	AMP/CTX/FOX/STR/SUL/TET/KAN	I	180	IncP	1	AmpC
B	AMP/CTX/FOX/STR/SUL/TET	I	180	IncP	7	AmpC
C	AMP/CTX/STR/SUL/TET/OFX	II	180, 50	IncP, Non-typable	4	ESBL
D	AMP/CTX/STR/SUL/TET/KAN	II	180,50	IncP, Non-typable	2	ESBL
E	AMP/CTX/STR/SUL/TET	I	180	IncP	2	ESBL
	AMP/CTX/STR/SUL/TET	II	180, 50	IncP, Non-typable	11	ESBL
	AMP/CTX/STR/SUL/TET	III	180, 125, 50	IncP, IncA/C, Non-typable	1	ESBL
F	AMP/CTX	II	180, 50	IncP, Non-typable	5	ESBL
G	AMP/STR/SUL/TET	I	180	IncP	1	-
H	STR/SUL/TET/OFX	I	180	IncP	7	-
I	STR/SUL/TET/KAN	I	180	IncP	7	-
J	STR/SUL/TET	I	180	IncP	43	-
K	KAN	I	180	IncP	2	_

AMP, ampicillin; CTX, cefotaxime; FOX, cefoxitin; CHL, chloramphenicol; STR, streptomycin; SUL, sulfamethoxazole; TET, oxytetracycline; KAN, kanamycin; OFX, ofloxacin.

Table 3 | Chronological change of β-lactamase genes in serovar Infantis

β-lactamase gene *(bla)*	No. of isolates during the isolation period		
	1998–2003[a] (178 isolates)	2004–2006[b] (120 isolates)	2007–2008[c] (93 isolates)
TEM-1	1 (0.7%)	17 (14.2%)	0 (0%)
TEM-52	0 (0%)	11 (9.2)	22 (24.4%)[d]
TEM-20	0 (0%)	0 (0%)	1 (1.8%)
CTX-M-25	0 (0%)	0 (0%)	1 (1.8%)
CMY-2	0 (0%)	0 (0%)	8 (8.6%)

[a] *Cited from the previous study (Shahada et al., 2006).*
[b] *Cited from the previous study (Shahada et al., 2010b).*
[c] *This study.*
[d] *CTX-M-25 and TEM-52 were simultaneously identified in one isolate.*

In the present study, we identified one *S.* Infantis isolate harboring the bla_{TEM-20} gene while other isolates had bla_{TEM-52}. It's worth noting that the wild-type bla_{TEM-1} gene was not detected during this study suggesting the likelihood of occurrence of point mutations which led to the emergence of observed variants, bla_{TEM-20} and bla_{TEM-52}. This hypothesis is supported by deduced amino acid sequence analysis which revealed that the bla_{TEM-20} gene differs from bla_{TEM-1} by two substitutions, Met182→Thr and Gly238→Ser; whereas the bla_{TEM-52} gene differs from bla_{TEM-1} by three substitutions, Glu104 Lys, Met182→Thr, and Gly238→Ser (Arlet et al., 1999; Weill et al., 2004). This phenomenon has the implications for bacterial adaptation mechanism because bla_{TEM-1} seems to have lost its fitness as a potential resistance trait necessary for survival of *Salmonella.* Thus, point mutations have taken place as the evolutionary adaptation mechanism crucial for successful colonization of the broiler chicken intestinal tract.

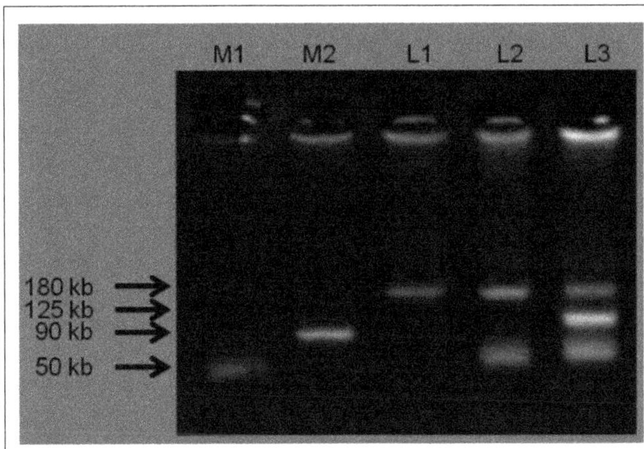

FIGURE 1 | Three plasmid profiles obtained from *S.* Infantis isolates. Lane M1 and M2 shows standard sizes of plasmids extracted from *S. Choleraesuis* ATCC 7001 (50 kbp) and *S.* Typhimurium DT104 strain 300-98 (90 kbp), respectively. L1: IncP (ca. 180 kbp), L2: IncP (ca. 180 kbp) and Untypable plasmid (ca. 50 kbp), L3: IncP (ca. 180 kbp), IncA/C (ca. 125 kbp), and Untypable plasmid (ca. 50 kbp).

In Japan, CTX-M-type ESBL-producing *Enterobacteriaceae* are important nosocomial infectious agents raising considerable concern in the public health community. Similarly, the detection of CTX-M-2 and CTX-M-25 ESBL-producing *E. coli* isolates from chickens affected with colibacillosis has raised concerns in the veterinary public health community (Kojima et al., 2005; Asai et al., 2011). We report for the first time one *S.* Infantis isolate harboring $bla_{CTX-M-25}$ on IncA/C plasmid and bla_{TEM-52} on non-typable plasmid. Because $bla_{CTX-M-25}$ was initially demonstrated in *E. coli* (Asai et al., 2011) a comprehensive molecular study is required to determine the likely source and elucidate mechanisms involved in collecting antimicrobial resistance traits and mobilizing them across taxonomical borders.

To date, several reports have described the emergence of AmpC β-lactamase-producing *Salmonella* derived from farm animals affected with salmonellosis. One of the studies involving *Salmonella enterica* serovar Typhimurium (*S.* Typhimurium) identified bla_{CMY-2} associated with self-transmissible IncI1-Iγ and A/C plasmids (Sugawara et al., 2011). Another study revealed a novel chromosomally integrated multi-drug resistance genomic island harboring bla_{CMY-2} among clonally related *S.* Typhimurium isolates (Shahada et al., 2011). Consequently, the detection of bla_{CMY-2} in several *S.* Infantis isolates from broilers poses another challenge in the veterinary public health community. Carriers of bla_{CMY-2} harbored IncP plasmids initially demonstrated in *Pseudomonas* bacteria (Shintani et al., 2011).

Antimicrobial susceptibility data indicate a gradual decrease of OFX resistance to 11.8 from 20.8% previously reported (Shahada et al., 2010b). Fluoroquinolones (e.g., OFX) are broad-spectrum antimicrobial agents widely used in clinical medicine. Emergence of fluoroquinolone resistance was attributed to overuse of this group of drugs in domestic animals either therapeutically or for the purpose of growth promotion (Asai et al., 2007a). Since 1991, the Japanese Ministry of Agriculture, Forestry and Fisheries (JMAFF) approved this class of antimicrobials in veterinary medicine for therapeutic purposes and prohibited its use as feed additives. Fluoroquinolones might have been prescribed prudently among antimicrobial agents used in broiler farms in Japan. This likely has contributed to the decline of resistance to OFX observed in the present study.

Taken together, these results show increased resistance against ESCs mediated by both ESBLs and AmpC β-lactamases. It seems these resistance traits have spread among farm animals in Japan while their likely source remains largely unknown. The probability that resistance to ESCs may continue to spread among members of the *Enterobacteriaceae* family poses another public health challenge because ESBLs and AmpC β-lactamases limit the effectiveness of cephalosporin therapy.

ACKNOWLEDGMENT

This study was partly supported by a Grants-in-Aid for Scientific Research (No.23580426) from the Japan Society for the Promotion of Science.

REFERENCES

Arlet, G., Barrett, T. J., Butaye, P., Cloeckaert, A., Mulvey, M. R., and White, D. G. (2006). *Salmonella* resistant to extended-spectrum cephalosporins: prevalence and epidemiology. *Microbes Infect.* 8, 1945–1954.

Arlet, G., Goussard, S., Courvalin, P., and Philippon, A. (1999). Sequences of the genes for the TEM-20, TEM-21, TEM-22, and TEM-29 extended-spectrum beta-lactamases. *Antimicrob. Agents Chemother.* 43, 969–971.

Asai, T., Harada, K., Ishihara, K., Kojima, A., Sameshima, T., Tamura, Y., et al. (2007a). Association of antimicrobial resistance in *Campylobacter* from food-producing animals with antimicrobial use on farms. *Jpn. J. Infect. Dis.* 60, 290–294.

Asai, T., Ishihara, K., Harada, K., Kojima, A., Tamura, Y., Sato, S., et al. (2007b). Long-term prevalence of antimicrobial-resistant *Salmonella enterica* subspecies *enterica* serovar Infantis in the broiler chicken industry in Japan. *Microbiol. Immunol.* 51, 111–115.

Asai, T., Masani, K., Sato, C., Hiki, M., Usui, M., Baba, K., et al. (2011). Phylogenetic groups and cephalosporin resistance genes of Escherichia coli from diseased food-producing animals in Japan. *Acta Vet. Scand.* 53, 52.

Bonnet, R. (2004). Growing group of extended-spectrum beta-lactamases: the CTX-M enzymes. *Antimicrob. Agents Chemother.* 48, 1–14.

Carattoli, A., Bertini, A., Villa, L., Falbo, V., Hopkins, K. L., and Threlfall, E. J. (2005). Identification of plasmids by PCR-based replicon typing. *J. Microbiol. Methods* 63, 219–228.

Chittick, P., Sulka, A., Tauxe, R. V., and Fry, A. M. (2006). A summary of national reports of foodborne outbreaks of *Salmonella* Heidelberg infections in the United States: clues for disease prevention. *J. Food Prot.* 69, 1150–1153.

Clinical and Laboratory Standards Institute. (2012). *Performance Standards for Antimicrobial Susceptibility Testing: 22th Information Supplement M100-S22*, Wayne, PA.

Dahshan, H., Chuma, T., Shahada, F., Akiba, M., Fujimoto, H., Akasaka, K., et al. (2010). Characterization of antibiotic resistance and the emergence of AmpC-producing *Salmonella* Infantis from pigs. *J. Vet. Med. Sci.* 72, 1437–1442.

Hohmann, E. L. (2001). Nontyphoidal salmonellosis. *Clin. Infect. Dis.* 32, 263–269.

Iwabuchi, E., Yamamoto, S., Endo, Y., Ochiai, T., and Hirai, K. (2011). Prevalence of *Salmonella* isolates and antimicrobial resistance patterns in chicken meat throughout Japan. *J. Food Prot.* 74, 270–273.

Kado, C. I., and Liu, S. T. (1981). Rapid procedure for detection and isolation of large and small plasmids. *J. Bacteriol.* 145, 1365–1373.

Kimura, A. C., Reddy, V., Marcus, R., Cieslak, P. R., Mohle-Boetani, J. C., Kassenborg, H. D., et al. (2004). Chicken consumption is a newly identified risk factor for sporadic *Salmonella enterica* serotype Enteritidis infections in the United States: a case-control study in FoodNet sites. *Clin. Infect. Dis.* 38, S244–S252.

Kojima, A., Ishii, Y., Ishihara, K., Esaki, H., Asai, T., Oda, C., et al. (2005). Extended-spectrum-beta-lactamase-producing *Escherichia coli* strains isolated from farm animals from 1999 to 2002: report from the Japanese Veterinary Antimicrobial Resistance Monitoring Program. *Antimicrob. Agents Chemother.* 49, 3533–3537.

Majowicz, S. E., Musto, J., Scallan, E., Angulo, F. J., Kirk, M., O'Brien, S. J., et al. (2010). The global burden of nontyphoidal *Salmonella* gastroenteritis. *Clin Infect Dis.* 50, 882–889.

National Committee for Clinical Laboratory Standards. (2001). *Performance Standards for Antimicrobial Disk and Dilution Susceptibility Test for Bacteria Isolated from Animals-Second Edition: Approved Standard M31-A2*, Wayne, PA.

Shahada, F., Chuma, T., Tobata, T., Okamoto, K., Sueyoshi, M., and Takase, K. (2006). Molecular epidemiology of antimicrobial resistance among *Salmonella enterica* serovar Infantis from poultry in Kagoshima, Japan. *Int. J. Antimicrob. Agents* 28, 302–307.

Shahada, F., Chuma, T., Okamoto, K., and Sueyoshi, M. (2008). Temporal distribution and genetic fingerprinting of *Salmonella* in broiler flocks from southern Japan. *Poult. Sci.* 87, 968–972.

Shahada, F., Chuma, T., Dahshan, H., Akiba, M., Sueyoshi, M., and Okamoto, K. (2010a). Detection and characterization of extended-spectrum beta-lactamase (TEM-52)-producing *Salmonella* serotype Infantis from broilers in Japan. *Foodborne Pathog. Dis.* 7, 515–521.

Shahada, F., Sugiyama, H., Chuma, T., Sueyoshi, M., and Okamoto, K. (2010b). Genetic analysis of multi-drug resistance and the clonal dissemination of beta-lactam resistance in *Salmonella* Infantis isolated from broilers. *Vet. Microbiol.* 140, 136–141.

Shahada, F., Sekizuka, T., Kuroda, M., Kusumoto, M., Ohishi, D., Matsumoto, A., et al. (2011). Characterization of *Salmonella enterica* serovar Typhimurium isolates harboring a chromosomally encoded CMY-2 beta-lactamase gene located on a multidrug resistance genomic island. *Antimicrob. Agents Chemother.* 55, 4114–4121.

Shintani, M., Tokumaru, H., Takahashi, Y., Miyakoshi, M., Yamane, H., Nishida, H., et al. (2011). Alterations of RNA maps of IncP-7 plasmid pCAR1 in various *Pseudomonas* bacteria. *Plasmid* 66, 85–92.

Sugawara, M., Komori, J., Kawakami, M., Izumiya, H., Watanabe, H., and Akiba, M. (2011). Molecular and phenotypic characteristics of CMY-2 beta-lactamase-producing *Salmonella enterica* serovar Typhimurium isolated from cattle in Japan. *J. Vet. Med. Sci.* 73, 345–349.

Weill, F. X., Demartin, M., Fabre, L., and Grimont, P. A. (2004). Extended-spectrum-beta-lactamase (TEM-52)-producing strains of *Salmonella enterica* of various serotypes isolated in France. *J. Clin. Microbiol.* 42, 3359–3362.

Who possesses drug resistance genes in the aquatic environment?: sulfamethoxazole (SMX) resistance genes among the bacterial community in water environment of Metro-Manila, Philippines

Satoru Suzuki[1]*, Mitsuko Ogo[1], Todd W. Miller[1], Akiko Shimizu[2], Hideshige Takada[2] and Maria Auxilia T. Siringan[3]

[1] Center for Marine Environmental Studies, Ehime University, Matsuyama, Japan
[2] Laboratory of Organic Geochemistry, Tokyo University of Agriculture and Technology, Fuchu, Japan
[3] Microbiological Research and Services Laboratory, Natural Sciences Research Institute, College of Science, University of the Philippines Diliman, Manila, Philippines

Edited by:
Marilyn C. Roberts, University of Washington, USA

Reviewed by:
Timothy LaPara, University of Minnesota, USA
Veljo Kisand, University of Tartu, Estonia

***Correspondence:**
Satoru Suzuki, Center for Marine Environmental Studies, Science Bldg. 2, Ehime University, Bunkyo-3, Matsuyama, Ehime 790-8577, Japan.
e-mail: ssuzuki@ehime-u.ac.jp

Recent evidence has shown that antibiotic resistant bacteria (ARB) and antibiotic resistance genes (ARGs) are ubiquitous in natural environments, including sites considered pristine. To understand the origin of ARGs and their dynamics, we must first define their actual presence in the natural bacterial assemblage. Here we found varying distribution profiles of *sul* genes in "colony forming bacterial assemblages" and "natural bacterial assemblages." Our monitoring for antibiotic contamination revealed that sulfamethoxazole (SMX) is a major contaminant in aquatic environments of Metro-Manila, which would have been derived from human and animal use, and subsequently decreased through the process of outflow from source to the sea. The SMX-resistant bacterial rate evaluated by the colony forming unit showed 10 to 86% of the total colony numbers showed higher rates from freshwater sites compared to marine sites. When *sul* genes were quantified by qPCR, colony-forming bacteria conveyed *sul1* and *sul2* genes in freshwater and seawater (10^{-5}–10^{-2} copy/16S) but not *sul3*. Among the natural bacterial assemblage, all *sul1*, *sul2*, and *sul3* were detected (10^{-5}–10^{-3} copy/16S), whereas all *sul* genes were at an almost non-detectable level in the freshwater assemblage. This study suggests that *sul1* and *sul2* are main *sul* genes in culturable bacteria, whereas *sul3* is conveyed by non-culturable bacteria in the sea. As a result marine bacteria possess *sul1*, *sul2* and *sul3* genes in the marine environment.

Keywords: sulfonamide resistance, sul gene, non-culturable, marine, aquatic environment

INTRODUCTION

Antibiotic resistant bacteria (ARB) are selected under low concentrations of antibiotics (Gullberg et al., 2011), in which the mutant selection window (MSW) comprising a range of concentrations where resistant bacteria can be selectable is designated (Drlica, 2001). Low concentrations of antibiotics selects for low-level ARB due to an adaptive mutation, which can sometimes result in high-level resistance (Baquero, 2001). Such a situation can be found in natural aquatic environments. Thus, the bacterial response to very low concentrations of antibiotics in the environment has been of particular focus (Gullberg et al., 2011), and the response behavior of environmental bacteria under MSW has been reviewed (Andersson and Hughes, 2011). However, a majority of environmental bacteria, especially in the ocean, are non-culturable (Colwell and Grimes, 2000), and hence it is necessary to study ARB including the non-culturable community while simultaneously monitoring antibiotic concentrations.

Antibiotics used in human and animal medicine are released through manure, wastewater and subsequently to rivers, lakes, and oceans, the culmination of which is a major concern in the development of ARB. Although the released antibiotics are diluted and degraded in the ocean, trace level concentrations can potentially select for and preserve ARB, even in areas considered to be pristine. Our previous studies have shown the potential for ARB and antibiotic resistance genes (ARGs) to be reserved in natural aquatic environments and even in non-contaminated areas (Rahman et al., 2008; Tamminen et al., 2011). It is generally understood that clinically derived ARGs are a risk to patients; however, whether the ARGs found in the environment are a risk to humans is not understood. To clarify the origin, movement and preservation of ARGs in natural environments and to assess risk, it is necessary to quantitatively track ARGs from terrestrial water ways to the ocean. Moreover, concentrations of antibiotics in various water ways should be quantified as a baseline to see correlation between antibiotic contamination and the occurrence of ARGs.

Among antibiotics used throughout tropical Asia, sulfonamides have been widely applied in human and animal medicine, with previous studies showing their bacterial resistance rate to be higher (2–90%; Hoa et al., 2011) than tetracycline (0.07–0.18%; Kobayashi et al., 2007) and quinolone (0.1–15%; Takasu et al., 2011). Sulfonamides have a low chelating ability, low binding constants, high water solubility, and stability (Sukul and Spiteller, 2006). Therefore, once sulfonamides are released into the aquatic environment, they remain active against bacteria due to their chemical characteristics, and can furthermore accelerate the development of ARB in natural microbial communities.

Although contamination by antibiotics and ARB in Vietnam, Thailand and other countries of Indochina has recently been summarized (Suzuki and Hoa, 2012), the extent to which this occurs in other tropical Asian areas is not known. As for aquatic environments in the Philippines, the occurrence of ARB has previously been reported (Tendencia and de la Peña, 2001; Kim et al., 2003), however, despite the frequent use of sulfonamides in humans and animals, sulfonamide resistance has not been addressed.

As mentioned above, to clarify the role of the environmental bacterial assemblage on the dynamics of ARGs, the full community including non-culturable bacteria should be targeted. Here we monitored antibiotic concentrations and sulfonamide resistance genes through a lake, river and bay system within Metro-Manila. Furthermore, comparison of culturable to the total bacterial assemblage provided new evidence that the possession profile of ARGs (*sul*) in bacteria varied between freshwater and marine bacteria.

MATERIALS AND METHODS

SAMPLING

Water samples were taken at four sites in Laguna Lake (st. MNL-1 ~4), two sites in the Pasig River (st. MNR-1 and 2) and four sites in Manila Bay (st. MNB-1 ~4), in November 3–4, 2009, in Metro-Manila, the Philippines (**Figure 1**). Among the lake sites, MNL-4 was closes to land relative to the other MNL sites.

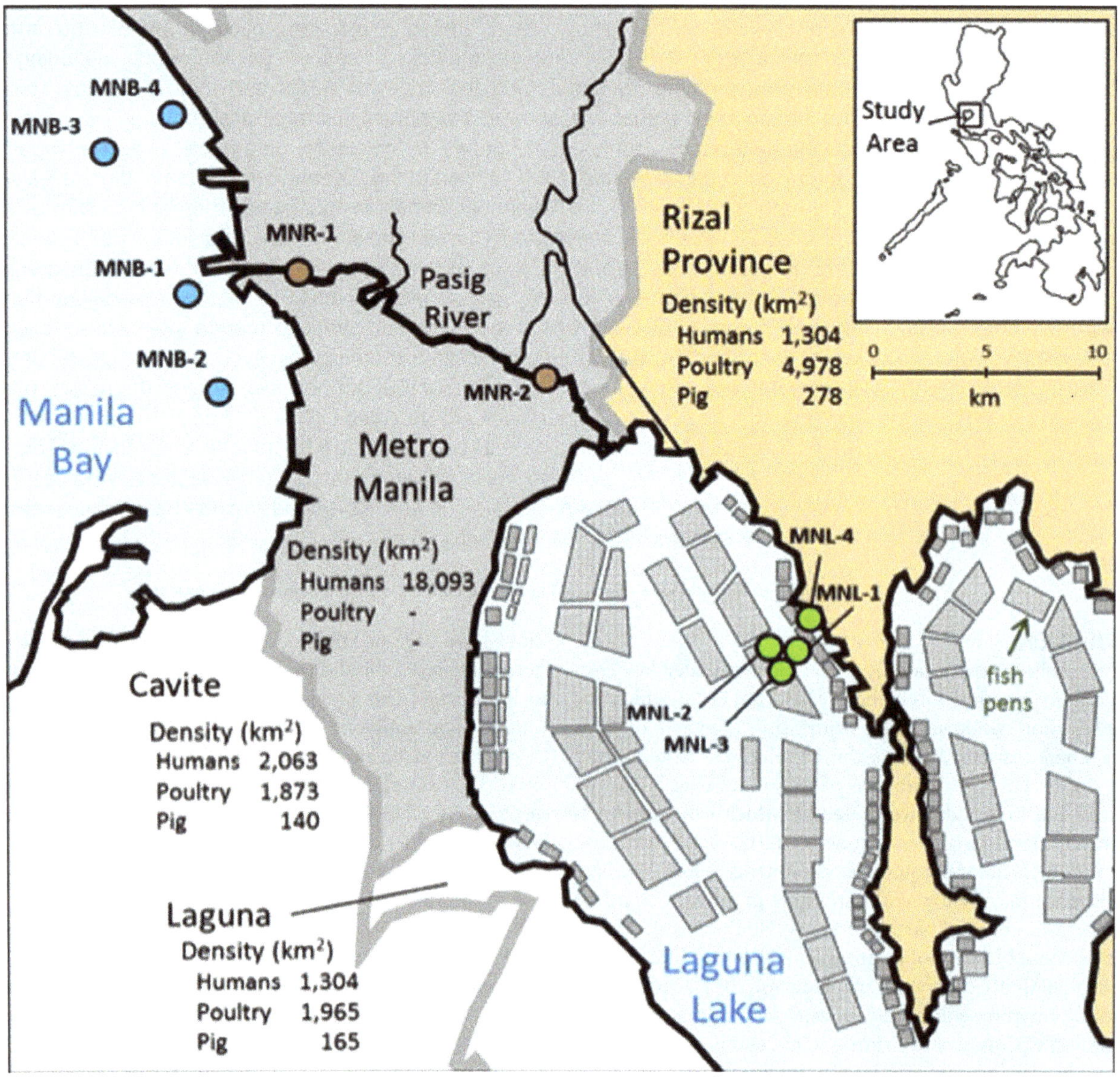

FIGURE 1 | Map of sampling sites in Metro-Manila. Surface water was taken from four sites (MNL-1~4) in Laguna Lake, two sites (MNR-1, 2) in the Pasig River, and four sites (MNB-1~4) in Manila Bay. Conditions in surrounding are inserted on map. Squares in Laguna Lake denote areas of aquaculture net pens.

From the river sites, MNR-2 was in the upper river location closest to Laguna Lake and –1 was the lower site closer to Manila Bay. The marine Manila Bay site MNB-1 was near the mouth of the Pasig River whereas MNB-4 was closer to land with a very high density of people with low capacity for wastewater control. For the entire study area, information on human population densities and agriculture activities are shown in **Figure 1**. Sampling occurred one month after Typhoon Ondoy, and there was still substantial high-flood levels in Laguna Lake that flooded well within the surrounding towns. For all sites, surface water was taken by alcohol-sterilized bucket, and stored in a sterilized polypropylene bottle for the bacterial experiment and a glass bottle for antibiotic analysis. All samples were transported on ice and taken to the lab within several hours for the experiment. At each site environment measurements of salinity, pH and temperature were taken by a pH/conductivity meter (Horiba D-54, Horiba, Kyoto, Japan). Total suspended solids (TSS) were measured by filtering 50 ml of subsurface water samples through a pre-weighed 47 mm glass fiber filter (GF/F, retention >0.7 μm), then drying in a drying oven at 60°C for 24 h. The filter was then allowed to cool and be reweighed in a temperature/humidity controlled room. The TSS was calculated as the added weight in mg to the filter divided by the total volume of water filtered (mg/ml).

ANTIBIOTIC CONCENTRATIONS

Target antibiotics of oxytetracycline (OTC), sulfamethoxazole (SMX), sulfamethazine, trimethoprim, and lincomycin, were all analyzed according to Ye et al. (2006). Briefly, the antibiotics were solid-phase extracted by using Oasis HLB (200 mg; Waers) and the extracts were analyzed by liquid chromatograph (Agilent series 1100, Tokyo, Japan) equipped with a tandem mass spectrometer (LC-MS/MS; TSQ Quantum 7000, Thermo Finnigan, Japan). The antibiotics quantified by LC-MS/MS were separated in a Xterra MS C18 (2.1 mm i.d. × 50 mm; particle size: 2.5 μm; Waters) with a guard column (Xterra MS C18; 2.1 mm i.d. 20 mm; particle size: 3.5 μm; Waters) by using a binary gradient system (solvent A: 1% formic acid in H_2O; solvent B: acetonitrile) at a flow rate of 0.2 ml/min. The run started at 5% B for 5 min, followed by a 11-min linear gradient to 95% B, then the initial conditions were reestablished and the column was equilibrated for 17 min. Analytes were quantified in selected reaction monitoring mode on positive electrospray, ESI positive mode. This procedure was used for other cases reported in Managaki et al. (2007) and Hoa et al. (2011).

BACTERIAL COUNTS

The colony-forming bacteria were counted on nutrient agar (NA) plates. Organic nutrients may affect the sensitivity on SMX. We have confirmed that nutrient concentration in NA did not have an effect on susceptibility of bacteria using a sensitive strain (*E. coli* AG1). Each water sample (0.5 ml) was 10-fold serially diluted with 4.5 ml of phosphate-buffered saline (PBS, pH 7.4). A 100-μl of aliquot was spread on Nutrient Broth (Difco Laboratories, Detroit, MI) plus 1.5% agar and 0.5% NaCl plate, and incubated at 30°C for 7 days in duplicates. NA plates containing 60 μg/ml of SMX or oxytetracycine (OTC) were used to enumerate SMX-resistant (SMX^r) and OTC-resistant bacteria. For total cell count, glutaraldehyde was added to 1 ml of sample to a final concentration of 2% to fix the cells. After filtration with a black polycarbonate filter (0.2 μm pore size, Millipore, Billerica, MA, USA), bacterial cells were stained with 5 μg/ml ethidium bromide. The bacteria were enumerated by epifluorescence microscopy (BX60, Olympus Co., Tokyo, Japan). More than 300 cells were enumerated, and a minimum of 20 fields were randomly selected. However, appropriate enumeration could not be done from lake and river (upper reach) samples due to interference by small clay particles.

DNA PREPARATION

Extraction of DNA was performed from filters and from mixtures of colonies on plates. To obtain DNA from the total bacterial assemblage, an appropriate amount of water samples (30–200 ml) was filtered through 47-mm polycarbonate filters (0.2 μm pore size, Millipore), which were kept at −20°C and transported to the laboratory. Triplicate filters were used for DNA extraction. All colonies that appeared on agar plates with SMX were suspended in PBS and cells were harvested by centrifugation. The cells were kept at −80°C until DNA extraction. The DNA of culturable SMX^r bacteria was obtained from this sample. The extraction of DNA from filters and mixtures of colonies was carried out according to the cethyltrimethylammonium bromide (CTAB)-method (Wilson, 1987) with some modification. Briefly, thawed filters were dipped in TE buffer (10 mM Tris-HCl, 1 mM EDTA, pH 8.0) containing sodium dodecyl sulfate (SDS, 0.5%), Proteinase K (0.1 mg/ml, TaKaRa, Otsu, Japan) and RNase A (0.05 mg/ml, SIGMA-ALDRICH, St. Louis, MO, USA). The filter was incubated at 37°C for 1 h. To remove polysaccharides, a CTAB/NaCl solution (10% CTAB and 0.7 M NaCl) was added, and the samples were incubated at 65°C for 10 min. The freeze-thawing was repeated with three cycles of freezing at −80°C and thawing at 65°C to increase the recovery of DNA from bacterial cells. Subsequently, an equal volume of phenol-chloroform-iso amyl alcohol (25:24:1) was added, and the tubes were inverted and centrifuged at 2100 ×g at 4°C for 10 min. The supernatant was divided between two 1.5-ml tubes, and an equal volume of chloroform-iso amyl alcohol (24:1) was added. The tubes were inverted and centrifuged at 21,600 ×g for 10 min at 4°C, and supernatant was collected in another 1.5-ml tube. The samples were precipitated with an addition of 0.1 volume of 3 M sodium acetate and then a 0.6 volume of iso-propanole. The precipitated pellets were dried under vacuum and dissolved in 50 μl of sterilized Milli-Q water. The recovered DNA was quantified by ultraviolet absorption meter (DU640, BECKMAN COULTER, Orange County, CA, USA), and the quality of the DNA was checked by electrophoresis on 1.0% agarose gel with ethidium bromide staining.

DENATURED GRADIENT GEL ELECTROPHORESIS (DGGE)

Community structure was estimated by DGGE targeting 16S rRNA gene, and the dominant microbial diversity was compared with banding profile (Boon et al., 2002; Takasu et al., 2011). Total DNA was purified from a filter (as environmental DNA) and pooled-colony on NA plate (as culturable bacterial DNA). PCR and electrophoresis conditions were the same as Muyzer et al. (1993). The representative bands, common ones and specific ones, on the DGGE gel were cut out from the gel and were sequenced.

QUANTITATIVE PCR

Quantitative PCR was performed using a CFX 96 Real-Time system (BioRad Laboratories, Hercules, CA, USA) to detect an increase of double-stranded DNA with an increase in fluorescence. PCR amplifications were performed in a 20 μl reaction volume containing 1× Sso Fast EvaGreen Supermix (BioRad), 500 nM of each primer and 1 μl of sample DNA. Quantitative PCR was performed using previously designed primers; bacterial 16S rRNA genes (Suzuki et al., 2000), *sul*1 (Heuer and Smalla, 2007), *sul*2 (Heuer et al., 2008), and *sul*3 (Pei et al., 2006). Serial 1:10 dilutions of plasmids constructed from the pGEM-T Easy vector (Promega, Madison, WI, USA) and 16S rRNA gene from *E. coli* K12, *sul*1 from plasmid R388, *sul*2 from plasmid RSF1010 and *sul*3 from plasmid pUVP4401 fragments were used as standards for quantification (Heuer and Smalla, 2007). The qPCR program consisted of an initial denaturation of 30 s at 95°C and 40 cycles of 5 s at 95°C (denaturation) and 10 s at 50°C for 16S rRNA gene and 10 s at 51°C for *sul*1 and *sul*2 and 20 s at 60°C (extension) for *sul*3 respectively. Melting curves for the amplicons were measured by raising the temperature slowly from 60°C and 65°C to 95°C for 16S rRNA gene, *sul1, sul2,* and *sul3*, respectively, while monitoring fluorescence (**Figure A1**). Each sample was measured in triplicate. The copy numbers of *sul1, sul2,* and *sul3* were normalized by dividing by the 16S rRNA gene copy number at the respective time points to take into account any temporal variation in bacterial cell numbers. Unit of the copy number is described as copies/16S through text. The results were analyzed using a Big Dye terminator kit on a 3130 ABI Prism sequencer (Applied Biosystems, Foster City, CA, USA). PCR products were sequenced and phylogenetic relationship among *sul1, sul2,* and *sul3* was analyzed.

DNA SEQUENCING

PCR product of *sul* genes and 16S rRNA genes on DGGE were sequenced to show phylogenicity of these genes. Purified PCR products were sequenced on an ABI Genetic Analyzer 3130 (Applied Biosystems) with BigDye Terminator, version 3.1. The sequencing primers for *sul* gene were the same as above and 341f was for 16S rRNA gene. Sequences were aligned with known sequences in the DDBJ database using BLAST. Phylogenetic relationships were inferred by pairwise comparison and the neighbor joining method using Clustal X (Thompson et al., 1997). Phylogenetic trees were edited using Treebiew (Page, 1996), and out groups were *E. coli* dihydropteroate synthase (DHPS) (accession number: CP001637) for *sul* genes and *Ketogulonigenium vulgrum* WSH-001 (accession number: NC-17384) for 16S rRNA gene. The accession numbers of the newly sequenced *sul* genes were shown in **Figure 3**.

RESULTS AND DISCUSSION

ENVIRONMENTAL CONDITION

We systematically sampled water from Laguna Lake to Manila Bay (**Figure 1**). Laguna Lake is the largest freshwater body in the Philippines (911 km^2) and the extensive area is used for fish pen-aquaculture as shown in **Figure 1**. The north side of Laguna Lake is Rizal Province, where the density of animal farms is high. Water from Laguna Lake flows out through the Pasig River to Manila Bay, with the Pasig River running through and receiving wastewater from Metro-Manila, the highest populated area of the Philippines. Physico-chemical conditions of sampling sites are summarized in **Table 1**. In Manila Bay, we collected surface water from four sites. The MNB-1 site is located near the mouth of the Pasig River, where salinity was lower than the other bay sites (**Table 1**). Since the sampling period was only one month after Typhoon Ondoy, surface seawater salinity indicated freshwater flow into the bay. The lake and river water samples contained clay particles, which interfered with cell counting under the microscope, whereas this was extensively lower in the bay samples due to dilution, aggregation and sedimentation.

ANTIBIOTICS CONTAMINATION

It has been reported that more developed countries frequently use macrolides as major antibiotics for humans and animals, whereas

Table 1 | Environmental and microbial data at sampling sites.

Site	Water temp (°C)	pH	Salinity	Suspended solid (mg/l)	EtBr* count (cells/ml)	Viable count (cells/ml)	SMX^r count (cells/ml) (%)***
MNL-1	27.0	8.10	0	86.5	CI**	1.6×10^4	2.7×10^3 (16.9)
MNL-2	27.4	8.16	0	94.6	CI	2.1×10^4	3.8×10^3 (18.1)
MNL-3	27.4	8.09	0	92.5	CI	1.5×10^4	2.8×10^3 (18.7)
MNL-4	27.2	7.49	0	72.3	CI	4.7×10^4	1.2×10^4 (25.5)
MNR-2	27.0	7.81	0	66.8	CI	5.5×10^4	2.2×10^4 (40.0)
MNR-1	26.0	7.80	0	114.2	3.37×10^5	3.4×10^5	7.1×10^4 (20.9)
MNB-1	25.0	8.09	16	54.7	1.04×10^6	1.4×10^5	4.9×10^4 (35.0)
MNB-2	25.4	8.11	25	16.3	9.98×10^5	1.3×10^4	2.6×10^3 (13.0)
MNB-3	25.3	7.85	27	24.3	1.66×10^6	1.8×10^4	1.9×10^3 (10.6)
MNB-4	25.4	7.74	27	13.4	1.61×10^6	3.0×10^4	2.6×10^4 (86.7)

*Ethidium bromide.

**Count impossible due to clay particles having self-fluorescence.

***% was calculated by SMX^r count/viable count × 100.

Asian developing counties use more inexpensive drugs such as sulfonamides (Managaki et al., 2007; Luo et al., 2011). We monitored OTC, SMX, sulfamethazine, trimethoprim and lincomycin in this study. As shown in **Table 2**, OTC was not detected from all of the sites, whereas SMX was a major antibiotic in all sites followed by sulfamethazine. Trimethoprim, which is usually used as a combination drug with SMX, and lincomycin were lower in concentration than sulfonamides. This profile is the same as that observed from Vietnam (Managaki et al., 2007) and China (Luo et al., 2011). The concentration gradient was the same for all antibiotics, i.e., concentration was highest in the river mouth (MNB-1) and the lower reach of the river (MNR-1), Laguna Lake (MNL-1 ~4) showed similar concentrations among sites (27.8–41.6 ng/l for SMX), and the open Manila Bay marine sites MNB-2 to MNB-4 showed similar concentrations (7.8–17.7 ng/l for SMX). The SMX concentrations detected at the ng/l level in Laguna Lake and Pasig River sites were much lower than the inhibition concentration for susceptible bacteria. For sulfonamide antibiotics, concentrations of 10–400 mg/l could inhibit microbial activity, which is found in activated sludge by more than 20% (Ingerslev and Halling-Sørensen, 2000).

MICROBIAL NUMBER AND DIVERSITY

The total cell number was enumerated by ethidium bromide staining, showing 10^5–10^6/ml from the Pasig River and Manila Bay sites (**Table 1**). As mentioned above, microscope cell counts were impossible for the Laguna Lake and the upper reach of the Pasig River due to interference from clay particles. Viable cell numbers by colony counting showed that lake and bay sites were 10^4-levels/ml, and one order of magnitude larger in river-related sites (MNR-2, -1 and MNB-1) (**Table 1**). Microbial diversity was estimated in the DGGE method. The DGGE profiles of all colonies pooled from NA agar plate (**Figure 2A**) and of the water assemblage from filters (**Figure 2B**) was obtained. Representative common and specific bands were sequenced (**Figure 3**). Among the cultured colony, common species of γ-Proteobacteria closed to *Pseudomonas* (band number 1, 2, 3, 7, 11, 12, and 13) and *Alteromonas* (band number 5, 6, 8, 10, and 15) were detected through the lake, river, and bay system. These genera could be detected as an abundant group in the water column by the culture method (Fuhrman and Hagström, 2008). Environmental assemblage samples showed different profiles. Cyanobacteria related bands were commonly detected through Laguna Lake, Pasig River and Manila Bay (band number 16, 18, 21, 22, 24, 28, and 31). Abundant common species from the DGGE profiles varied between culturable bacteria and the assemblage. This suggests that culturable bacteria are not a major component of the natural assemblage, which are selected by the culture method. Thus, the detection of ARB by culture further suggests selection of ARGs from the total community. Enteric bacteria can be commonly detected from freshwater systems (Hoa et al., 2008, 2011; Hu et al., 2008), suggesting freshwater ARB most likely occur from aquatic, terrestrial and enteric species. Although the present study did not show enteric species among the sequenced band of DGGE, we still cannot ignore the possibility of horizontal gene transfer (HGT) across the bacterial community including enteric/terrestrial bacteria. In-part this is because of the high survival of enteric bacteria in water over time (Vital et al., 2008). We have previously suggested that species diversity may relate to a high ARG reserving potential (Suzuki et al., 2008). If physical turbulent mixing is occurring, the community may be resilient to the event and may recover over a short period, such as on a scale of days (Shade et al., 2012). Turbulence may also have an effect on ARG transfer among the community by quick HGT, which can occur within as short of a period as 60 min (Andrup and Anderson, 1999).

SMX^r BACTERIA

SMX^r rate is shown in **Table 1**. Laguna Lake sites (MNL-1~4) showed an SMX^r rate of 16.0–25.5%, which increased to 20.9–40.0% in the Pasig River sites (MNR-2, -1, and MNB-1). Manila Bay sites (MNB-2 and -3) showed rates of 10.6–13.0% with the exception at MNB-4 of 86.7%. The notably higher percentage at MNB-4 may have been due to the fact that this site was very close to a land area with high-density housing and poor wastewater control, where unknown substances and/or human derived bacteria may have contaminated the sample water. From SMX^r rate (**Table 1**) and drug concentration (**Table 2**), it can be seen that SMX was likely urban wastewater runoff (point and non-point sources) to the river and subsequently diluted in the sea. The SMX^r bacterial rate was highest from lake and river sites,

Table 2 | Antibiotic concentrations at sampling sites.

Site	OTC (ng/l)	SMX (ng/l)	Sulfamethazine (ng/l)	Trimethoprim (ng/l)	Lincomycin (ng/l)
MNL-1	<LOQ*	37.8	8.6	1.7	2.4
MNL-2	<LOQ	28.8	8.3	2.3	2.6
MNL-3	<LOQ	27.8	9.2	2.1	2.2
MNL-4	<LOQ	41.6	16.2	2.5	2.6
MNR-2	n.d.	46.6	12.0	2.3	5.5
MNR-1	<LOQ	79.8	73.1	9.2	7.4
MNB-1	<LOQ	93.8	61.1	18.3	6.7
MNB-2	n.d.	11.7	2.4	2.3	0.83
MNB-3	n.d.	7.8	3.9	1.6	0.80
MNB-4	n.d.	17.7	4.6	5.8	6.5

**LOQ, limit of quantitation, where compound was detected as a peak but not quantitative concentration; n.d., not detectable.*

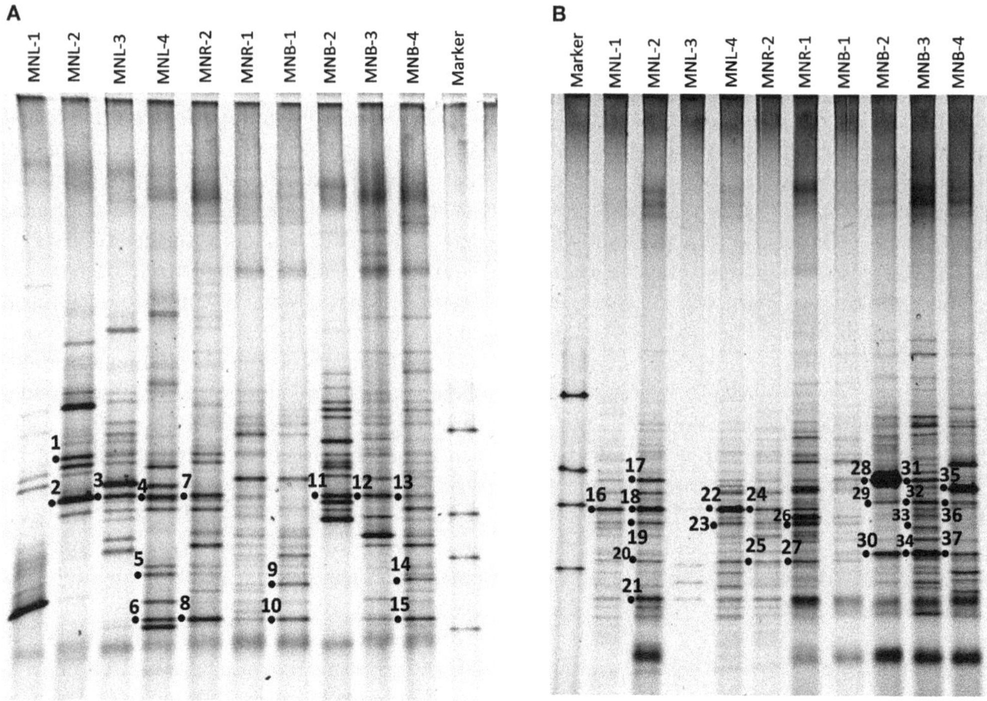

FIGURE 2 | DGGE analysis of each site using a primer set for 16S rRNA gene. (A) Cultured bacterial community, and **(B)** Natural environmental assemblage. Numbers are sequenced bands.

suggesting that SMX^r-culturable bacteria were minor in seawater. Correlation between concentrations of antibiotics and ARG (*sul1*) has been reported for wastewater treatment plants, WWTP (Gao et al., 2012b), suggesting that higher concentrations select ARB in the case of sulfonamides. In the WWTP reported by Gao et al. (2012b), 191 ng/l SMX was detected even in effluent, which is possibly an effective concentration for bacteria. Bacteria continuously exposed to higher concentrations of antibiotics should contain higher copies of *sul* genes, which spread among the community. The *sul* genes were reported from enteric and environmental bacteria, being mostly culturable species. However, particular attention should be given to non-culturable bacteria as an AGR reservoir. The present study examined the distribution of *sul* genes with qPCR among waters as well as colony forming assemblages as shown below.

QUANTIFICATION OF *sul* GENES

Total DNA was recovered from "SMX^r-colony forming bacterial assemblages" and "natural bacterial assemblages" which were purified from 0.2 µm Nuclepore filters. Detection of *sul* genes is shown in **Figure 4**. Colony forming bacteria possessed *sul1* as the major *sul* gene from Laguna Lake samples, and *sul2* was detected at a similar level from Pasig River and Manila Bay samples (**Figure 4A**). The *sul3* was not detected from all sites with the exception of MNR-1. Exceptionally high copies found in MNR-1 may have been due to colony formation of *sul3* possessing bacteria. The present study and other studies indicated that *sul3* is a minor sulfonamide resistance determinant in bacterial isolates in the aquatic environment (Hoa et al., 2008; Su et al., 2011). The origin of *sul3* is suspected to be human (Grape et al., 2003), however, Su et al. (2012) recently reported a high incidence (<40%) of *sul3* in environmental SMX-trimethoprim^r *E. coli*, suggesting that the distribution of *sul3* varies among environments. On the other hand, *sul* detection profiles from natural assemblages were quite different. Both *sul1* and *sul2* were mostly under the detection limit from lake and river sites (**Figure 4B**). This suggests that although *sul* genes are a minor gene in lake and river bacterial communities, the cultivation procedure effectively selected the *sul* possessing bacteria from the total assemblage. Gao et al. (2012a) recently reported that a natural assemblage from an aquaculture site and measured for several isolates, showed that SMX^r bacteria were found in a relatively wide group whereas *sul1* and *sul2* were detected in restricted species. In contrast to freshwater lake and river sites, bay site samples showed 10^{-5} to 10^{-3} copies/16S for all *sul1*, *sul2*, and *sul3*. The quantitative detection of *sul* genes in the marine environment has not been reported, and the present results are the first to indicate that the total bacterial assemblage possesses not only *sul1* and *sul2* but also *sul3*. It is thus clear that *sul* genes including *sul3* are relatively abundant in the marine bacterial assemblage, the majority of which are the non-culturable bacteria.

We sequenced *sul* genes from culturable bacteria and an environmental assemblage. Results showed no difference among each *sul1* and *sul2* gene (**Figure 5**). The *sul3* from culturable bacteria in MNR-1 and the seawater sample in MNB-4 were slightly different. This suggests that each *sul* group is possibly homogenous around this area.

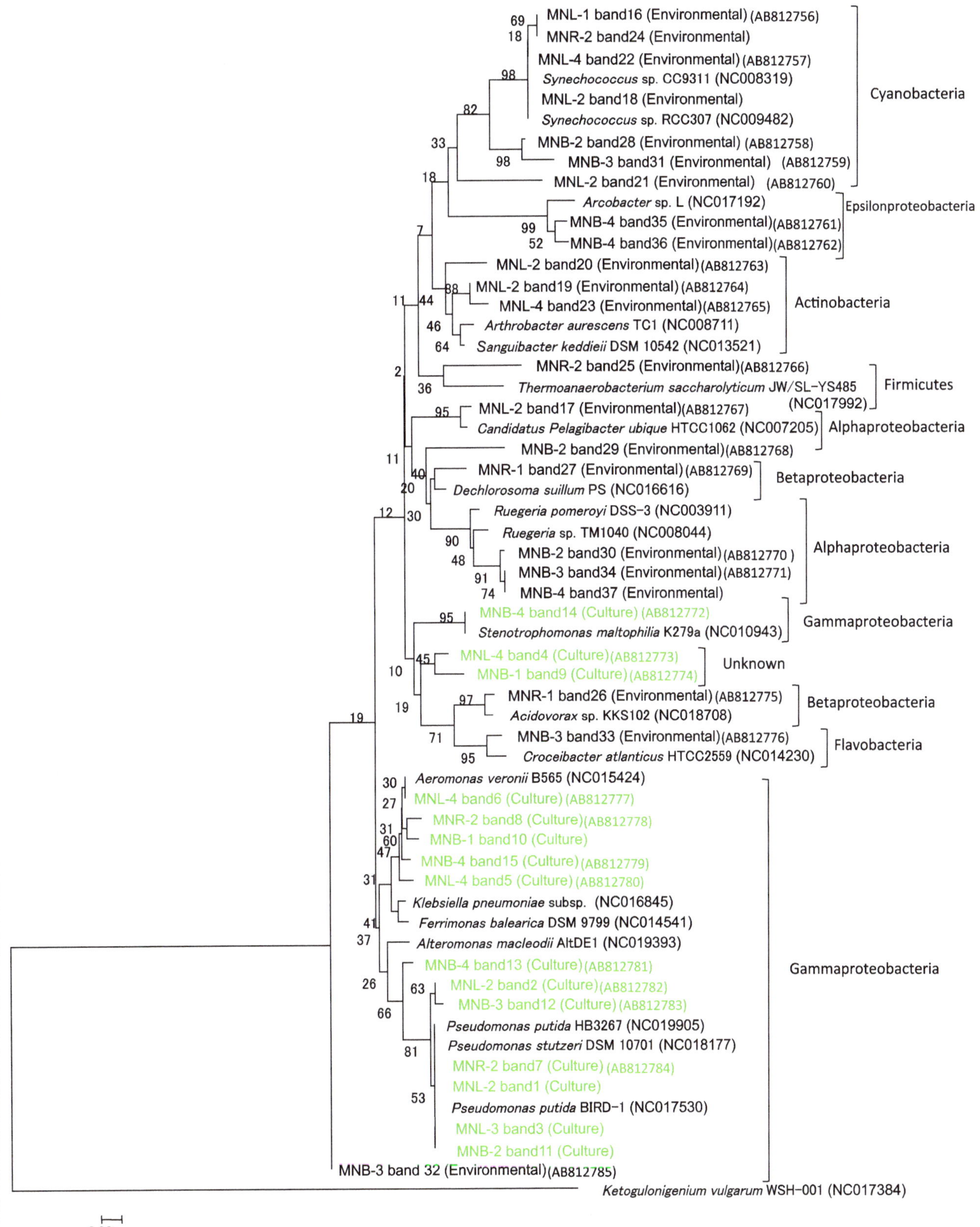

FIGURE 3 | Phylogenetic tree of 16S rRNA gene in DGGE (Figure 2). Representative common and specific 37 bands were sequenced. Green color is DNA of the pooled colony (Culture) and red color is DNA of the environmental water assemblage (Environmental).

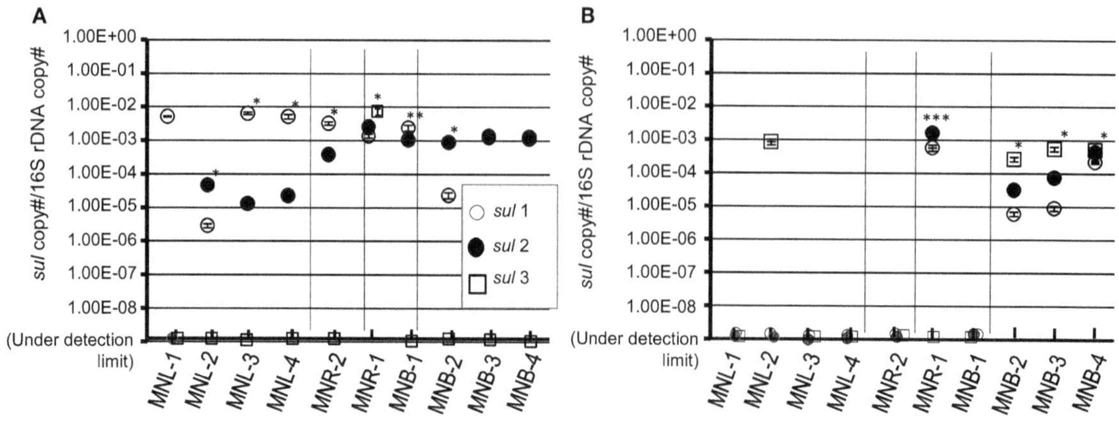

FIGURE 4 | Copy number of *sul* genes in a pooled-colony of SMX^r bacteria (A) and that of a natural total assemblage (B). Copy number was normalized by 16S rRNA gene (16S). Symbols are denoted as: open circle is *sul1*, closed circle is *sul2* and open square is *sul3*. SD from triplicate experiments is shown with vertical bar with symbol. *, significantly different three genes (ANOVA, $p < 0.001$) or two genes (*t*-test, $p < 0.001$); **, significantly different two genes (*t*-test, $p = 0.013$); ***, significantly different two genes (*t*-test, $p = 0.002$); no asterisk, not significantly different or only single gene was detected.

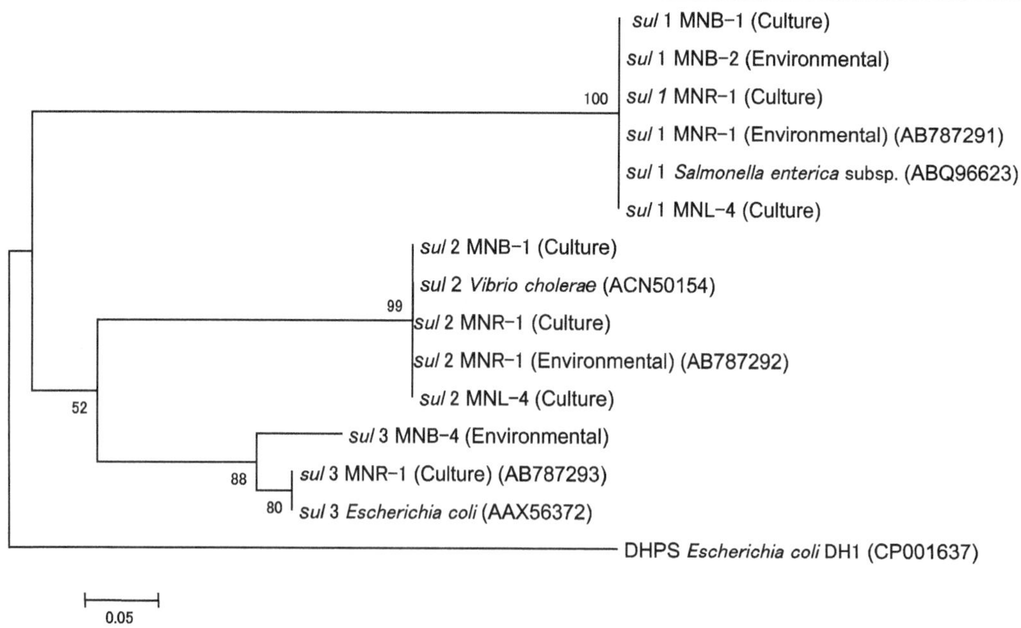

FIGURE 5 | Phylogenetic tree of *sul1*, *sul2*, and *sul3* from culturable bacteria (Culture) and the environmental water assemblage (Environmental).

The *sul* genes are frequently found on plasmids with integrons, suggesting these are transferable among bacteria (Sholz et al., 1989; Hall and Collis, 1998), although SMX^r based on chromosomal mutation is also known (Gibreel and Sköld, 1999). The present study used known PCR-primers to detect *sul* genes, suggesting the *sul* genes in seawater are the same as those genes prevalent among enteric and soil bacteria (Pei et al., 2006; Heuer and Smalla, 2007; Heuer et al., 2008). Thus, the origin(s) of the genes are suspected to be human and terrestrial bacteria, and the genes have a pathway and potential to be transferred to marine bacteria. The opposite HGT can be occurred from marine *Vibrio* to *E. coli* in OTC resistance gene (Neela et al., 2008). Generally ARGs are thought to originate within antibiotic producing bacteria, which are horizontally transferred to environmental microbes; known as the "producer hypothesis" based on Benveniste and Davies (1973). However, since sulfonamides are synthetic small molecules and there are no producers in the environment, the sulfonamide case does not fit the "producer hypothesis." Sulfonamide resistance genes have been suggested to be a fixed-mutation, which have been proposed to be a reservoir of ARGs (Sköld, 2010), although the *in situ* HGT between environmental bacteria and human pathogenic/enteric bacteria is unclear.

Recent evidence shows that enteric bacteria can survive and grow in aquatic environments by biofilm formation (Soreira et al., 2012) and also in soil (Byappanahalli et al., 2012). The bacteria conveying the *sul* genes with class 1 and 2 integrons predominantly originate from the discharge of wastewater (Su et al., 2012). Therefore, the contaminated bacteria having *sul* genes are mainly of human, animal and terrestrial origin, which transfer the genes to marine bacteria including non-culturable ones. The *sul1, sul2,* and *sul3* found in the seawater assemblage thus should flow into the sea and eventually accumulate in the marine bacteria community.

It is known that ARGs are circulated among animals and humans (Wooldridge, 2012). Once ARGs have become fixed in a bacterium, they are difficult to eliminate (Andersson and Hughes, 2011). We have reported that the OTC resistance gene *tet*(M) is distributed even in pristine ocean sediments (Rahman et al., 2008). This evidence also supports that ARGs in the marine environment would be of human and terrestrial origin, and ultimately fixed into the marine bacterial assemblage. Our study focusing on non-culturable bacteria in relation to ARGs is a useful approach to reveal potential reservoirs of ARGs in natural environments, with the potential of including different hosts in different environments.

ACKNOWLEDGMENTS

This work was supported in part by the GCOE Program, Ehime University, and KAKENHI (22241014, 22254001, 19405004), Japan Society for the Promotion of Science. Authors thank Mr. T. Ogawa and Dr. T. Yokokawa for their technical support.

REFERENCES

Andersson, D. I., and Hughes, D. (2011). Persistence of antibiotic resistance in bacterial populations. *FEMS Microb. Rev.* 35, 901–911.

Andrup, L., and Anderson, K. (1999). A comparison of the kinetics of plasmid transfer in the conjugation systems encoded by the F plasmid from *Escherichia coli* and plasmid pCF10 from *Enterococcus faecalis*. *Microbiology* 145, 2001–2009.

Baquero, F. (2001). Low-level antibacterial resistance: a gateway to clinical resistance. *Drug Resist. Updat.* 4, 93–105.

Benveniste, R., and Davies, J. (1973). Aminoglycoside antibiotic-inactivating enzymes in Actinomycetes similar to those present in clinical isolates of antibiotic-resistant bacteria. *Proc. Nat. Acad. Sci. U.S.A.* 70, 2276–2280.

Boon, N., De Windt, W., Verstraete, W., and Top, E. M. (2002). Evaluation of nested PCR-DGGE (denaturing gradient gel electrophoresis) with group-specific 16S rRNA primers for the analysis of bacterial communities from different wastewater treatment plants. *FEMS Microbiol. Ecol.* 39, 101–112.

Byappanahalli, M., Roll, B. M., and Fujioka, R. (2012). Evidence for occurrence, persistence, and growth potential of *Escherichia coli* and Enterocossi in Hawaii's soil environments. *Microbes Environ.* 27, 164–170.

Colwell, R. R., and Grimes, D. J. (eds.). (2000). *Nonculturable Microorganisms in the Environment*, Washington, DC: ASM Press.

Drlica, K. (2001). A strategy for fighting antibiotic resistance. *ASM News* 67, 27–33.

Fuhrman, J. A., and Hagström, A. (2008). "Bacterial and Archaeal community structure and its patterns," in *Microbial Ecology of the Ocean*, ed D. L. Kirchman (Hoboken, NJ: John Wiley and Sons, Inc.), 45–90.

Gao, P., Mao, D., Lui, Y., Wang, L., Xu, B., and Xu, L. (2012a). Occurrence of sulfonamide and tetracycline-resistant bacteria and resistance genes in aquaculture environment. *Wat. Res.* 46, 2355–2364.

Gao, P., Munir, M., and Xagoraraki, I. (2012b). Correlation of tetracycline and sulfonamide antibiotics with corresponding resistance genes and resistant bacteria in a conventional municipal wastewater treatment plant. *Sci. Total Environ.* 421–422, 173–183.

Gibreel, A., and Sköld, O. (1999). Sulfonamide resistance in clinical isolates of *Campylobacter jejuni:* mutational changes in the chromosomal dihydropteroate synthase. *Antimicrob. Agents Chemother.* 43, 2156–2160.

Grape, M., Sundström, L., and Kronvall, G. (2003). Sulphonamide resistance gene *sul3* in *Escherichia coli* isolated from human sources. *J. Antimicrob. Chemother.* 52, 1022–1024.

Gullberg, E., Cao, S., Berg, O. G., Ilback, C., Sandergren, L., Hughes, D., et al. (2011). Seletion of resistant bacteria at very low antibiotic concentrations. *PLoS Pathog.* 7:e1002158. doi: 10.1371/journal.ppat.1002158

Hall, R. M., and Collis, C. M. (1998). Antibiotic resistance in gram-negative bacteria: the role of gene cassettes and integrons. *Drug Resist. Updat.* 1, 109–119.

Heuer, H., Focks, A., Lamshoft, M., and Smalla, K. (2008). Fate of sulfadiazine administered to pigs and its quantitative effect on the dynamics of bacterial resistance genes in manure and manured soil. *Soil Biol. Biochem.* 40, 1892–1900.

Heuer, H., and Smalla, K. (2007). Manure and sulfadiazine synergistically increased bacterial antibiotic resistance in soil over at least two months. *Environ. Microbiol.* 9, 657–666.

Hoa, P. T. P., Managaki, S., Nakada, N., Takada, H., Shimizu, A., Anh, D. H., et al. (2011). Antibiotic contamination and occurrence of antibiotic-resistant bacteria in aquatic environments of northern Vietnam. *Sci. Total Environ.* 409, 2894–2901.

Hoa, P. T. P., Nonaka, L., Viet, P. H., and Suzuki, S. (2008). Detection of the sul1, sul2 and sul3 genes in sulfonamide-resistant bacteria from wastewater and shrimp ponds of North Vietnam. *Sci. Total Environ.* 405, 377–384.

Hu, J. Y., Shi, J. C., Chang, H., Li, D., Yang, M., and Kamagata, Y. (2008). Phenotyping and gebotyping of antibiotic-resistant *Escherichia coli* isolated from a natural river basin. *Environ. Sci. Technol.* 42, 3415–3420.

Ingerslev, F., and Halling-Sørensen, B. (2000). Biodegradation properties of sulfonamides in activated sludge. *Environ. Toxicol. Chem.* 19, 2467–2473.

Kobayashi, T., Suehiro, F., Tuyen, B. C., and Suzuki, S. (2007). Distribution and diversity of tetracycline resistance genes encoding ribosomal protection proteins in Mekong River sediments in Vietnam. *FEMS Microbiol. Ecol.* 59, 729–737.

Kim, S.-R., Nonaka, L., Oh, M.-J., Lavilla-Pitogo, C., and Suzuki, S. (2003). Distribution of an oxytetracycline resistance determinant *tet*(34) among marine bacterial isolates of a *Vibrio* species. *Microbes Environ.* 18, 74–81.

Luo, Y., Xu, L., Rysz, M., Wang, Y., Zhang, H., and Alvarez, P. J. J. (2011). Occurrence and transport of tetracycline, sulfonamide, quinolone, and macrolide antibiotics in the Haihe River basin, China. *Environ. Sci. Technol.* 45, 1827–1833.

Managaki, S., Murata, A., Takada, H., Tuyen, B. C., and Chiem, N. H. (2007). Distribution of macrolides, sulfonamides and trimethoprim in tropical waters: ubiquitous occurrence of veterinary antibiotics in the Mekong delta. *Environ. Sci. Technol.* 41, 8004–8010.

Muyzer, G., de Waal, E. C., and Uitterlinden, A. G. (1993). Profiling of complex microbial populations by denaturing gradient gel electrophoresis analysis of polymerase chain reaction-amplified genes coding for 16S rRNA. *Appl. Environ. Microbiol.* 59, 695–700.

Neela, F. A., Nonaka, L., Rahman, M. H., and Suzuki, S. (2008). Transfer of the chromosomal encoded tetracycline resistance gene *tet*(M) from marine bacteria to *Escherichia coli*. *World J. Microbiol. Biotechnol.* 25, 1095–1101.

Page, R. D. M. (1996). Tree view: an application to display phylogenetic trees on personal computers. *Comput. Appl. Biosci.* 12, 357–358.

Pei, R., Kim, S.-C., Carlson, K. H., and Pruden, A. (2006). Effect of river landscape on the sediment concentrations of antibiotics and corresponding antibiotic resistance genes (ARG). *Wat. Res.* 40, 2427–2435.

Rahman, H. M., Nonaka, L., Tago, R., and Suzuki, S. (2008). Occurrence of two genotypes of tetracycline (TC) resistance gene *tet*(M) in the TC-resistant bacteria in marine sediments of Japan. *Environ. Sci. Technol.* 42, 5055–5061.

Shade, A., Read, J. S., Youngblut, N. D., Fierer, N., Knight, R., Kratz, T. K., et al. (2012). Lake microbial communities are resilient after a whole-ecosystem disturbance. *ISME J.* 6, 2153–2167.

Sholz, P., Haring, V., Wittmannliebold, B., Ashman, K., Bagdasarian, M., and Scherzinger, E. (1989). Complete nucleotide-sequence and gene organization of the broad-host-range plasmid RSF1010. *Gene* 75, 271–288.

Sköld, O. (2010). Sulfonamides and trimethoprim. *Expert Rev. Anti Infect. Ther.* 8, 1–6.

Soreira, S., Brown, A., Ha, R., Iserhoff, K., Yim, M., Yang, J., et al. (2012). Persistence of Escherichia coli in freshwater periphyton: biofilm-forming capacity as a selective advantage. *FEMS Microbiol. Ecol.* 79, 608–618.

Su, H.-C., Ying, G.-G., Tao, R., Zhang, R.-Q., Reynolds, L., Fogarty, L. R., et al. (2011). Occurrence of antibiotic resistance and characterization of resistance genes and integrons in Enterobacteriaceae isolated from integrated fish farms in south China. *J. Environ. Monit.* 13, 3229–3236.

Su, H.-C., Ying, G.-G., Tao, R., Zhang, R.-Q., Zhao, J.-L., and Liu, Y.-S. (2012). Class 1 and 2 integrons, *sul* resistance genes and antibiotic resistance in *Escherichia coli* isolated from Dongjiang River, South China. *Environ. Pollut.* 169, 42–49.

Sukul, P., and Spiteller, M. (2006). Sulfonamides in the environment as veterinary drugs. *Rev. Environ. Contam. Toxicol.* 187, 67–101.

Suzuki, M. S., Taylor, L. T., and Delong, E. F. (2000). Quantitative analysis of small-subunit rRNA genes in mixed microbial populations via 5′-nuclease assays. *Appl. Environ. Microbiol.* 66, 4605–4614.

Suzuki, S., and Hoa, P. T. P. (2012). Distribution of quinolone, sulfonamides, tetracyclines in aquatic environment and antibiotic resistance in Indochina. *Front. Microbio.* 3:67. doi: 10.3389/fmicb.2012.00067

Suzuki, S., Kobayashi, T., Suehiro, F., Tuyen, B. C., and Tana, T. S. (2008). High occurrence rate of tetracycline (TC)-resistant bacteria and TC resistance genes relates to microbial diversity in sediment of Mekong river main waterway. *Microbes Environ.* 23, 149–152.

Takasu, H., Suzuki, S., Reungsang, A., and Viet, P. H. (2011). Fluoroquinolone (FQ) contamination does not correlate with occurrence of FQ-resistant bacteria in aquatic environments of Vietnam and Thailand. *Microbes Environ.* 26, 135–143.

Tamminen, M., Karkman, A., Lõhmus, A., Muziasari, W. I., Takasu, H., Wada, S., et al. (2011). Tetracycline resistance genes persist at aquaculture farms in the absence of selection pressure. *Environ. Sci. Technol.* 45, 386–391.

Tendencia, E. A., and de la Peña, L. D. (2001). Antibiotic resistance of bacteria from shrimp ponds. *Aquaculture* 195, 193–204.

Thompson, J. D., Gibson, T. J., Plewniak, F., Jeanmougin, F., and Higgins, D. G. (1997). The Clustal X windows interface: flexible strategies for multiple sequence alignment aided by quality analysis tools. *Nucl. Acids Res.* 25, 4876–4882.

Vital, M., Hammes, F., and Egli, T. (2008). *Escherichia coli* O157 can grow in natural freshwater at low carbon concentration. *Environ. Microbiol.* 10, 2387–2396.

Wilson, K. (1987). "Preparation of genomic DNA from bacteria," in *Current Protocols in Molecular Biology*, eds F. M. Ausubel, R. Brent, R. E. Kingston, D. D. Moore, J. D. Seidman, J. A. Smith, and K. Atruhl (New York, NY: Jhon Wiley and Sons), 2.4.1–2.4.5.

Wooldridge, M. (2012). Evidence for the circulation of antimicrobial-resistant strains and genes in nature and especially between humans and animals. *Rev. Sci. Tech.* 31, 231–247.

Ye, Z., Weinberg, H. S., and Meyer, M. T. (2006). Trace analysis of trimethoprim and sulfonamide, macrolide, quinolone, and tetracycline antibiotics in chlorinated drinking water using liquid ch matography electrospray tande mass spectrometry. *Anal. Chem.* 7 1135–1144.

APPENDIX

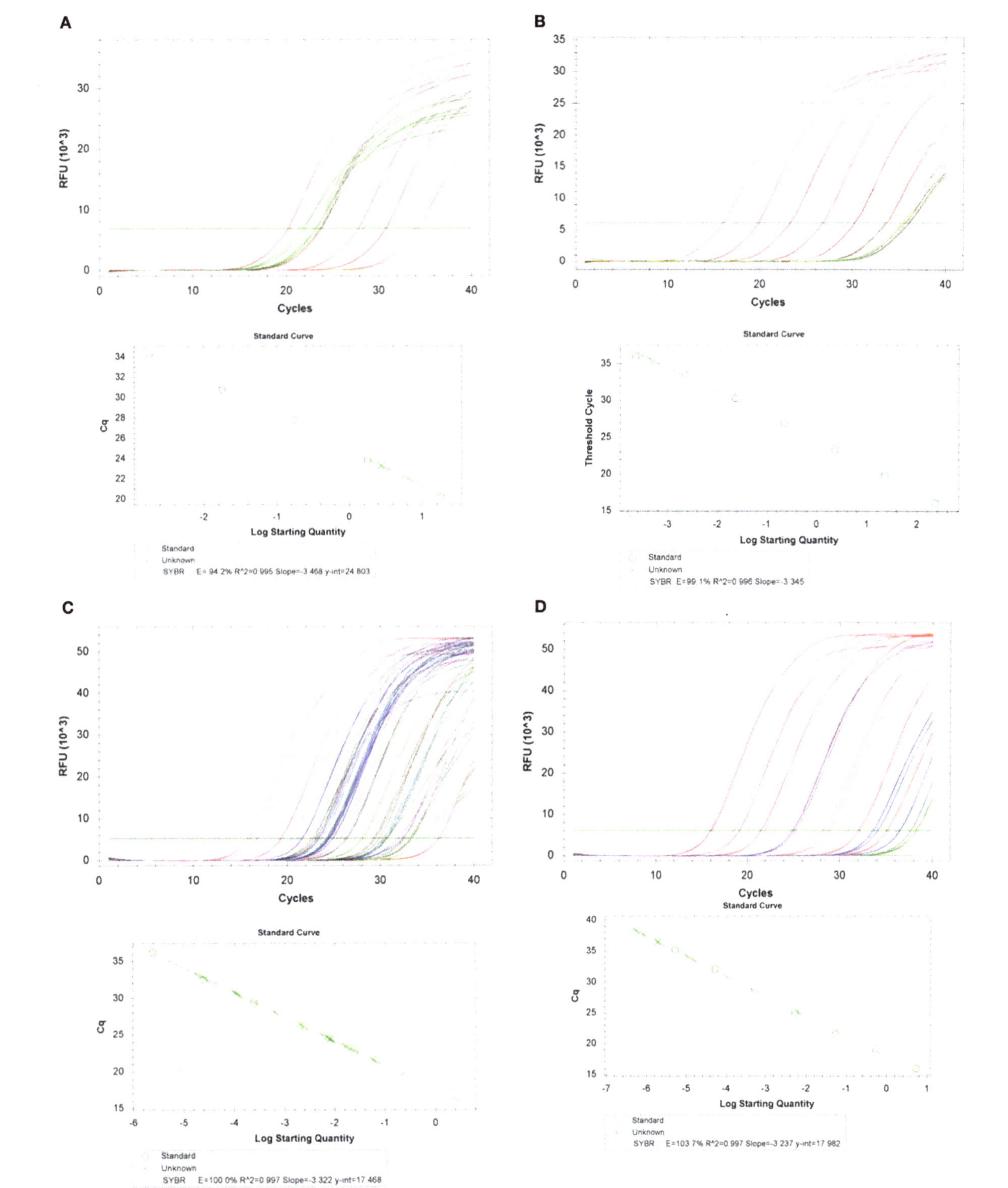

FIGURE A1 | (A) qPCR standard curve, 16S rRNA gene (Colony DNA) Amplification efficiency = 94.2%, Linearity (R^2) = 0.995. **(B)** qPCR standard curve, 16S rRNA gene (Filter DNA) Amplification efficiency = 99.1%, linearity (R^2) = 0.996. **(C)** qPCR standard curve, sul1 gene (Colony DNA) Amplification efficiency = 100.0%, linearity (R^2) = 0.997. **(D)** qPCR standard curve, sul1 gene (Filter DNA) Amplification efficiency = 103.7%, linearity (R^2) = 0.997.

(Continued)

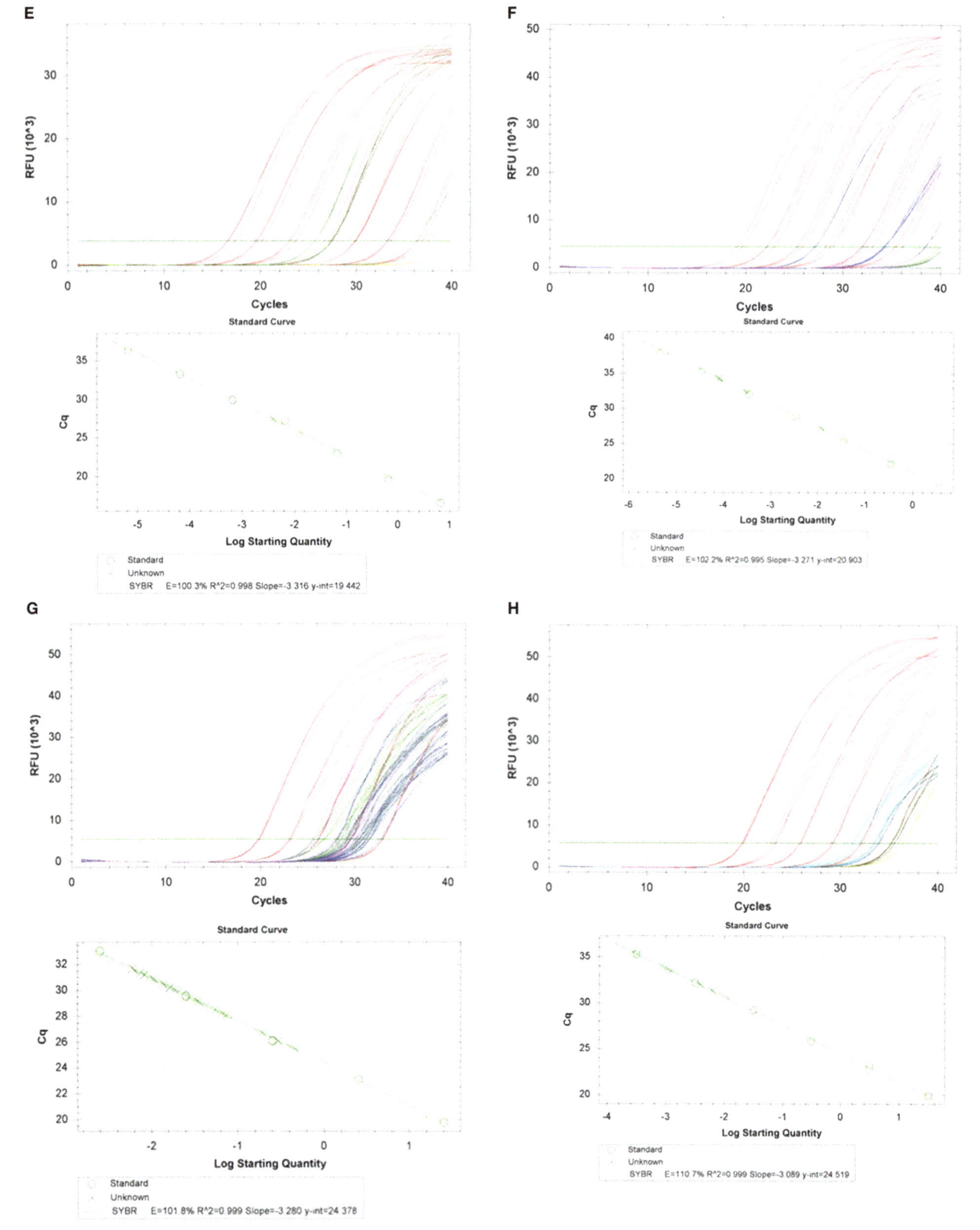

FIGURE A1 | Continued

(E) qPCR standard curve, sul2 gene (Colony DNA) Amplification efficiency = 100.3%, linearity (R^2) = 0.998. **(F)** qPCR standard curve, sul2 gene (Filter DNA) Amplification efficiency = 102.2%, linearity (R^2) = 0.995. **(G)** qPCR standard curve, sul3 gene (Colony DNA) Amplification efficiency = 101.8%, linearity (R^2) = 0.999. **(H)** qPCR standard curve, sul3 gene (Filter DNA) Amplification efficiency = 110.7%, linearity (R^2) = 0.999.

12

Anaerobic expression of the *gadE-mdtEF* multidrug efflux operon is primarily regulated by the two-component system ArcBA through antagonizing the H-NS mediated repression

Ziqing Deng, Yue Shan, Qing Pan, Xiang Gao and Aixin Yan*

School of Biological Sciences, The University of Hong Kong, Hong Kong, China

Edited by:
Kunihiko Nishino, Osaka University, Japan

Reviewed by:
Yuji Morita, Aichi Gakuin University, Japan
Hidetada Hirakawa, Gunma University, Japan

****Correspondence:***
Aixin Yan, School of Biological Sciences, The University of Hong Kong, Pokfulam Road, Hong Kong Special Administrative Region, Hong Kong Island, Hong Kong, China
e-mail: ayan8@hku.hk

The *gadE-mdtEF* operon encodes a central acid resistance regulator GadE and two multidrug efflux proteins MdtEF. Although transcriptional regulation of *gadE* in the context of acid resistance under the aerobic growth environment of *Escherichia coli* has been extensively studied, regulation of the operon under the physiologically relevant environment of anaerobic growth and its effect on the expression of the multidrug efflux proteins MdtEF in the operon has not been disclosed. Our previous study revealed that anaerobic induction of the operon was dependent on ArcA, the response regulator of the ArcBA two-component system, in the M9 glucose minimal medium. However, the detailed regulatory mechanism remains unknown. In this study, we showed that anaerobic activation of *mdtEF* was driven by the 798 bp unusually long *gadE* promoter. Deletion of *evgA*, *ydeO*, *rpoS*, and *gadX* which has been shown to activate the *gadE* expression during acid stresses under aerobic condition did not have a significant effect on the anaerobic activation of the operon. Rather, anaerobic activation of the operon was largely dependent on the global regulator ArcA and a GTPase MnmE. Under aerobic condition, transcription of *gadE* was repressed by the global DNA silencer H-NS in M9 minimal medium. Interestingly, under anaerobic condition, while Δ*arcA* almost completely abolished transcription of *gadE-mdtEF*, further deletion of *hns* in Δ*arcA* mutant restored the transcription of the full-length P*gadE-lacZ*, and P1- and P3-*lacZ* fusions, suggesting an antagonistic effect of ArcA on the H-NS mediated repression. Taken together, we conclude that the anaerobic activation of the *gadE-mdtEF* was primarily mediated by the two-component system ArcBA through antagonizing the H-NS mediated repression.

Keywords: multidrug efflux pump, acid resistance, anaerobic adaptation, H-NS, ArcBA two-component system, antagonization

INTRODUCTION

Drug efflux constitutes an important mechanism in bacterial drug resistance. Efflux activity is mediated by a class of membrane protein transporters called multidrug efflux pumps, which actively extrude a variety of cytotoxic substances including antibiotics out of bacterial cells (Li and Nikaido, 2009; Allen et al., 2010). Based on phylogenetic analysis and functional properties, drug efflux pumps of bacteria are classified into five families: the ATP-binding cassette (ABC), the major facilitator (MFS), the multidrug and toxic compound extrusion (MATE), the small multidrug resistance (SMR), and the resistance nodulation division (RND) family (Piddock, 2006). Among them, the tripartite RND pumps are particularly noteworthy in gram-negative bacteria owing to their capability of exporting a broad range of structurally diverse drugs directly to the outside of bacterial cells (Poole, 2008). The three components of RND efflux pumps include cytoplasmic membrane transporter component of RND family, outer membrane factor (OMF) component, and periplasmic component belonging to the membrane fusion protein (Murakami et al., 2006; Piddock, 2006). The constitutive activity of these efflux systems, such as the AcrAB-TolC pump in *Escherichia coli* and the MexAB-OprM and MexXY-OprM systems in *Pseudomonas aeruginosa*, renders the bacteria a low level, intrinsic resistance to a wide range of toxic substances (Poole, 2005).

Previous genome wide studies revealed that there are 20 efflux systems encoded in the *E. coli* K-12 genome (Nishino and Yamaguchi, 2001). However, except for the housekeeping AcrAB-TolC pump, the expression of other 19 pumps is largely inactive under ordinary laboratory growth condition, i.e., at 37°C in rich medium with aeration (Nishino and Yamaguchi, 2001). Increasing evidence suggests that bacterial stress response, i.e., bacterial growth in the adverse environment of their natural ecological niches and human host, induces the expression of specific efflux pumps (Piddock, 2006; Li and Nikaido, 2009; Poole, 2012a). Indeed, our previous studies revealed that MdtEF (previously known as YhiUV), an RND family pump, is activated during the anaerobic growth of *E. coli*, a signature environment of human gut where the bacterium primarily colonizes (Zhang et al., 2011). The pump was shown to expel the cytotoxic indole nitrosative compounds from *E. coli* cells accumulated during the anaerobic respiration of nitrate and thus protect the bacterium from nitrosative stress under this physiological condition (Zhang et al., 2011). Activation of MdtEF under this condition was shown to be dependent on ArcA, the response regulator of the ArcBA two-component system, which is a global regulatory system dedicated to the anaerobic adaptation of *E. coli* (Green and Paget, 2004), but the detailed regulatory mechanism remains unknown.

MdtEF forms an RND type multidrug efflux system with the common outer membrane channel TolC in which MdtF forms the cytoplasmic membrane transporter and is connected to TolC by the periplasmic protein MdtE (Nishino and Yamaguchi, 2002). Over-expression of the pump from a multicopy plasmid has been shown to confer resistance to a broad range of antimicrobial agents such as some β-lactams (e.g., oxacillin, cloxacillin, and nafcillin), macrolide antibiotic erythromycin, as well as doxorubicin, crystal violet, ethidium bromide, rhodamine 6G, tetraphenylphosphonium bromide (TPP), benzalkonium, SDS, deoxycholate, suggesting that MdtEF is a multidrug resistance determinant (Nishino and Yamaguchi, 2001; Nishino et al., 2003; Lennen et al., 2013). Recently, MdtEF was also found to be involved in the efflux of physiological substance fatty acids (Lennen et al., 2013), and their expression can be induced by various of environmental and physiological signals, such as the entry of the stationary growth phase, N-acetyl-glucosomine, indole, as well as the combined environmental challenges of oxygen limitation and acid stress (Hirakawa et al., 2005, 2006; Hayes et al., 2006; Kobayashi et al., 2006), highlighting the physiological relevance of the MdtEF-TolC efflux pump.

MdtEF genes are located in the *gadE-mdtEF* operon where *mdtE* is 339 bp downstream of the *gadE* gene (Keseler et al., 2011). Interestingly, the *gadE* gene in this operon encodes a key regulator of the major acid resistance system in *E. coli* which is composed of the glutamate decarboxylase isoenzymes GadA and GadB, and a dedicated glutamic acid/γ-aminobutyrate (GABA) antiporter GadC (Hommais et al., 2004). During bacterial response to acid stresses, GadA and GadB catalyze the decarboxylation of glutamic acid, yielding GABA, which is subsequently exported by GadC in exchange for another molecule of glutamic acid (Foster, 2004). Since the reaction consumes a proton and releases CO_2, it effectively limits the intracellular acidification during acid stresses, thus plays an important role in the adaptation and survival of *E. coli* in certain host niches, such as the extremely low pH environment (pH = 2) of gastric acid (Foster, 2004). The expression of this system is primarily subject to the control of the acid resistance regulator GadE in the *gadE-mdtEF* operon (Masuda and Church, 2003).

Owing to its significant roles in acid resistance, transcriptional regulation from the *gadE* promoter has been extensively studied. It was demonstrated that the *gadE* promoter encompasses an unusually large 798 bp intergenic region between the *hdeD* and *gadE* gene (Ma et al., 2004), representing one of the eight similarly large intergenic regions in the entire *E. coli* genome (Tjaden et al., 2002). Transcription from at least four starting sites which are located at -21 (T), -124 (T1), -324/-317 (T2), and -566 (T3) relative to the *gadE* start codon have been identified (Ma et al., 2004; Itou et al., 2009; Sayed and Foster, 2009). More than ten transcription regulators including EvgA, YdeO, GadE, TorR, H-NS, PhoP, RpoS, CRP, MnmE, GadX, and GadW have been found to participate in the regulation of *gadE* during various circumstances of acid stresses through at least five different regulatory circuits (Ma et al., 2004; Sayed and Foster, 2009). Involvement of EvgA, YdeO, H-NS, CRP, GadX, as well as a small RNA DsrA in the regulation of the *mdtEF* gene in the same operon has also been reported (Nishino and Yamaguchi, 2002, 2004; Oshima et al., 2006; Nishino et al., 2008a,b, 2009, 2011). However, little is known about the regulation of the *gadE-mtEF* expression in the anaerobic physiological condition of *E. coli* which is the predominant environmental challenge encountered by the *Entericbacteria* family of bacteria when they are being transmitted from the status of free living to human intestinal tract, except for the involvement of the global transcription regulator ArcA as shown in our previous study (Zhang et al., 2011). Moreover, it remains unclear whether the various of regulatory circuits that activate the expression of *gadE* in the context of acid resistance also lead to the expression of the multidrug efflux genes *mdtEF* present in the same operon.

In the current study we set out to investigate the detailed regulatory circuits governing the anaerobic transcription from the *gadE* promoter in *E. coli* and examine its effect on the expression of the multidrug efflux proteins MdtEF present in the operon. We found that unlike the regulatory patterns occurred during aerobic acid stresses, anaerobic activation of the *gadE-mdtEF* operon is primarily mediated by ArcA through its antagonization of the H-NS mediated repression.

MATERIALS AND METHODS

BACTERIAL STRAINS AND PLASMIDS

The bacteria strains and plasmids used in this study are listed in **Table 1**. Gene deletion mutants were constructed either by P1 phage transduction from the Keio collection (Baba et al., 2006) or using the method described by Datsenko and Wanner (2000). All of the constructed strains were verified by colony PCR and DNA sequencing (BGI, Hong Kong). *E. coli* was cultured in Luria Bertani (LB) broth (USB) or M9 minimum medium supplemented with 0.2% glucose (USB), 0.2% casamino acids (CAA) (USB), 4 μg/ml thiamin (Sigma), 0.1 mM $CaCl_2$, 1 mM $MgCl_2$, 10 μg/ml ferric ammonium citrate (Sigma), and 0.5 μM $(NH_4)_6Mo_7O_{24}$ (Sigma). Without specific indication, exponential phase cells were harvested when A_{600} of cultures reached around 0.3. Antibiotic concentrations used for bacterial culture or colony screening were 100 μg/ml ampicillin (USB), 20 μg/ml kanamycin (USB), or 25 μg/ml chloramphenicol (USB). All other chemicals without specification were purchased from USB.

CONSTRUCTION OF PROMOTER-*lacZ* TRANSCRIPTION REPORTER IN pNN387

Promoter-*lacZ* fusions were constructed based on the methods described previously (Zhang et al., 2011). Firstly, DNA fragments corresponding to the desired promoter regions were amplified using iProof High Fidelity DNA polymerase (Bio-Rad). The PCR condition and program is as follows: initial

Table 1 | Bacterial strains and plasmids used in this study.

Constructs	Genotype	Source
STRAIN		
MG1655	Wild type *Escherichia coli*	Mettert and Kiley, 2007
AY0416	MG1655 Δ*lacZ::kan*	Zhang et al., 2011
AY0433	MG1655 Δ*lacZ::kan* Δ*arcA::bla*	Zhang et al., 2011
AY0451	MG1655 Δ*arcA::cat mdtE-FLAG::kan*	Zhang et al., 2011
AY0452	MG1655 *mdtE-FLAG::kan*	Zhang et al., 2011
AY1543	MG1655 Δ*gadE* Δ*lacZ::Km*	This study
AY1603	MG1655 Δ*gadX::cat mdtE-FLAG::kan*	This study
AY1611	MG1655 Δ*rpoS mdtE-FLAG::kan*	This study
AY1612	MG1655 Δ*evgA mdtE-FLAG::kan*	This study
AY1613	MG1655 Δ*crp::cat, mdtE-FLAG::kan*	This study
AY2304	MG1655 Δ*mnmE mdtE-FLAG::kan*	This study
AY2305	MG1655 Δ*ydeO mdtE-FLAG::kan*	This study
AY2306	MG1655 Δ*ydeO* Δ*lacZ::kan*	This study
AY2311	MG1655 Δ*mnmE* Δ*lacZ::kan*	This study
AY2312	MG1655 Δ*evgA* Δ*lacZ::kan*	This study
AY2313	MG1655 Δ*rpoS* Δ*lacZ::kan*	This study
AY2400	MG1655 Δ*hns* Δ*lacZ::kan*	This study
AY2401	MG1655 Δ*crp* Δ*lacZ::kan*	This study
AY2420	MG1655 Δ*hns mdtE-FLAG::kan*	This study
AY2421	MG1655 P*icdA-lacZ* Δ*mnmE*	This study
AY2422	MG1655 P*lpdA-lacZ* Δ*mnmE*	This study
AY2426	MG1655 Δ*hns* Δ*arcA::bla* Δ*lacZ::kan*	This study
AY2442	MG1655 Δ*hns* Δ*arcA::cat* mdtE-FLAG::kan	This study
PK9460	MG1655 P*lpdA-lacZ*	Gift from Prof. Patricia J. Kiley (University of Wisconsin-Madison)
PK9463	MG1655 P*lpdA-lacZ* Δ*arcA*	Gift from Prof. Patricia J. Kiley
PK9483	MG1655 P*icdA-lacZ*	Gift from Prof. Patricia J. Kiley
PK9484	MG1655 P*icdA-lacZ* Δ*arcA*	Gift from Prof. Patricia J. Kiley
PLASMID		
pNN387	Single-copy vector, Cm^r, a NotI-HindIII cloning site upstream of promoterless *lacZ*	Kobayashi et al., 2006
pNN387mdtE	pNN387 (P*gadE-lacZ*)	Nishino and Yamaguchi, 2001
pAY1633	pNN387 (P*mdtE-lacZ*)	This study
pAY1655	pNN387 (P2/P4+P1+P-*lacZ*)	This study
pAY1656	pNN387 (P4+P1+P-*lacZ*)	This study
pAY1657	pNN387 (P1+P-*lacZ*)	This study
pAY1658	pNN387 (P-*lacZ*)	This study
pAY2401	pNN387 (P3-*lacZ*)	This study
pAY2402	pNN387 (P3+P2/P4-*lacZ*)	This study
pAY2403	pNN387 (P3+P2/P4+P1-*lacZ*)	This study
pAY2404	pNN387 (P2/P4-*lacZ*)	This study
pAY2405	pNN387 (P2/P4+P1-*lacZ*)	This study
pAY2406	pNN387 (P1-*lacZ*)	This study
pAY2409	pNN387 (P*mnmE-lacZ*)	This study

denaturation at 98°C for 30 s followed by 35 cycles of denaturation, annealing, and extension which are achieved by the program of: 98°C for 10 s, 60°C for 30 s, 72°C for 45 s, and the final extension at 72°C for 5 min. The pair of primers used in PCR includes protective bases (lowercase), restriction enzyme site (NotI or HidIII), followed by ~20 bp homologous to the 5′- and 3′-end of the desirable promoter regions respectively (e.g., PgadE-F: 5′-aaggaaaaaaGCGGCCGCTTACCC CGGTTGTCACCCGGAT-3′; PgadE-R: 5′-cccAAGCTTAACTT GCTCCTTAGCCGTTATC-3′). Primers for construction of other *promoter-lacZ* fusions were designed similarly and the detailed sequences are available upon request. The PCR fragments were purified using illustra GFX PCR DNA and Gel Band Purification Kit (GE) followed by NotI/HindIII (NEB) digestion, and then were ligated into NotI/HindIII (NEB) digested single copy plasmid pNN387 using Quick Ligase (NEB). Colonies were screened by chloramphenicol resistance and then verified by colony PCR and DNA sequencing (BGI, Hong Kong).

CONSTRUCTION OF CHROMOSOMAL *mdtE-FLAG* BY P1 vir TRANSDUCTION

Construction of *chromosomal mdtE-FLAG* in various of deletion mutants was achieved by P1 phage transduction using the lysate from the strain AY0451 (Zhang et al., 2011). To prepare the lysate of the donor strain, AY0451 was grown in 2 ml LB medium till A_{600} achieved 0.1–0.2, and then 40 μl P1vir and 10 mM $CaCl_2$ was added to the culture. The mixture was shaken at 37°C for ~3 h or till cells lysed. 2 drops of chloroform per ml of culture was then added to the lysate to diminish any chance of cell viability. After a vortex and centrifugation at 16,000 g for 2 min, the supernatant was transferred to a fresh tube and stored at 4°C in the presence of couple of drops of chloroform. Culture of the recipient strain was prepared as follows: the recipient strain was grown in LB medium till A_{600} exceeded 0.7. 10 mM $CaCl_2$ was then added followed by continuing growth for 15 min. 200 μl of the culture was then mixed with 100 μl lysate of the donor strain and incubated at 37°C for 20 min. Following the incubation, 100 μl of 1 M citrate was added to terminate the infection. Following the addition of 600 μl LB medium, the transductant was incubated at 37°C for 1 h before being spread onto LB agar plates containing kanamycin and 4 mM citrate. Desirable colonies were screened by colony PCR and were verified by DNA sequencing (BGI, Hong Kong).

β-GALACTOSIDASE ACTIVITY ASSAY

β-galactosidase activity assay was performed based on the method by Miller (1972) and detailed experimental procedure has been described previously (Zhang et al., 2011). Briefly, cells were grown anaerobically by inoculating a small number of cell cultures (initial cell density of 10^3 cells/ml) into screw-capped culture tubes filled with M9 medium, and subsequently cultured in 37°C water bath without aeration. When A_{600} of the cultures reached ~0.3, tetracycline (10 μg/ml) was added to terminate protein synthesis and cell growth, and the cultures were placed on ice until assayed. The assays were performed in triplicate, and results were presented as the mean in either Miller unit or the percentages relative to the activity of full length promoter-*lacZ* fusion in WT (wild type) strain. Error bars indicate the standard deviation.

TOTAL RNA EXTRACTION

8 ml anaerobically grown (the same condition as used in β-galactosidase activity assay) culture of *E. coli* MG1655 was mixed with 1.25 ml ice-cold ethnol/phenol stop solution (5% water-saturated phenol pH 4.5 in ethanol) and placed on ice for 10 min before being harvested by centrifugation at 4000 g for 9 min at 4°C. After removing supernatant, the cell pellet was frozen in liquid nitrogen and stored at −80°C to aid lysis. Cells were lysed by resuspending in 800 μl TE buffer (pH 8.0) containing 1.4 μl 36 kU μl^{-1} lysozyme (epicenter), and then placed in 64°C water bath for 2 min. After incubation, 88 μl 3M NaOAc (pH 5.2) was added to adjust the pH and ion strength of the lysate solution. Subsequently, acid-phenol/chloroform extraction followed by ethanol precipitation was performed to obtain the total RNA following the manufacturer's instruction. To remove trace amount of genomic DNA contamination, the extracted RNA was subject to DNase I treatment using the turbo DNA Free Kit (Amibion). Absence of genomic DNA contamination was confirmed by PCR suing the prepared RNA as template. The quantity of RNA was determined using NanoDrop 2000 (Thermo Scientific).

RNA LIGASE-MEDIATED RAPID AMPLIFICATION OF 5′ cDNA ENDS (5′ RLM-RACE)

1 μg of RNA which was treated with the turbo DNA Free Kit (Amibion) as above and shown as tight, no smearing band on the agrose gel (following the instructions of the FirstChoice RLM-RACE Kit (Ambion)) was treated with the Tobacco Acid Pyrophosphatase (TAP), ligated to the 5′ RACE adapter, and reverse transcripted with reagents supplied in the FirstChoice RLM-RACE Kit (Ambion) following the manufacturer's instruction. The obtained cDNA was subsequently utilized to perform outer (primer: PgadEout: 5′-TCCAGAAAT TTAATCGCTTCTTCATC-3′) and inner (primer: PgadEin: 5′-GTACTCGAGGTGATTATCTTTCAACTGCCAAAAGC-3′) PCR using Fastart Taq (Roche) DNA polymerase. The PCR products were gel band purified using PCR DNA and Gel Band Purification Kit (GE) and cloned into BamHI and XhoI sites of pPK7035 (Kang et al., 2005) followed by DNA sequencing. The first nucleotide being sequenced following the 5′ RACE adapter sequence was determined as the transcription start site.

SODIUM DODECYL SULFATE-POLYACRYLAMIDE GEL ELECTROPHORESIS (SDS-PAGE) AND WESTERN BLOT

E. coli strains containing chromosomal FLAG tagged MdtE were grown anaerobically (the same condition as used in β-galactosidase activity assay) to log phase ($A_{600} = 0.3$) in M9 minimal medium supplemented with 0.2% glucose, 0.2% CAA, 4 μg/ml thiamin, 0.1 mM $CaCl_2$, 1 mM $MgCl_2$, 10 μg/ml ferric ammonium citrate, and 0.5 μM $(NH_4)_6Mo_7O_{24}$. Cells were harvested by centrifugation at 3800 g at 4°C for 10 min. Cell pellet was resuspended in lysis mix (BugBuster reagent (Merck) supplemented with 2.5 mg/mL lysozyme and 10 U/mL DNase I (Invitrogen)). Following the cell lysis, a small fraction of the lysis was subject to the *Dc* Protein Assay kit (BioRad) to measure the concentration of total proteins in the lysate. The volumes of the cell lysis loaded onto the SDS-PAGE were then determined based on the concentrations of each of the samples such that each of the lanes contains the same amount of total protein. The lysis was then heated at 55°C for 25 min prior to being subjected to sodium dodecyl sulfate-polyacrylamide gel electrophoresis (SDS-PAGE). Separated proteins were electrically (Wet/Tank Blotting Systems, Bio-Rad; 110V) transferred to a nitrocellulose membrane (Bio-Rad) for 1.5 h. After blocking with 5% non-fat milk in 1% TBST (*T*ris *B*uffered *S*aline with *T*ween 20, 0.1 M Tris, 0.15 M NaCl, 0.1% Tween 20, and pH was adjusted with HCl to 7.6), the membrane was incubated with monoclonal anti-FLAG antibody (Sigma), and then secondary antibody (goat anti-mouse IgG HRP conjuate, Bio-Rad). After treatment of the membrane by the ECL Plus Western Blotting Detection Reagents (GE health), the protein bands were visualized by X-ray film development. Signals corresponding to MdtE-FLAG proteins were quantified using ImageJ (National Institutes of Health) and are presented as percentages relative to the level of MdtE-FLAG in the wild type strain.

EB STAINED ELECTROPHORESIS GEL MOBILITY SHIFT ASSAY (EMSA)

Purification and subsequent *in vitro* phosphorylation of His_6-ArcA protein was following the method described previously (Bekker et al., 2010). Briefly, *E. coli* strain BL21 transformed with pET-His_6ArcA were grown in LB to A_{600} of 0.4 before adding 1 mM isopropyl-β-D-thiogalactopyranoside (IPTG) to induce the overexpress of His_6-ArcA. After grown for additional 2.5 h, cells were harvested by centrifugation. Cell pellet was then resuspended in 4 ml of buffer A (0.5 MNaCl, 20 mMTris-HCl, pH 7.9) containing 1.3 mg/ml lysozyme, 30 g/ml DNase and RNase. Cells were then incubated at room temperature for 30 min followed by sonication to lyse the cells. Cell lysate was obtained by centrifugation at 15,000 g for 30 min and then was subjected to a 1.5-ml Ni-nitrilotriacetic acid–agarose column (Qiagen) equilibrated with buffer A. Following washing the column with 10 ml buffer A containing 10 mM imidazole, His_6-ArcA was eluted with buffer A containing 50 mM imidazole. Purified His_6-ArcA protein was phosphorylated by incubating the protein in TEGD buffer (50 mM Tris-HCl [pH 7.5], 0.5 mM EDTA, 10% glycerol) supplemented with 5 mM $MgCl_2$ and 50 mM (final concentration) carbamoyl phosphate. The mixture was incubated for 90 min at 25°C, and then the phosphorylated ArcA was used immediately for DNA-binding reaction. To initiate the DNA binding reaction, various concentration of DNA probes and phosphorylated proteins were mixed and subsequently incubated at 37°C for 20 min in EMSA binding buffer (pH 7.2, 20 mM Tris, 50 mM NaCl, 10 mM EDTA, 4 mM DTT, 5% glycerol, 0.5 mg/mL BSA). The reaction mixture was then subjected to 6% non-denaturing polyacrylamide gel electrophoresis in 0.5× TBE buffer. The polyacrylamide gel was visualized under UV light (254–366 nm) following the staining in 0.5× TBE buffer containing 0.5 μg/ml ethidium bromide (EB) for 10 min.

RESULTS

ANAEROBIC TRANSCRIPTION OF *mdtEF* IS INITIATED FROM THE *gadE* PROMOTER

MdtEF are located downstream of the *gadE* gene, which encodes a central regulator of the glutamic acid dependent acid resistance system in *E. coli* (Nishino and Yamaguchi, 2002). Previous RT-PCR analysis revealed that *mdtEF* were co-transcribed with *gadE*, thus were annotated in the operon of *gadE-mdtEF* (Hirakawa et al., 2006). However, an EMSA study by Nishino et al. showed that EvgA, one of the regulators that can activate the expression of *mdtEF*, could bind to the intergenic region between *gadE* and *mdtEF*, indicating that this region might serve as a potential promoter of *mdtEF* under certain conditions (Nishino and Yamaguchi, 2002). Thus, we first examined whether this intergenic region (namely P*mdtE*) is involved in the transcription of *mdtEF* under anaerobic condition. To address this, we constructed *lacZ* fusion of the intergenic region (denoted as P*mdtE-lacZ*) in the single copy plasmid pNN387 and performed β-galactosidase activity assay. It was shown that no transcription from P*mdtE-lacZ* was detected under either aerobic or anaerobic condition, while transcription from P*gadE-lacZ* constructed in the same vector was significantly induced under anaerobic condition (data not shown). These results suggested that anaerobic transcription of *mdtEF* was primarily initiated from the *gadE* promoter. Therefore we focused on the 798 bp P*gadE* region in the following investigation to examine its contribution to the expression of *mdtEF* under anaerobic condition.

TRANSCRIPTION FROM THE SAME FOUR STARTING SITES OF *gadE* WERE IDENTIFIED IN THE ANAEROBICALLY GROWN *E. coli*

In previous studies, three transcription starting sites, located at -124 (T1), -324/-317 (T2), and -566 (T3) relative to the *gadE* start codon respectively, have been identified in *E. coli* grown in LB glucose to early stationary phase ($A_{600} = 1.75$) (Sayed and Foster, 2009) and one transcription starting site located at the -21 position was detected from *E. coli* grown in the EG minimal buffer at pH 5.5 (Ma et al., 2004). To examine whether transcription from all these starting sites, and whether transcription from additional starting site, is active under anaerobic growth condition, we performed 5′ RLM-RACE using RNA isolated from *E. coli* grown anaerobically in M9 glucose medium which has been shown to significantly induce the expression of MdtEF in our previous study (Zhang et al., 2011). 5′-RACE revealed that transcription from the three starting sites identified previously was detected from several clones (data not shown). Transcription starting site of -21 was identified from one clone, but a weak -35 and -10 element was present upstream of this starting site. Two putative new transcription starting sites were also detected, however, since no recognizable -35 and -10 elements were present upstream of the sites, they are probably the digestive products from the established four transcripts. This result suggested that transcription from all four starting sites of *gadE-mdtEF* operon, -21 (T), -124 (T2/T4), -566 (T3), is active under anaerobic conditions. We next investigated the transcription regulatory mechanism of *gadE-mdtEF* from all these sites under anaerobic condition.

THE P3 REGION IS IMPORTANT IN THE ANAEROBIC ACTIVATION OF THE *gadE-mdtEF* OPERON

Following the designation of the P*gadE* region in previous studies (Sayed and Foster, 2009), the four transcription starting sites from 5′- to 3′-end of the 798 bp intergenic region between *hdeD* and *gadE* are designated as T3, T2, T4, T1, and T, respectively (**Figure 1A**) (Ma et al., 2004; Itou et al., 2009; Sayed and Foster, 2009), and the promoter regions immediately upstream of these transcription start sites are designated as P3, P2, P4, P1, and P accordingly. To examine which promoter regions are important for the anaerobic transcription of the *gadE-mdtEF* operon, we first constructed three P*gadE* truncations which lacked P3, P2/P4, P1 from 5′-end of the region successively, resulting in the promoter-*lacZ* fusion containing the intact P2/P4+P1+P, P1+P, and P regions, respectively (the upper four constructs in **Figure 1A**). Transcription activity assay showed that promoter-*lacZ* fusions lacking the P3 region, i.e., *lacZ* fusions of P2/P4+P1+P, and P1+P, displayed only ~1/3 activity of that of the full length P*gadE-lacZ* fusion (**Figure 1B**), and that of P region showed almost no activity. These results suggested that the P3 region is important in anaerobic activation of the *gadE-mdtEF* operon and that transcription from the P promoter region is not active under this condition. This result also indicated that the -21 transcription starting site (driven by the P promoter) detected from the RACE analysis might be a digestive product from the transcripts initiated from the other three sites.

To dissect the contribution of each of these promoter regions, we performed another series of truncation on P*gadE*, resulting in *lacZ* fusions containing individual or combined promoters (the lower six constructs in **Figure 1A**). Transcription activities of these truncations showed that promoter-*lacZ* fusions containing the P3 region, i.e., P3, P3+P2/P4 and P3+P2/P4+P1, displayed similar or even higher activity than that of the full length, whereas promoter-*lacZ* fusions lacking the P3 region, i.e., P2/P4, P2/P4+P1, and P1, displayed very low activities (**Figure 1B**), confirming the important role of the P3 region in the up-regulation of *gadE-mdtEF* operon under anaerobic condition. This result indicated that a strong activator binding site may exist at the P3 region. Furthermore, transcription of *lacZ* fusion containing the P2/P4 promoter region was almost undetectable, suggesting that similar as the transcription starting site T which is driven by the individual P promoter region, transcription from the individual P2/P4 promoter is also inactive under anaerobic conditions. These results combined explained the observed very low activities of the promoter-*lacZ* fusions of P2/P4+P1, P1, P2/P4+P1+P and P1+P (**Figure 1B**).

INVOLVEMENT OF DIFFERENT REGULATORS IN THE ANAEROBIC EXPRESSION OF *mdtEF* FROM THAT OF AEROBIC CONDITION

Previous studies focusing on the expression of *gadE-mdtEF* operon during acid resistance have revealed that several regulators, such as EvgA, YdeO, MnmE, GadE, GadX, CRP, and H-NS, are involved in the regulation of *gadE-mdtEF* operon (Gong et al., 2004; Ma et al., 2004; Hirakawa et al., 2006; Tramonti et al., 2008). However, all those studies were carried out under aerobic condition and primarily focused on the transcription of the *gadE* gene. A previous study from our group focusing on the

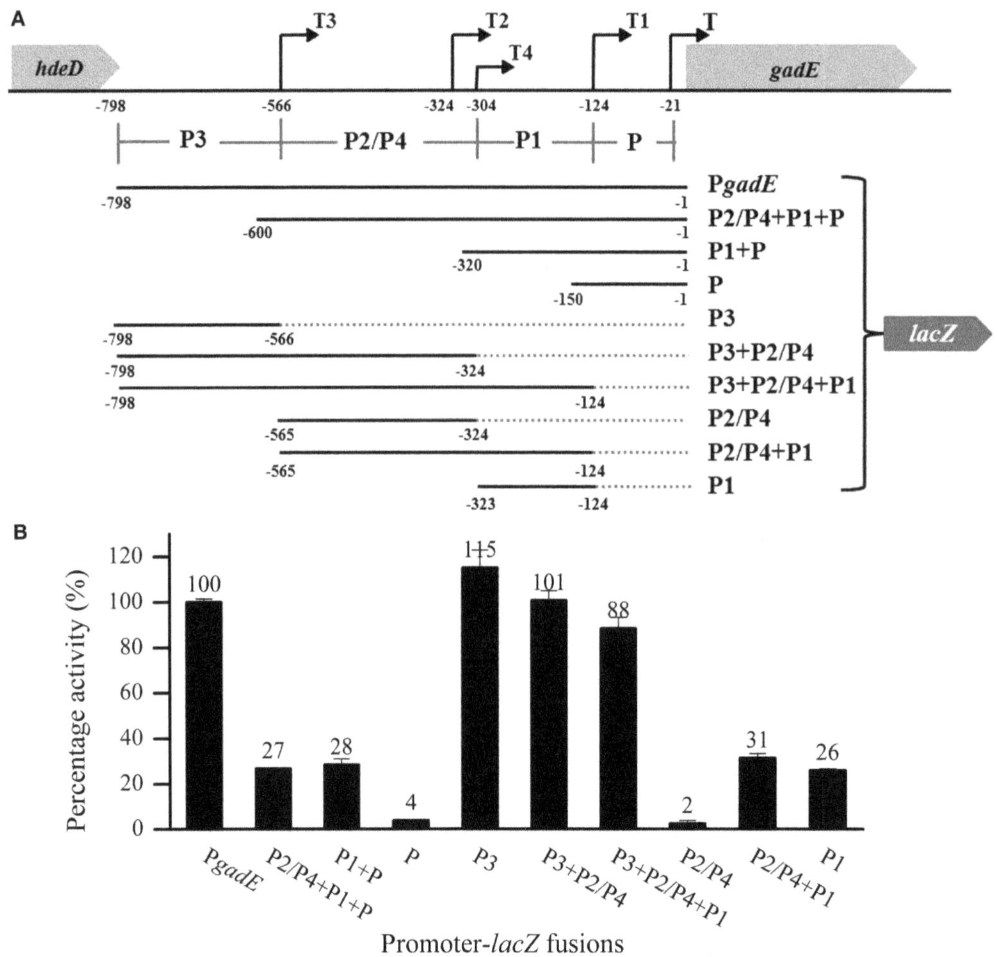

FIGURE 1 | The P3 region is important in the anaerobic up-regulation of *gadE-mdtEF*. (A) Schematic diagram of the constructed promoter-*lacZ* fusions. P*gadE* is defined as the 798 bp intergenic region between the *hdeD* and *gadE* genes. Labeled numbers indicate the nucleotides positions relative to the ATG start codon of *gadE*. Transcription starting sites are indicated as black arrows, and the regions upstream of each of the transcription starting sites are designated as its individual promoters, labeled as P3, P2/P4, P1, and P, respectively. **(B)** Promoter activity of all P*gadE* truncations determined by β-galactosidase activity of corresponding *lacZ* fusions. Cells were grown anaerobically to exponential phase ($A_{600} = 0.3$) in minimal M9 glucose medium. Results are presented as percentages relative to that of full length *gadE* promoter activity (100%), and error bars represent the standard errors of triplicate experiments ($n = 3$).

expression of the multidrug efflux genes *mdtEF* present in the same operon showed that under anaerobic condition the global regulator ArcA activates the expression of *mdtEF*, since Δ*arcA* caused significant decrease of both transcription and protein levels of *mdtE* and *mdtF* (Zhang et al., 2011). However, whether other regulators also participate in the regulation of *mdtEF* under this condition is unknown. Thus, in the present study, we first examined whether previously identified regulators, such as EvgA, YdeO, MnmE, GadE, GadX, and H-NS, also participate in the anaerobic activation of *mdtEF*. Since our previous finding on the anaerobic activation of *mdtEF* occurred in M9 glucose minimal medium in which the effect of CRP on gene expression is minimal, we focused on the effect of other regulators in the current study.

We constructed strains containing deletion of each of these genes and measured β-galactosidase activities of P*gadE-lacZ* in these strains. As shown in **Figure 2A**, deletion of *arcA* caused dramatic decrease of the β-galactosidase activity of P*gadE-lacZ*, confirming the role of ArcA in activating the *gadE-mdtEF* expression under anaerobic condition. Interestingly, except for *mnmE*, deletion of the regulators previously shown to participate in the regulation of *mdtEF* under aerobic condition, such as EvgA, YdeO, GadE, and GadX, caused no or only a moderate decrease (17–40%) of the transcription of P*gadE-lacZ*, and deletion of H-NS caused a moderate increase of P*gadE-lacZ* activity, suggesting that these regulators are not responsible for the activation of *mdtEF* under anaerobic condition. Interestingly, deletion of the GTPase MnmE caused a significant decrease of the transcription of *gadE-mdtEF*, suggesting that MnmE may also contribute to the activation of *gadE-mdtEF* under this condition. Since the current study focuses on the regulation of the multidrug efflux genes *mdtEF* present in the

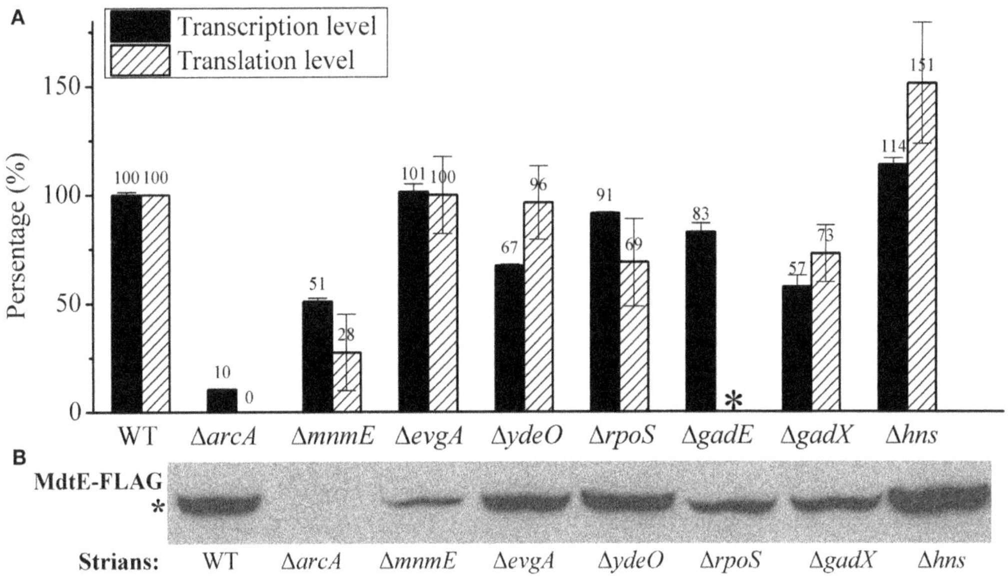

FIGURE 2 | *MdtEF* expression in various mutants at both transcription and translation level under anaerobic condition. (A) Transcription of *gadE-mdtEF* was determined by β-galactosidase activity of P*gadE-lacZ*, and translation of the gene is determined by Western blot to detect the production of MdtE-FLAG. **(B)** Production of chromosomal MdtE-FLAG in various mutants. Cells were grown anaerobically to exponential phase (A_{600} = 0.3) in minimal M9 glucose medium. All results were presented as percentages relative to the transcription of P*gadE-lacZ* or production of MdtE-FLAG in wild type strain. Error bars represent the standard errors of triplicate experiments (n = 3). **mdtE-flag* in Δ*gadE* mutant was not constructed because of the close proximity of *gadE* and *mdtEF* which is not applicable by the P1 phage transduction.

same operon, we next examined whether deletion of these genes caused alteration of MdtEF protein levels. We constructed chromosomal *mdtE-flag* in these strains (except for Δ*gadE*) and performed Western blot to examine the level of MdtE-FLAG. As shown in **Figure 2B**, production of MdtE-FLAG in the corresponding deletion mutants showed a similar pattern as that of β-galactosidase activity assay except Δ*mnmE*, which caused a more significant reduction of MdtE expression at translational level. Together these results confirmed that ArcA and MnmE are primarily responsible for the anaerobic activation of *mdtEF*.

As a control, we also measured the effect of deletion of these regulators on the aerobic expression of *gadE-mdtEF* in *E. coli* grown in M9 glucose medium at log phase. As shown in **Figure 3**, P*gadE-lacZ* activities in wild type strain, and in Δ*arcA*, Δ*mnmE*, Δ*evgA*, Δ*ydeO*, Δ*gadE*, Δ*gadX* mutants are very low (around 20 Miller units), consistent with the fact that ArcA is not active under this condition. However, in Δ*hns* mutants, the P*gadE-lacZ* activities increased more than 10-fold to about 250 Miller units, suggesting H-NS strongly represses the expression of *gadE-mdtEF* under aerobic condition in the M9 glucose minimal medium. This result is consistent with previous findings that H-NS represses the transcription from P*gadE* through its interaction with various sites in the *gadE* promoter region (Sayed and Foster, 2009). It is noted that deletion of *evgA*, *ydeO*, *gadE*, and *gadX* did not show obvious effect on the transcription of P*gadE-lacZ* in this assay. This is not unexpected as previous studies on the regulation of *gadE-mdtEF* by these regulators was found to be effective in the acidified minimal medium (pH 5.5) containing glucose or during stationary phase in rich medium (Ma et al., 2004), whereas the current study is carried out in the neutral M9 minimal medium with glucose, the identical culture medium as in our previous assay which showed increased expression of MdtEF under anaerobic condition. These results together suggested that the regulatory network of *mdtEF* expression under anaerobic condition is different from that under aerobic condition, and anaerobic activation of *mdtEF* is largely dependent on ArcA and MnmE.

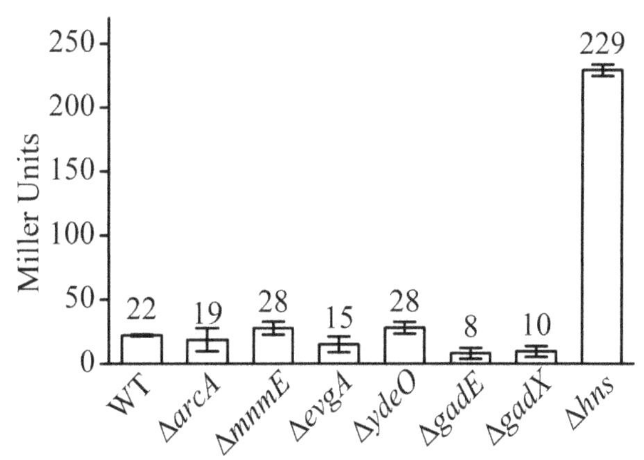

FIGURE 3 | β-galactosidase activity of P*gadE-lacZ* fusion in WT (MG1655 Δ*lacZ*), Δ*arcA*, Δ*mnmE*, Δ*evgA*, Δ*ydeO*, Δ*gadE*, Δ*gadX*, and Δ*hns* mutant strains under aerobic condition.

DELETION OF EvgA, YdeO, H-NS DOES NOT HAVE OBVIOUS EFFECT ON THE TRANSCRIPTION FROM INDIVIDUAL PROMOTERS UNDER ANAEROBIC CONDITION

Our investigation above showed that ArcA and MnmE are the major activators responsible for the expression of *gadE-mdtEF* under anaerobic condition, whereas other regulators tested did not show obvious regulatory effects. However, since four promoter regions (P, P1, P2/P4, and P3) are involved in the transcription initiation of *gadE-mdtEF*, we cannot rule out the possibility that they might participate in the regulation of individual promoters contained in the complete 798 bp promoter of *gadE*. For example, it is possible that a certain regulator activates the transcription from one promoter region while represses transcription from another promoter, consequently cancels its effect on the transcription from the full promoter in our assay. To verify this, we examined the anaerobic transcription activity of those P*gadE* truncations in the deletion mutants constructed in this study except for GadX and GadW since they were indicated to be active in low pH, complex medium or stationary phase (Ma et al., 2003). It was shown that deletion of *evgA*, *ydeO*, and *hns* did not cause significant changes on the transcription activity from each of the individual promoters (data not shown), indicating that these regulators had no effect on the transcript from the individual promoters contained in the 798 bp full promoter of *gadE* either under anaerobic condition.

GadE AUTOREGULATES TRANSCRIPTION FROM P1 REGION UNDER ANAEROBIC CONDITION

Interestingly, deletion of *gadE* caused different effects on the transcription from different promoters contained in the full 798 bp P*gadE* region, which is dissimilar from that observed in the case of Δ*evgA*, Δ*ydeO*, and Δ*hns*. As shown in **Figure 4** (stripe bars), while *gadE* deletion had no significant effect on the transcription from the *lacZ* fusions of the full length, P3, P3+P2/P4, as well as P3+P2/P4+P1, deletion of *gadE* caused almost complete abolishment of transcription from the P2/P4+P1 and the P1 promoters. This observation combined with the results above which showed that individual P2/P4 was not active under anaerobic conditions suggested that GadE autoactivates the transcription of *gadE-mdtEF* from its P1 promoter. This result is consistent with a previous truncation study performed under aerobic condition, where deletion of *gadE* caused decrease of transcription from P2/P4+P1 and P1 promoters (Sayed and Foster, 2009), and the presence of a conserved GAD box to which GadE binds in the P1 region (Ma et al., 2004). Moreover, the fact that deletion of *acrA* and *mnmE* caused decrease of transcription from P1 at variable degrees whereas deletion of *gadE* almost completely abolished transcription from this promoter suggested that activation of P1 is dependent on the production of GadE which is transcribed from the ArcA and MnmE activated other promoters, such as P3, in the case of the full length, native promoter in the cell.

ArcA DIRECTLY BINDS TO MULTIPLE SITES AT THE *gadE* PROMOTER TO ACTIVATE THE EXPRESSION OF THE *gadE-mdtEF*

Since ArcA and MnmE were identified as transcription activators of the *gadE-mdtEF* operon, we next asked how these two regulators activate *gadE* expression, i.e., through which promoters these two regulators affect the transcription of the *gadE-mdtEF* operon under anaerobic conditions. To address this, we measured the transcription of promoter-*lacZ* fusions containing various lengths of the P*gadE* region in Δ*arcA* and Δ*mnmE* strains, respectively (**Figure 4**). Surprisingly, deletion of *arcA* (grid bars) or *mnmE* (gray bars) caused decrease of transcription from the full length and all the truncation mutants with variable promoter lengths, indicating ArcA and MnmE might affect transcription from multiple promoters, especially the P3 and P1 regions, since P2/P4 and P individual promoters were not active under this condition as shown above. Considering that the activation of the P1 promoter is dependent on GadE, it is possible that ArcA and MnmE primarily activate the P3 promoter.

To examine whether the ArcA dependent activation of P*gadE* is through its direct binding on the *gadE* promoter region, we

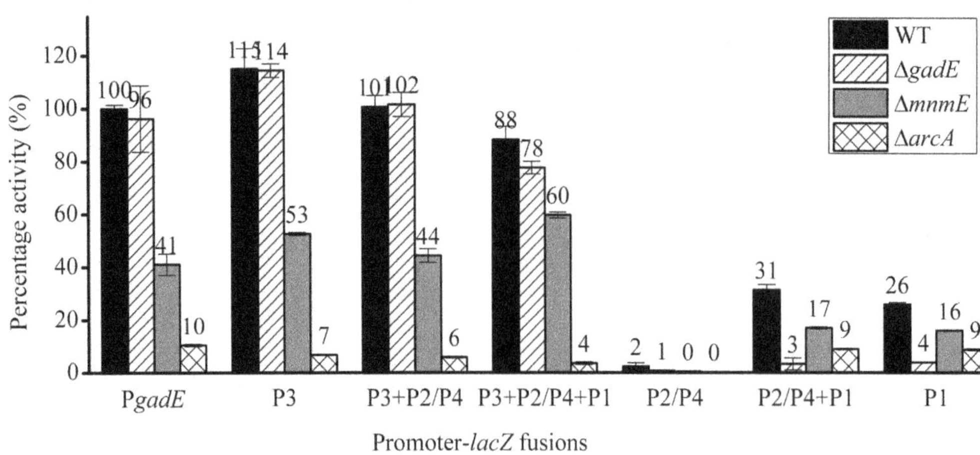

FIGURE 4 | β-galactosidase activity of P*gadE* truncations in WT (black bars), Δ*gadE* (stripe bars), Δ*mnmE* (gray bars) and Δ*arcA* (grid bars) strains under anaerobic growth condition.

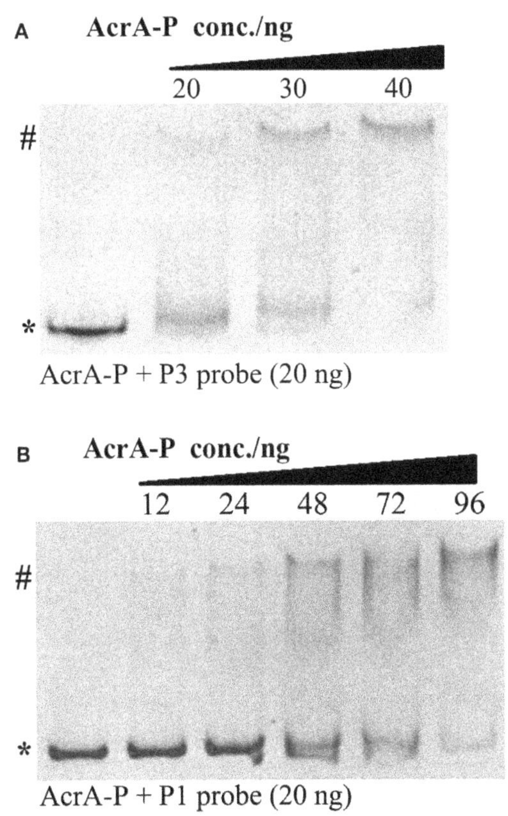

FIGURE 5 | Binding of ArcA-P to P1 and P3 promoters using EB stained EMSA assay. Various concentrations of AcrA-P were incubated with P3 **(A)** or P1 **(B)**. AcrA-P refers to phosphorylated His_6-ArcA protein. Asterisk indicates free DNA probe and pound indicates protein–DNA complex.

performed EMSA to measure the direct binding of ArcA-P (phosphorylated His_6-ArcA) to the P1 and P3 promoters. As shown in **Figure 5**, retarded bands corresponding to the DNA-protein complexes of ArcA-P with both P3 and P1 were observed, suggesting AcrA-P binds to multiple sites at the *gadE* promoter encompassed in the individual P1 and P3 promoters and activates the expression of *gadE* under anaerobic condition. Genome wide CHIP-chip (Chromatin immunoprecipitation with microarray) and CHIP-seq study which determines all the ArcA binding sites across the *E. coli* K-12 MG1655 genome under anaerobic conditions in glucose minimum media also identified two broad ArcA binding peaks in the *gadE* promoter. Furthermore, the presence of the ArcA peaks correlated with the presence of a strong σ^{70} peak comparing with the very low σ^{70} peak on this region under aerobic condition (Park and Kiley, et al., unpublished data, pers. communication), further confirming the ArcA dependent activation of the *gadE-mdtEF* operon through its direct binding of multiple sites on the *gadE* promoter.

ArcA ANTAGONIZES THE H-NS MEDIATED REPRESSION OF *gadE-mdtEF* DURING THE TRANSITION FROM AEROBIC TO ANAEROBIC GROWTH

Our results above showed that the expression of *gadE-mdtEF* is largely repressed by the DNA silencer H-NS under aerobic conditions in M9 glucose medium, whereas under anaerobic condition in the same medium its expression is activated primarily in an ArcA dependent manner. This led us to ask how the H-NS mediated repression is replaced by the ArcA dependent activation during the transition of the facultative bacterium *E. coli* from its aerobic to anaerobic growth. To answer this question, we first examined which individual promoter region is responsible for the H-NS mediated repression under aerobic condition. As shown in **Figure 6A**, in addition to the full length promoter P*gadE*, deletion of *hns* caused de-repression of transcription from the P1 and P3 promoters, but no effect on the transcription from the P2/P4 and P promoters, indicating that H-NS represses the transcription of P*gadE* from both the P1 and P3 promoters under aerobic condition in the M9 glucose medium. This pattern is similar to that of how ArcA achieves its activation of P*gadE* under anaerobic condition which is also through its interaction with the P3 and P1 promoters.

Two possibilities may explain the transition from H-NS mediated repression to ArcA mediated activation of *gadE-mdtEF* during the transition from aerobic to anaerobic growth. One possibility is that H-NS is inactive under anaerobic conditions and it disassembles from the *gadE* promoter, allowing ArcA which is active under this condition to bind the promoter of *gadE* and initiate gene transcription. Alternatively, under anaerobic conditions H-NS can still bind to the *gadE* promoter, however, its binding is antagonized by the activated ArcA, resulting in the recruitment of RNAP and transcript initiation of the operon under this condition. To differentiate these two possibilities, we constructed Δ*arcA* Δ*hns* double deletion and examined transcription of P*gadE-lacZ* in this strain. If H-NS is inactive under anaerobic condition and is disassembled from the *gadE* promoter, then transcription of P*gadE-lacZ* in Δ*arcA* Δ*hns* should be similar to that of Δ*arcA* alone. However, if H-NS was not inactivated, rather, it can still bind to the promoter but its binding was antagonized by ArcA, then its binding to the *gadE* promoter should be resumed when ArcA is absent and an increase of P*gadE-lacZ* activity should be observed in Δ*hns* Δ*arcA* than Δ*arcA* single deletion strain. As shown in **Figure 6B**, transcription of P*gadE-lacZ* in Δ*arcA* Δ*hns* double deletion did display significantly higher activity than that in Δ*arcA* strain, suggesting that the anaerobically up-regulated *gadE-mdtEF* expression was through the antagonization of H-NS mediated repression by ArcA. Western blot analysis of chromosomal MdtE-FLAG showed the same pattern as that of transcription assay (**Figure 6C**). More interestingly, the increased transcription of *lacZ* fusions in Δ*arcA* Δ*hns* double deletion strain than that in Δ*arcA* single deletion strain was also observed in the case of individual P3 and P1 promoters, suggesting that ArcA antagonization of H-NS takes place at multiple sites in the P*gadE* promoter, consistent with the notion that both H-NS and ArcA can oligomerize and bind to a broad region in its regulated gene promoters (Green and Paget, 2004; Dorman, 2006). CHIP-chip data of H-NS and ArcA are also consistent with this proposal, as characterized by a broad peak of H-NS binding to PgadE under aerobic conditions and the replacement of this broad peak by that of ArcA under anaerobic conditions (Park and Kiley et al., unpublished data, pers. communication).

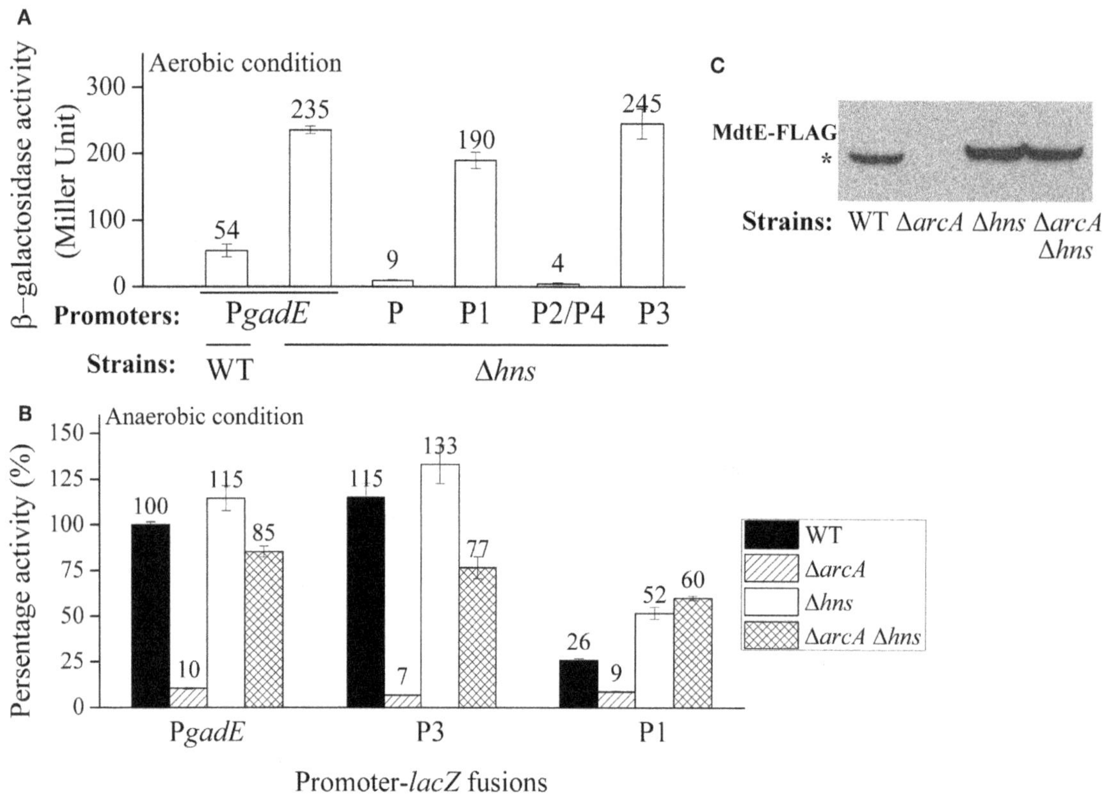

FIGURE 6 | ArcA antagonizes the H-NS mediated repression of *gadE* under anaerobic growth. **(A)** Promoter activity of P*gadE* and its truncations under aerobic condition determined by β-galactosidase activity of corresponding *lacZ* fusions in WT and Δ*hns* strains; **(B)** Promoter activity of P*gadE* and its truncations under anaerobic condition determined by β-galactosidase activity of corresponding *lacZ* fusions in WT, Δ*arcA*, Δ*hns*, and Δ*arcA* Δ*hns* strains; **(C)** Protein level of MdtE-FLAG in WT, Δ*arcA*, Δ*hns* and Δ*arcA* Δ*hns* strains determined by Western blot. Cells used for all assays were grown anaerobically in M9minimal glucose medium to exponential phase (A_{600} = 0.3). Results of β-galactosidase activity assay are presented in Miller unit or percentage activity to that of wild type strain, error bars represent the standard errors of triplicate experiments (n = 3). * indicates the band of MdtE-FLAG.

THE EFFECT OF MnmE ON THE ANAEROBIC ACTIVATION OF *gadE-mdtEF* IS NOT THROUGH ArcA

As shown in **Figure 4**, Δ*mnmE* caused a very similar pattern on the transcription activities of the various P*gadE* truncations as that caused by Δ*arcA*, only to a less extent. This, combined with the fact that MnmE itself does not have DNA binding property whereas ArcA was shown to directly bind to P*gadE* and activate its expression, led us to speculate that the effect of Δ*mnmE* on *gadE-mdtEF* expression may be indirect, i.e., MnmE may affect the translation and/or activity of ArcA (such as through affecting its phosphorylation). To address this, we tested the effect of Δ*mnmE* on the transcription of two ArcA dependent promoters, P*lpdA* and the mutated P*icdA*. Transcription of *lpdA* gene has been shown to be mediated by the repression of ArcA under anaerobic conditions. In the case of *icdA*, it contains two known promoters, P_I and P_{II}, in which P_I is the primary promoter and is repressed only by ArcA. In the mutated P*icdA-lacZ*, transcription from P_{II} was eliminated by removal of its −10 element such that transcription repression of this P*icdA-lacZ* is exclusively ArcA dependent (Park and Kiley et al., unpublished work, pers. communication). If MnmE affects either the production or phosphorylation of ArcA (which affects the regulatory activity of ArcA), Δ*mnmE* should cause full or partial de-repression of these two promoters under anaerobic condition. As shown in **Figure 7**, as expected, transcription of P*icdA-lacZ* and P*lpdA-lacZ* fusions were significantly repressed by ArcA under anaerobic condition, since Δ*arcA* caused de-repression of their transcription under anaerobic condition in M9 glucose medium, the same condition used in this study. However, Δ*mnmE* had little or no effect on the transcription of these two promoters, suggesting that MnmE does not affect the production or phosphorylation of ArcA *in vivo*. Therefore, the observed MnmE mediated anaerobic activation of *gadE-mdtEF* was not due to its potential effects on ArcA.

DISCUSSION

DIFFERENT REGULATORY CIRCUITS ON THE EXPRESSION OF THE *gadE-mdtEF* OPERON UNDER DIFFERENT PHYSIOLOGICAL CONDITIONS

Owing to the important roles of GadE and MdtEF in acid resistance and drug efflux respectively in *E. coli*, transcriptional regulation of the *gadE-mdtEF* operon under various of growth phases and conditions has been extensively investigated. While previous

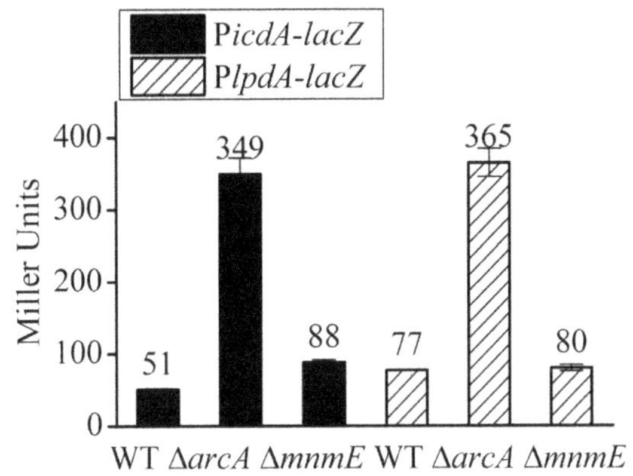

FIGURE 7 | MnmE has no effect on the transcription of P*icdA-lacZ* and P*lpdA-lacZ*, two ArcA dependent promoters. β-galactosidase activities of chromosomal P*icdA-lacZ* (black bars) and P*lpdA-lacZ* (stripe bars) fusions were measured from cells grown anaerobically to exponential phase (A_{600} = 0.3) in minimal M9 glucose medium. Results are presented in Miller unit and error bars represent the standard errors of triplicate experiments (*n* = 3).

studies largely focused on its relevance in bacterial acid resistance under aerobic growth environment, the current study aimed to dissect the up-regulation of the operon under the physiologically relevant environment of anaerobic growth and its effect on the production of the multidrug efflux protein MdtEF.

Several well-characterized regulatory circuits that activate *gadE* expression in the context of acid resistance have been disclosed. These include the EvgA-YdeO-GadE feed forward regulatory loop which is effective in minimal glucose medium under aerobic condition (Ma et al., 2004), the conditional activation of the operon in a MnmE dependent manner in LB containing glucose (LBG) (Gong et al., 2004), as well as the GadX or GadW dependent activation which functions primarily in rich media in stationary growth phase (Sayed et al., 2007). Here we show that the anaerobic activation of the operon, particularly the expression of the multidrug efflux protein MdtEF, is also dependent on the 798 bp *gadE* promoter and the activation is primarily dependent on the anaerobic global regulator ArcA, adding yet another regulatory circuit to the existing complex regulatory loops of the operon. These results reinforced the important role of the promoter region of *gadE* in integrating various of environmental and physiological signals to facilitate the adaptation of *E. coli*.

We also measured the transcription of *PgadE-lacZ* under anaerobic condition in stationary phase and examined whether the previously identified regulators, such as RpoS and GadE, participate in the regulation of the *gadE-mdtEF* expression under this growth phase anaerobically. Surprisingly, while a slightly higher transcription of *PgadE-lacZ* in stationary phase than in log phase (~700 Miller units vs. ~480 Miller units in log phase) was observed, deletion of *rpoS* or *gadE* did not have any effect on the transcription of *PgadE-lacZ* in this growth phase (data not shown), whereas Δ*arcA* still caused significant decrease of the *gadE-mdtEF* expression in the same growth phase. These results suggested that anaerobic expression of the *gadE-mdtEF* operon is primarily regulated by ArcA in both log phase and stationary phase under anaerobic condition. It is noted that previously a putative ArcA binding site located at the P2 region was proposed (Zhang et al., 2011), whereas in the current study, the P3 and P1 region of the *gadE* promoter was shown to be bound by ArcA and they play an important role in the anaerobic activation of the operon. This inconsistency is likely due to the inaccuracy of the bioinformatic search which utilized a sequence motif of "(5′ [A/T]GTTAATTA[A/T] 3′)" as the template and the motif was proposed as the ArcA binding site by Lynch and Lin (1996) following the DNA foot-printing analysis of a limited number of ArcA regulated promoters. Indeed, a genome-wide search of all the ArcA regulated promoters and subsequent characterization of them suggest a motif (Kiley et al., unpublished work, pers. communication) that deviates from the previously proposed ArcA binding site.

Interestingly, we demonstrated that the ArcA dependent activation of the operon is through its antagonistic effect on the H-NS mediated repression of the operon. This regulatory model explains the dynamic process taking place during the transition of *E. coli* from its aerobic to anaerobic growth, which mimics the transition of the bacterium from free living status to the anaerobic environment of the human host. H-NS mediated repression of the operon has also been implicated in previous studies (Ma et al., 2004; Sayed and Foster, 2009). However, the inter-relationship of this repression and gene activation mediated by other regulators has not been revealed. Our findings demonstrating that ArcA activates the expression of the operon through antagonizing the H-NS mediated repression probably provide a common model that underlies the dynamic and coordinated regulation of *gadE-mdtEF* in response to different environmental signals. Perhaps under unstressed conditions when the expression of the operon is unnecessary, the promoter of *gadE* is primarily occupied by H-NS and transcription from the various promoters in this region is repressed. Upon the activation of different transcription activators in response to different environmental or physiological conditions that presage acid stresses or efflux of certain metabolic by-products, the activators then displace H-NS binding on the promoter, resulting in the activation of the operon. Several lines of evidence support this proposal: first, bioinformatics have suggested the presence of an efficient DNA helix locking mechanism by H-NS in the promoter of *gadE* (Hommais et al., 2004); Second, H-NS mediated repression has been found to be common among acquired gene clusters which is consistent with the functions of these gene clusters in conferring the survival and adaptation of bacteria in various adverse growth environments (Oshima et al., 2006). The acid resistant island including the *gadE-mdtEF* operon indeed is one of the acquired gene clusters in *E. coli* with different GC content from the rest of *E. coli* genome; Third, the interplay between the H-NS mediated repression and ArcA mediated antagonizing of the repression is also observed in the case of another gene *cydAB* which is also involved in adapting *E. coli* to the microaerobic and anaerobic growth (Govantes et al., 2000). Thus, anaerobic activation of *gadE-mdtEF* through antagonizing the H-NS mediated repression by ArcA provides a regulatory model that is relevant to the dynamic lifestyle of the facultative bacterium *E. coli*. A model to explain this dynamic regulation is presented in **Figure 8**.

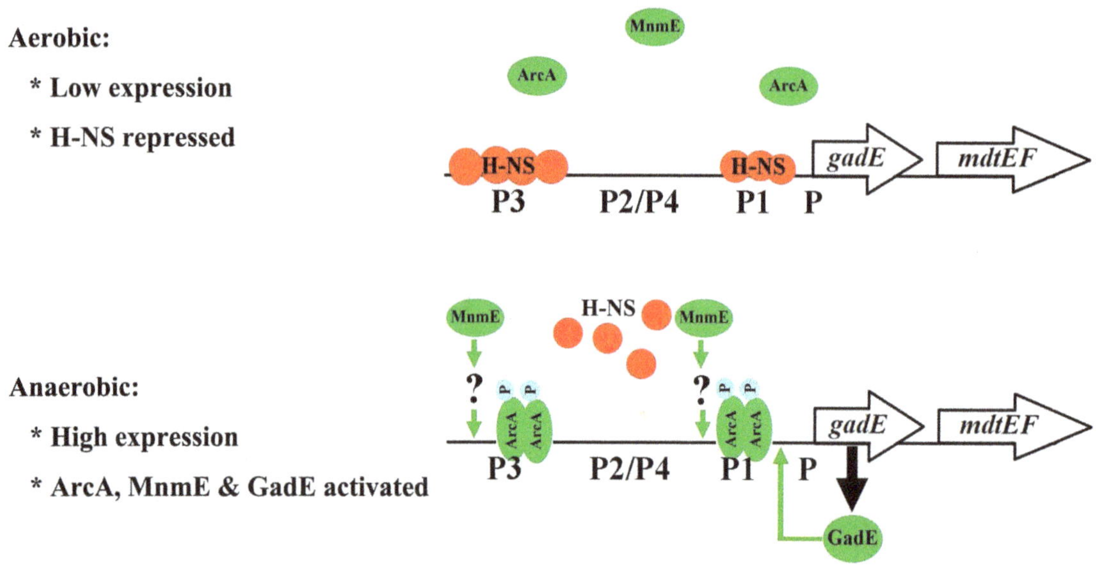

FIGURE 8 | A regulatory model for the transcriptional regulation of *gadE-mdtEF* operon during the transition from aerobic to anaerobic growth in minimal M9 glucose medium. During aerobic growth, the *gadE-mdtEF* is expressed at a very low level due to the strong repression by H-NS. Upon transition to anaerobiosis, the response regulator ArcA is phosphorylated and activated by its sensor kinase ArcB. Phosphorylated ArcA (ArcA-P) antagonizes H-NS binding to *gadE* promoter, resulting in the relief of repression. ArcA-P also directly binds to the *gadE* promoter and activates the expression of *gadE-mdtEF*. ArcA-P activated *gadE* expression produces GadE, which activates the transcription from the P1 promoter and further up-regulate the *gadE-mdtEF* expression. MnmE also participates in the anaerobic activation of *gadE-mdtEF*, but in a yet uncharacterized manner.

ROLES OF THE *gadE-mdtEF* OPERON IN BOTH ACID RESISTANCE AND DRUG EFFLUX

It is interesting that the drug efflux genes *mdtEF* exist in the same operon with the central acid resistance regulator *gadE*, and their expression is driven by the same unusually long 798 bp promoter region upstream of the *gadE* gene. While functions of GadE in controlling the expression of the major acid resistant system GadA and GadBC is well established, the relevance of MdtEF to acid resistance has not been fully recognized. Our previous studies showed that MdtEF functions to expel indole nitrosative by-products accumulated during nitrate respiration under anaerobic condition (Zhang et al., 2011). It is known that anaerobic metabolism often causes pH reduction in growth medium, especially during glucose fermentation by *E. coli* which leads to the production of various organic acids. Although anaerobic induction of *gadE-mdtEF* occurs at a fairly neutral pH (6.9 at the log phase culture when the cells were harvested for transcription and Western blot analyses), significant accumulation of the indole nitrosative by-product occurred when pH dropped to 5.8 or below (Weiss, 2006). Thus, it seems that MdtEF does contribute to the detoxification of acid induced metabolic by-products. Yet, its activation does not necessarily depend on the occurrence of acid stresses. This is consistent with the findings from previous studies which propose that the *gadE-mdtEF* operon is rigged to be induced under many different circumstances that could presage an encounter with acid stresses (Hommais et al., 2004).

This raises the interesting question of whether the housekeeping pump AcrAB is also involved in the nitrosative and/or acid resistance by expelling metabolic by-products under anaerobic conditions. Although the broad substrate specificity of AcrAB-TolC was established in terms of its capability of exporting antibiotics, we speculate that the same degree of broad substrate specificity may not apply in terms of its capability of exporting physiological substances, since it has been well recognized that expression of certain efflux pump genes other than the housekeeping AcrAB pump is activated by specific environmental or physiological conditions (Piddock, 2006; Li and Nikaido, 2009; Poole, 2012b). We recently performed metabolic profiling of the WT vs. Δ*mdtEF* under the growth condition of anaerobic nitrate respiration and it was shown that Δ*mdtEF* cells accumulated more indole nitrosative by-products than the WT (data not shown) in the presence of the *acrAB* genes, suggesting that the MdtEF pump exhibits at least certain degree of substrate specificity even in the presence of the housekeeping pump AcrAB. It is highly likely that MdtEF also expels other metabolic by-products accumulated during acid stresses. If that is the case, there are probably more extensive relevance between MdtEF mediated drug efflux and the physiology of *E. coli* during acid resistance. This relevance probably can be disclosed through metabolic profiling by comparing the total metabolites in Δ*mdtEF* and WT strain grown during acid stresses.

THE UNRESOLVED ROLE OF MnmE IN THE UP-REGULATION OF *mdtEF* EXPRESSION

MnmE is a GTP binding protein that is involved in tRNA modification (Cabedo et al., 1999). This protein was found to be in cytoplasm but can partially associate with the inner membrane (Cabedo et al., 1999). Its involvement in the conditional activation of *gadE* at exponential growth in LB medium with glucose (LBG) or stationary growth of *E. coli* in unbuffered LBG under aerobic condition has been reported (Gong et al., 2004). However, the detailed regulatory mechanism remains elusive. Since MnmE itself does not have DNA binding property, it was speculated that MnmE affects the *gadE* expression by controlling an unknown regulator which can bind to *gadE* promoter and mediate its transcription. Since Δ*mnmE* resulted in a similar pattern of decreased transcription from both full length and various truncation promoter fusions as in Δ*arcA* strain except to a less extent, and ArcA was shown to directly bind to P*gadE*, we had speculated that MnmE regulation of the *gadE* expression was through its effect on ArcA, i.e., through its mediation of the translation and/or phosphorylation of ArcA. However, our β-galactosidase activity results showing that Δ*mnmE* does not have any effect on two different ArcA dependent promoters (P*icdA* and P*lpdA*) suggested that MnmE does not affect the production and/or activity of ArcA under anaerobic conditions, and thus the observed reduction of *gadE-mdtEF* expression in Δ*mnmE* strain was not due to its potential effect on ArcA.

Studies also indicated that MnmE dependent conditional expression of *gadE* mainly depends on the P2 promoter region (Sayed and Foster, 2009). However, our study showed that the P2 region is not active under anaerobic condition at log growth phase; instead, the MnmE dependent *gadE* activation was likely through its effect on the P3 region, which is indispensable in the anaerobic activation of *gadE*. Furthermore, we found that MnmE dependent activation of the *gadE-mdtEF* expression also occurred in non-glucose media, such as LB and glycerol supplemented with nitrate (data not shown). This observation is not in agreement with a previous finding which suggested that MnmE dependent *gadE* expression was induced only in the presence of glucose. Thus, although several studies support the notion that the GTPase MnmE participates in the transcriptional activation of the *gadE-mdtEF* operon under certain growth conditions and phases, how exactly MnmE is involved in the process is still ambiguous. This is largely due to the fact that the exact biological function of MnmE itself is still elusive. Obviously, further studies of MnmE protein is needed before we can reveal its role in the up-regulation of *gadE-mdtEF* under the physiologically relevant conditions.

It is noteworthy that the 798 bp sensory integration region of the *gadE-mdtEF* promoter is highly conserved among the pathogenic *E. coli* strains, including pathogenic strains O157:H7, 2369, RS128 and CFT073 and Shigella (96–99% identity), and GadE has been demonstrated to be indispensable for the survival of *E. coli* O157::H7 in a simulated gastric environment (Kailasan Vanaja et al., 2009), underlying the importance of the *gadE-mdtEF* operon to the physiology of *E. coli*. Since both low pH, such as that of gastric acid, and oxygen limitation (anaerobic environment) activates the expression of the *gadE-mdtEF* operon, it is conceivable that synergetic activation of the system by both regulatory circuits may occur during the transition of *E. coli* to human host, particularly the passage of the gastrointestinal tract, thus greatly facilitate the adaptation and survival of this neutrophilic bacterium in its host niches.

ACKNOWLEDGMENTS

We are grateful for Dr. Patricia J. Kiley (Department of Biomolecular Chemistry, University of Wisconsin-Madison) and Mr. Dan Park in the Kiley lab to share the unpublished data and the strains of P*icdA-lacZ* and P*lpdA-lacZ*. We appreciate Dr. Kunihiko Nishino (Institute of Scientific and Industrial Research, Osaka University) for the pNN387 vector and the P*gadE-lacZ* strain. This work was supported by the Hong Kong Research Fund for the Control of Infectious Diseases 11100982 (to Aixin Yan).

REFERENCES

Allen, H. K., Donato, J., Wang, H. H., Cloud-Hansen, K. A., Davies, J., and Handelsman, J. (2010). Call of the wild: antibiotic resistance genes in natural environments. *Nat. Rev. Microbiol.* 8, 251–259. doi: 10.1038/nrmicro2312

Baba, T., Ara, T., Hasegawa, M., Takai, Y., Okumura, Y., Baba, M., et al. (2006). Construction of *Escherichia coli* K-12 in-frame, single-gene knockout mutants: the Keio collection. *Mol. Syst. Biol.* 2. doi: 10.1038/msb4100050

Bekker, M., Alexeeva, S., Laan, W., Sawers, G., Teixeira De Mattos, J., and Hellingwerf, K. (2010). The ArcBA two-component system of *Escherichia coli* is regulated by the redox state of both the ubiquinone and the menaquinone pool. *J. Bacteriol.* 192, 746–754. doi: 10.1128/JB.01156-09

Cabedo, H., Macián, F., Villarroya, M., Escudero, J. C., Martínez-Vicente, M., Knecht, E., et al. (1999). The *Escherichia coli* trmE (mnmE) gene, involved in tRNA modification, codes for an evolutionarily conserved GTPase with unusual biochemical properties. *EMBO J.* 18, 7063–7076. doi: 10.1093/emboj/18.24.7063

Datsenko, K. A., and Wanner, B. L. (2000). One-step inactivation of chromosomal genes in *Escherichia coli* K-12 using PCR products. *Proc. Natl. Acad. Sci. U.S.A.* 97, 6640–6645. doi: 10.1073/pnas.120163297

Dorman, C. J. (2006). H-NS, the genome sentinel. *Nat. Rev. Microbiol.* 5, 157–161. doi: 10.1038/nrmicro1598

Foster, J. W. (2004). *Escherichia coli* acid resistance: tales of an amateur acidophile. *Nat. Rev. Microbiol.* 2, 898–907. doi: 10.1038/nrmicro1021

Gong, S., Ma, Z., and Foster, J. W. (2004). The Era-like GTPase TrmE conditionally activates gadE and glutamate-dependent acid resistance in *Escherichia coli*. *Mol. Microbiol.* 54, 948–961. doi: 10.1111/j.1365-2958.2004.04312.x

Govantes, F., Orjalo, A. V., and Gunsalus, R. P. (2000). Interplay between three global regulatory proteins mediates oxygen regulation of the *Escherichia coli* cytochrome d oxidase (*cydAB*) operon. *Mol. Microbiol.* 38, 1061–1073. doi: 10.1046/j.1365-2958.2000.02215.x

Green, J., and Paget, M. S. (2004). Bacterial redox sensors. *Nat. Rev. Microbiol.* 2, 954–966. doi: 10.1038/nrmicro1022

Hayes, E. T., Wilks, J. C., Sanfilippo, P., Yohannes, E., Tate, D. P., Jones, B. D., et al. (2006). Oxygen limitation modulates pH regulation of catabolism and hydrogenases, multidrug transporters, and envelope composition in *Escherichia coli* K-12. *BMC Microbiol.* 6:89. doi: 10.1186/1471-2180-6-89

Hirakawa, H., Inazumi, Y., Masaki, T., Hirata, T., and Yamaguchi, A. (2005). Indole induces the expression of multidrug exporter genes in *Escherichia coli*. *Mol. Microbiol.* 55, 1113–1126. doi: 10.1111/j.1365-2958.2004.04449.x

Hirakawa, H., Inazumi, Y., Senda, Y., Kobayashi, A., Hirata, T., Nishino, K., et al. (2006). N-acetyl-d-glucosamine induces the expression of multidrug exporter genes, mdtEF, via catabolite activation in *Escherichia coli*. *J. Bacteriol.* 188, 5851–5858. doi: 10.1128/JB.00301-06

Hommais, F., Krin, E., Coppée, J.-Y., Lacroix, C., Yeramian, E., Danchin, A., et al. (2004). GadE (YhiE): a novel activator involved in the response to acid environment in *Escherichia coli*. *Microbiology* 150, 61–72. doi: 10.1099/mic.0.26659-0

Itou, J., Eguchi, Y., and Utsumi, R. (2009). Molecular mechanism of transcriptional cascade initiated by the EvgS/EvgA system in *Escherichia coli* K-12. *Biosci. Biotechnol. Biochem.* 73, 870–878. doi: 10.1271/bbb.80795

Kailasan Vanaja, S., Bergholz, T. M., and Whittam, T. S. (2009). Characterization of the *Escherichia coli* O157:H7 Sakai GadE regulon. *J. Bacteriol.* 191, 1868–1877. doi: 10.1128/JB.01481-08

Kang, Y., Weber, K. D., Qiu, Y., Kiley, P. J., and Blattner, F. R. (2005). Genome-wide expression analysis indicates that FNR of *Escherichia coli* K-12 regulates a large number of genes of unknown function. *J. Bacteriol.* 187, 1135–1160. doi: 10.1128/JB.187.3.1135-1160.2005

Keseler, I. M., Collado-Vides, J., Santos-Zavaleta, A., Peralta-Gil, M., Gama-Castro, S., Muñiz-Rascado, L., et al. (2011). EcoCyc: a comprehensive database of *Escherichia coli* biology. *Nucleic Acids Res.* 39, D583–D590.

Kobayashi, A., Hirakawa, H., Hirata, T., Nishino, K., and Yamaguchi, A. (2006). Growth phase-dependent expression of drug exporters in *Escherichia coli* and its contribution to drug tolerance. *J. Bacteriol.* 188, 5693–5703. doi: 10.1128/JB.00217-06

Lennen, R. M., Politz, M. G., Kruziki, M. A., and Pfleger, B. F. (2013). Identification of transport proteins involved in free fatty acid efflux in *Escherichia coli. J. Bacteriol.* 195, 135–144. doi: 10.1128/JB.01477-12

Li, X. Z., and Nikaido, H. (2009). Efflux-mediated drug resistance in bacteria: an update. *Drugs* 69, 1555–1623.

Lynch, A. S., and Lin, E. C. (1996). Transcriptional control mediated by the ArcA two-component response regulator protein of *Escherichia coli*: characterization of DNA binding at target promoters. *J. Bacteriol.* 178, 6238–6249.

Ma, Z., Masuda, N., and Foster, J. W. (2004). Characterization of EvgAS-YdeO-GadE branched regulatory circuit governing glutamate-dependent acid resistance in *Escherichia coli. J. Bacteriol.* 186, 7378–7389. doi: 10.1128/JB.186.21.7378-7389.2004

Ma, Z., Richard, H., and Foster, J. W. (2003). pH-Dependent modulation of cyclic AMP levels and GadW-dependent repression of RpoS affect synthesis of the GadX regulator and *Escherichia coli* acid resistance. *J. Bacteriol.* 185, 6852–6859. doi: 10.1128/JB.185.23.6852-6859.2003

Masuda, N., and Church, G. M. (2003). Regulatory network of acid resistance genes in *Escherichia coli. Mol. Microbiol.* 48, 699–712. doi: 10.1046/j.1365-2958.2003.03477.x

Mettert, E. L., and Kiley, P. J. (2007). Contributions of [4Fe-4S]-FNR and integration host factor to *fnr* transcriptional regulation. *J. Bacteriol.* 189, 3036–3043. doi: 10.1128/JB.00052-07

Miller, J. H. (1972). *Experiments in Molecular Genetics.* Cold Spring Harbor, NY: Cold Spring Harbor Laboratory Press.

Murakami, S., Nakashima, R., Yamashita, E., Matsumoto, T., and Yamaguchi, A. (2006). Crystal structures of a multidrug transporter reveal a functionally rotating mechanism. *Nature* 443, 173–179. doi: 10.1038/nature05076

Nishino, K., Senda, Y., Hayashi-Nishino, M., and Yamaguchi, A. (2009). Role of the AraC-XylS family regulator YdeO in multidrug resistance of *Escherichia coli. J. Antibiot. (Tokyo)* 62, 251–257. doi: 10.1038/ja.2009.23

Nishino, K., Senda, Y., and Yamaguchi, A. (2008a). The AraC-family regulator GadX enhances multidrug resistance in *Escherichia coli* by activating expression of mdtEF multidrug efflux genes. *J. Infect. Chemother.* 14, 23–29. doi: 10.1007/s10156-007-0575-y

Nishino, K., Senda, Y., and Yamaguchi, A. (2008b). CRP regulator modulates multidrug resistance of *Escherichia coli* by repressing the mdtEF multidrug efflux genes. *J. Antibiot. (Tokyo)* 61, 120–127. doi: 10.1038/ja.2008.120

Nishino, K., Yamada, J., Hirakawa, H., Hirata, T., and Yamaguchi, A. (2003). Roles of TolC-dependent multidrug transporters of *Escherichia coli* in resistance to beta-lactams. *Antimicrob. Agents Chemother.* 47, 3030–3033. doi: 10.1128/AAC.47.9.3030-3033.2003

Nishino, K., and Yamaguchi, A. (2001). Analysis of a complete library of putative drug transporter genes in *Escherichia coli. J. Bacteriol.* 183, 5803–5812. doi: 10.1128/JB.183.20.5803-5812.2001

Nishino, K., and Yamaguchi, A. (2002). EvgA of the two-component signal transduction system modulates production of the YhiUV multidrug transporter in *Escherichia coli. J. Bacteriol.* 184, 2319–2323. doi: 10.1128/JB.184.8.2319-2323.2002

Nishino, K., and Yamaguchi, A. (2004). Role of histone-like protein H-NS in multidrug resistance of *Escherichia coli. J. Bacteriol.* 186, 1423–1429. doi: 10.1128/JB.186.5.1423-1429.2004

Nishino, K., Yamasaki, S., Hayashi-Nishino, M., and Yamaguchi, A. (2011). Effect of overexpression of small non-coding DsrA RNA on multidrug efflux in *Escherichia coli. J. Antimicrob. Chemother.* 66, 291–296. doi: 10.1093/jac/dkq420

Oshima, T., Ishikawa, S., Kurokawa, K., Aiba, H., and Ogasawara, N. (2006). *Escherichia coli* histone-like protein H-NS preferentially binds to horizontally acquired DNA in association with RNA polymerase. *DNA Res.* 13, 141–153. doi: 10.1093/dnares/dsl009

Piddock, L. J. V. (2006). Multidrug-resistance efflux pumps - not just for resistance. *Nat. Rev. Microbiol.* 4, 629–636. doi: 10.1038/nrmicro1464

Poole, K. (2005). Efflux-mediated antimicrobial resistance. *J. Antimicrob. Chemother.* 56, 20–51. doi: 10.1093/jac/dki171

Poole, K. (2008). Bacterial multidrug efflux pumps serve other functions. *Microbe Wash DC* 3, 179.

Poole, K. (2012a). Bacterial stress responses as determinants of antimicrobial resistance. *J. Antimicrob. Chemother.* 67, 2069–2089. doi: 10.1093/jac/dks196

Poole, K. (2012b). Stress responses as determinants of antimicrobial resistance in Gram-negative bacteria. *Trends Microbiol.* 20, 227–234. doi: 10.1016/j.tim.2012.02.004

Sayed, A. K., and Foster, J. W. (2009). A 750 bp sensory integration region directs global control of the *Escherichia coli* GadE acid resistance regulator. *Mol. Microbiol.* 71, 1435–1450. doi: 10.1111/j.1365-2958.2009.06614.x

Sayed, A. K., Odom, C., and Foster, J. W. (2007). The *Escherichia coli* AraC-family regulators GadX and GadW activate gadE, the central activator of glutamate-dependent acid resistance. *Microbiology* 153, 2584–2592. doi: 10.1099/mic.0.2007/007005-0

Tjaden, B., Saxena, R. M., Stolyar, S., Haynor, D. R., Kolker, E., and Rosenow, C. (2002). Transcriptome analysis of *Escherichia coli* using high-density oligonucleotide probe arrays. *Nucleic Acids Res.* 30, 3732–3738. doi: 10.1093/nar/gkf505

Tramonti, A., De Canio, M., and De Biase, D. (2008). GadX/GadW-dependent regulation of the *Escherichia coli* acid fitness island: transcriptional control at the gadY–gadW divergent promoters and identification of four novel 42 bp GadX/GadW-specific binding sites. *Mol. Microbiol.* 70, 965–982.

Weiss, B. (2006). Evidence for mutagenesis by nitric oxide during nitrate metabolism in *Escherichia coli. J. Bacteriol.* 188, 829–833. doi: 10.1128/JB.188.3.829-833.2006

Zhang, Y., Xiao, M., Horiyama, T., Zhang, Y., Li, X., Nishino, K., et al. (2011). The multidrug efflux pump MdtEF protects against nitrosative damage during the anaerobic respiration in *Escherichia coli. J. Biol. Chem.* 286, 26576–26584. doi: 10.1074/jbc.M111.243261

13

Reclaimed water as a reservoir of antibiotic resistance genes: distribution system and irrigation implications

Nicole Fahrenfeld[1], Yanjun Ma[1], Maureen O'Brien[2] and Amy Pruden[1]*

[1] Department of Civil and Environmental Engineering, Virginia Tech, Blacksburg, VA, USA
[2] Department of Civil and Environmental Engineering, Colorado School of Mines, Golden, CO, USA

Edited by:
Jun Lin, The University of Tennessee, USA

Reviewed by:
Timothy LaPara, University of Minnesota, USA
Paul D. Brown, University of the West Indies, Jamaica

***Correspondence:**
Amy Pruden, Department of Civil and Environmental Engineering, Virginia Tech, 418 Durham Hall, Blacksburg, VA 24060, USA.
e-mail. apruden@vt.edu

Treated wastewater is increasingly being reused to achieve sustainable water management in arid regions. The objective of this study was to quantify the distribution of antibiotic resistance genes (ARGs) in recycled water, particularly after it has passed through the distribution system, and to consider point-of-use implications for soil irrigation. Three separate reclaimed wastewater distribution systems in the western U.S. were examined. Quantitative polymerase chain reaction (qPCR) was used to quantify ARGs corresponding to resistance to sulfonamides (*sul*1, *sul*2), macrolides (*erm*F), tetracycline [*tet*(A), *tet*(O)], glycopeptides (*van*A), and methicillin (*mec*A), in addition to genes present in waterborne pathogens *Legionella pneumophila* (L*mip*), *Escherichia coli* (*gad*AB), and *Pseudomonas aeruginosa* (*ecf*x, *gyr*B). In a parallel lab study, the effect of irrigating an agricultural soil with secondary, chlorinated, or dechlorinated wastewater effluent was examined in batch microcosms. A broader range of ARGs were detected after the reclaimed water passed through the distribution systems, highlighting the importance of considering bacterial re-growth and the overall water quality at the point of use (POU). Screening for pathogens with qPCR indicated presence of L*mip* and *gad*AB genes, but not *ecf*x or *gyr*B. In the lab study, chlorination was observed to reduce 16S rRNA and *sul*2 gene copies in the wastewater effluent, while dechlorination had no apparent effect. ARGs levels did not change with time in soil slurries incubated after a single irrigation event with any of the effluents. However, when irrigated repeatedly with secondary wastewater effluent (not chlorinated or dechlorinated), elevated levels of *sul*1 and *sul*2 were observed. This study suggests that reclaimed water may be an important reservoir of ARGs, especially at the POU, and that attention should be directed toward the fate of ARGs in irrigation water and the implications for human health.

Keywords: antibiotic resistance genes, water reuse, reclaimed water distribution systems, irrigation

INTRODUCTION

Water reuse is an increasingly common sustainable water management practice motivated by climate change, urbanization, energy efficiency, and environmental protection (US Environmental Protection Agency [USEPA], 2012). Reclaimed or recycled wastewater is treated by municipalities for a variety of purposes, including non-potable urban reuse (Grant et al., 2012; USEPA, 2012). In the United States Environmental Protection Agency (USEPA) guidelines on water reuse, the presence of antibiotics as trace organic contaminants in wastewater is noted and a need for more information is acknowledged to reduce the proliferation of antibiotic resistance and protect public health (USEPA, 2012).

Antibiotic resistance proliferation is currently outpacing the development of novel antibiotics, calling for effective strategies to mitigate the spread of antibiotic resistance (Carlet et al., 2012). Bacterial resistance to antibiotics is partially conferred through antibiotic resistance genes (ARGs), which code for specific antimicrobial functions such as efflux pumps (Webber and Piddock, 2003). ARG contamination has been quantified in a variety of environmentally relevant matrices, including wastewater treatment plant (WWTP) effluent, which is known to contribute to ARG loadings in surface waters (Pruden et al., 2013; Storteboom et al., 2010; LaPara et al., 2011). Some states require chlorine or UV disinfection for reused water (USEPA, 2012) and certain disinfectants (free chlorine, O_3, and UV) are capable of reacting with nucleic acids during treatment and therefore may potentially reduce ARGs, as recently reviewed by Dodd (2012). However, McKinney and Pruden (2012) recently demonstrated in a controlled lab study that typical UV doses applied at WWTPs are capable of reducing antibiotic resistant strains of bacteria, but not ARGs. Others have noted little reduction in ARGs following UV effluent treatment in full-scale WWTPs (Auerbach et al., 2007; Kim et al., 2010).

While WWTPs are now well-established as a reservoir of ARGs (Auerbach et al., 2007; Kim et al., 2010; Czekalski et al., 2012), and some have considered effect of irrigation with reclaimed water (McLain and Williams, 2012; Negreanu et al., 2012), there is a void of studies focused on the potential for re-growth in treated wastewater distribution systems ("purple" pipes). In one study examining soil irrigated with treated wastewater, no differences in the microbiome or ARG levels were observed compared to soil irrigated with fresh water (Negreanu et al., 2012). In fact, in Llobregat (NE Spain), reclaimed water emitted to a river had lower concentrations of indicator organisms than the stream water (Rubiano et al., 2012). In contrast, re-growth of indicator organisms has been observed between the point of entry (POE) and point of use (POU) in reclaimed water systems (Ryu et al., 2005), raising the question of whether ARGs can also increase during distribution. In a study examining drinking water distribution systems, antibiotic resistant bacteria were shown to decrease between POE and POU, but ARGs were observed to increase (Xi et al., 2009).

In this study, ARG occurrence patterns were evaluated in the POU water in three arid western U.S. recycled water distribution systems using quantitative polymerase chain reaction (qPCR). Depending on access, POE, POU biofilm, and soil irrigated with recycled water were also examined. Samples were also screened by qPCR for the potential presence of known waterborne pathogenic bacteria and indicators, *Legionella pneumophila, Escherichia coli,* and *Pseudomonas aeruginosa.* To simulate the effect of reused water for irrigation, a series of batch laboratory soil microcosm studies were performed to compare irrigation with secondary, chlorinated, and dechlorinated effluent from a representative conventional WWTP.

MATERIALS AND METHODS

WATER REUSE SYSTEMS

Samples were collected from three non-potable reclaimed wastewater distribution systems in the western U.S., together served by four WWTPs (**Table 1**). Water samples (-POE or -POU) were collected in sterile centrifuge tubes. Biofilm (-F) was collected with a sterile swab, and packed in a sterile centrifuge tube. A soil sample was collected from a field irrigated with reclaimed wastewater (-S), in a sterile centrifuge tube. All samples were shipped overnight on ice and stored frozen until extraction. Water samples were freeze-dried prior to DNA extraction (FreeZone Plus, Labconco, Kansas City, MO, USA).

BATCH MICROCOSMS

Aerobic, batch microcosms were prepared to investigate two water reuse scenarios on historically manured soil: (1) a single irrigation event ("batch irrigation") and (2) repeated irrigation events ("periodic irrigation"). Soil was collected (upper 7.5–10 cm) in winter from historically manured corn fields near Virginia Tech campus using a soil probe. Soil was air dried and sieved (2 mm), and an aliquot was preserved for DNA extraction. For each study, microcosms were prepared in 250 mL flasks in triplicate with 50 g of soil and incubated at room temperature on a shaking table to maintain aerobic conditions. Slurry samples were collected weekly without sacrifice. Secondary, chlorinated, and dechlorinated WWTP effluents were collected before each irrigation treatment event from a representative 4.5 Mgd Domestic WWTP.

Batch irrigation soil was initially treated with 80 mL of freshly collected WWTP effluent fractions. Slurry samples (~0.4 g wet) were collected and an equal volume of deionized (DI) water was added to each flask to maintain soil moisture. WWTP effluent fractions (2–4 L) were filtered through 0.22 μm membrane and total DNA was extracted from the filter, as described below. The periodic irrigation soil was initially treated with 100 mL of freshly collected WWTP effluent fractions. Slurry samples (10 mL) were collected, centrifuged at 3,300 × *g* for 5 min, and 0.4 g of the pellet was used for DNA extraction. Fresh WWTP effluent fractions were added to the flasks to replace the volume removed during each sampling. WWTP effluent fractions (60 mL) were freeze-dried, as above, and DNA was extracted from the residuals.

Table 1 | Summary of reclaimed WWTP tertiary treatment characteristics.

	Aa[1]	Ab[1]	B	C
Capacity (Mgd)	6	4	1.1	0.6
Filtration	Media	Dual media	Carbon filter	Sand + activated carbon
Disinfection	Chlorine	UV	Chlorine	Chlorine

All WWTPs studied use conventional primary and secondary treatment processes.
[1] *Aa and Ab are separate WWTPs that emit water to a commingled distribution system.*

MOLECULAR TECHNIQUES

DNA was extracted from freeze-dried water/slurry, 0.4 g soil, or swabs using a FastDNA® SPIN Kit for Soil (MP Biomedicals, Solon, OH, USA) and diluted 1:50 or 1:100 for the water reuse field study and 1:30 for the irrigation studies prior to downstream analysis. qPCR was performed to quantify 16S rRNA (Suzuki et al., 2000), *sul*1 (Aminov et al., 2001), *sul*2 (Aminov et al., 2001), *tet*(A) (Aminov et al., 2002), *tet*(O) (Aminov et al., 2001), *erm*F (Chen et al., 2007), *van*A (Dutka-Malen et al., 1995), *mec*A (McKinney and Pruden, 2012), *L. pneumophila*-specific *mip* (Nazarian et al., 2008), *E. coli*-specific *gad*AB (Chen et al., 2006), and *P. aeruginosa*-specific *ecfX*/*gyr*B (Anuj et al., 2009) genes for the water reuse field study. Reaction matrix and PCR protocols were as previously described (Ma et al., 2011; Wang et al., 2012). For the irrigation study, 16S rRNA, *sul*1, *sul*2, *tet*(O), and *tet*(W) genes were monitored. All standard curves of qPCR were constructed from serial dilutions of cloned genes ranging from 10^8 to 10^2 gene copies/μL. Samples were analyzed in triplicate with a standard curve and negative control included in each run. Limits of quantification with respect to sample volume varied depending on the volume processed and the dilution of DNA extract, ranging from −1.4 to 0.6 $\log_{10}$ gene copies/mL, 3.1–5.1 $\log_{10}$ gene copies per swab, and 0.5–2.5 $\log_{10}$ gene copies/g of soil. Additionally, cloning and sequencing of qPCR product was performed for assays that had not been validated previously (*van*A) to demonstrate specificity of PCR product (GenBank accession number KC792557–KC792573).

STATISTICS

Cluster analysis was performed on transformed (square root) 16S rRNA gene normalized ARG profiles from the reclaimed wastewater systems and significance testing was carried out using the SimProf test in PrimerE (Plymouth, UK). To compare between wastewater treatment effluent fractions and treatments in the irrigation study, data was Box–Cox transformed. Transformed data were compared using ANOVA, and significant differences

($p < 0.05$) were determined using Tukey's honest significance test, as implemented in R (http://www.r-project.org/). Multiple comparisons for the distribution system and irrigation studies were performed on Box–Cox transformed data using least square means comparison with a Satterthwaite estimation of degrees of freedom in SAS, again using Tukey adjustment for multiple comparisons. Linear modeling for the irrigation study data was performed in Microsoft Excel.

RESULTS

ARG OCCURRENCE PATTERNS IN RECYCLED WATER

Antibiotic resistance genes were detected in all water reuse samples (**Figures 1** and **2**). The most frequently detected ARGs were *van*A, *erm*F, and *sul*2 with frequencies of detection of 100, 73, and 65% ($n = 23$), respectively. *tet*(O) had the lowest frequency of detection (17%, $n = 23$) other than *mec*A, which was not detected in any of the samples. For System A, significant differences in ARG

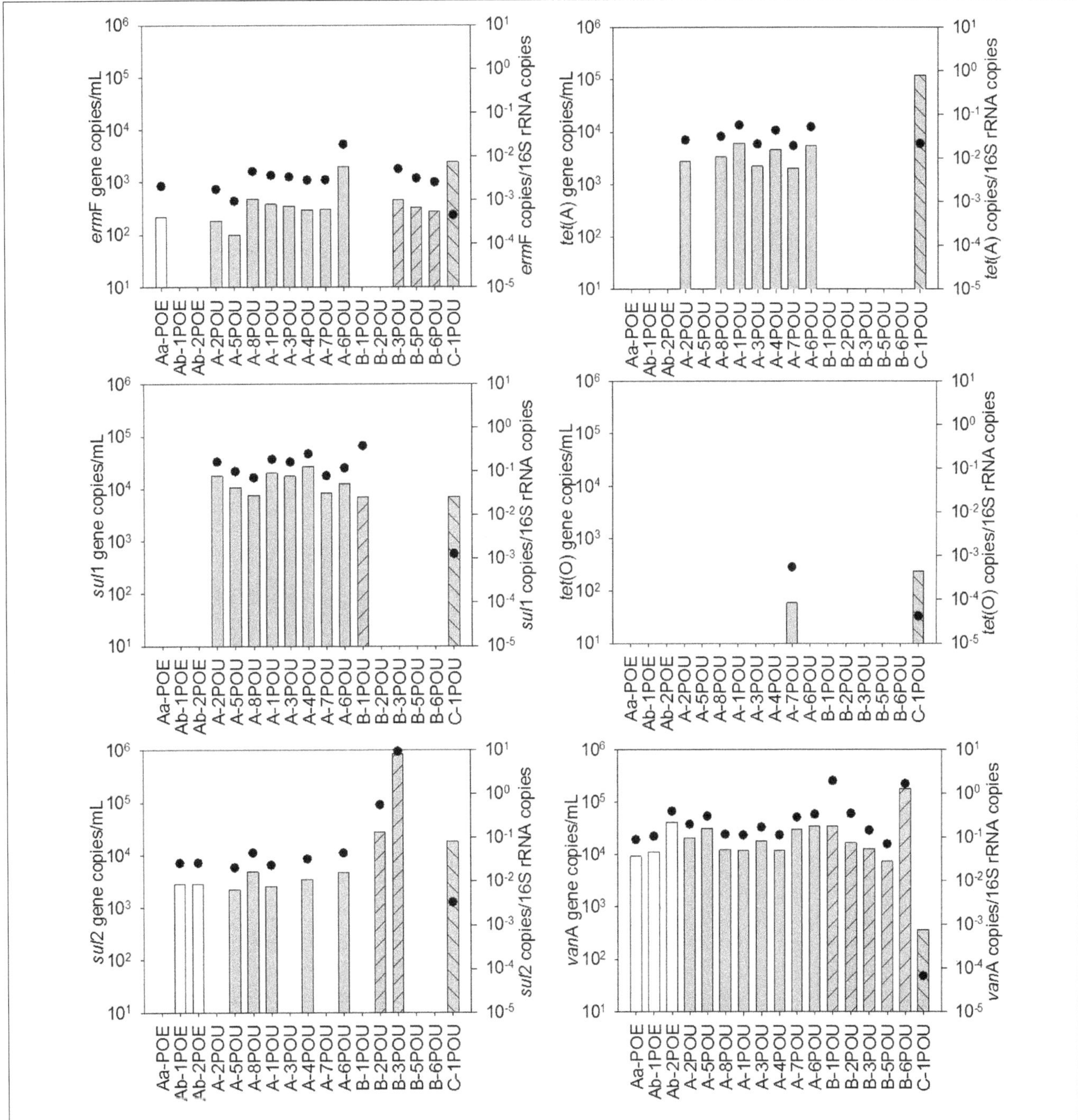

FIGURE 1 | Absolute (bars) and 16S rRNA gene-normalized (symbols) levels of ARGs in water samples collected at point of entry (POE) for WWTPs Aa and Ab and at point of use (POU) for systems A, B, and C, numbers differentiate between sample locations.

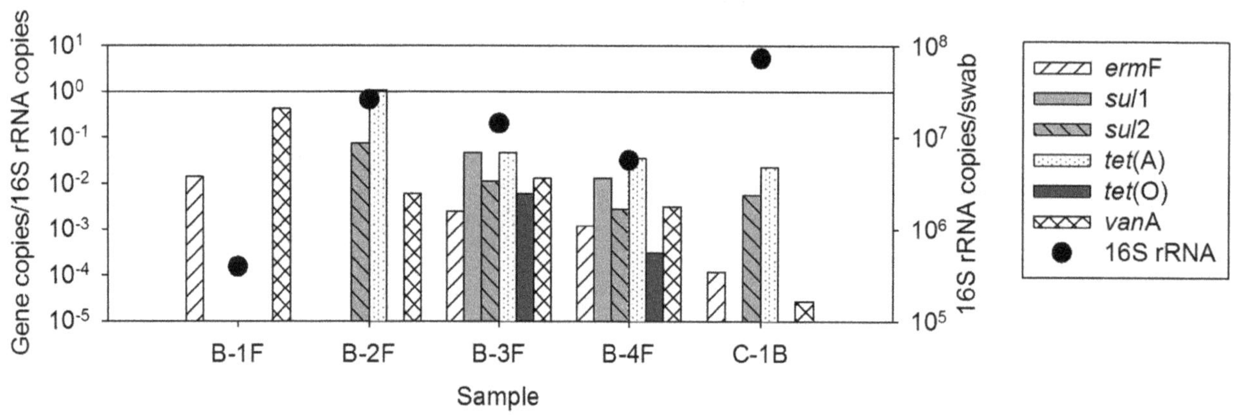

FIGURE 2 | Quantification of ARGs in biofilm samples available from recycled water distribution systems B and C. Bars represent absolute ARG copies per swab, symbols represent 16S rRNA gene copies per swab.

concentrations were observed between POE and POU for *sul*1 and *tet*(A), $p < 0.001$ for both. Concentrations of *van*A, *erm*F, and *sul*2, 16S rRNA, and *tet*(O) were not significantly different between POE and POU ($p = 0.33$–0.99).

In the irrigated soil sample (B-7S), 9.5, 7.3, 7.2, and 5.6 $\log_{10}$ gene copies/g of soil were quantified for 16S rRNA, *sul*1, *sul*2, and *van*A, respectively; *erm*F, *tet*(A), and *tet*(O) were below detection. Normalizing ARGs to 16S rRNA gene copy numbers indicated that *sul*1 and *sul*2 were one to two orders of magnitude lower and *van*A three to five orders of magnitude lower in the soil sample than observed in water and biofilm samples.

The occurrence of ARGs varied among the five biofilm samples examined, ranging from two to six classes of ARGs (**Figure 2**). However, individual ARG levels in the biofilm did not correlate with corresponding bulk water ARGs among the available paired samples (**Figure 3**). For example, the most abundant ARG, *tet*(A), in B-2F was below detection in B-2POU.

Cluster analysis performed on 16S rRNA gene normalized ARG profiles considered both the kinds of ARGs detected and their frequencies and resulted in several significantly different sample clusters (**Figure 4**). Generally, three distinct clusters were formed primarily by POE, WWTP-A POU, and WWTP-C POU samples, while the WWTP-B POU samples were interspersed among the three clusters, and a fourth cluster consisting only of WWTP-B samples. The three WWTP-A POE samples formed a significantly different cluster from POU samples in its corresponding distribution system (50% similarity). POU samples from System A ($n = 7$) formed a cluster with 78–96% similarity, except A-5POU which was significantly different (71%) and clustered with some samples from System B ($n = 5$). No patterns were observed in the biofilm and water clustering patterns for paired samples ($n = 4$). Biofilms did not cluster with one another nor did biofilm samples cluster with paired water sample with similarities ranging from 16% for F2 and F3 (significantly different) to 100% for F1 (no difference). The soil sample (B-7S) clustered with other B system biofilm and water samples, which were only 20% similar to the remainder of the samples selected.

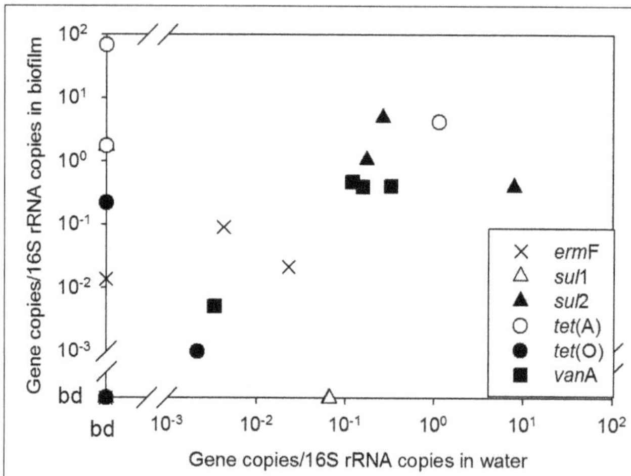

FIGURE 3 | Biofilm versus bulk water ARG copies normalized to 16S rRNA gene copies in available paired biofilm and water samples. ARGs were below detection in several samples, indicated on the *x* and *y* axes as bd.

WATERBORNE PATHOGEN AND FECAL INDICATOR SCREENING

Quantitative PCR screening for *E. coli* and *L. pneumophila* through *gad*AB and *mip* resulted in positive detections for 48% of samples: 35 and 17% for *gad*AB and *mip*, respectively (**Table 2**). *ecrfX*/*gyr*B, corresponding to *P. aeruginosa*, were below detection in all samples.

ARGs DURING SIMULATED LAND APPLICATION

WWTP effluent fraction ARG loads

Levels of ARGs in secondary, chlorinated, and dechlorinated WWTP effluent are compared in **Figure 5**. *sul*1 was the most frequently detected ARG (100%), followed by *sul*2 (71%), *tet*(W) (71%), and *tet*(O) (61%; $n = 21$). Comparing the ARGs and 16S rRNA gene levels across effluent fractions, secondary effluent was significantly higher than chlorinated and dechlorinated (both $p < 0.0001$) effluents, which were not significantly different from each other ($p = 0.45$). Comparing by gene across effluent fractions,

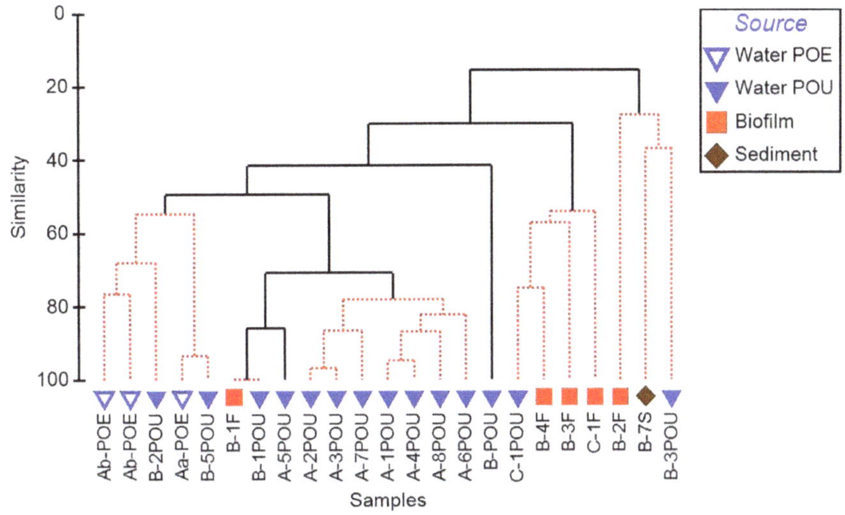

FIGURE 4 | Cluster analysis of 16S rRNA gene normalized ARG copy numbers, considerate of class and relative abundance of each ARG measured in the distribution systems (Aa, Ab, B, C) and across environmental matrices (POE, point of entry water; POU, point of use water; F, biofilm; S, soil). Solid branches indicate significantly different clusters ($p < 0.05$).

Table 2 | Log copies of *E. coli* (*gad*AB) and *L. pneumophila* (*mip*) specific genes per milliliter (POE and POU's), swab (F's), or gram soil (S).

Sample	*gad*AB	*mip*
Ab-POE	3.7	bd*
A-1POU	4.2	bd
A-2POU	5.1	1.8
A-3POU	4.4	bd
A-8POU	5.3	bd
B-1POU	bd	1.4
C-1POU	6.6	bd
B-1F	bd	4.6
B-2F	6.0	bd
C-1F	6.9	bd
B-7S	bd	5.6

** bd, below detection.*

secondary effluent and chlorinated effluent were significantly different in terms of 16S rRNA and *sul*2 gene copies ($p < 0.0001$ for both). Interestingly, when ARGs were normalized to 16S rRNA gene copies, significant differences were not observed among the secondary, chlorinated, or dechlorinated effluents ($p = 0.29$–0.91). This suggests no preferential destruction of specific gene types by chlorination.

Irrigation studies

Results of the batch irrigation study (**Figure 6**) indicated no difference between soil irrigated with secondary, chlorinated, or dechlorinated effluent, or DI water in terms of ARG concentration with time for *sul*1, *sul*2, *tet*(O), or *tet*(W) ($p > 0.405$ for all, except for *sul*2 deionized $p = 0.05$ and secondary effluent $p = 0.006$).

Soil periodically irrigated resulted in a significant increase in *sul*2 when receiving secondary effluent, compared to irrigation with the other water types (p ranging from 0.032 to $p < 0.0001$; **Figure 7**). Additionally, soil irrigated with secondary effluent had significantly higher *sul*1 copies than that irrigated with chlorinated effluent, dechlorinated effluent, or DI water (all $p < 0.0001$). No significant difference across time was observed among the irrigation water types for *tet*(O) ($p = 0.13$–1.0) or *tet*(W) ($p = 0.74$–1.0). Linear modeling of gene copies versus time revealed an increasing trend of *sul*2 copies with time in soil irrigated with secondary effluent ($R^2 = 0.92$).

DISCUSSION

This study explored the occurrence of several ARGs in three reclaimed water distribution systems in the U.S. Given limited access to such systems, only one sampling event was possible. Nonetheless, the results provide important baseline information to support future research, including insight into the kinds of ARGs, bacteria, and applications that may be of concern. To the knowledge of the authors, this is the first study specifically investigating the potential for ARGs to persist or amplify within the reclaimed water distribution pipes.

ARG OCCURRENCE IN RECYCLED WATER DISTRIBUTION SYSTEMS

Several ARGs were detected at the POU in this study, many of which were below detection at the POE. This highlights the need to consider microbiological processes occurring in reclaimed water distribution systems that may be contributing to ARG amplification and suggests that focus on the water quality at the POU may be the most appropriate for assessing risk. Re-growth is a well-known

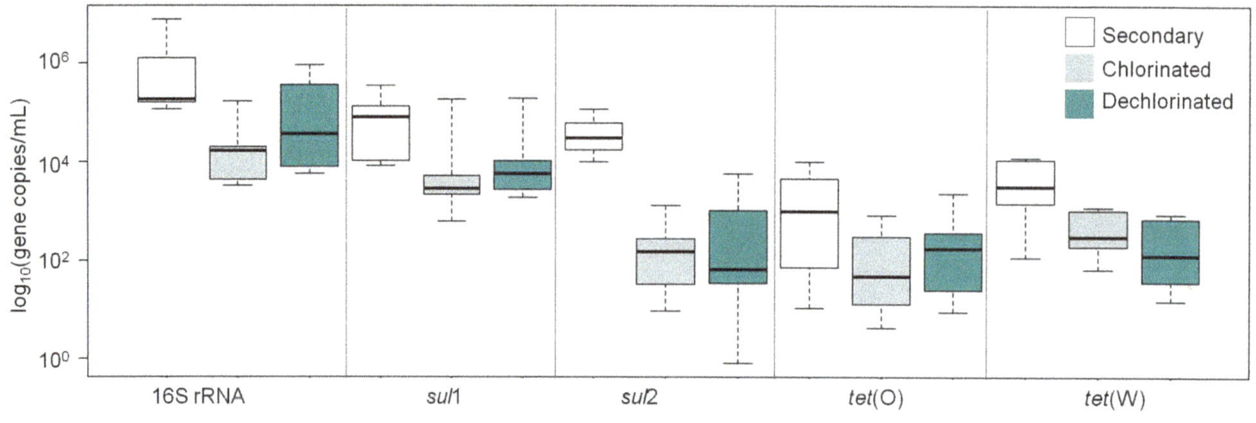

FIGURE 5 | Censored boxplot of 16S rRNA genes, *sul*1, *sul*2, *tet*(O), and *tet*(W) gene copies per milliliter in secondary (no fill), chlorinated (gray), and dechlorinated (blue) domestic WWTP effluents applied in the batch (2–4 L 0. 22 μm filtered) and periodic (60 mL freeze-dried) irrigation study (*n* = 6 *tet* genes, 7 *sul* and 16S rRNA genes).

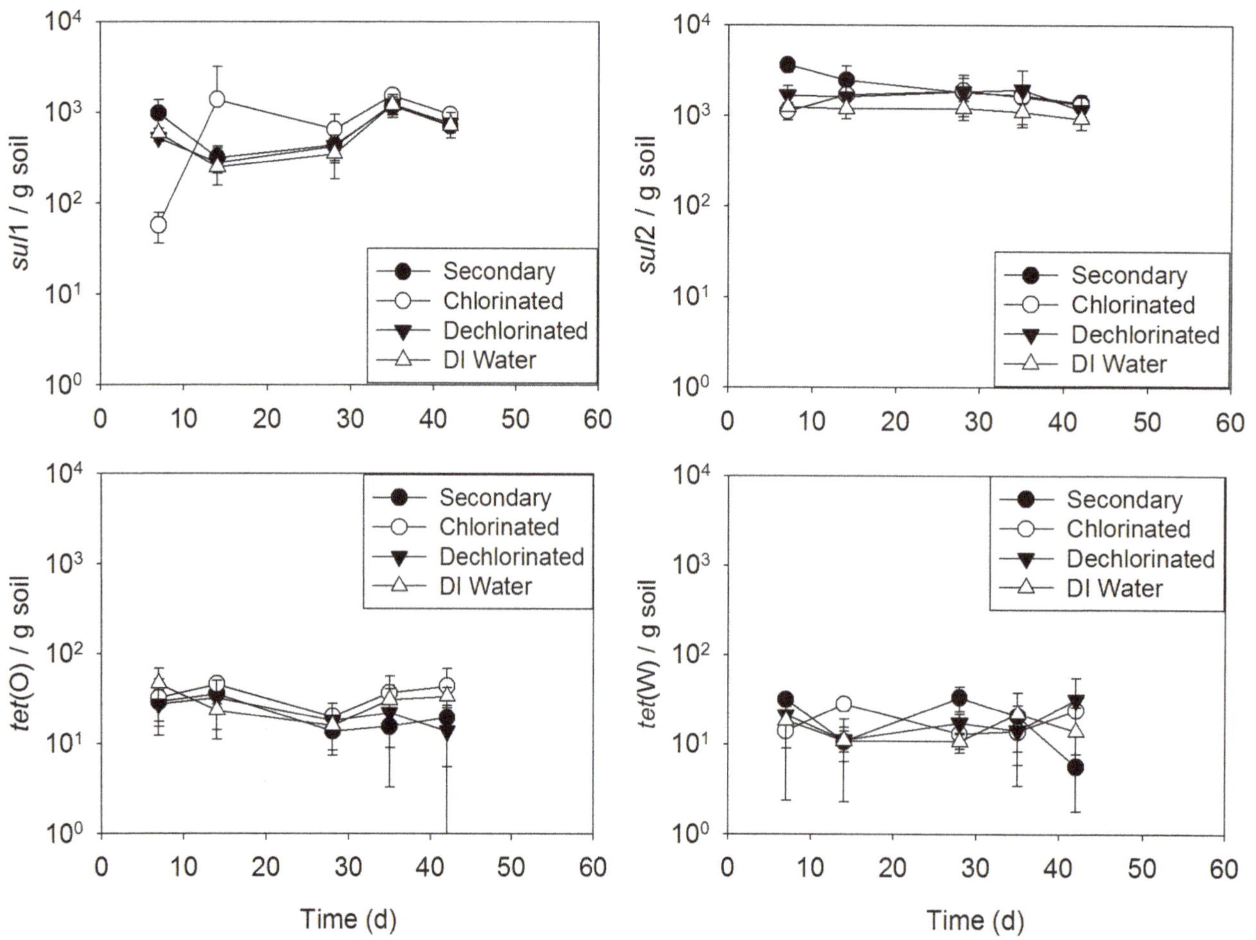

FIGURE 6 | *sul*1, *sul*2, *tet*(O), and *tet*(W) genes in soils subject to one time (batch) irrigation with secondary, chlorinated, dechlorinated domestic WWTP effluents and deionized (DI) water, per gram of soil (slurry). Error bars represent standard deviation of triplicate microcosms.

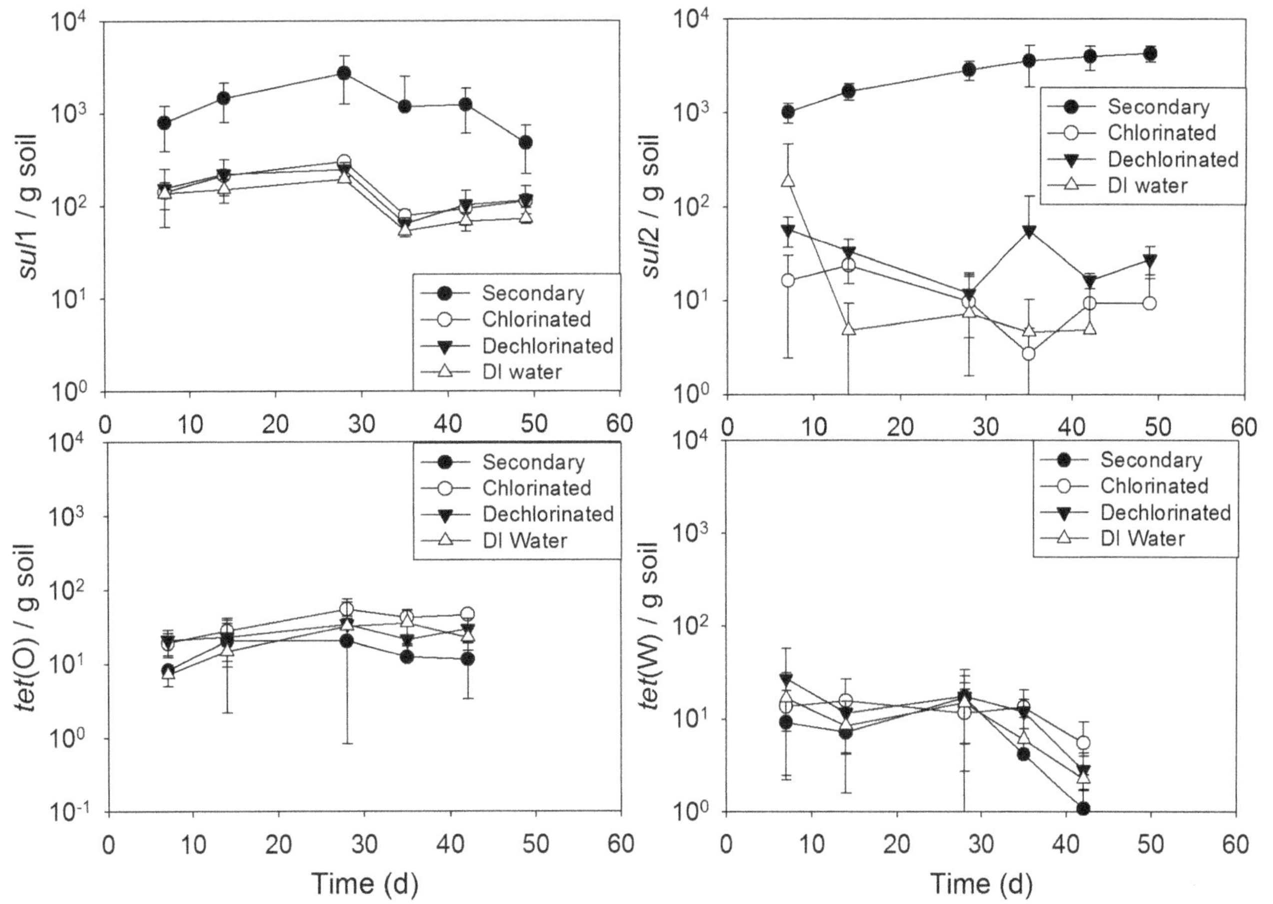

FIGURE 7 | *sul1*, *sul2*, *tet*(O) and *tet*(W) genes in soils periodically irrigated with secondary, chlorinated, dechlorinated domestic WWTP effluents and deionized (DI) water, normalized to soil mass (wet weight). Error bars represent standard deviation of triplicate microcosms.

phenomenon even in drinking water distribution systems (Xi et al., 2009), and has also recently been documented in a recycled water system (Ryu et al., 2005).

Several studies have documented levels of ARGs in WWTP effluents, providing a reference for comparison. Generally, *erm*F, *sul*1, *sul*2, *tet*(A), and *tet*(O) levels measured in the POE, POU, and WWTP effluent applied in the irrigation study were below or at the lower end of ranges reported by others in WWTP effluents (Kim et al., 2010; Czekalski et al., 2012; Negreanu et al., 2012). However, the irrigated soil in this study carried higher levels of *sul*1 (7.3 $\log_{10}$ copies/g) and *sul*2 (7.2 $\log_{10}$ copies/g) than reported by others in a field study of irrigation with recycled water (5.1–6.7 and 3.5–4.7 $\log_{10}$ copies/g, respectively; Negreanu et al., 2012).

The occurrence of *van*A is of particular interest given that it confers resistance to vancomycin, a last-resort life-saving antibiotic. Vancomycin is commonly prescribed to treat methicillin-resistant *Staphylococcus aureus* (MRSA) infections, but has been losing effectiveness due to increased resistance among staphylococci (Stevens, 2006). *van*A was detected in every sample in this study using primers targeting a 732-bp product. Interestingly, using *van*A primers designed for longer target products (1030 bp; Clark et al., 1993), *van*A was detectable at several POU sites, but not in any POE samples (data not shown). Detection differences between the two PCR primer sets may indicate that *van*A was partially damaged during disinfection, preventing amplification of longer PCR products. Long-amplicon PCR has recently been demonstrated to provide enhanced detection of DNA damage events (McKinney and Pruden, 2012). Few studies have reported detection of *van*A in environmental samples, providing little reference for comparison. However, *van*A has been reported in drinking water biofilms and wastewater (Schwartz et al., 2003), but was below detection in wastewater reclaimed for groundwater recharge environments (Böckelmann et al., 2009). To the knowledge of the authors, this is the first report of the presence of *van*A in distributed recycled water.

MOLECULAR DETECTION OF WATERBORNE PATHOGENS AND INDICATORS

Opportunistic pathogens residing in water systems, such as *L. pneumophila* and *P. aeruginosa*, are now the primary source of waterborne disease outbreak in developed countries (Brunkard et al., 2011). However, there is a need for epidemiological studies to better quantify the precise contributions of various water systems to human disease (Pruden et al., 2013). Of interest to the present study was whether such organisms may be present in recycled water, which could be of special concern for bacterial pathogens because they are capable of developing antibiotic resistance. *P. aeruginosa* is an example of an opportunistic pathogen that colonizes taps and is prone to multi-antibiotic resistant forms (Trautmann et al., 2005). *E. coli* was also of interest as a fecal indicator.

The *mip* gene, specific to *L. pneumophila*, was detectable at levels comparable to those recently observed in chloraminated drinking water distribution systems (Wang et al., 2012). Thus, there could be concern for aerosolization of *L. pneumophila* during spray irrigation. Future research is suggested to more closely examine this potential transmission pathway. *gad*AB, specific to *E. coli*, detected at POU in this study, was comparable to levels previously observed in manure runoff (4.6–4.9 $\log_{10}$ copies/mL, assuming one gene copy per cell) and higher than previously observed in WWTP effluent (2.74 $\log_{10}$ copies/mL) (Grant et al., 2001). This combined with the observation of *gad*AB below detection at POE, but detectable at POU, is further evidence of bacterial re-growth within reclaimed water distribution systems.

EFFECT OF DISINFECTION ON ARGs

Chlorination is commonly applied to WWTP effluents during warm seasons, in which case the effluent must be dechlorinated prior to discharge. Chlorination had a significant impact on 16S rRNA and *sul*2 gene copies, which is consistent with the expectation that chlorination would have a moderate reactivity with nucleic acids (Dodd, 2012). Although occasionally ARGs detected in dechlorinated effluent were not detected in chlorinated effluent, the levels of detected genes were not significantly different. The levels of ARGs in secondary, chlorinated, and dechlorinated WWTP effluent fractions were comparable to those detected at the POU in the field study (**Figure 5**).

ARG FATE DURING WWTP EFFLUENT LAND APPLICATION

In the lab study, periodic irrigation with secondary effluent increased the prevalence of *sul*1 and *sul*2 in historically manured soil compared to soil irrigated with chlorinated, dechlorinated, or DI water. This could be due to direct inputs of extracellular ARGs, intracellular ARGs, or horizontal gene transfer to native soil bacteria (Dodd, 2012). Interestingly, *tet*(O) or *tet*(W) levels in the soil slurry were not affected by irrigation. This highlights that different ARGs have different environmental fates, as has been observed recently with respect to *sul*1 and *tet*(W) in a watershed-scale study (Storteboom et al., 2010; Pruden et al., 2012). Differences in ARG fate likely relate to host properties and their overall propensity for horizontal gene transfer. Because 16S rRNA gene copy levels were relatively consistent with time across the soil irrigation treatments (data not shown), changes in total bacterial population sizes were not likely a factor in the observed differences.

A recent field study carried out in Israel suggested that irrigation does not significantly affect the soil microbiome, and increases were not observed in *sul*1, *sul*2, *tet*(O), *erm*F, or *erm*B in soil subjected to long-term (6–12 years) irrigation with secondary effluent compared to freshwater irrigation (Negreanu et al., 2012). Given the difference in controls, irrigation frequency, soil type, climate, and wastewater chemistry, direct comparison between the studies is difficult. It is suspected that the difference in soil moisture and incubation time may likely be an important difference. Negreanu et al. (2012) irrigated with 4 L of water/m^2 soil/day which experienced a combination of infiltration, run off, and evaporation. In this study, soil-water slurries were used with irrigation waters that incubated with soil rather than infiltrating, allowing for greater contact time. Therefore, the microcosm results presented here may indicate that irrigating at high rates with secondary effluent may still result in amplified soil ARGs. The present study is consistent with the observation of increased ARG copies directly under irrigation drippers compared to soils 50 m from drippers (Negreanu et al., 2012). Further, soil type has been noted to be a critical factor in determining the level of impact of land application of biosolids containing ARGs (Munir and Xagoraraki, 2011), and may also affect the fate of ARGs applied by irrigation.

Understanding land use scenarios that affect soil ARGs is of utmost importance given that the resistome of multi-drug resistant soil bacteria was recently shown to match that from diverse human pathogens (Forsberg et al., 2012). Heavy irrigation with secondary effluent is shown here to be capable of increasing soil ARGs. In practice, given that ARG prevalence can increase between POE and POU within distribution systems, increased ARG levels in irrigation waters and therefore soils are expected. Given that spray irrigation of recreational fields with treated wastewater is common practice, there is considerable potential for human contact with aerosols and soil.

CONCLUSION

This study brings to light the occurrence of ARGs at the POU in recycled water irrigation systems, including *van*A, which is of significant concern to human health. Differences between POE and POU ARG occurrences underscore the need to take into consideration re-growth that occurs in the distribution system when estimating overall exposure and risk. Based on the lab microcosm study, amplified levels of ARGs in soil irrigated with recycled water is possible. Molecular data in this study also indicates the potential presence of waterborne bacterial pathogens, such as *L. pneumophila*. As ARGs are emerging contaminants, risk assessment is in its infancy and no guidance yet exists on safe levels (Pruden, 2011). In addition to direct contact with water and aerosols during recreational activity, a greater concern may be overall contribution to the global pool of antibiotic resistance and ultimately reducing the effectiveness of available antibiotics for treating human disease.

ACKNOWLEDGMENTS

This work was funded by the Virginia Tech Institute for Critical Technology and Applied Science Award TSTS 11-26 and NSF Research Experience for Undergraduates site award #1062860. Any opinions, findings, and conclusions or recommendations expressed in this paper are those of the author(s) and do not necessarily reflect the views of the sponsors. Gratitude is also extended to Chad McKinney and Mark Mazzochette for laboratory assistance and Andrew Hoegh for assistance with statistics.

REFERENCES

Aminov, R., Garrigues-Jeanjean, N., and Mackie, R. (2001). Molecular ecology of tetracycline resistance: development and validation of primers for detection of tetracycline resistance genes encoding ribosomal protection proteins. *Appl. Environ. Microbiol.* 67, 22–32.

Aminov, R. I., Chee-Sanford, J. C., Garrigues, N., Teferedegne, B., Krapac, I. J., White, B. A., et al. (2002). Development, validation, and application of PCR primers for detection of tetracycline efflux genes of Gram-negative bacteria. *Appl. Environ. Microbiol.* 68, 1786–1793.

Anuj, S. N., Whiley, D. M., Kidd, T. J., Bell, S. C., Wainwright, C. E., Nissen, M. D., et al. (2009). Identification of *Pseudomonas aeruginosa* by a duplex real-time polymerase chain reaction assay targeting the *ecfX* and the *gyrB* genes. *Diagn. Microbiol. Infect. Dis.* 63, 127–131.

Auerbach, E. A., Seyfried, E. E., and McMahon, K. D. (2007). Tetracycline resistance genes in activated sludge wastewater treatment plants. *Water Res.* 41, 1143–1151.

Böckelmann, U., Dörries, H.-H., Ayuso-Gabella, M. N., Salgot de Marçay, M., Tandoi, V., Levantesi, C., et al. (2009). Quantitative PCR monitoring of antibiotic resistance genes and bacterial pathogens in three European artificial groundwater recharge systems. *Appl. Environ. Microbiol.* 75, 154–163.

Brunkard, J. M., Ailes, E., Roberts, V. A., Hill, V., Hilborn, E. D., Craun, G. F., et al. (2011). Surveillance for waterborne disease outbreaks associated with drinking water – United States. *MMWR Surveill. Summ.* 60, 38–75.

Carlet, J., Jarlier, V., Harbarth, S., Voss, A., Goossens, H., and Pittet, D. (2012). Ready for a world without antibiotics? The pensières antibiotic resistance call to action. *Antimicrob. Resist. Infect. Control* 1, 11.

Chen, J., Yu, Z., Michel, F. C., Wittum, T., and Morrison, M. (2007). Development and application of real-time PCR assays for quantification of *erm* genes conferring resistance to macrolides–lincosamides–streptogramin B in livestock manure and manure management systems. *Appl. Environ. Microbiol.* 73, 4407–4416.

Chen, Y.-C., Higgins, M. J., Maas, N. A., and Murthy, S. N. (2006). DNA extraction and *Escherichia coli* quantification of anaerobically digested biosolids using the competitive touchdown PCR method. *Water Res.* 40, 3037–3044.

Clark, N. C., Cooksey, R. C., Hill, B. C., Swenson, J. M., and Tenover, F. C. (1993). Characterization of glycopeptide-resistant enterococci from U.S. hospitals. *Antimicrob. Agents Chemother.* 37, 2311–2317.

Czekalski, N., Berthold, T., Caucci, S., Egli, A., and Buergmann, H. (2012). Increased levels of multiresistant bacteria and resistance genes after wastewater treatment and their dissemination into Lake Geneva, Switzerland. *Front. Microbiol.* 3:106. doi: 10.3389/fmicb.2012.00106

Dodd, M. C. (2012). Potential impacts of disinfection processes on elimination and deactivation of antibiotic resistance genes during water and wastewater treatment. *J. Environ. Monit.* 14, 1754–1771.

Dutka-Malen, S., Evers, S., and Courvalin, P. (1995). Detection of glycopeptide resistance genotypes and identification to the species level of clinically relevant enterococci by PCR. *J. Clin. Microbiol.* 33, 24–27.

Forsberg, K. J., Reyes, A., Wang, B., Selleck, E. M., Sommer, M. O. A., and Dantas, G. (2012). The shared antibiotic resistome of soil bacteria and human pathogens. *Science* 337, 1107–1111.

Grant, M. A., Weagant, S. D., and Feng, P. (2001). Glutamate decarboxylase genes as a prescreening marker for detection of pathogenic *Escherichia coli* groups. *Appl. Environ. Microbiol.* 67, 3110–3114.

Grant, S. B., Saphores, J.-D., Feldman, D. L., Hamilton, A. J., Fletcher, T. D., Cook, P. L. M., et al. (2012). Taking the "waste" out of "wastewater" for human water security and ecosystem sustainability. *Science* 337, 681–686.

Kim, S., Park, H., and Chandran, K. (2010). Propensity of activated sludge to amplify or attenuate tetracycline resistance genes and tetracycline resistant bacteria: a mathematical modeling approach. *Chemosphere* 78, 1071–1077.

LaPara, T. M., Burch, T. R., McNamara, P. J., Tan, D. T., Yan, M., and Eichmiller, J. J. (2011). Tertiary-treated municipal wastewater is a significant point source of antibiotic resistance genes into Duluth–Superior harbor. *Environ. Sci. Technol.* 45, 9543–9549.

Ma, Y., Wilson, C. A., Novak, J. T., Riffat, R., Aynur, S., Murthy S., et al. (2011). Effect of various sludge digestion conditions on sulfonamide, macrolide, and tetracycline resistance genes and class I Integrons. *Environ. Sci. Technol.* 45, 7855–7861.

McKinney, C. W., and Pruden, A. (2012). Ultraviolet disinfection of antibiotic resistant bacteria and their antibiotic resistance genes in water and wastewater. *Environ. Sci. Technol.* 46, 13393–13400.

McLain, J. T., and Williams, C. (2012). Assessing environmental impacts of treated wastewater through monitoring of fecal indicator bacteria and salinity in irrigated soils. *Environ. Monit. Assess.* 184, 1559–1572.

Munir, M., and Xagoraraki, I. (2011). Levels of antibiotic resistance genes in manure, biosolids, and fertilized soil. *J. Environ. Qual.* 40, 248–255.

Nazarian, E. J., Bopp, D. J., Saylors, A., Limberger, R. J., and Musser, K. A. (2008). Design and implementation of a protocol for the detection of *Legionella* in clinical and environmental samples. *Diagn. Microbiol. Infect. Dis.* 62, 125–132.

Negreanu, Y., Pasternak, Z., Jurkevitch, E., and Cytryn, E. (2012). Impact of treated wastewater irrigation on antibiotic resistance in agricultural soils. *Environ. Sci. Technol.* 46, 4800–4808.

Pruden, A. (2011). "Unique challenges in the health risk assessment of antibiotic resistance genes in the environment," in *Society for Environmental Toxicology and Chemistry (SETAC) 32nd Annual Meeting*, November 13–16, Boston, MA.

Pruden, A., Arabi, M., and Storteboom, H. N. (2012). Correlation between upstream human activities and riverine antibiotic resistance genes. *Environ. Sci. Technol.* 46, 11541–11549.

Pruden, A., Edwards, M., and Falkinham, J. O. III. (2013). "State of the Science of opportunistic pathogens in premise plumbing: methodology, microbial ecology, and epidemiology," in *Water Research Foundation Project 4379 Final Report*. Denver, CO: Water Research Foundation.

Pruden, A., Pei, R., Storteboom, H., and Carlson, K. H. (2006). Antibiotic resistance genes as emerging contaminants: studies in Northern Colorado. *Environ. Sci. Technol.* 40, 7445–7450.

Rubiano, M.-E., Agulló-Barceló, M., Casas-Mangas, R., Jofre, J., and Lucena, F. (2012). Assessing the effects of tertiary treated wastewater reuse on a Mediterranean river (Llobregat, NE Spain), part III: pathogens and indicators. *Environ. Sci. Pollut. Res.* 19, 1026–1032.

Ryu, H., Alum, A., and Abbaszadegan, M. (2005). Microbial characterization and population changes in nonpotable reclaimed water distribution systems. *Environ. Sci. Technol.* 39, 8600–8605.

Schwartz, T., Kohnen, W., Jansen, B., and Obst, U. (2003). Detection of antibiotic-resistant bacteria and their resistance genes in wastewater, surface water, and drinking water biofilms. *FEMS Microbiol. Ecol.* 43, 325–335.

Stevens, D. L. (2006). The role of vancomycin in the treatment paradigm. *Clin. Infect. Dis.* 42, S51–S57.

Storteboom, H., Arabi, M., Davis, J. G., Crimi, B., and Pruden, A. (2010). Tracking antibiotic resistance genes in the South Platte River basin using molecular signatures of urban, agricultural, and pristine sources. *Environ. Sci. Technol.* 44, 7397–7404.

Suzuki, M. T., Taylor, L. T., and DeLong, E. F. (2000). Quantitative analysis of small-subunit rRNA genes in mixed microbial populations via 5′-nuclease assays. *Appl. Environ. Microbiol.* 66, 4605–4614.

Trautmann, M., Lepper, P. M., and Haller, M. (2005). Ecology of *Pseudomonas aeruginosa* in the intensive care unit and the evolving role of water outlets as a reservoir of the organism. *Am. J. Infect. Control* 33, S41–S49.

US Environmental Protection Agency (USEPA). (2012). *Guidelines for Water Reuse*. Washington, DC: USEPA.

Wang, H., Edwards, M., Falkinham, J. O., and Pruden, A. (2012). Molecular survey of the occurrence of *Legionella* spp., *Mycobacterium* spp., *Pseudomonas aeruginosa*, and *Amoeba* hosts in two chloraminated drinking water distribution systems. *Appl. Environ. Microbiol.* 78, 6285–6294.

Webber, M. A., and Piddock, L. J. V. (2003). The importance of efflux pumps in bacterial antibiotic resistance. *J. Antimicrob. Chemother.* 51, 9–11.

Xi, C., Zhang, Y., Marrs, C. F., Ye, W., Simon, C., Foxman, B., et al. (2009). Prevalence of antibiotic resistance in drinking water treatment and distribution systems. *Appl. Environ. Microbiol.* 75, 5714–5718.

14

Resistance in tuberculosis: what do we know and where can we go?

Keith D. Green and Sylvie Garneau-Tsodikova*

Department of Pharmaceutical Sciences, University of Kentucky, Lexington, KY, USA

Edited by:
Jun Lin, The University of Tennessee, USA

Reviewed by:
Nicholas Allenby, Demuris Ltd, UK
Michael J. Hall, Newcastle University, UK

***Correspondence:**
Sylvie Garneau-Tsodikova, Department of Pharmaceutical Sciences, University of Kentucky, BioPharm Complex, Room 423, 789 South Limestone Street, Lexington, KY 40536-0596, USA
e-mail: sylviegtsodikova@uky.edu

Tuberculosis (TB) has become a worldwide threat, mainly due to the emergence of multidrug-resistant (MDR) and extensively drug-resistant (XDR) strains of *Mycobacterium tuberculosis* (*Mtb*). This mini-review is focused on the various mechanisms of resistance to the currently available anti-TB drugs and provides perspective on novel strategies and lead scaffolds/compounds aimed at inhibiting/overcoming these resistance mechanisms.

Keywords: antibiotics, inhibitors, mechanisms of resistance, new drug targets, synergistic drug therapy

INTRODUCTION

Approximately 1.4 million deaths were attributed to *Mtb* infections in 2012. When compared to other infectious agents, only HIV claims more lives (WHO, 2012). While recent efforts have resulted in a global decline in TB incidence and mortality (WHO, 2011), the number of individuals infected with drug-resistant isolates continues to increase, presenting a serious global health threat. Generally, drug-susceptible *Mtb* infections are treated with a combination of four compounds; rifampicin (RIF), ethambutol (EMB), pyrazinamide (PZA), and isoniazid (INH) for 2 months, followed by treatment with RIF and INH for 4 additional months (Lienhardt et al., 2012) (**Figure 1A**). By definition, MDR-TB is resistant to the most potent first-line drugs, RIF and INH. The WHO reports that ~60,000 cases of MDR-TB were diagnosed in 2011, likely an underestimate. To treat MDR-TB, second-line drugs including fluoroquinolones (FQs), amikacin (AMK), kanamycin (KAN), and capreomycin (CAP) are employed. These drugs are administered for ~20 months and can be toxic, poorly tolerated, and difficult to procure. Approximately 95% of MDR-TB is XDR-TB, having additional resistance to at least one FQ and one injectable drug (AMK, KAN, or CAP), and for which treatment options are limited. Therefore, new therapeutics are critically needed to overcome drug resistance and to eliminate TB as a public health threat.

Herein we briefly discuss the drugs currently used to treat TB and the respective mechanisms of resistance followed by a review of approaches aimed toward overcoming TB drug resistance.

CURRENT DRUGS AND RESISTANCE

Mtb is intrinsically resistant to many antibiotics due to the low permeability of its mycolic acid-rich waxy cell envelope, the action of efflux pumps (Banerjee et al., 1996; Silva et al., 2001; Singh et al., 2011), and the presence of chromosomally encoded resistance genes. Drug resistance in *Mtb* has been emerging due to the accumulation of chromosomal mutations and not acquisition of mobile genetic elements. The major mechanisms of acquired drug resistance in *Mtb* can be broken down into several categories: (1) mutations or modifications (e.g., RNA methylation) of the drug targets (RIF, EMB, KAN, AMK, CAP, and the FQs), (2) the inability to activate a prodrug [INH, PZA, ethionamide (ETH)] due to mutations leading to a loss of function, and (3) enzymatic inactivation of the drug (KAN).

MUTATIONS OR MODIFICATIONS OF THE DRUG TARGETS

Mutations

Antibiotics target cellular processes that are vital in bacteria by binding their targets at a specific site, often directly interacting with key functional residues of the target. The most common mechanism of resistance in *Mtb* is the alteration of the target's binding site through the accumulation of mutations. These mutations decrease the binding affinity of the drug to its target and typically occur in a very defined region of the gene termed the resistance-determining region. This mechanism is used by *Mtb* to confer resistance to RIF, EMB, and FQs by altering the binding site of their respective targets: the β-subunit of RNA polymerase (Campbell et al., 2001), a glycosyltransferase (Telenti et al., 1997), and DNA gyrase (Takiff et al., 1994). Similarly, ribosomal mutations (e.g., A1401G) in the 16S rRNA have been found to confer resistance to AMK, KAN, and CAP (Wachino et al., 2010).

Modifications

An alternative mode of resistance in *Mtb* is the inactivation of rRNA methyltransferase enzymes. Mutations in TlyA hindering the methylation activity of rRNA 2′-*O*-methyltransferase at nucleotides C1409 of 16S rRNA and C1920 of 23S rRNA have been linked to resistance to the ribosome-targeting drugs CAP and viomycin (VIO) (Johansen et al., 2006). Mutations in a putative 16S rRNA methyltransferase, GidB, were found to confer low-level resistance to the aminoglycoside (AG) streptomycin (STR) (Spies et al., 2011; Wong et al., 2011).

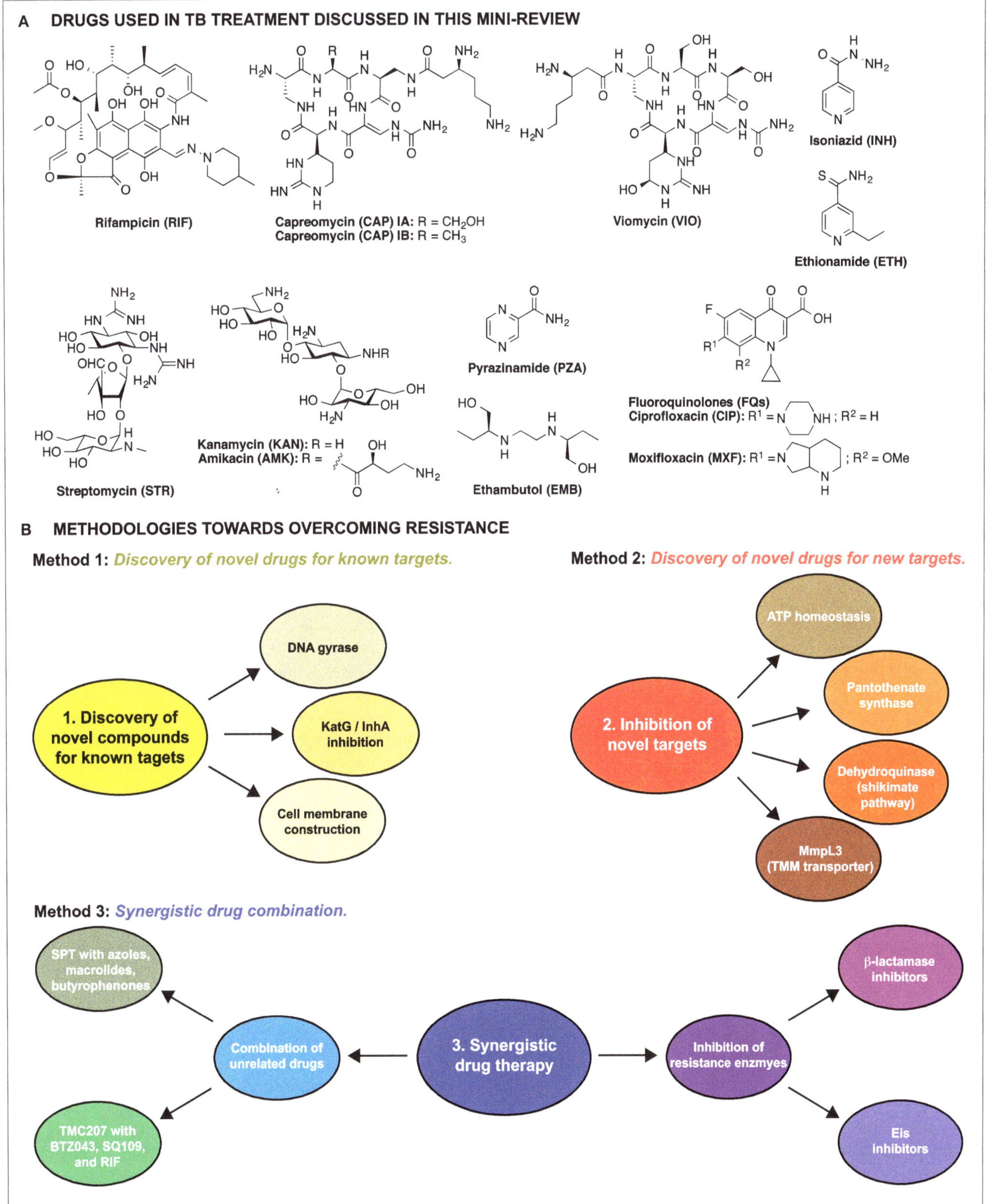

FIGURE 1 | (A) Structures of the anti-TB drugs discussed in this mini-review. **(B)** Schematic representation of the three methodologies explored to overcome resistance in *Mtb*.

INABILITY TO ACTIVATE A PRODRUG

Three first-line drugs, INH, PZA, and ETH, are prodrugs that must be metabolized to be active against *Mtb*. INH is activated by the catalase-peroxidase, KatG, and produces isonicotinic-acyl radicals that react with NADH to form an INH-NADH adduct. The adduct binds its main target, enoyl-acyl carrier protein reductase (InhA), and inhibits mycolic acid biosynthesis. ETH is a structural analog of INH and is activated by the monooxygenase EthA, which oxidizes ETH to its active form, 2-ethyl-4-amidopyridine. This activated compound also targets InhA and blocks mycolic acid biosynthesis similarly to INH. PZA is activated by pyrazinamidase/nicotinamidase, PncA, to pyrazinoic acid (POA). The proposed targets of POA range from cell membrane energy to fatty acid synthesis, but the exact killing mechanism of POA remains unclear. Resistance to any of the prodrugs can arise due to reduced metabolism by their corresponding activator. Structural mutations that lower or abolish the enzymatic activity of KatG (Ramaswamy et al., 2003; Hazbon et al., 2006), EthA (Baulard et al., 2000; Debarber et al., 2000; Morlock et al., 2003), and PncA (Stoffels et al., 2012; Rajendran and Sethumadhavan, 2013) were found to lead to INH, ETH, and PZA resistance, respectively. Mutations in InhA causing overexpression of the target (Baulard et al., 2000; Debarber et al., 2000; Larsen et al., 2002) or preventing binding of the active form of INH and ETH to the target (Banerjee et al., 1994; Vilcheze et al., 2008) also confer cross-resistance to these drugs.

INACTIVATION OF THE DRUG

Drug modification is perhaps the most prevalent and well-studied resistance mechanism employed by bacteria. Many bacteria either degrade or modify the offending compound thereby generating an inactive molecule. Resistance to penicillin is mediated by a class of enzymes known as the β-lactamases, which inactivate the antibiotic by destroying the β-lactam ring. *Mtb* naturally harbors a chromosomally encoded class A β-lactamase, BlaC, which is constitutively expressed providing intrinsic resistance to penicillin (Hugonnet and Blanchard, 2007). One mechanism of acquired resistance to AGs, such as KAN and AMK, is their modification and inactivation by a family of enzymes known as AG-modifying enzymes (AMEs) (Ramirez and Tolmasky, 2010; Labby and Garneau-Tsodikova, 2013). *Mtb* expresses two AMEs, the AG 2′-*N*-acetyltransferace AAC(2′)-Ic (Hegde et al., 2001) and the enhanced intracellular survival (Eis) protein (Zaunbrecher et al., 2009). Both enzymes acetylate AGs, reducing the ability of these drugs to inhibit the ribosome. In the case of Eis, increased expression due to mutations in the *eis* promoter or the 5′-untranslated region of the transcriptional activator WhiB7 leads to clinically relevant, low-level resistance to KAN (Zaunbrecher et al., 2009; Reeves et al., 2013). A unique feature of Eis resides in its ability to modify AGs at multiple sites *in vitro*, completely inactivating these compounds (Chen et al., 2011). A recent report has shown that Eis also acetylates CAP at its β-lysine side chain *in vitro*, but the clinical relevance of this finding remains unclear (Houghton et al., 2013).

METHODOLOGIES TO OVERCOME RESISTANCE

Three major strategies have been explored to overcome resistance in TB: (1) identification of novel drugs for well-established targets, (2) identification and characterization of novel compounds that target unexplored vital cell processes or enzymes, thus killing the cell by preventing regular metabolism, and (3) identification of compounds that behave synergistically with current anti-TB drugs (**Figure 1B**).

DISCOVERY OF NOVEL DRUGS FOR KNOWN TARGETS

DNA gyrase

Among the known *Mtb* drug targets, DNA gyrase remains attractive for development of inhibitors interacting with either GyrA or GyrB subunits. To overcome the FQ resistance of DNA gyrase mutants, a series of 30 ofloxacin derivatives with various substituents *ortho* to the fluoro moiety of the FQ scaffold were synthesized (Dinakaran et al., 2008). These compounds displayed MIC_{99} values $<10\,\mu M$ and retained anti-mycobacterial activity against MDR-*Mtb* strains. While ofloxacin displayed a 17-fold lower activity against MDR-*Mtb* relative to susceptible *Mtb* strains, its derivatives displayed at most a 4-fold lower activity and, in some cases, higher activity against MDR-*Mtb*. The toxicity of selected compounds in mammalian Vero cells displayed a range of IC_{50} values (60 to $>150\,\mu M$), 6-fold higher than the highest MIC_{99} value. When tested in culture, the compound with the best MIC_{99} value showed reduction in *Mtb* colonies similar to that observed with ofloxacin.

While many efforts have been directed toward the development of FQ analogs to target the GyrA subunit of DNA gyrase, development of inhibitors targeting GyrB has also been pursued. A series of aminopyrazinamides were found to target the ATPase site of GyrB and inhibit the growth of *Mtb* in the low micromolar/high nanomolar range (Shirude et al., 2013). A variety of naphthoquinones were also discovered to inhibit the ATPase domain of the GyrB subunit of *Mtb* DNA gyrase with IC_{50} values between 15 and $>200\,\mu M$ (Karkare et al., 2013). The most promising naphthoquinone, diospyrin, was tested against DNA gyrase from other bacterial species and found to be a broad spectrum DNA gyrase inhibitor. The aminobenzimidazole AB-1 was also investigated for its inhibitory properties of GyrB and compared to the well-characterized GyrB inhibitor novobiocin (Chopra et al., 2012). AB-1 displayed lower MIC values than novobiocin with *Mtb* strains resistant to STR, INH, CIP, and *p*-aminosalicylic acid. AB-1 also displayed improved activity in aerobic and anaerobic conditions while not interfering with RIF or INH mechanisms.

KatG/InhA inhibition

To overcome mutations of KatG and other mechanisms of INH resistance, analogs of INH have been synthesized. Early generations of INH analogs incorporated aryloxyacetonitriles onto the hydrazide of the INH scaffold (Bukowski et al., 1999). These compounds were then evolved into 1,2,3-triazole derivatives with MIC values slightly higher than those of INH (Boechat et al., 2011).

As an alternative strategy to overcoming KatG mutations or deletion, InhA inhibitors, not needing KatG activation, have been investigated. Triclosan (Parikh et al., 2000) served as a lead compound for the design of a series of 5-alkyl-diphenyl ethers (Sullivan et al., 2006). These ethers displayed IC_{50} values for InhA ranging from 5 nM to $2\,\mu M$, displayed higher bactericidal activity than the parent triclosan, and were further optimized to slow the release time from the InhA active site (Luckner et al., 2010). More recently, from screening 300 molecules, CD117 was identified as an InhA inhibitor that likely targets other enzymes (Vilcheze et al., 2011). CD117 was active against hypoxic *Mtb* and yielded 80% Vero cell viability at the highest concentration tested. This year, virtual screening efforts led to the identification of 7 potential InhA inhibitors (Kinjo et al., 2013). In model *Mycobacterium* species the top hit compounds displayed similar growth inhibition to that of INH and directly inhibited *Mtb* InhA.

Cell membrane construction

The inhibition of cell membrane construction also remains a target of choice for the development of new drugs. Nitroimidazoles such as PA-824 and OPC-67683 have been found to inhibit the synthesis of membrane proteins and lipids (Mukherjee and Boshoff, 2011). Much like INH and PZA, PA-824 is a prodrug that requires activation by reduction of its nitro group (Stover et al., 2000). PA-824 and OPC-67683 have demonstrated activity against both susceptible and resistant-*Mtb* strains (Stover et al., 2000; Rivers and Mancera, 2008a,b). PA-824 showed activity in the high ng/mL range for both susceptible and resistant-*Mtb* (Ginsberg et al., 2009) and OPC-67683 displayed better MIC values in the low ng/mL range (Matsumoto et al., 2006).

Benzothiazinones (BTZs) (Makarov et al., 2006), such as BTZ043, have also been shown to interfere with cell membrane construction. Like EMB, these compounds disrupt arabinan's biosynthesis by targeting decaprenylphosphoryl-β-D-ribose 2′-epimerase (DprE) (Makarov et al., 2009). In infected macrophages, BTZ043 showed a faster decrease in percentage of infected cells and bacterial load compared to INH or RIF. BTZ043 has also been tested in 240 clinical isolates of *Mtb* from European hospitals and was active against all strains (Pasca et al., 2010).

DISCOVERY OF NOVEL DRUGS FOR NEW TARGETS

ATP homeostasis

One of the challenges in treating TB is the organism's extended period(s) of dormancy. One key difference in the states of growing and hypoxic non-growing *Mtb* is a reduced, but significant, ATP pool in the non-growing organism (Rao et al., 2008). A plausible way to attack the non-growing bacilli is to affect their ATP storage by inactivating ATP synthase to deplete the ATP and eventually kill the bacilli (Andries et al., 2005). This strategy led to the identification of the ATP synthase inhibitor TMC207 (bedaquiline or sirturo), which was approved by the FDA in December 2012 for TB treatment (Diacon et al., 2009; Avorn, 2013). TMC207 is the first FDA-approved anti-TB drug in 40 years (Mahajan, 2013). TMC207 targets the C-subunit of ATP synthase proton pump and mutations are known that are resistant to this novel compound (Segala et al., 2012). There are also some mycobacterial strains that are naturally resistant to TMC207. Because of the potential risks associated with this drug, it is recommended that it be utilized only in patients for which other treatment options have failed. A high-throughput screen (HTS) to identify additional compounds that block ATP synthesis and kill dormant *Mtb* resulted in 0.5% hit rate from a library of 600,000 compounds (Mak et al., 2012).

Pantothenate synthetase

Pantothenate synthetase has also been explored as an antibiotic target of *Mtb*. Actinomycin D was identified *via* HTS as an inhibitor of this *de novo* synthesis enzyme (Yang et al., 2011). Futher *in silico* HTS led to the discovery of two compounds that inhibit the panthothenate synthesis 10× more efficiently than actinomycin D does. These compounds displayed identical MIC values against susceptible and MDR-*Mtb* strains. Analogs of the pantothenate synthetase reaction intermediate were shown to bind the enzyme more tightly than the nucleotide substrate (Ciulli et al., 2008). Another essential enzyme, pantothenate kinase (CoaA) has also been considered as a target. Three classes of compounds were found to target CoaA: triazoles, quinoline carboxamides, and biaryl acetic acids (Venkatraman et al., 2012). All compounds inhibited CoaA with IC_{50} values ranging from 70 nM to 8.4 μM with various modes of inhibition.

Dehydroquinase of the shikimate pathway

The essential shikimate pathway, responsible for the biosynthesis of aromatic amino acids, folate, and vitamins E/K, is also an antibacterial target (Gonzalez-Bello and Castedo, 2007; Payne et al., 2007a,b; Tran et al., 2011). Recently, inhibitors of the dehydroquinase enzyme of the shikimate pathway have been optimized against *Mtb* and a series of 3,4-dihydroxyacetophenone and acetonide cores with MIC values in the low-micromolar range were identified (Tran et al., 2012). Similarly, a series of anhydroquinones were synthesized and found to be low-micromolar to high-nanomolar *Mtb* dehydroquinase inhibitors (Payne et al., 2007a; Prazeres et al., 2007). Other studies have focused on generating dehydroquinic acid derivatives (Lence et al., 2013) or 3-alkyl enol mimics (Blanco et al., 2012) to inhibit dehydroquinase and disrupt the shikimate pathway. Dehydroquinic acid analogs showed IC_{50} values in the mid-nanomolar range (26–100 nM), while the 3-alkyl enol mimics had a broader nanomolar range (28–780 nM).

MmpL3 (TMM transporter)

SQ109 is an EMB analog with an adamantyl moiety that targets cell well-biosynthesis. SQ109 was discovered in a screen of ~63,000 compounds and showed high ng/mL MIC values (Sacksteder et al., 2012). Recent studies revealed that SQ109 acts on MmpL3, the trehalose monomycolate (TMM) transporter of *Mtb* (Tahlan et al., 2012). Adamantyl ureas, discovered by high-throughput screening, also displayed anti-tubercular activity (Brown et al., 2011) by targeting MmpL3 (Grzegorzewicz et al., 2012). Since their discovery, the structure of organic ureas has undergone several optimizations for solubility (Scherman et al., 2012) and pharmacokinetic properties (North et al., 2013). Additional scaffolds based on the structure of the pyrrole derivative BM212 have also recently emerged as MmpL3 inhibitors (Poce et al., 2013).

SYNERGISTIC DRUG COMBINATION

Combination of unrelated drugs

In an effort to reduce emerging resistance, combinations of small molecules have been explored. In a search for compounds that would work synergistically with spectinomycin (SPT), a high-throughput synergy screen (HTSS) was performed with a library of molecules with known pharmacological properties. Three structural cores were found to enhance the antibiotic activity of SPT: the macrolides, azoles, and butyrophenones (Ramon-Garcia et al., 2011). Bromperidol displayed bactericidal activity, was effective against *Mtb* in a macrophage model, and displayed similar enhancement of the activities of RIF, STR, clofazimine, and clarithromycin. In addition to its anti-TB activity, TMC207 has also been shown to speed up treatment with the first-line anti-TB drugs (Diacon et al., 2009). Lechartier et al. combined BTZ043 with known and experimental TB treatments (Lechartier et al., 2012). In most cases additive interactions of BTZ043 with the second TB treatment were observed. However, BTZ043 was shown to act synergistically with TMC207. Both drugs used at one-quarter of the MIC concentration showed more significant growth retardation than TMC207 at its MIC value alone. The authors suggest that BTZ043 inhibits DprE1 leading to weaker cell walls allowing transmission of TMC207 across the cell membrane. In a recent study, SQ109 acted synergistically with RIF and TMC207 (Reddy et al., 2010).

Inhibition of resistance enzymes

The use of inhibitors of drug-modifying enzymes along with currently approved anti-TB drugs complements the drug combination strategy described above. Perhaps the best-known combination of this type is a β-lactam and a β-lactamase inhibitor. A combination of clavulanate and meropenem proved to be active against both susceptible and XDR-*Mtb* strains (Hugonnet et al., 2009) A novel β-lactamase inhibitor, NXL104, was recently reported and found to bind BlaC in a 1:1 molar ratio (Xu et al., 2012). Recently, inhibitors of the AG-resistance enzyme Eis were discovered (Green et al., 2012). These compounds encompass a wide variety of chemical structures and offer a plethora of scaffolds to be studied for development of novel anti-TB drug adjuvants. While these compounds have not yet been tested in AG-resistant *Mtb* strains, combinations of inhibitors with AGs are predicted to restore the antibacterial activity of AGs in cells.

CONCLUSION

Even though current TB treatments are still broadly employed, the rapid spread of MDR-TB and XDR-TB is a rising threat. Based on our current understanding of the resistance mechanisms, contemporary strategies are focused on generating compounds that will avoid or overcome the defenses of *Mtb*. Research is being carried out to find novel compounds that will disrupt DNA, cell membrane biosynthesis, and general cellular metabolism. Other lines of inquiry are focusing on pathways currently not used to treat TB: cellular energetics, cellular transport, and other aspects of cellular metabolism. A third facet relies on current TB treatment and combines drugs to achieve synergistic effects, either blocking two separate pathways or inhibiting a drug-modifying enzyme. While many of the compounds discussed herein are far from being approved as drugs, the recent approval of TMC207 and the multitude of efforts in searching for novel antibiotics give hope for the discovery of novel TB treatments.

ACKNOWLEDGMENTS

Work on TB in our group is supported by NIH Grant AI090048 (Sylvie Garneau-Tsodikova). We thank James Posey and Melisa Willby (Centers for Disease Control and Prevention) and Oleg Tsodikov (University of Kentucky) for critical proof-reading of this mini-review.

REFERENCES

Andries, K., Verhasselt, P., Guillemont, J., Gohlmann, H. W., Neefs, J. M., Winkler, H., et al. (2005). A diarylquinoline drug active on the ATP synthase of *Mycobacterium tuberculosis*. *Science* 307, 223–227. doi: 10.1126/science.1106753

Avorn, J. (2013). Approval of a tuberculosis drug based on a paradoxical surrogate measure. *JAMA* 309, 1349–1350. doi: 10.1001/jama.2013.623

Banerjee, A., Dubnau, E., Quemard, A., Balasubramanian, V., Um, K. S., Wilson, T., et al. (1994). InhA, a gene encoding a target for isoniazid and ethionamide in *Mycobacterium tuberculosis*. *Science* 263, 227–230. doi: 10.1126/science.8284673

Banerjee, S. K., Bhatt, K., Rana, S., Misra, P., and Chakraborti, P. K. (1996). Involvement of an efflux system in mediating high level of fluoroquinolone resistance in *Mycobacterium smegmatis*. *Biochem. Biophys. Res. Commun.* 226, 362–368. doi: 10.1006/bbrc.1996.1362

Baulard, A. R., Betts, J. C., Engohang-Ndong, J., Quan, S., McAdam, R. A., Brennan, P. J., et al. (2000). Activation of the prodrug ethionamide is regulated in mycobacteria. *J. Biol. Chem.* 275, 28326–28331.

Blanco, B., Sedes, A., Peon, A., Lamb, H., Hawkins, A. R., Castedo, L., et al. (2012). Synthesis of 3-alkyl enol mimics inhibitors of type II dehydroquinase: factors influencing their inhibition potency. *Org. Biomol. Chem.* 10, 3662–3676. doi: 10.1039/c2ob07081b

Boechat, N., Ferreira, V. F., Ferreira, S. B., De Lourdes, G. F. M., De, C. D. S. F., Bastos, M. M., et al. (2011). Novel 1,2,3-triazole derivatives for use against *Mycobacterium tuberculosis* H37Rv (ATCC 27294) strain. *J. Med. Chem.* 54, 5988–5999. doi: 10.1021/jm2003624

Brown, J. R., North, E. J., Hurdle, J. G., Morisseau, C., Scarborough, J. S., Sun, D., et al. (2011). The structure-activity relationship of urea derivatives as anti-tuberculosis agents. *Bioorg. Med. Chem.* 19, 5585–5595. doi: 10.1016/j.bmc.2011.07.034

Bukowski, L., Janowiec, M., Zwolska-Kwiek, Z., and Andrzejczyk, Z. (1999). Synthesis and some reactions of 2-acetylimidazo[4,5-b]pyridine. Antituberculotic activity of the obtained compounds. *Pharmazie* 54, 651–654.

Campbell, E. A., Korzheva, N., Mustaev, A., Murakami, K., Nair, S., Goldfarb, A., et al. (2001). Structural mechanism for rifampicin inhibition of bacterial RNA polymerase. *Cell* 104, 901–912. doi: 10.1016/S0092-8674(01)00286-0

Chen, W., Biswas, T., Porter, V. R., Tsodikov, O. V., and Garneau-Tsodikova, S. (2011). Unusual regioversatility of acetyltransferase Eis, a cause of drug resistance in XDR-TB. *Proc. Natl. Acad. Sci. U.S.A.* 108, 9804–9808. doi: 10.1073/pnas.1105379108

Chopra, S., Matsuyama, K., Tran, T., Malerich, J. P., Wan, B., Franzblau, S. G., et al. (2012). Evaluation of gyrase B as a drug target in *Mycobacterium tuberculosis*. *J. Antimicrob. Chemother.* 67, 415–421. doi: 10.1093/jac/dkr449

Ciulli, A., Scott, D. E., Ando, M., Reyes, F., Saldanha, S. A., Tuck, K. L., et al. (2008). Inhibition of *Mycobacterium tuberculosis* pantothenate synthetase by analogues of the reaction intermediate. *Chembiochem* 9, 2606–2611. doi: 10.1002/cbic.200800437

Debarber, A. E., Mdluli, K., Bosman, M., Bekker, L. G., and Barry, C. E. 3rd. (2000). Ethionamide activation and sensitivity in multidrug-resistant *Mycobacterium tuberculosis*. *Proc. Natl. Acad. Sci. U.S.A.* 97, 9677–9682. doi: 10.1073/pnas.97.17.9677

Diacon, A. H., Pym, A., Grobusch, M., Patientia, R., Rustomjee, R., Page-Shipp, L., et al. (2009). The diarylquinoline TMC207 for multidrug-resistant tuberculosis. *N. Engl. J. Med.* 360, 2397–2405. doi: 10.1056/NEJMoa0808427

Dinakaran, M., Senthilkumar, P., Yogeeswari, P., China, A., Nagaraja, V., and Sriram, D. (2008). Novel ofloxacin derivatives: synthesis, antimycobacterial and toxicological evaluation. *Bioorg. Med. Chem. Lett.* 18, 1229–1236. doi: 10.1016/j.bmcl.2007.11.110

Ginsberg, A. M., Laurenzi, M. W., Rouse, D. J., Whitney, K. D., and Spigelman, M. K. (2009). Safety, tolerability, and pharmacokinetics of PA-824 in healthy subjects. *Antimicrob. Agents Chemother.* 53, 3720–3725. doi: 10.1128/AAC.00106-09

Gonzalez-Bello, C., and Castedo, L. (2007). Progress in type II dehydroquinase inhibitors: from concept to practice. *Med. Res. Rev.* 27, 177–208. doi: 10.1002/med.20076

Green, K. D., Chen, W., and Garneau-Tsodikova, S. (2012). Identification and characterization of inhibitors of the aminoglycoside resistance acetyltransferase Eis from *Mycobacterium tuberculosis*. *ChemMedChem* 7, 73–77. doi: 10.1002/cmdc.201100332

Grzegorzewicz, A. E., Pham, H., Gundi, V. A., Scherman, M. S., North, E. J., Hess, T., et al. (2012). Inhibition of mycolic acid transport across the *Mycobacterium tuberculosis* plasma membrane. *Nat. Chem. Biol.* 8, 334–341. doi: 10.1038/nchembio.794

Hazbon, M. H., Brimacombe, M., Bobadilla Del Valle, M., Cavatore, M., Guerrero, M. I., Varma-Basil, M., et al. (2006). Population genetics study of isoniazid resistance mutations and evolution of multidrug-resistant *Mycobacterium tuberculosis*. *Antimicrob. Agents Chemother.* 50, 2640–2649. doi: 10.1128/AAC.00112-06

Hegde, S. S., Javid-Majd, F., and Blanchard, J. S. (2001). Overexpression and mechanistic analysis of chromosomally encoded aminoglycoside 2′-N-acetyltransferase (AAC(2′)-Ic) from *Mycobacterium tuberculosis*. *J. Biol. Chem.* 276, 45876–45881. doi: 10.1074/jbc.M108810200.

Houghton, J. L., Green, K. D., Pricer, R. E., Mayhoub, A. S., and Garneau-Tsodikova, S. (2013). Unexpected N-acetylation of capreomycin by mycobacterial Eis enzymes. *J. Antimicrob. Chemother.* 68, 800–805. doi: 10.1093/jac/dks497

Hugonnet, J. E., and Blanchard, J. S. (2007). Irreversible inhibition of the *Mycobacterium tuberculosis* beta-lactamase by clavulanate. *Biochemistry* 46, 11998–12004. doi: 10.1021/bi701506h

Hugonnet, J. E., Tremblay, L. W., Boshoff, H. I., Barry, C. E. 3rd, and Blanchard, J. S. (2009). Meropenem-clavulanate is effective against extensively drug-resistant *Mycobacterium tuberculosis*. *Science* 323, 1215–1218. doi: 10.1126/science.1167498

Johansen, S. K., Maus, C. E., Plikaytis, B. B., and Douthwaite, S. (2006). Capreomycin binds across the ribosomal subunit interface using tlyA-encoded 2′-O-methylations in 16S and 23S rRNAs. *Mol. Cell* 23, 173–182. doi: 10.1016/j.molcel.2006.05.044

Karkare, S., Chung, T. T., Collin, F., Mitchenall, L. A., McKay, A. R., Greive, S. J., et al. (2013). The naphthoquinone diospyrin is an inhibitor of DNA gyrase with a novel mechanism of action. *J. Biol. Chem.* 288, 5149–5156. doi: 10.1074/jbc.M112.419069

Kinjo, T., Koseki, Y., Kobayashi, M., Yamada, A., Morita, K., Yamaguchi, K., et al. (2013). Identification of compounds with potential antibacterial activity against *Mycobacterium* through structure-based drug screening. *J. Chem. Inf. Model.* 53, 1200–1212. doi: 10.1021/ci300571n

Labby, K. J., and Garneau-Tsodikova, S. (2013). Methods to identify compounds to overcome the action of aminoglycoside-modifying enzymes for treating resistant bacteria. *Future. Med. Chem.* [Epub ahead of print].

Larsen, M. H., Vilcheze, C., Kremer, L., Besra, G. S., Parsons, L., Salfinger, M., Jr. et al. (2002). Overexpression of inhA, but not kasA, confers resistance to isoniazid and ethionamide in *Mycobacterium smegmatis*, *M. bovis* BCG and *M. tuberculosis*. *Mol. Microbiol.* 46, 453–466. doi: 10.1046/j.1365-2958.2002.03162.x

Lechartier, B., Hartkoorn, R. C., and Cole, S. T. (2012). *In vitro* combination studies of benzothiazinone lead compound BTZ043 against *Mycobacterium tuberculosis*. *Antimicrob. Agents Chemother.* 56, 5790–5793. doi: 10.1128/AAC.01476-12

Lence, E., Tizon, L., Otero, J. M., Peon, A., Prazeres, V. F., Llamas-Saiz, A. L., et al. (2013). Mechanistic basis of the inhibition of type II dehydroquinase by (2S)- and (2R)-2-benzyl-3-dehydroquinic acids. *ACS Chem. Biol.* 8, 568–577. doi: 10.1021/cb300493s

Lienhardt, C., Raviglione, M., Spigelman, M., Hafner, R., Jaramillo, E., Hoelscher, M., et al. (2012). New drugs for the treatment of tuberculosis: needs, challenges, promise, and prospects for the future. *J. Infect. Dis.* 205, S241–S249. doi: 10.1093/infdis/jis034

Luckner, S. R., Liu, N., Am Ende, C. W., Tonge, P. J., and Kisker, C. (2010). A slow, tight binding inhibitor of InhA, the enoyl-acyl carrier protein reductase from *Mycobacterium tuberculosis*. *J. Biol. Chem.* 285, 14330–14337. doi: 10.1074/jbc.M109.090373

Mahajan, R. (2013). Bedaquiline: First FDA-approved tuberculosis drug in 40 years. *Int. J. Appl. Basic Med. Res.* 3, 1–2. doi: 10.4103/2229-516X.112228

Mak, P. A., Rao, S. P., Ping Tan, M., Lin, X., Chyba, J., Tay, J., et al. (2012). A high-throughput screen to identify inhibitors of ATP homeostasis in non-replicating *Mycobacterium tuberculosis*. *ACS Chem. Biol.* 7, 1190–1197. doi: 10.1021/cb2004884

Makarov, V., Manina, G., Mikusova, K., Mollmann, U., Ryabova, O., Saint-Joanis, B., et al. (2009). Benzothiazinones kill *Mycobacterium tuberculosis* by blocking arabinan synthesis. *Science* 324, 801–804. doi: 10.1126/science.1171583

Makarov, V., Riabova, O. B., Yuschenko, A., Urlyapova, N., Daudova, A., Zipfel, P. F., et al. (2006). Synthesis and antileprosy activity of some dialkyldithiocarbamates. *J. Antimicrob. Chemother.* 57, 1134–1138. doi: 10.1093/jac/dkl095

Matsumoto, M., Hashizume, H., Tomishige, T., Kawasaki, M., Tsubouchi, H., Sasaki, H., et al. (2006). OPC-67683, a nitro-dihydro-imidazooxazole derivative with promising action against tuberculosis *in vitro* and in mice. *PLoS Med.* 3:e466. doi: 10.1371/journal.pmed.0030466

Morlock, G. P., Metchock, B., Sikes, D., Crawford, J. T., and Cooksey, R. C. (2003). ethA, inhA, and katG loci of ethionamide-resistant clinical *Mycobacterium tuberculosis* isolates. *Antimicrob. Agents Chemother.* 47, 3799–3805. doi: 10.1128/AAC.47.12.3799-3805.2003

Mukherjee, T., and Boshoff, H. (2011). Nitroimidazoles for the treatment of TB: past, present and future. *Future. Med. Chem.* 3, 1427–1454. doi: 10.4155/fmc.11.90

North, E. J., Scherman, M. S., Bruhn, D. F., Scarborough, J. S., Maddox, M. M., Jones, V., et al. (2013). Design, synthesis and anti-tuberculosis activity of 1-adamantyl-3-heteroaryl ureas with improved *in vitro* pharmacokinetic properties. *Bioorg. Med. Chem.* 21, 2587–2599. doi: 10.1016/j.bmc.2013.02.028

Parikh, S. L., Xiao, G., and Tonge, P. J. (2000). Inhibition of InhA, the enoyl reductase from *Mycobacterium tuberculosis*, by triclosan and isoniazid. *Biochemistry* 39, 7645–7650. doi: 10.1021/bi0008940

Pasca, M. R., Degiacomi, G., Ribeiro, A. L., Zara, F., De Mori, P., Heym, B., et al. (2010). Clinical isolates of *Mycobacterium tuberculosis* in four European hospitals are uniformly susceptible to benzothiazinones. *Antimicrob. Agents Chemother.* 54, 1616–1618. doi: 10.1128/AAC.01676-09

Payne, R. J., Peyrot, F., Kerbarh, O., Abell, A. D., and Abell, C. (2007a). Rational design, synthesis, and evaluation of nanomolar type II dehydroquinase inhibitors. *ChemMedChem* 2, 1015–1029. doi: 10.1002/cmdc.200700032

Payne, R. J., Riboldi-Tunnicliffe, A., Kerbarh, O., Abell, A. D., Lapthorn, A. J., and Abell, C. (2007b). Design, synthesis, and structural studies on potent biaryl inhibitors of type II dehydroquinases. *ChemMedChem* 2, 1010–1013. doi: 10.1002/cmdc.200700062.

Poce, G., Bates, R. H., Alfonso, S., Cocozza, M., Porretta, G. C., Ballell, L., et al. (2013). Improved BM212 MmpL3 inhibitor analogue shows efficacy in acute murine model of tuberculosis infection. *PLoS ONE* 8:e56980. doi: 10.1371/journal.pone.0056980

Prazeres, V. F., Sanchez-Sixto, C., Castedo, L., Lamb, H., Hawkins, A. R., Riboldi-Tunnicliffe, A., et al. (2007). Nanomolar competitive inhibitors of *Mycobacterium tuberculosis* and Streptomyces coelicolor type II dehydroquinase. *ChemMedChem* 2, 194–207. doi: 10.1002/cmdc.200600208

Rajendran, V., and Sethumadhavan, R. (2013). Drug resistance mechanism of PncA in *Mycobacterium tuberculosis*. *J. Biomol. Struct. Dyn.* doi: 10.1080/07391102.2012.759885. [Epub ahead of print].

Ramaswamy, S. V., Reich, R., Dou, S. J., Jasperse, L., Pan, X., Wanger, A., et al. (2003). Single nucleotide polymorphisms in genes associated with isoniazid resistance in *Mycobacterium tuberculosis*. *Antimicrob. Agents Chemother.* 47, 1241–1250. doi: 10.1128/AAC.47.4.1241-1250.2003

Ramirez, M. S., and Tolmasky, M. E. (2010). Aminoglycoside modifying enzymes. *Drug. Resist. Updat.* 13, 151–171. doi: 10.1016/j.drup.2010.08.003

Ramon-Garcia, S., Ng, C., Anderson, H., Chao, J. D., Zheng, X., Pfeifer, T., et al. (2011). Synergistic drug combinations for tuberculosis therapy identified by a novel high-throughput screen. *Antimicrob. Agents Chemother.* 55, 3861–3869. doi: 10.1128/AAC.00474-11

Rao, S. P., Alonso, S., Rand, L., Dick, T., and Pethe, K. (2008). The protonmotive force is required for maintaining ATP homeostasis and viability of hypoxic, nonreplicating *Mycobacterium tuberculosis*. *Proc. Natl. Acad. Sci. U.S.A.* 105, 11945–11950. doi: 10.1073/pnas.0711697105

Reddy, V. M., Einck, L., Andries, K., and Nacy, C. A. (2010). *In vitro* interactions between new antitubercular drug candidates SQ109 and TMC207. *Antimicrob. Agents Chemother.* 54, 2840–2846. doi: 10.1128/AAC.01601-09

Reeves, A. Z., Campbell, P. J., Sultana, R., Malik, S., Murray, M., Plykaytis, B. B., et al. (2013). Aminoglycoside cross-resistance in *Mycobacterium tuberculosis* due to mutations in the 5'-untranslated region of whiB7. *Antimicrob. Agents Chemother.* 57, 1857–1865. doi: 10.1128/AAC.02191-12

Rivers, E. C., and Mancera, R. L. (2008a). New anti-tuberculosis drugs in clinical trials with novel mechanisms of action. *Drug. Discov. Today* 13, 1090–1098. doi: 10.1016/j.drudis.2008.09.004

Rivers, E. C., and Mancera, R. L. (2008b). New anti-tuberculosis drugs with novel mechanisms of action. *Curr. Med. Chem.* 15, 1956–1967. doi: 10.2174/092986708785132906

Sacksteder, K. A., Protopopova, M., Barry, C. E., 3rd, Andries, K., and Nacy, C. A. (2012). Discovery and development of SQ109a new antitubercular drug with a novel mechanism of action. *Future Microbiol.* 7, 823–837. doi: 10.2217/fmb.12.56

Scherman, M. S., North, E. J., Jones, V., Hess, T. N., Grzegorzewicz, A. E., Kasagami, T., et al. (2012). Screening a library of 1600 adamantyl ureas for anti-*Mycobacterium tuberculosis* activity *in vitro* and for better physical chemical properties for bioavailability. *Bioorg. Med. Chem.* 20, 3255–3262. doi: 10.1016/j.bmc.2012.03.058

Segala, E., Sougakof, W., Nevejans-Chauffour, A., Jarlier, V., and Petrella, S. (2012). New mutations in the mycobacterial ATP synthase: new insights into the binding of the diarylquinoline TMC207 to the ATP synthase C-ring structure. *Antimicrobial. Agents Chemother.* 56, 2326–2334. doi: 10.1128/AAC.06154-11.

Shirude, P. S., Madhavapeddi, P., Tucker, J. A., Murugan, K., Patil, V., Basavarajappa, H., et al. (2013). Aminopyrazinamides: novel and specific GyrB inhibitors that kill replicating and nonreplicating *Mycobacterium tuberculosis*. *ACS Chem. Biol.* 8, 519–523. doi: 10.1021/cb300510w

Silva, P. E., Bigi, F., Santangelo, M. P., Romano, M. I., Martin, C., Cataldi, A., et al. (2001). Characterization of P55, a multidrug efflux pump in *Mycobacterium bovis* and *Mycobacterium tuberculosis*. *Antimicrob. Agents Chemother.* 45, 800–804. doi: 10.1128/AAC.45.3.800-804.2001

Singh, M., Jadaun, G. P. S., Srivastava, R. K., Chauhan, V., Mishra, R., Gupta, K., et al. (2011). Effect of efflux pump inhibitors on drug susceptibility of ofloxacin ressitant *Mycobacterium tuberculosis* isolates. Indian *J. Med. Res.* 133, 535–540.

Spies, F. S., Ribeiro, A. W., Ramos, D. F., Ribeiro, M. O., Martin, A., Palomino, J. C., et al. (2011). Streptomycin resistance and lineage-specific polymorphisms in *Mycobacterium tuberculosis* gidB gene. *J. Clin. Microbiol.* 49, 2625–2630. doi: 10.1128/JCM.00168-11

Stoffels, K., Mathys, V., Fauville-Dufaux, M., Wintjens, R., and Bifani, P. (2012). Systematic analysis of pyrazinamide-resistant spontaneous mutants and clinical isolates of *Mycobacterium tuberculosis*. *Antimicrob. Agents Chemother.* 56, 5186–5193. doi: 10.1128/AAC.05385-11

Stover, C. K., Warrener, P., Vandevanter, D. R., Sherman, D. R., Arain, T. M., Langhorne, M. H., et al. (2000). A small-molecule nitroimidazopyran drug candidate for the treatment of tuberculosis. *Nature* 405, 962–966. doi: 10.1038/35016103

Sullivan, T. J., Truglio, J. J., Boyne, M. E., Novichenok, P., Zhang, X., Stratton, C. F., et al. (2006). High affinity InhA inhibitors with activity against drug-resistant strains of *Mycobacterium tuberculosis*. *ACS Chem. Biol.* 1, 43–53. doi: 10.1021/cb0500042

Tahlan, K., Wilson, R., Kastrinsky, D. B., Arora, K., Nair, V., Fischer, E., et al. (2012). SQ109 targets MmpL3, a membrane transporter of trehalose monomycolate involved in mycolic acid donation to the cell wall core of *Mycobacterium tuberculosis*. *Antimicrob. Agents Chemother.* 56, 1797–1809. doi: 10.1128/AAC.05708-11

Takiff, H. E., Salazar, L., Guerrero, C., Philipp, W., Huang, W. M., Kreiswirth, B., et al. (1994). Cloning and nucleotide sequence of *Mycobacterium tuberculosis* gyrA and gyrB genes and detection of quinolone resistance mutations. *Antimicrob. Agents Chemother.* 38, 773–780. doi: 10.1128/AAC.38.4.773

Telenti, A., Philipp, W. J., Sreevatsan, S., Bernasconi, C., Stockbauer, K. E., Wieles, B., et al. (1997). The emb operon, a gene cluster of *Mycobacterium tuberculosis* involved in resistance to ethambutol. *Nat. Med.* 3, 567–570. doi: 10.1038/nm0597-567

Tran, A. T., Cergol, K. M., West, N. P., Randall, E. J., Britton, W. J., Bokhari, S. A., et al. (2011). Synthesis and evaluation of potent ene-yne inhibitors of type II dehydroquinases as tuberculosis drug leads. *ChemMedChem* 6, 262–265. doi: 10.1002/cmdc.201000399

Tran, A. T., West, N. P., Britton, W. J., and Payne, R. J. (2012). Elucidation of *Mycobacterium tuberculosis* type II dehydroquinase inhibitors using a fragment elaboration strategy. *ChemMedChem* 7, 1031–1043. doi: 10.1002/cmdc.201100606.

Venkatraman, J., Bhat, J., Solapure, S. M., Sandesh, J., Sarkar, D., Aishwarya, S., et al. (2012). Screening, identification, and characterization of mechanistically diverse inhibitors of the *Mycobacterium tuberculosis* enzyme, pantothenate kinase (CoaA). *J. Biomol. Screen* 17, 293–302. doi: 10.1177/1087057111423069

Vilcheze, C., Av-Gay, Y., Attarian, R., Liu, Z., Hazbon, M. H., Colangeli, R., Jr. et al. (2008). *Mycothiol biosynthesis* is essential for ethionamide susceptibility in *Mycobacterium tuberculosis*. *Mol. Microbiol.* 69, 1316–1329. doi: 10.1111/j.1365-2958.2008.06365.x

Vilcheze, C., Baughn, A. D., Tufariello, J., Leung, L. W., Kuo, M., Basler, C. F., Jr. et al. (2011). Novel inhibitors of InhA efficiently kill *Mycobacterium tuberculosis* under aerobic and anaerobic conditions. *Antimicrob. Agents Chemother.* 55, 3889–3898. doi: 10.1128/AAC.00266-11

Wachino, J., Shibayama, K., Kimura, K., Yamane, K., Suzuki, S., and Arakawa, Y. (2010). RmtC introduces G1405 methylation in 16S rRNA and confers high-level aminoglycoside resistance on Gram-positive microorganisms. *FEMS Microbiol. Lett.* 311, 56–60. doi: 10.1111/j.1574-6968.2010.02068.x

World Heath Organization (WHO). (2011). *Global Tuberculosis Control.* ISBN: 978-92-4-156438-0

World Heath Organization (WHO). (2012). *Global Tuberculosis Report.* ISBN: 978-92-4-156450-2

Wong, S. Y., Lee, J. S., Kwak, H. K., Via, L. E., Boshoff, H. I., and Barry, C. E. 3rd. (2011). Mutations in gidB confer low-level streptomycin resistance in *Mycobacterium tuberculosis*. *Antimicrob. Agents Chemother.* 55, 2515–2522. doi: 10.1128/AAC.01814-10

Xu, H., Hazra, S., and Blanchard, J. S. (2012). NXL104 irreversibly inhibits the beta-lactamase from *Mycobacterium tuberculosis*. *Biochemistry* 51, 4551–4557. doi: 10.1021/bi300508r

Yang, Y., Gao, P., Liu, Y., Ji, X., Gan, M., Guan, Y., et al. (2011). A discovery of novel *Mycobacterium tuberculosis* pantothenate synthetase inhibitors based on the molecular mechanism of actinomycin D inhibition. *Bioorg. Med. Chem. Lett.* 21, 3943–3946. doi: 10.1016/j.bmcl.2011.05.021

Zaunbrecher, M. A., Sikes, R. D. Jr., Metchock, B., Shinnick, T. M., and Posey, J. E. (2009). Overexpression of the chromosomally encoded aminoglycoside acetyltransferase eis confers kanamycin resistance in *Mycobacterium tuberculosis*. *Proc. Natl. Acad. Sci. U.S.A.* 106, 20004–20009.

Novel β-lactamase inhibitors: a therapeutic hope against the scourge of multidrug resistance

Richard R. Watkins[1,2] *, Krisztina M. Papp-Wallace[3,4], Sarah M. Drawz[5] and Robert A. Bonomo[3,4,6,7] *

[1] Department of Internal Medicine, Northeast Ohio Medical University, Rootstown, OH, USA
[2] Division of Infectious Diseases, Akron General Medical Center, Akron, OH, USA
[3] Research Service, Louis Stokes Cleveland Department of Veterans Affairs Medical Center, Cleveland, OH, USA
[4] Department of Medicine, Case Western Reserve University, Cleveland, OH, USA
[5] Department of Lab Medicine and Pathology, University of Minnesota, Minneapolis, MN, USA
[6] Pharmacology, Case Western Reserve University, Cleveland, OH, USA
[7] Molecular Biology and Microbiology, Case Western Reserve University, Cleveland, OH, USA

Edited by:
Marcelo Tolmasky, California State University Fullerton, USA
Reviewed by:
Marcelo Tolmasky, California State University Fullerton, USA
Gabriel Gutkind, Universidad de Buenos Aires, Argentina
***Correspondence:**
Richard R. Watkins, Division of Infectious Diseases, Akron General Medical Center, 224 West Exchange Street, Suite 290, Akron, OH 44302, USA
e-mail: richard.watkins@akrongeneral.org;
Robert A. Bonomo, Research Service, Louis Stokes Cleveland Department of Veterans Affairs Medical Center, Cleveland, OH 44106, USA
e-mail: robert.bonomo@va.gov

The increasing incidence and prevalence of multi-drug resistance (MDR) among contemporary Gram-negative bacteria represents a significant threat to human health. Since their discovery, β-lactam antibiotics have been a major component of the armamentarium against these serious pathogens. Unfortunately, a wide range of β-lactamase enzymes have emerged that are capable of inactivating these powerful drugs. In the past 30 years, a major advancement in the battle against microbes has been the development of β-lactamase inhibitors, which restore the efficacy of β-lactam antibiotics (e.g., ampicillin/sulbactam, amoxicillin/clavulanate, ticarcillin/clavulanate, and piperacillin/tazobactam). Unfortunately, many newly discovered β-lactamases are not inactivated by currently available inhibitors. Is there hope? For the first time in many years, we can anticipate the development and introduction into clinical practice of novel inhibitors. Although these inhibitors may still not be effective for all β-lactamases, their introduction is still welcome. This review focuses on the novel β-lactamase inhibitors that are closest to being introduced in the clinic.

Keywords: antibiotic resistance, β-lactamase inhibitors

INTRODUCTION

The ongoing dissemination of multi-drug resistant (MDR) bacteria is a serious threat to global health. Microbiological and epidemiological surveys commissioned by public and private institutions paint a frightening portrait of the emergence of β-lactam resistance in both the community and the hospital setting. A major mechanism for antibiotic resistance among Gram-negative bacteria is the production of β-lactamases. β-lactamases are enzymes that inactivate β-lactam antibiotics by hydrolyzing the amide bond of the β-lactam ring. β-lactamases are bacterial resistance determinants that have been known for more than seventy years, yet the details of their evolution, dissemination and hydrolytic capacity still remains a great scientific challenge.

Two classification systems are presently used to categorize β-lactamases. Introduced more than thirty years ago, the Ambler classification system divides β-lactamases into four classes (A, B, C, and D) based on their amino acid sequences (Ambler, 1980). The Bush-Medeiros-Jacoby classification system groups β-lactamases according to functional properties; this classification system uses substrate and inhibitor profiles in an attempt to organize the enzymes in ways that can be correlated with their phenotype in clinical isolates (Bush and Jacoby, 2010). For purposes of simplicity in this review, we will refer to the Ambler classification system.

Class A enzymes include both plasmid-mediated and chromosomally-encoded β-lactamases that demonstrate broad-spectra (e.g., TEM-1 and SHV-1), extended-spectra (e.g., CTX-M-15), and carbapenemase activity (e.g., KPC-2). Class B enzymes are metallo-β-lactamases (MBLs) which can hydrolyze penicillins, cephalosporins, and carbapenems such as the recently described New Delhi metallo-β-lactamase (NDM-1) found in *Klebsiella pneumoniae* and *Escherichia coli* (Kumarasamy et al., 2010). Class C enzymes are cephalosporinases that are chromosomally-encoded for example the inducible *Pseudomonas aeruginosa* AmpC and P99 β-lactamase of *Enterobacter* spp., or plasmid-mediated such as CMY-2, first found in *Escherichia coli.* Class D enzymes have a substrate preference for oxacillin and are referred to as oxacillinases (e.g., OXA-1). Recent surveys have shown that class D enzymes are a rapidly expanding class of β-lactamases and have enzymes that can hydrolyze extended-spectrum cephalosporins (e.g., OXA-10) and carbapenems (e.g., OXA-23). Several class D enzymes are often found in non-fermenting bacteria such as *P. aeruginosa* and *Acinetobacter baumannii* and occasionally in *E. coli* and *K. pneumoniae.*

At present, there are three commercially available β-lactamase inhibitors: clavulanic acid, sulbactam and tazobactam (**Figure 1**). These are mechanism-based inhibitors that share a common β-lactam structure. As a group, they are best active against most

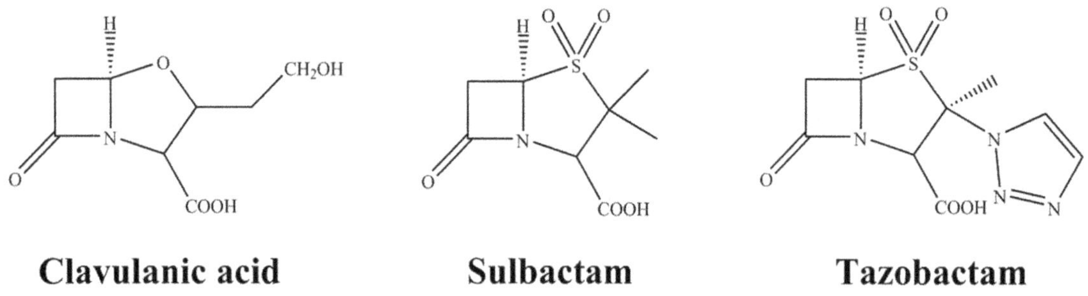

FIGURE 1 | Chemical structures of the clinically available β-lactamase inhibitors.

class A β-lactamases, exceptions include KPC-2 carbapenemase and inhibitor resistant TEMs (IRTs) and SHVs. Clavulanate, sulbactam, and tazobactam have less effect on class C enzymes, and are essentially inactive against class B and most class D enzymes (Bush and Jacoby, 2010).

Encouragingly, pharmaceutical companies are aggressively developing and bringing to market new combinations of β-lactam antibiotics with β-lactamase inhibitors. Several of these are now close to clinical availability. A promising new design for β-lactamase inhibitors has been to focus on scaffolds that can rapidly acylate a wide range of β-lactamases while minimizing hydrolysis. This review will focus on recent data regarding the mechanisms of inhibition of these novel agents, their antimicrobial activity, and the progress in their clinical trials. Specifically, avibactam and MK-7655 are members of a new class of non-β-lactam-β-lactamase inhibitors called diazabicyclooctanes (DBOs) with a broader spectrum of activity than other inhibitors. Recent modifications to boronic acid (BA) compounds have led to very potent *E. coli* AmpC inhibitors that are eagerly awaited. Finally, the discovery of a "universal" β-lactamase inhibitor has been an important goal of both academia and the pharmaceutical industry but has proven to be quite challenging. Emerging data show this ideal might not be feasible and researchers investigating mechanisms of β-lactamase inhibition will likely need to develop alternative strategies.

DIAZABICYCLOOCTANES

AVIBACTAM

Avibactam (AVI) is a non-β-lactam compound in the class of DBOs (**Figure 2**). As a β-lactamase inhibitor, AVI inactivates β-lactams by a reversible fast acylation and relatively slow deacylation reaction. Against most class A and class C β-lactamases this results in a low turnover ratio (Ehmann et al., 2012). The β-lactamase inhibition by AVI is mostly reversible and AVI demonstrates a half-life of 16 min for TEM-1 which closely approaches one generation time of *E. coli* (Ehmann et al., 2012). Thus despite reversibly of AVI, AVI is predicted to remain bound to TEM-1 during most of an entire generation cycle of *E. coli*; thus keeping the enzyme inactive. Unlike clavulanic acid and like sulbactam, AVI does not induce β-lactamase production (Coleman, 2011). In addition to TEM-1 and SHV-1, clinically important β-lactamases that are readily inhibited by AVI include the serine carbapenemase KPC-2, the ESBL CTX-M-15, class C β-lactamases such as the AmpC and some class D enzymes (OXA-48).

An interesting development is the combination of this DBO inhibitor with a number of β-lactam antibiotics that have traditionally been used to treat Gram-negative bacteria. Despite the tendency of this class of antibiotics to select ESBLs, expanded-spectrum cephalosporins are seen as potential partners because they have a broader spectrum of activity. As a result, the combination of ceftazidime-AVI has potent activity against *K. pneumoniae*

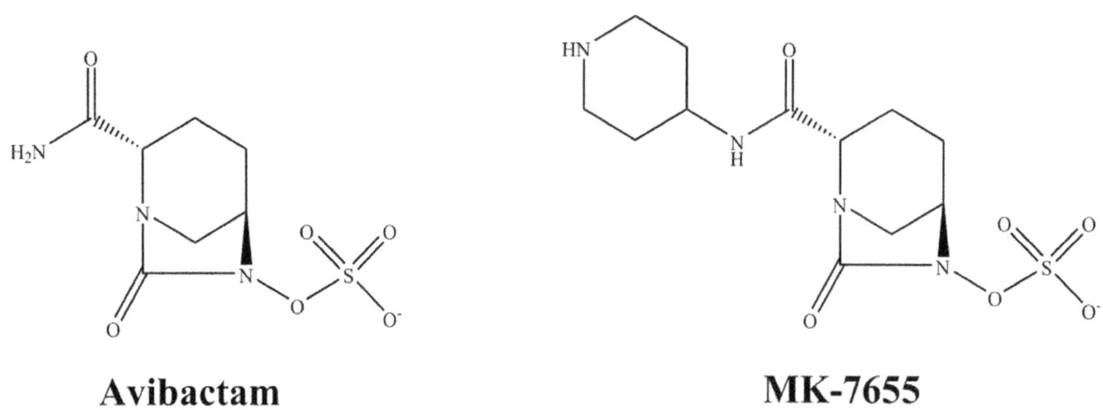

FIGURE 2 | Chemical structures of diazabicyclooctanes.

carrying ESBLs such as SHV-5, other ESBLs and AmpC enzymes and also against most *Klebsiella* spp. harboring the KPC enzyme (Livermore et al., 2011). Against *P. aeruginosa*, AVI reverses AmpC-mediated ceftazidime resistance, reducing MICs for fully derepressed mutants and isolates to ≤8 mg/L (Mushtaq et al., 2010). Unfortunately, ceftazidime-AVI lacks activity against *A. baumannii* and most species of anaerobic bacteria (Citron et al., 2011; Zhanel et al., 2013).

Emerging data from clinical trials that are registered show that ceftazidime-AVI is as effective as carbapenem therapy for complicated urinary tract infections (UTIs) and complicated intra-abdominal infections (cIAI), including those caused by expanded-spectrum cephalosporin-resistant Gram-negative organisms (Zhanel et al., 2013). Furthermore, a recent trial of ceftazidime-AVI plus metronidazole in the treatment of cIAIs found a favorable clinical response rate when compared to meropenem (Lucasti et al., 2013).

Ceftaroline is a novel semisynthetic anti-methicillin-resistant *Staphylococcus aureus* (MRSA) cephalosporin with broad-spectrum activity. The combination of ceftaroline-AVI is active against *Enterobacteriaceae* that produce KPC, various ESBLs (CTX-M types), and AmpC (chromosomally derepressed or plasmid-mediated enzymes), as well as against those producing more than one of these β-lactamase types (Castanheira et al., 2012b). However, ceftaroline's activity against *Acinetobacter* spp. and *P. aeruginosa* is limited. In a clinical study of diabetic foot infections (which are often polymicrobial), ceftaroline-AVI reduced ceftaroline MICs for strains of resistant *Enterobacter* spp. and one strain of *Morganella*, as well as for the anaerobes *Bacteroides fragilis* and *Prevotella* spp. (Goldstein et al., 2013a). A Phase 2 clinical trial comparing ceftaroline-AVI to doripenem in adults with complicated UTIs is in progress[1].

Monobactams resist hydrolysis by MBLs, thus another promising partner for AVI is aztreonam. For example, if any *Enterbacteriaceae* and *P. aeruginosa* strains carrying MBLs and co-produce ESBLs or AmpC, the aztreonam would target the MBLs, while the avibactam would inhibit the ESBLs and AmpC (Livermore et al., 2011; Crandon et al., 2012). As such, this combination will be a very welcome addition to the antibiotic formulary as the safety and efficacy of aztreonam are already established in clinical practice.

MK-7655

MK-7655, a novel DBO that is structurally similar to AVI except for an additional piperidine ring, exhibits synergy in combination with imipenem against KPC-producing *K. pneumoniae* and *P. aeruginosa* expressing AmpC (**Figure 2**; Mangion et al., 2011; Hirsch et al., 2012). Studies show that at a concentration of 4 mg/L, MK-7655 lowers imipenem MICs for *Enterobacteriaceae* with KPC carbapenemases from 16–64 mg/L to 0.12–1 mg/L (Livermore et al., 2013). Interestingly, synergy is also seen for *Enterobacteriaceae* with carbapenem resistance mediated by porin loss. Among strains of *P. aeruginosa*, 4 mg/L of MK-7655 reduces the MIC of imipenem for all isolates, except those with MBLs.

Two separate Phase 2 clinical trials of two doses (125 mg or 250 mg) of MK-7655 plus imipenem-cilastatin vs. imipenem-cilastatin alone for treatment of complicated UTIs or cIAIs began in early 2012[1]. Results from these trials are eagerly awaited.

BAs

The inhibitory effects of BAs on β-lactamases have been known for several decades. Boron forms a reversible bond with β-lactamases. Recent studies have shown that different BAs are high affinity inhibitors of the AmpC β-lactamase of *E. coli*, class A β-lactamases TEM-1, CTX-M, and SHV-1, and class C β-lactamase, ADC-7 from *Acinetobacter* spp. and *P. aeruginosa* (Drawz et al., 2010a; Winkler et al., 2013). Many BAs are in early developmental stages, however the progress of these compounds is rapidly advancing.

Despite the large number of BAs in development, only one so far is approaching clinical trials. First introduced at the 2012 Interscience Conference on Antimicrobial Agents and Chemotherapy, RPX7009 is a new boron-based inhibitor being developed in combination with biapenem (RPX2003; **Figure 3**; Castanheira et al., 2012a; Hecker et al., 2012; Sabet et al., 2012). RPX7009 lacks direct antibacterial activity but it does enhance the activity of biapenem against class A carbapenemase-producing *Enterobacteriaceae* (e.g., KPC, SME, or IMI/NMC-A; Livermore and Mushtaq, 2013). Moreover, RPX7009 lowers the MICs of biapenem against *Enterobacteriaceae* with complex β-lactamase backgrounds (AmpC or ESBL activity) and porin losses. Unfortunately, RPX7009 does not inhibit class B MBLs and class D carbapenemases. Against *Bacteroides* and other select anaerobes, biapenem and RPX7009 demonstrates comparable activity to meropenem alone (Goldstein et al., 2013b). Regarding other anaerobes (*Fusobacterium* spp and *Prevotella*) biapenem and RPX7009 are reasonable active. *Clostridia* are a notable exception with the range extending up to 8 mg/L. As expected against MBL-producing *Bacteroides*, activity is poor.

BAL30072 AND BAL30376

BAL30072 (**Figure 4**) is a novel siderophore monosulfactam similar to aztreonam. BAL30072 demonstrates activity against a broad range of Gram-negative bacilli including *Acinetobacter* spp., *P. aeruginosa*, *Burkholderia cepacia*, and some MDR *Enterobacteriaceae* (Page et al., 2010; Russo et al., 2011; Higgins et al., 2012). BAL30072 shows potency against carbapenem-resistant *Enterobacteriaceae* including those with AmpC, ESBL, and KPC enzymes, *P. aeruginosa* including most strains with MBLs and most isolates of *A. baumannii* except those producing OXA-58 (Mushtaq et al., 2013). However, resistance is still observed with the *K. pneumoniae* ST258 isolates carrying KPC. The addition of meropenem to BAL30072 increases activity against certain individual isolates of *A. baumannii*. BAL30072 is currently in a Phase 1 study and will likely be combined with meropenem in future clinical development[1].

In addition to BAL30072, researchers have also developed another compound with broad activity against β-lactamases called BAL30376, which combines three β-lactams: the siderophore monobactam BAL19764, the bridged monobactam class C β-lactamase inhibitor BAL29880 for class C cephalosporinases, and clavulanic acid to inhibit class A enzymes (Bush and Macielag,

[1]www.clinicaltrials.gov

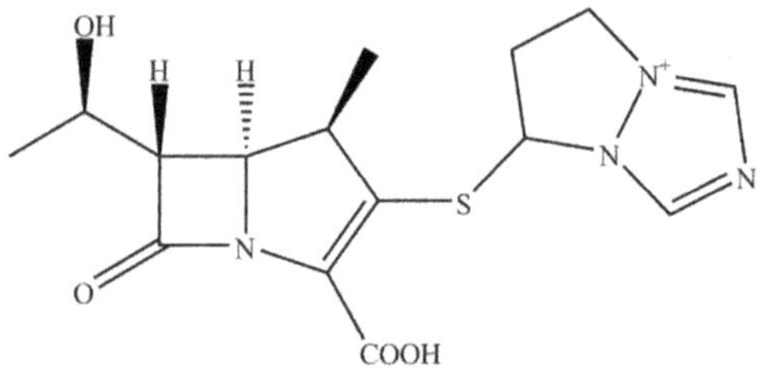

Biapenem

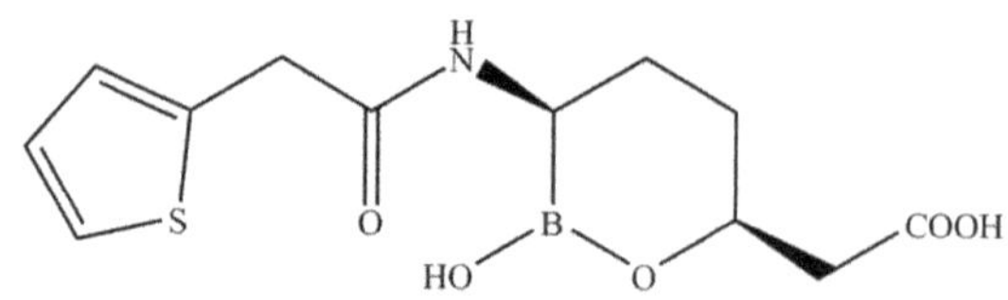

RPX7009

FIGURE 3 | Chemical structures of a novel combination: a carbapenem (left) with a new boron-based β-lactamase inhibitor (right).

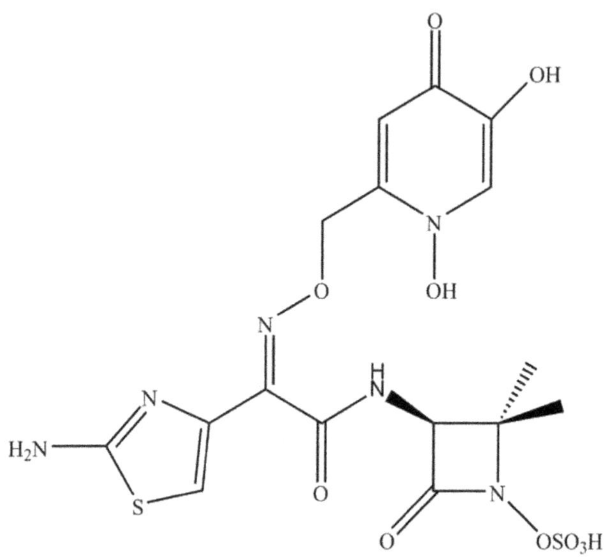

BAL30072

FIGURE 4 | Chemical structure of a novel siderophore monosulfactam.

2010). Further *in vitro* analysis and animal studies of BAL30376 will be necessary before its developmental pathway is clear.

NEW CARBAPENEMS AND BEYOND

Originally developed in the 1970s, carbapenems are among the most broad-spectrum antibiotics in clinical use. One major advantage of this class of agents is their stability against hydrolysis by many ESBLs and class C cephalosporinases. The unique property of carbapenems that merits their inclusion in this review is their ability to inhibit both class A and class C β-lactamases (Drawz and Bonomo, 2010; Papp-Wallace et al., 2011) and their high affinity for the bacterial transpeptidases and carboxypeptidases that synthesize the peptidoglycan-based cell wall. The carbapenem class of β-lactams act as a "slow substrates." Crystallographic analyses show how these compounds inactivate the serine-based class A and C enzymes by adopting unique conformations in the active site that disfavor hydrolysis (carbonyl oxygen outside of the oxyanion hole). The remaining parts of this section will examine the promise of some of these carbapenems that are apart from imipenem, meropenem, ertapenem, and doripenem.

Biapenem has been available in Japan since 2002 and is currently in Phase 2 clinical study in the USA. Biapenem achieves high concentration in respiratory tissue making it an attractive choice for pulmonary infections (Bassetti et al., 2011). Biapenem is hydrolyzed by MBLs and its bicyclic derivative has significant affinity for these enzymes (Garau et al., 2005). Recent experimental evidence shows it might be possible to obtain new competitive inhibitors of B2 MBLs by modification of this bicyclic compound (Gatti, 2012).

Razupenem (SMP-601; **Figure 5**) is a β-methyl carbapenem with activity against MRSA, enterococci including *Enterococcus faecium* and many species of Enterobacteriaceae. The activity of razupenem is not abrogated by ESBLs but AmpC and class A carbapenemases seem to affect it more than ertapenem or imipenem (Livermore et al., 2009). Pharmacodynamic data suggest razupenem can be dosed the same for *E. coli*, *Proteus mirabilis* and *Klebsiella* spp. as for MRSA (MacGowan et al., 2011). However, the development of razupenem has been discontinued.

LK-157 is a novel tricyclic carbapenem with potent inhibitory activity against serine β-lactamases (**Figure 5**; Plantan et al., 2007). LK-157 is a close structural analog to sanfetrinem, an oral, broad-spectrum antibiotic whose development was stopped after Phase 2 clinical trials (Babini et al., 1998). LK-157 restores the diminished activity of β-lactam antibiotics against a number of bacterial strains producing class A ESBLs (excluding CTX-M and KPC) as well as class C β-lactamases (Paukner et al., 2009). Of note, data from a rat jejunum model suggest the compound has good bioavailability, raising the exciting possibility of an oral broad-spectrum agent active against class A and C enzymes (Iglicar et al., 2009).

S-649266 is a novel cephem antibiotic that promises to be stable against MBLs[2]. Details are still forthcoming about this compound, but early reports indicate S-649266 is stable against MBL producing strains and is effective against *A. baumannii*, *Stenotrophomonas maltophilia*, and *Burkholderia* spp. This is not a new β-lactamase inhibitor, but the activity against MBLs merits close attention.

[2]www.shionogi.com/pdf/RDmeeting2012.pdf

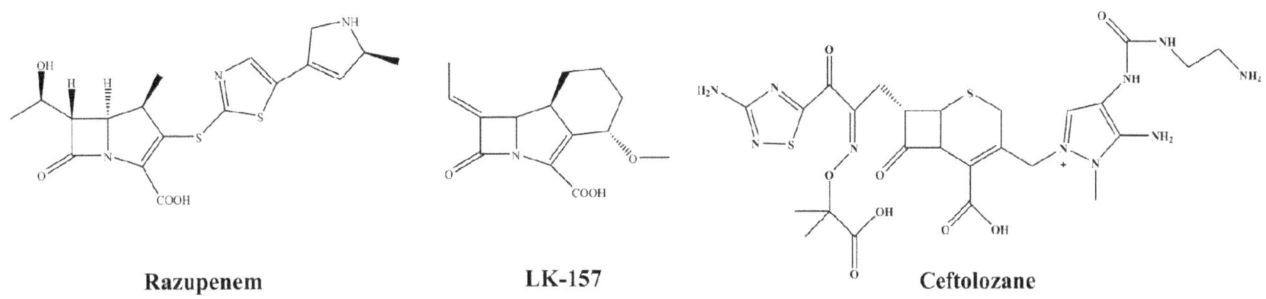

Razupenem LK-157 Ceftolozane

FIGURE 5 | Chemical structures of novel β-lactams with β-lactamase inhibitor activity.

CXA-202 is the combination of ceftolozane (CXA-201) with tazobactam (**Figure 5**). This formulation is targeted for *P. aeruginosa* and other MDR strains and has advanced into Phase 3 trials. *Per se*, this is not a novel β-lactamase inhibitor but is a new partner. The enhanced activity of the cephalosporin partner will be examined closely as this combination represents a novel testing paradigm in this area.

INHIBITORS OF CLASS B ENZYMES

Except for aztreonam-AVI, BAL30072, and S-649266, none of the other aforementioned experimental β-lactams and β-lactamase inhibitors have significant activity against isolates expressing MBLs. This is problematic because MBLs can spread rapidly through mobile genetic elements, as seen with the global emergence of NDM-1 (Liu et al., 2013).

The hydrolytic mechanisms of MBLs are significantly different from other classes of β-lactamases, requiring one or two zinc atoms depending on the subclass. Our understanding of MBLs is emerging as compared to the better studied class A and C enzymes (Dubus et al., 1995; Powers and Shoichet, 2002; Chen et al., 2006, 2009; Fisher and Mobashery, 2009). One class of agents that appear promising against MBLs is the thiol derivatives. Thiols, including the anti-hypertensive medication captopril, effectively inhibit several MBLs including NDM-1 and subclass B1, B2, and B3 enzymes (Heinz et al., 2003; King et al., 2012). Thiol compounds utilize the same mechanisms of zinc chelation and hydrolytic displacement. Additional clinical studies using these compounds in combination with antibiotics seem warranted.

CHALLENGES OF INHIBITING CLASS D ENZYMES

Similar to MBLs in their diversity, class D β-lactamases are designated OXA-type because of their ability to hydrolyze oxacillin. Their substrate profiles range from narrow to broad-spectrum, including carbapenems (Nazik et al., 2012). At present, β-lactamase inhibitors effective against class D enzymes are not available but promising data are emerging.

Several class D enzyme inhibitors are in development. For instance, substituted penicillin sulfones demonstrate efficacy against a number of OXA enzymes including OXA-24/40, a clinically relevant enzyme found in *A. baumannii* (Bou et al., 2010; Drawz et al., 2010b). A compound in development, 4,7-dichloro-1-benzothien-2-yl sulfonylaminomethyl BA (DSABA), is the first BA-based class D enzyme inhibitor. DSABA inhibits class A and C enzymes as well and demonstrates synergy with imipenem against *A. baumannii* (Tan et al., 2010). A series of thiophenyl oxime phosphonate β-lactamase inhibitors with potency against OXA-24/40 have also been discovered (Tan et al., 2011). Of interest, one compound reduces the MIC of imipenem against a highly imipenem-resistant strain of OXA-24/40 producing *A. baumannii.*

CHOOSING THE RIGHT PARTNER ANTIBIOTIC AND THE CHALLENGES AHEAD

Determining the ideal β-lactam for a given β-lactamase inhibitor and defining the ratio of the inhibitor to that β-lactam is a complex process. Indeed, it has been suggested that several considerations should be taken into account: (1) the ability of the inhibitor to protect the β-lactam ring from hydrolysis by key target enzymes; (2) the quantity of inhibitor needed to protect the β-lactam ring; (3) the feasibility and stability of the formulation; (4) pharmacokinetic and dosing parameters; and (5) cost (Shlaes, 2013). However, it is difficult to use standard pharmacokinetic and pharmacodynamic indices with inhibitors because they have weak to no intrinsic antimicrobial activity and they are usually partnered with an active antimicrobial agent. Mathematical modeling is one approach to these challenges. Using mathematical systems in pharmacodynamic models may help define regimens for inhibitors to prevent false labeling of a drug as ineffective because of dosing failures (Bush, 2012).

The report of a single isolate of *K. pneumoniae* producing a serine carbapenemase, a MBL, an ESBL and a plasmid-encoded AmpC carbapenemase underscores the challenge of using β-lactam antibiotics in the clinical setting (Pournaras et al., 2010). Treating this kind of pathogen with a β-lactam will likely require one with high stability to many common β-lactamases (e.g., aztreonam), together with two or more β-lactamase inhibitors that inhibit MBLs and serine β-lactamases. An example is the triple compound BAL30376 (Bush and Macielag, 2010; Livermore et al., 2010; Page et al., 2011). In addition to exerting a bactericidal effect against a wide range of β-lactamase-producing organisms including strains that were resistant to other β-lactams (except for KPC carbapenemases); BAL30376 is also relatively refractory toward selection of resistant mutants (Page et al., 2011).

FUTURE PERSPECTIVE

The majority of the compounds reviewed in this paper are in preclinical stages and (with the exception of AVI and MK-7655) are years away from availability. Thus, the pace of drug development must increase in order to meet the Infectious Diseases Society of America's goal of 10 new systemic drugs to treat infections caused by resistant bacteria by 2020 (Infectious Diseases Society of America, 2010; Boucher et al., 2013). The lack of drug candidates potentially active against MBLs is a great concern. For infections caused by bacteria harboring MBLs, treatment options are limited to polymyxins, tigecycline, and fosfomycin. Moreover, new β-lactamases are reported worldwide with alarming frequency, which continues to put strain on our existing antibiotic armamentarium (Lamoureaux et al., 2013). While novel β-lactamase inhibitors with new mechanisms of action provide substantial advances compared to currently available agents, incremental advances to existing classes are also valuable and should be encouraged (Page and Heim, 2009). The long quest for a universal β-lactamase inhibitor is becoming increasing quixotic with more pragmatic approaches, such as drug combinations, now a leading paradigm.

A plethora of strategies to invigorate drug development have been recently proposed (Infectious Diseases Society of America, 2012; Spellberg et al., 2013). These include conducting superiority and organism-specific clinical trials, transparency through public reporting of antibiotic usage tied to reimbursement, using molecular techniques for diagnostic confirmation of antibiotic indications, and investigating agents that modify host immune responses to pathogens to circumvent resistance selection. We also suggest that attention be given to alternative agents with activity against β-lactamases. Additional research studies are warranted especially since MBLs are important drivers of pan-resistant phenotypes. We remain positive in our outlook as the progress to date merits confidence that new drugs will be available very soon.

ACKNOWLEDGMENTS

Dr. R. Watkins is supported by a research grant from the Akron General Foundation. He reports no financial conflicts of interest. No writing assistance was utilized in the production of this manuscript. This work was supported in part by funds and/or facilities provided by the Cleveland Department of Veterans Affairs, the Veterans Affairs Career Development Program to Dr. K. M. Papp-Wallace, the Veterans Affairs Merit Review Program and the Geriatric Research Education and Clinical Center Veterans Integrated Service Network 10 to Dr. R. A. Bonomo. The National Institute of Allergy and Infectious Diseases of the National Institutes of Health under Award Numbers R01 AI100560 and R01 AI063517 to Dr. R. A. Bonomo also supported this work. The content is solely the responsibility of the authors and does not necessarily represent the official views of the National Institutes of Health. Drs. K. M. Papp-Wallace and R. A. Bonomo have research funding from AstraZeneca and Dr. R. A. Bonomo is also supported by research grants from Merck and Rib-X.

REFERENCES

Ambler, R. P. (1980). The structure of β-lactamases. *Philos. Trans. R. Soc. Lond. B Biol. Sci.* 289, 321–331. doi: 10.1098/rstb.1980.0049

Babini, G. S., Yuan, M., and Livermore, D. M. (1998). Interactions of β-lactamases with sanfetrinem (GV 104326) compared to those with imipenem and with oral β-lactams. *Antimicrob. Agents Chemother.* 42, 1168–1175.

Bassetti, M., Ginocchio, F., and Mikulska, M. (2011). New treatment options against Gram-negative organisms. *Crit. Care* 15, 215. doi: 10.1186/cc9997

Bou, G., Santillana, E., Sheri, A., Beceiro, A., Sampson, J. M., Kalp, M., et al. (2010). Design, synthesis, and crystal structures of 6-alkylidene-2'-substituted penicillanic acid sulfones as potent inhibitors of *Acinetobacter baumannii* OXA-24 carbapenemase. *J. Am. Chem. Soc.* 132, 13320–13331. doi: 10.1021/ja104092z

Boucher, H. W., Talbot, G. H., Benjamin, D. K. Jr., Bradley, J., Guidos, R. J., Jones, R. N., et al. (2013). 10 x '20 Progress–development of new drugs active against gram-negative bacilli: an update from the Infectious Diseases Society of America. *Clin. Infect. Dis.* 56, 1685–1694. doi: 10.1093/cid/cit152

Bush, K. (2012). Improving known classes of antibiotics: an optimistic approach for the future. *Curr. Opin. Pharmacol.* 12, 527–534. doi: 10.1016/j.coph.2012. 06.003

Bush, K., and Jacoby, G. A. (2010). Updated functional classification of β-lactamases. *Antimicrob. Agents Chemother.* 54, 969–976. doi: 10.1128/AAC.01009-09

Bush, K., and Macielag, M. J. (2010). New β-lactam antibiotics and β-lactamase inhibitors. *Expert Opin. Ther. Pat.* 20, 1277–1293. doi: 10.1517/ 13543776.2010.515588

Castanheira, M., Becker, H., Rhomberg, P., and Jones, R. (2012a). "Pre-clinical evalu- ation of a carbapenem/β-lactamase inhibitor combination (RPX2003/ RPX7009) tested against serine-carbapenemase-producing pathogens, abstr. F-856," in *Interscience Conference on Antimicrobial Agents and Chemotherapy* (San Francisco, CA).

Castanheira, M., Sader, H. S., Farrell, D. J., Mendes, R. E., and Jones, R. N. (2012b). Activity of ceftaroline-avibactam tested against Gram-negative organ- ism populations, including strains expressing one or more β-lactamases and methicillin-resistant *Staphylococcus aureus* carrying various staphylococcal cas- sette chromosome mec types. *Antimicrob. Agents Chemother.* 56, 4779–4785. doi: 10.1128/AAC.00817-12

Chen, Y., McReynolds, A., and Shoichet, B. K. (2009). Re-examining the role of Lys67 in class C β-lactamase catalysis. *Protein Sci.* 18, 662–669. doi: 10.1002/pro.60

Chen, Y., Minasov, G., Roth, T. A., Prati, F., and Shoichet, B. K. (2006). The deacylation mechanism of AmpC β-lactamase at ultrahigh resolution. *J. Am. Chem. Soc.* 128, 2970–2976. doi: 10.1021/ja056806m

Citron, D. M., Tyrrell, K. L., Merriam, V., and Goldstein, E. J. (2011). In vitro activity of ceftazidime-NXL104 against 396 strains of β-lactamase-producing anaerobes. *Antimicrob. Agents Chemother.* 55, 3616–3620. doi: 10.1128/AAC.01682-10

Coleman, K. (2011). Diazabicyclooctanes (DBOs): a potent new class of non- β-lactam β-lactamase inhibitors. *Curr. Opin. Microbiol.* 14, 550–555. doi: 10.1016/j.mib.2011.07.026

Crandon, J. L., Schuck, V. J., Banevicius, M. A., Beaudoin, M. E., Nichols, W. W., Tanudra, M. A., et al. (2012). Comparative in vitro and in vivo efficacies of human simulated doses of ceftazidime and ceftazidime-avibactam against *Pseudomonas aeruginosa*. *Antimicrob. Agents Chemother.* 56, 6137–6146. doi: 10.1128/AAC.00851-12

Drawz, S. M., Babic, M., Bethel, C. R., Taracila, M., Distler, A. M., Ori, C., et al. (2010a). Inhibition of the class C β-lactamase from *Acinetobacter* spp.: insights into effective inhibitor design. *Biochemistry* 49, 329–340. doi: 10.1021/bi9015988

Drawz, S. M., Bethel, C. R., Doppalapudi, V. R., Sheri, A., Pagadala, S. R., Hujer, A. M., et al. (2010b). Penicillin sulfone inhibitors of class D β-lactamases. *Antimicrob. Agents Chemother.* 54, 1414–1424. doi: 10.1128/AAC.00743-09

Drawz, S. M., and Bonomo, R. A. (2010). Three decades of β-lactamase inhibitors. *Clin. Microbiol. Rev.* 23, 160–201. doi: 10.1128/CMR.00037-09

Dubus, A., Normark, S., Kania, M., and Page, M. G. (1995). Role of asparagine 152 in catalysis of β-lactam hydrolysis by *Escherichia coli* AmpC β-lactamase studied by site-directed mutagenesis. *Biochemistry* 34, 7757–7764. doi: 10.1021/bi00023a023

Ehmann, D. E., Jahic, H., Ross, P. L., Gu, R. F., Hu, J., Kern, G., et al. (2012). Avibactam is a covalent, reversible, non-β-lactam β-lactamase inhibitor. *Proc. Natl. Acad. Sci. U.S.A.* 109, 11663–11668. doi: 10.1073/pnas.1205073109

Fisher, J. F., and Mobashery, S. (2009). Three decades of the class A β-lac - tamase acyl- enzyme. *Curr. Protein Pept. Sci.* 10, 401–407. doi: 10.2174/138920309789351967

Garau, G., Bebrone, C., Anne, C., Galleni, M., Frere, J. M., and Dideberg, O. (2005). A metal - lo-β-lactamase enzyme in action: crystal structures of the monozinc car- bapenemase CphA and its complex with biapenem. *J. Mol. Biol.* 345, 785–795. doi: 10.1016/j.jmb.2004.10.070

Gatti, D. L. (2012). Biapenem in - activation by B2 metallo β-lact - amases: energy land- scape of the post-hydrolysis reactions. *PLoS ONE* 7:e30079. doi: 10.1371/journal.pone.0030079

Goldstein, E. J., Citron, D. M., Mer - riam, C. V., and Tyrrell, K. L. (2013a). Comparative in vitro activity of ceftaroline, ceftaro - line-avibactam, and other antimi - crobial agents against aerobic and anaerobic bacteria cultured from infected diabetic foot wounds. *Diagn. Microbiol. Infect. Dis.* 76, 347–351. doi: 10.1016/j.diagmi - crobio.2013.03.019

Goldstein, E. J., Citron, D. M., Tyrrell, K. L., and Merriam, C. V. (2013b). In vitro activity of Biapenem plus RPX7009, a carbapenem com - bined with a serine β- lactamase inhibitor, against anaerobic bac - teria. *Antimicrob. Agents Chemother.* 57, 2620–2630. doi: 10.1128/AAC.02418-12

Hecker, S., Reddy, K., Totrov, M., Hirst, G., Sabet, M., Tarazi, Z., et al. (2012). "Dis- covery of RPX7009, a broad-spectrum β-lactamase in - hibitor with utility vs. class A ser - ine carbapenemase, abstr F-848," in *Interscience Conference on Antimicrobial Agents and Chemotherapy* (San Francisco, CA).

Heinz, U., Bauer, R., Wommer, S., Meyer-Klaucke, W., Papamichaels, C., Bateson, J., et al. (2003). Coordination geometries of metal ions in d- or l- captopril-inhibit - ed metallo-β-lactamases. *J. Biol. Chem.* 278, 20659–20666. doi: 10.1074/jbc.M212581200

Higgins, P. G., Stefanik, D., Page, M. G., Hackel, M., and Seifert, H. (2012). In vitro activity of the siderophore monosulfactam BAL30072 against meropen - em-non- susceptible *Acinetobacter baumannii*. *J. Antimicrob. Chemother.* 67, 1167-1169. doi: 10.1093/jac/dks009

Hirsch, E. B., Ledesma, K. R., Chang, K. T., Schwartz, M. S., Motyl, M. R., and Tam, V. H. (2012). In vi - tro activity of MK-7655, a novel β-lactamase inhibitor, in com- bination with imipenem against carbapenem-resistant Gram-negative bacteria. *Antimicrob. Agents Chemother.* 56, 3753–3757. doi: 10.1128/AAC.05927-11

Iglicar, P., Legen, I., Vilfan, G., Selic, L., and Prezelj, A. (2009). Perme - ability of a novel β-lactamase in - hibitor LK-157 and its ester pro - drugs across rat jejunum in vitro. *J. Pharm. Pharmacol.* 61, 1211–1218. doi: 10.1211/jpp/61.09.0011

Infectious Diseases Society of America. (2010). The 10 x '20 initiative: pursuing a global commitment to develop 10 new antibacterial drugs by 2020. *Clin. Infect. Dis.* 50, 1081–1083. doi: 10.1086/652237

Infectious Diseases Society of America. (2012). White paper: recom - mendations on the conduct of superiority and organism-specific clinical trials of antibac- terial agents for the treatment of in - fections caused by drug-resistant bacterial pathogens. *Clin. Infect. Dis.* 55, 1031–1046. doi: 10.1093/cid/cis688

King, D. T., Worrall, L. J., Gruninger, R., and Strynadka, N. C. (2012). New Delhi metallo-β-lactamase: structural insights into β-lactam recognition and inhibition. *J. Am. Chem. Soc.* 134, 11362–11365. doi: 10.1021/ja303579d

Kumarasamy, K. K., Toleman, M. A., Walsh, T. R., Bagaria, J., Butt, F., Balakrishnan, R., et al. (2010). Emergence of a new antibiotic re - sistance mechanism in India, Paki - stan, and the UK: a molecular, bio - logical, and epidemiological study. *Lancet Infect. Dis.* 10, 597–602. doi: 10.1016/S1473-3099(10)70143-2

Lamoureaux, T. L., Vakulenko, V., Toth, M., Frase, H., and Vakulen - ko, S. B. (2013). A novel extend - ed-spectrum β-lactamase, SGM-1, from an environmental iso- late of Sphingobium sp. *Antimicrob. Agents Chemother.* 57, 3783–3788. doi: 10.1128/AAC.00808-13

Liu, Z., Li, W., Wang, J., Pan, J., Sun, S., Yu, Y., et al. (2013). Identifica - tion and characterization of the first *Escherichia coli* strain carry- ing NDM-1 gene in China. *PLoS ONE* 8:e66666. doi: 10.1371/journal.pone.0066666

Livermore, D. M., and Mushtaq, S. (2013). Activity of biapenem (RPX2003) combined with the boronate β-lactamase inhibitor RPX7009 against carbapenem-resistant Enterobacteriaceae. *J. Antimicrob. Chemother.* 68, 1825–1831. doi: 10.1093/jac/dkt118

Livermore, D. M., Mushtaq, S., and Warner, M. (2009). Activity of the anti-MRSA carbapenem razupenem (PTZ601) against Enterobacteriaceae with defined resistance mechanisms. *J. Antimicrob. Chemother.* 64, 330–335. doi: 10.1093/jac/dkp187

Livermore, D. M., Mushtaq, S., and Warner, M. (2010). Activi - ty of BAL30376 (monobactam BAL19764 + BAL29880 + clavu - lanate) versus Gram-negative bac- teria with characterized resis - tance mechanisms. *J. Antimicrob. Chemother.* 65, 2382–2395. doi: 10.1093/jac/dkq310

Livermore, D. M., Mushtaq, S., Warner, M., Zhang, J., Maharjan, S., Doumith, M., et al. (2011). Ac - tivities of NXL104 combinations with ceftazidime and aztre- onam against carbapenemase-produc - ing Enterobacteriaceae. *Antimicrob. Agents Chemother.* 55, 390–394. doi: 10.1128/AAC.00756-10

Livermore, D. M., Warner, M., and Mushtaq, S. (2013). Activity of MK-7655 com- bined with imi - penem against Enterobacteriaceae and *Pseudomonas aeruginosa*. *J. Antimicrob. Chemother.* 68, 2286–2290. doi: 10.1093/jac/dkt178

Lucasti, C., Popescu, I., Ramesh, M. K., Lipka, J., and Sable, C. (2013). Comparative study of the efficacy and safety of ceftazidime/avibac - tam plus metronidazole versus meropenem in the treatment of complicated intra-abdominal in - fections in hospitalized adults: results of a randomized, dou - ble-blind, Phase II trial. *J. Antimicrob. Chemother.* 68, 1183–1192. doi: 10.1093/jac/dks523

MacGowan, A. P., Noel, A., Tomasel - li, S., Elliott, H., and Bowker, K. (2011). Pharmacodynamics of razupenem (PZ601) studied in an in vitro pharmacoki- netic model of infection. *Antimicrob. Agents Chemother.* 55, 1436–1442. doi: 10.1128/AAC.00936-10

Mangion, I. K., Ruck, R. T., Rivera, N., Huffman, M. A., and Shevlin, M. (2011). A concise synthesis of a β-lactamase inhibitor. *Org. Lett.* 13, 5480–5483. doi: 10.1021/ol202195n

Mushtaq, S., Warner, M., and Liver - more, D. M. (2010). In vitro ac - tiv- ity of ceftazidime+NXL104 against *Pseudomonas aeruginosa* and other non- fermenters. *J. Antimicrob. Chemother.* 65, 2376–2381. doi: 10.1093/jac/dkq306

Mushtaq, S., Woodford, N., Hope, R., Adkin, R., and Livermore, D. M. (2013). Activity of BAL30072 alone or combined with β-lact - amase inhibitors or with mero - penem against carbapenem-re - sistant Enterobacteriaceae and non- fermenters. *J. Antimicrob. Chemother.* 68, 1601–1608. doi: 10.1093/jac/ dkt050

Nazik, H., Ongen, B., Ilktac, M., Aydin, S., Kuvat, N., Sahin, A., et al. (2012). Carbapenem resistance due to blaOXA-48 among ES - BL-producing *Escherichia coli* and *Klebsiella pneumoniae* isolates in a univesity hospital, Turkey. *Southeast Asian J. Trop. Med. Public Health* 43, 1178–1185.

Page, M. G., Dantier, C., and Desar - bre, E. (2010). In vitro properties of BAL30072, a novel siderophore sulfactam with activity against multiresistant Gram-negative ba - cilli. *Antimicrob. Agents Chemother.* 54, 2291–2302. doi: 10.1128/AAC. 01525-09

Page, M. G., Dantier, C., Desarbre, E., Gaucher, B., Gebhardt, K., and Schmitt- Hoffmann, A. (2011). In vitro and in vivo properties of BAL30376, a β-lactam and dual β-lactamase inhibitor com - bination with enhanced activity against Gram- negative Bacilli that express multiple β-lactamas - es. *Antimicrob. Agents Chemother.* 55, 1510–1519. doi: 10.1128/AAC.01370-10

Page, M. G., and Heim, J. (2009). New molecules from old classes: revis - iting the development of β-lact - ams. *IDrugs* 12, 561–565.

Papp-Wallace, K. M., Endimiani, A., Taracila, M. A., and Bonomo, R. A. (2011). Carbapenems: past, present, and future. *Antimicrob. Agents Chemother.* 55, 4943–4960. doi: 10.1128/AAC.00296-11

Paukner, S., Hesse, L., Prezelj, A., Solmajer, T., and Urleb, U. (2009). In vitro activity of LK-157, a novel tricyclic carbapenem as broad-spectrum β-lactamase inhibitor. *Antimicrob. Agents Chemother.* 53, 505–511. doi: 10.1128/AAC.00085-08

Plantan, I., Selic, L., Mesar, T., An - derluh, P. S., Oblak, M., Prezelj, A., et al. (2007). 4-Substituted trinems as broad spectrum β-lact - amase inhibitors: structure-based design, synthesis, and biological activity. *J. Med. Chem.* 50, 4113–4121. doi: 10.1021/jm0703237

Pournaras, S., Poulou, A., Voulgari, E., Vrioni, G., Kristo, I., and Tsakris, A. (2010). Detection of the new metallo-β-lactamase VIM-19 along with KPC-2, CMY-2 and CTX-M-15 in *Klebsiella pneumoniae*. *J. Antimicrob. Chemother.* 65, 1604–1607. doi: 10.1093/jac/dkq190

Powers, R. A., and Shoichet, B. K. (2002). Structure-based approach for binding site identification on AmpC β-lactamase. *J. Med. Chem.* 45, 3222–3234. doi: 10.1021/jm020002p

Russo, T. A., Page, M. G., Beanan, J. M., Olson, R., Hujer, A. M., Hu - jer, K. M., et al. (2011). In vivo and in vitro activity of the sidero - phore monosulfactam BAL30072 against *Acinetobacter baumannii*. *J. Antimicrob. Chemother.* 66, 867–873. doi: 10.1093/jac/dkr013

Sabet, M., Tarazi, Z., Lomovskaya, O., Hecke, S., Dudley, M., and Griffith, (2012). "In vivo efficacy of the β-lactamase inhibitor RPX7009 combined with the carbapenem RPX2003 against KPC-producing K. pneumoniae, abstr F-858," in *Interscience Conference on Antimicrobial Agents and Chemotherapy* (San Francisco, CA).

Shlaes, D. M. (2013). New β-lactam-β-lactamase inhibitor combinations in clinical development. *Ann. N. Y. Acad. Sci.* 1277, 105–114. doi: 10.1111/nyas.12010

Spellberg, B., Bartlett, J. G., and Gilbert, D. N. (2013). The future of antibiotics and resistance. *N. Engl. J. Med.* 368, 299–302. doi: 10.1056/NEJMp1215093

Tan, Q., Ogawa, A. M., Painter, R. E., Park, Y. W., Young, K., and Dininno, F. (2010). 4,7-Dichloro benzothien-2-yl sulfonylaminomethyl boronic acid: first boronic acid-derived β-lactamase inhibitor with class A, C, and D activity. *Bioorg. Med. Chem. Lett.* 20, 2622–2624. doi: 10.1016/j.bmcl.2010.02.065

Tan, Q., Ogawa, A. M., Raghoobar, S. L., Wisniewski, D., Colwell, L., Park, Y. W., et al. (2011). Thiophenyl oxime-derived phosphonates as nano-molar class C β-lactamase inhibitors reducing MIC of imipenem against *Pseudomonas aerugi- nosa* and *Acinetobacter baumannii*. *Bioorg. Med. Chem. Lett.* 21, 4363–4365. doi: 10.1016/j.bmcl.2011.04.122

Winkler, M. L., Rodkey, E. A., Taracila, M. A., Drawz, S. M., Bethel, C. R., Papp-Wallace, K. M., et al. (2013). Design and exploration of novel boronic acid inhibitors reveals important interactions with a clavulanic acid-resistant sulfhydryl-variable (SHV) β-lactamase. *J. Med. Chem.* 56, 1084–1097. doi: 10.1021/jm301490d

Zhanel, G. G., Lawson, C. D., Adam, H., Schweizer, F., Zelenitsky, S., Lagace-Wiens, P. R., et al. (2013). Ceftazidime-avibactam: A novel cephalosporin/β-lactamase inhibitor combination. *Drugs* 73, 159–177. doi: 10.1007/s40265-013-0013-7

16

The antibiotic resistance "mobilome": searching for the link between environment and clinic

Julie A. Perry[1,2] and Gerard D. Wright[1,2]*

[1] *M. G. DeGroote Institute for Infectious Disease Research, McMaster University, Hamilton, ON, Canada*
[2] *Department of Biochemistry and Biomedical Sciences, McMaster University, Hamilton, ON, Canada*

Edited by:
Marilyn C. Roberts, University of Washington, USA

Reviewed by:
Rustam I. Aminov, University of the West Indies, Jamaica
Vincent Burrus, Université de Sherbrooke, Canada
Carlos F. Amábile-Cuevas, Fundación Lusara, Mexico

****Correspondence:***
Gerard D. Wright, M. G. DeGroote Institute for Infectious Disease Research, McMaster University, 1280 Main Street West, Hamilton, ON, Canada L8S4K1
e-mail: wrightge@mcmaster.ca

Antibiotic resistance is an ancient problem, owing to the co-evolution of antibiotic-producing and target organisms in the soil and other environments over millennia. The environmental "resistome" is the collection of all genes that directly or indirectly contribute to antibiotic resistance. Many of these resistance determinants originate in antibiotic-producing organisms (where they serve to mediate self-immunity), while others become resistance determinants only when mobilized and over-expressed in non-native hosts (like plasmid-encoded β-lactamases). The modern environmental resistome is under selective pressure from human activities such as agriculture, which may influence the composition of the local resistome and lead to gene transfer events. Beyond the environment, we are challenged in the clinic by the rise in both frequency and diversity of antibiotic resistant pathogens. We assume that clinical resistance originated in the environment, but few examples of direct gene exchange between the environmental resistome and the clinical resistome have been documented. Strong evidence exists to suggest that clinical aminoglycoside and vancomycin resistance enzymes, the extended-spectrum β-lactamase CTX-M and the quinolone resistance gene *qnr* have direct links to the environmental resistome. In this review, we highlight recent advances in our understanding of horizontal gene transfer of antibiotic resistance genes from the environment to the clinic. Improvements in sequencing technologies coupled with functional metagenomic studies have revealed previously underappreciated diversity in the environmental resistome, and also established novel genetic links to the clinic. Understanding mechanisms of gene exchange becomes vital in controlling the future dissemination of antibiotic resistance.

Keywords: antibiotic resistance, horizontal gene transfer, environmental resistome, evolution

INTRODUCTION

Griffith (1928) demonstrated the transformation of non-virulent *Streptococcus pneumoniae* with a heat-stable substance from a virulent strain. The "transforming principle" was later identified as DNA (Avery et al., 1944), and the notion that genetic material can flow both vertically (from parent to offspring), and horizontally (from siblings or peers) in bacteria continues to form the basis of modern-day molecular genetics. Also in 1928, Alexander Fleming discovered the antibiotic penicillin: arguably one of the most important discoveries in modern medicine, but one that is threatened today by the mechanisms discovered by Griffith and Avery. In this review, we highlight recent advances in our understanding of horizontal gene transfer of antibiotic resistance genes in the environment. The development and use of functional metagenomic techniques coupled with advances in sequencing technologies have revealed new diversity in the antibiotic resistome, and also established novel genetic links between the environment and the clinic.

ON THE ORIGINS OF RESISTANCE: EXPLORING THE ENVIRONMENTAL RESISTOME

The antibiotic "resistome" is the collection of all genes that directly or indirectly contribute to antibiotic resistance, both in the environment and the clinic. Antibiotic-producing bacteria of the genus *Streptomyces* are found abundantly in soils around the globe, and encode resistance genes against their own antibiotics [the so-called "producer hypothesis" (Cundliffe, 1989; Wright, 2007)]. Importantly, these organisms are often multi-drug resistant (D'Costa et al., 2006), which may reflect their ability to produce more than one antibiotic, or be a by-product of their evolution in proximity to antibiotic-producing neighbors in the soil. It is clear that the environmental "resistome" is a substantial source of resistance genes, and it has been theorized that antibiotic-producing organisms in the environment are the source of resistance genes found in clinical pathogens. Davies and colleagues demonstrated almost 40 years ago that the biochemical activity of aminoglycoside resistance enzymes encoded by producing organisms was identical to those found in pathogens (Benveniste and Davies, 1973). However, direct evidence of gene transfer between the environmental resistome and the clinic are rare as resistance genes may undergo many rounds of evolution between the soil and the clinic (Aminov and Mackie, 2007). The most cited examples of recent exchange between the environmental and clinical resistomes include the class-A extended-spectrum β-lactamase CTX-M, found on plasmids carried by major global pathogens and traced to environmental *Kluyvera* spp. (Humeniuk et al., 2002), and the quinolone resistance gene *qnr* (found on a broad-host range conjugative plasmid from a ciprofloxacin-resistant strain of *Klebsiella pneumoniae* and traced to several environmental water-borne species (Poirel et al., 2005a,b; Baquero et al., 2008). Still, the environmental resistome is so vast (and underexplored) that further links to the clinic are sure to surface.

SAMPLING THE ENVIRONMENT FOR RESISTANCE GENES

Two main approaches are used to study the environmental resistome: culture-based and metagenomic searches. Culture-based approaches involve growing all microorganisms resistant to a given antibiotic in the lab, and subsequently analyzing their genetics and associated biochemistry for resistance determinants. While the major disadvantage to this technique is that it is estimated that only a small fraction (~1%) of environmental organisms are readily grown in the lab (Amann et al., 1995), culture-based approaches allow detailed studies of the genomic context of resistance (including identification of host species, identification of multiple resistance determinants in a single genome, identification of antibiotic production capabilities of the host, etc.) that is not possible using culture-independent methods. Metagenomic studies are performed by culture-independent extraction of total microbial DNA from the environment, and subsequent analysis using either polymerase chain reaction (PCR)-based methods with specific primers or deep sequencing technologies. While a metagenomic approach has the obvious advantage of overcoming culture-based bias, it can be difficult to design oligonucleotide primers with both enough specificity and flexibility to capture sequences with minor deviation from the reference sequence. Metagenomic datasets can be difficult to assemble, and using bioinformatics alone to search for homologs of known resistance determinants may miss novel resistance determinants that are not sufficiently homologous to known genes. Functional metagenomic approaches (in which a metagenomic library is expressed in a heterologous host and screened for resistance) offer significant advantages over culture-based and metagenomic/PCR-based screens and are discussed in detail in the final section of this review.

NOVEL RESISTANCE DETERMINANTS AS A RESULT OF GENE MOBILIZATION

Perhaps one of the main reasons why resistance genes are missed in traditional metagenomic screens is that genes may not present as resistance genes in their native context. Often, resistance genes are expressed in low copy number in their native host because they form part of a tightly coordinated network (Martinez, 2008). However, if these genes are mobilized into a new genetic context where regulation is absent (or expression is strongly favored), they many function as novel resistance determinants. An excellent example of this type of resistance gene "repurposing" is the efflux pumps belonging to the resistance/nodulation/cell division (RND) family (reviewed in Dantas and Sommer, 2012). This family of small molecule pumps is found ubiquitously in all kingdoms of living organisms, where they function as transporters of toxic compounds. However, when mobilized and expressed at high levels in pathogens like *Campylobacter jejuni, Escherichia coli, Salmonella enterica* serotype Typhimurium or *Pseudomonas aeruginosa,* they are capable of conferring high level antibiotic resistance via drug efflux (reviewed in Piddock, 2006a,b; Dantas and Sommer, 2012). Gene mobilization can therefore contribute to the formation (as well as the dissemination) of antibiotic resistance.

THE ENVIRONMENTAL "MOBILOME"

Bacterial evolution occurs on an accelerated time scale compared to plant and animal species, due to the ease with which genes move between organisms. Gene transfer allows a bacterium to build on existing adaptations in order to invade a new niche or to be more successful in its current niche; the abundance of naturally transformable bacteria, transducing phage, and conjugative elements present in the environment are testament to the importance of horizontal gene transfer to bacterial evolution (Ochman et al., 2000).

WHAT DRIVES GENE TRANSFER IN THE ENVIRONMENT?

The modern environmental resistome is under selective pressure from human activities such as the use of antibiotics in agriculture, which may influence the composition of the local resistome and lead to gene transfer events. However, rough calculations suggest that 1 g of soil can contain ~580 different species of actinobacteria, which have the genetic capacity to produce 11,600 bioactive small molecules (Wright, 2010). Since these organisms also encode resistance elements to counteract the effects of the molecules they produce, the networks of selection and resistance that exist in soil are vast, and have evolved over millennia. In a carefully controlled study of 30,000-year old Beringian permafrost, D'Costa et al. (2011) showed that genes conferring resistance to β-lactams, tetracyclines, and glycopeptides existed in the environment well before the use of these antibiotics in the clinic. Structural and functional assays on the glycopeptide resistance element VanA demonstrated that the ancient soil resistance determinant was similar to the modern clinical resistance element. While this study showed that the origin of resistance to several natural product antibiotics is in the environment, a quantitative temporal study of resistance genes in agricultural soil from the Netherlands revealed that levels of all resistance genes investigated rose over time, from the pre-antibiotic era (1940s) to the present (Knapp et al., 2010). Moreover, plasmids isolated from pathogenic bacteria pre-dating the antibiotic era do not contain resistance genes (Hughes and Datta, 1983). While resistance to natural product antibiotics is undoubtedly ancient, anthropomorphic factors are clearly contributing to the mobilization, fixation, and dissemination of resistance genes in the present day. Although there is no direct evidence that antibiotics reach concentrations in the soil that approach the highly selective concentrations used therapeutically, antibiotic resistance genes may be necessary if that niche is affected by agricultural animals or humans frequently treated by antibiotics (Wiedenbeck and Cohan, 2011).

REQUIREMENTS FOR SUCCESSFUL GENE EXCHANGE

Regardless of mechanism or environment, the success of gene transfer depends first and foremost on the proximity of donor and recipient – they must be in physical proximity, and are generally assumed to share the same niche. Genetic exchange communities are variable in taxonomic composition but usually share vector types (plasmid or transposon) and do not contain strong restriction/modification systems such that genetic exchange is more frequent (Wiedenbeck and Cohan, 2011). DNA transferred via transformation is typically short (often the length of one to several genes), which limits the chances a restriction enzyme target sequence will occur, and increases the chances of recombination in deeply divergent bacterial species (Wiedenbeck and Cohan, 2011). Plasmids transferred via conjugation are often able to carry several resistance genes in tandem (reviewed in Barlow, 2009). Once inside the recipient cell, new DNA must replicate autonomously or integrate into the chromosome of the recipient (by homology or via insertion sequences). Recombination is heavily favored if the sequence is flanked by insertion sequences as integration is therefore independent of sequence homology (Vo et al., 2010).

Integrons and transposons are now widely recognized as playing important roles in the dissemination of antibiotic resistance. Integrons are composed of three key elements: the *intI* integrase, a specific recombination site *attI* and a promoter (expertly reviewed in Stalder et al., 2012). Integrons are found chromosomally, on plasmids and transposons, and are found widely distributed in both the clinic and the environment, especially in Gram-negative bacteria. Interestingly, a class 1 integron found in an isolate of *Pseudomonas* from 15,000- to 40,000-year-old Siberian permafrost contained all the elements characteristic of modern-day clinical class 1 integrons, including being located on a transposon and containing an antibiotic resistance gene (*aadA2*, encoding resistance to streptomycin and spectinomycin; Petrova et al., 2011).

The exchange of DNA can occur passively, but may also be actively controlled. Many naturally competent species of *Streptococcus* undergo autolysis to liberate cellular DNA using the same signaling molecule that triggers DNA uptake in the surviving population (Guiral et al., 2006; Perry et al., 2009). Some genera can actively secrete DNA, including *Acinetobacter, Alcaligenes, Azotobacter, Pseudomonas, Micrococcus, Bacillus,* and *Flavobacterium* (reviewed in Thomas and Nielsen, 2005). On the flip side, bacteria also express defense mechanisms to prevent invasion by foreign DNA elements. Viral infections are prevented at the level of adsorption, injection, or by abortive infection, while restriction–modification systems and the use of sugar-non-specific nucleases target invading nucleic acids. An area of intense research is immunity mediated by clustered regularly interspaced short palindromic repeats (CRISPR)/Cas motifs, present in most archeal and many bacterial genomes (reviewed in Horvath and Barrangou, 2010).

GENE TRANSFER IN THE SOIL

While gene exchange occurs in all environments, it has been best studied in the soil. The physical properties of soil (temperature, pH, concentration of nutrients and oxygen, etc.), combined with biological factors (diversity, nature, and total microbial biomass) dictate the frequency and nature of gene transfer in this environment (Aminov, 2011). Soil bacteria typically undergo higher rates of gene transfer in areas of higher nutritional content like the rhizosphere, the phyllosphere, decaying plant and animal tissues, and manure-applied soil (van Elsas and Bailey, 2002), and are capable of transformation, transduction, and conjugation.

Transformation is the uptake and incorporation of extracellular DNA from the environment (Chen et al., 2005). Not all bacteria can become "competent" for genetic transformation [although recent reports put the number of naturally transformable strains at more than 60 (Johnsborg et al., 2007)], but both environmental organisms and clinical pathogens use this method of gene acquisition. Environmental bacteria that undergo natural transformation include species of *Pseudomonas* (most studied of which is *P. stutzeri*), species of *Acinetobacter* (notably *A. baylyi*), and the plant pathogens *Ralstonia solanacearum* and *Xylella fastidiosa* (reviewed in Seitz and Blokesch, 2012). The mineral/particulate composition of soil has been implicated in protecting naked DNA against degradation on several occasions, making transformation a viable method of gene transfer in the environment (Aminov, 2011). Transformation may also play a role in the dissemination of integron-based resistance both in the environment and in the clinic: in a study using the naturally competent environmental organism *Acinetobacter baylyi*, Domingues et al. (2012) found that DNA from integron-carrying strains of *Acinetobacter, Citrobacter, Enterobacter, Escherichia, Pseudomonas,* and *Salmonella* could confer antibiotic resistance as well as transfer integrons and transposons in a 24 h period. Furthermore, the transformation of *Acinetobacter baylyi* occurred with equal efficiency using the supernatants from heat-killed bacterial cultures; DNA purity was not important for transformation. This study is important in that it demonstrates that environmental bacteria have the capacity to acquire and replicate genes from bacteria found in clinical settings; although it does not show an historical association between antibiotic producers and the origins of clinical resistance, it demonstrates the capacity for genetic exchange between these two communities.

Transduction involves the transfer of genes via bacteriophages, and is likely an important mechanism of HGT in the environment. Bacteriophage found in soil display local tropisms, and become highly adapted to the bacteria present in their immediate environment (Vos et al., 2009). Lysogenic phage are present in approximately 30% of cultivable soil bacteria, and estimates of prevalence range from 4 to 68% in culture-independent assessments of soil (Ghosh et al., 2008). Generalized transducing phages can be isolated from *Streptomyces* sp. (Burke et al., 2001), and Ghosh et al. (2008) demonstrated that viral preparations from soil carry hybrid 16S ribosomal ribonucleic acid (rRNA) genes indicative of horizontal transfer and recombination within the community. A study of the fecal virome of swine fed the common agricultural antibiotics carbadox and ASP250 revealed that in-feed antibiotics induced prophages from gut bacteria, and induced population shifts in both the bacterial and viral populations. However, metagenomic sequencing revealed that most viromes harbored few antibiotic resistance genes (0.01% of total reads; Allen et al., 2011). In a study of bacteriophage DNA isolated from environmental water samples (including both urban sewage and river water), Colomer-Lluch et al. (2011) found a relative abundance of *bla*(TEM) and *bla*(CTX-M). Interestingly, transduction has been linked to the transfer of pathogenicity islands and virulence traits more often than resistance genes in the clinic: sub-inhibitory concentrations of ciprofloxacin have been reported to promote the mobilization and transfer of the SaPIbov1 pathogenicity island in *Staphylococcus aureus* via SOS-response-mediated transduction (Ubeda et al., 2005), and fluoroquinolones trigger the expression and dissemination of prophage genes including Shiga toxin in *Escherichia coli* H57:0157, also via SOS (Zhang et al., 2000). Given the enormous diversity of environmental phage and the relatively few viromes that have been sequenced thus far, further metagenomic exploration will provide many more examples of phage-mediated transfer of resistance in both the environment and the clinic.

The most frequent mechanism of horizontal gene transfer for antibiotic resistance genes is on plasmids and integrative conjugative elements (ICEs or conjugative transposons) via conjugation. Conjugative transfer of DNA requires physical contact between donor and recipient cells, and the formation of a pore through which DNA can pass (Thomas and Nielsen, 2005). Plasmids are classified according to their replication and partitioning systems into specific incompatibility (Inc) groups, where two plasmids belonging to the same Inc group cannot co-exist in the same bacterial cell (Shintani et al., 2010b). Antibiotic resistance genes have been found on plasmids belonging to Inc groups P, Q, N, and W, all of which are characterized by a wide host range, including both environmental and pathogenic bacteria (Popowska and Krawczyk-Balska, 2013). Plasmids of subgroup IncP-1 are highly efficient in their ability to spread via conjugation, and are also able to replicate in virtually all Gram-negative bacteria (Shintani et al., 2010a; Popowska and Krawczyk-Balska, 2013). Plasmids belonging to this Inc group often also carry genes conferring resistance against heavy metals (including Ni, Cd, Co, Cu, Hg, Pb, Zn), which can co-select for antibiotic resistance genes. Due to all these factors combined, it has been suggested that spread of multidrug resistance in soil, water and wastewater treatment plants is mainly due to IncP-1 plasmids (Popowska and Krawczyk-Balska, 2013).

Integrative conjugative elements include all self-transmissible integrative and conjugative elements, regardless of their mechanism of integration or conjugation (Wozniak and Waldor, 2010). Unlike plasmids, however, ICEs must integrate into the chromosome to be maintained. They require little sequence specificity for integration, however, and are therefore considered capable of both intracellular and intercellular transfer (Wozniak and Waldor, 2010). Since ICEs are known carriers of antibiotic resistance genes [the first known mobile element with ICE-like properties was Tn*916* carrying tetracycline resistance (Franke and Clewell, 1981)] and have broad-host range, they are potentially important links between resistance in the environment and the clinic. For example, ICE elements have recently been characterized in the genus *Frankia*, a member of the actinobacteria (Ghinet et al., 2011). Members of the actinobacteria are prolific antibiotic producers, and usually also resistant to multiple antibiotics (D'Costa et al., 2006). Gene exchange across genera on broad-host range plasmids has been demonstrated to occur in nutrient rich environments like the rhizosphere: an IncP-1 plasmid was shown to undergo high frequency conjugal transfer in bacteria belonging to the alpha, beta, and gamma Proteobacteria, as well as to *Arthrobacter* sp., a member of the actinobacteria (Molbak et al., 2007). Several low %G+C conjugative plasmids conferring resistance to sulfonamides were recently discovered in manure-spread soil (Heuer et al., 2009). This study showed not only conjugative transfer to *Escherichia coli* from the soil-based host (postulated to be *Acinetobacter* sp.), but highlights gene transfer in an environment in which the soil mobilome mixes frequently with human and animal microbiota. Furthermore, *Acinetobacter baumannii* is an environmental organism and an emerging clinical pathogen (Howard et al., 2012). Plasmids found in environmental species that can also be found in the hospital setting offer a further potential link between the environment and the clinic.

DIVERSITY OF ANTIBIOTIC RESISTANCE ELEMENTS IN WATER ENVIRONMENTS

Antibiotic resistant marine bacteria have been found as far as 522 km offshore and at depths as extreme as 8,200 m (reviewed in Aminov, 2011). Not surprisingly, antibiotic resistance and the presence of plasmids in marine bacteria tends to correlate with the degree of pollution in the environment (Aminov, 2011). Marine environments have been studied both *in situ* using metagenomic sampling methods and under laboratory conditions simulating the natural environment, and undergo all three methods of gene exchange like their counterparts in the soil (for an excellent review, see Aminov, 2011). The importance of water environments for gene exchange is that they are mixing grounds for environmental and clinical organisms. In a study examining the diversity of integron-based resistance genes in freshwater floc, Drudge et al. (2012) used a combination of PCR-based amplification (targeting the conserved regions of type I integrons) and microarray-based detection of resistance genes from the amplicons. This protocol allowed the authors to increase the sensitivity of the assay as well as to provide genomic context to resistance. The effluent from wastewater treatment plants is well-studied for similar reasons, as environmental and clinical organisms mix in this environment in the presence of high levels of pollutants like pesticides, detergents, heavy metals, and antibiotics. Szczepanowski et al. (2009) used a PCR-based approach to identify 140 clinically relevant plasmid-based antibiotic resistance genes in the metagenome of a wastewater treatment plant. In a similar study of wastewater, Parsley et al. (2010) used sequence- and function-based metagenomic approaches to identify resistance determinants from bacterial chromosomes, on plasmids and in viral metagenomes found in activated sludge from a treatment plant. Although these authors did not identify as many resistance genes as Szczepanowski et al. (2009), the diversity of sources of resistance elements emphasizes the broad range of mobile genetic elements present in these environments, and the corresponding broad reach of target organisms.

A WORD ABOUT FITNESS COSTS

Acquiring resistance genes can incur fitness costs, such that a resistance gene may not become fixed in a population unless a positive selective pressure is present (Martinez, 2012). In many soil and water environments, selective pressures are abundant due to regrettable anthropomorphic activities. However, several studies have shown that the introduction of a resistance gene does not necessarily impose a metabolic burden (reviewed in Martinez, 2012). For example, AmpC β-lactamases are usually accompanied by repressors of their expression on *Salmonella* plasmids (Verdet et al., 2000) which minimize their fitness cost. Antibiotic resistance genes are often found in conjunction with other resistance genes, such that selection for one will maintain the others in the population. Heavy metal resistance genes, and genes coding for the production of siderophores, toxin/antitoxin systems, or bacteriocins are often found on the same mobile elements as resistance genes, which become fixed in the population due to the co-selection of their beneficial counterparts, even in the absence of antibiotic selection.

LINKING THE SOIL TO THE CLINIC

The mobility of resistance genes is well-documented in both the environment and in the clinic, but tangible links between the two remain elusive. The above-mentioned examples of aminoglycoside resistance (Benveniste and Davies, 1973), CTX-M in *Kluyvera* spp. (Humeniuk et al., 2002) and *qnr* in waterborne *Vibrio*, *Shewanella*, and *Aeromonas* (Poirel et al., 2005a,b; Baquero et al., 2008) are conclusive examples of recent exchange between the environmental and clinical resistomes. Comparing the amino acid sequence of the aminoglycoside phosphotransferase APH(3′) between transposons found in Gram-negative and Gram-positive pathogens and from environmental bacteria (*Bacillus circulans* and *Streptomyces fradiae*) also indicates that they have diverged from a common ancestor (Trieu-Cuot and Courvalin, 1986). These examples provide powerful evidence that resistance is able to move from the environment into pathogens, but given the prevalence of resistance genes in environmental reservoirs, certainly more examples of transfer exist?

The acquisition of antibiotic resistance by clinic pathogens from the environment must follow the same rules as all gene transfer events: the most likely place for gene exchange is a niche shared by pathogens and environmental organisms (Wiedenbeck and Cohan, 2011). Sommer et al. (2009) used functional genomics to clone and express DNA from the human microbiome and select for resistance to various antibiotics. The healthy human microbiome is presumably in constant contact with environmental organisms, but is also exposed to pathogenic microorganisms. This approach identified several new resistance factors, but importantly also identified a number of resistance genes harbored in the aerobic gut flora of healthy individuals that are also found in major pathogens (Sommer et al., 2009). Wiedenbeck and Cohan (2011) propose screening for resistance genes in the metagenomes of other organisms from which we frequently acquire pathogens, like agricultural animals, mice, ticks, and mosquitoes, as commensal microorganisms could provide an important link to pathogens.

The most recent evidence for transfer of resistance genes between the environment and the clinic is provided by Forsberg et al. (2012). Using an innovating approach, the authors cultured multi-drug resistant Proteobacteria from the soil to enrich for resistance genes, and a metagenomic library was constructed from the enriched cells (Forsberg et al., 2012). This library was transformed into *Escherichia coli*, and selected on media containing 1 or 12 antibiotics representing sulfonamides, aminoglycosides, phenicols, β-lactams, and tetracyclines at inhibitory concentrations. Resistance was detected against all 12 antibiotics, and 110 resistance genes were identified via homology. Of the genes identified, 18 had 100% identity to entries in GenBank, and a further 32 had ≥90% homology. Importantly, 54% of resistance genes identified by this method were previously unknown, and many of which would not have been predicted to encode resistance genes by sequence alone. Moreover, seven sequences were identified with 100% identity to resistance genes in clinical pathogens, including resistance against β-lactams, tetracyclines, aminoglycosides, sulfonamides, and chloramphenicol. Although the authors could not show definitively that these genes originated in soil organisms due to the nature of their metagenomic approach, these results emphasize the importance of the soil resistome regardless of the direction of gene flow (from soil to clinic, or vice versa).

CONCLUSION

Regardless of methodology, numerous studies have confirmed the fact that antibiotic resistance genes have an environmental reservoir. However, the number and diversity of resistance genes that are found in clinical pathogens is relatively small compared to the diversity in the environment (Martinez, 2012). Why is there such a diversity of resistance genes in the environment? How are they maintained (and what role do they play) outside the clinic? What is the bottleneck preventing transfer of environmental genes to clinical pathogens (and how can we maintain it)? Due to horizontal gene transfer, the microbial world should be considered in a pan-genomic sense, where the selective pressures applied on the environmental microbiome can result in the recruitment and dissemination of resistance genes in clinical pathogens. Mapping both the environmental resistome and the associated mobilome are important steps in slowing the rise of resistant pathogens in the clinic.

ACKNOWLEDGMENTS

Gerard D. Wright is funded by the Canadian Institutes of Health Research (CIHR) and by a Canada Research Chair in Biochemistry Julie A. Perry is the recipient of a CIHR Fellowship.

REFERENCES

Allen, H. K., Looft, T., Bayles, D. O., Humphrey, S., Levine, U. Y., Alt, D., et al. (2011). Antibiotics in feed induce prophages in swine fecal microbiomes. *MBio* 2, e00260-11. doi: 10.1128/mBio.00260-11

Amann, R. I., Ludwig, W., and Schleifer, K. H. (1995). Phylogenetic identification and in situ detection of individual microbial cells without cultivation. *Microbiol. Rev.* 59, 143–169.

Aminov, R. I. (2011). Horizontal gene exchange in environmental microbiota. *Front. Microbiol.* 2:158. doi: 10.3389/fmicb.2011.00158

Aminov, R. I., and Mackie, R. I. (2007). Evolution and ecology of antibiotic resistance genes. *FEMS Microbiol. Lett.* 271, 147–161.

Avery, O. T., Macleod, C. M., and Mccarty, M. (1944). Studies on the chemical nature of the substance inducing transformation of pneumococcal types: induction of transformation by a desoxyribonucleic acid fraction isolated from Pneumococcus type III. *J. Exp. Med.* 79, 137–158. doi: 10.1084/jem.79.2.137

Baquero, F., Martinez, J. L., and Canton, R. (2008). Antibiotics and antibiotic resistance in water environments. *Curr. Opin. Biotechnol.* 19, 260–265. doi: 10.1016/j.copbio.2008.05.006

Barlow, M. (2009). What antimicrobial resistance has taught us about horizontal gene transfer. *Methods Mol. Biol.* 532, 397–411. doi: 10.1007/978-1-60327-853-9_23

Benveniste, R., and Davies, J. (1973). Aminoglycoside

antibiotic-inactivating enzymes in actinomycetes similar to those present in clinical isolates of antibiotic-resistant bacteria. *Proc. Natl. Acad. Sci. U.S.A.* 70, 2276–2280. doi: 10.1073/pnas.70.8.2276

Burke, J., Schneider, D., and Westpheling, J. (2001). Generalized transduction in *Streptomyces coelicolor*. *Proc. Natl. Acad. Sci. U.S.A.* 98, 6289–6294. doi: 10.1073/pnas.101589398

Chen, I., Christie, P. J., and Dubnau, D. (2005). The ins and outs of DNA transfer in bacteria. *Science* 310, 1456–1460. doi: 10.1126/science.1114021

Colomer-Lluch, M., Imamovic, L., Jofre, J., and Muniesa, M. (2011). Bacteriophages carrying antibiotic resistance genes in fecal waste from cattle, pigs, and poultry. *Antimicrob. Agents Chemother.* 55, 4908–4911. doi: 10.1128/AAC.00535-11

Cundliffe, E. (1989). How antibiotic-producing organisms avoid suicide. *Annu. Rev. Microbiol.* 43, 207–233. doi: 10.1146/annurev.mi.43.100189.001231

Dantas, G., and Sommer, M. O. (2012). Context matters – the complex interplay between resistome genotypes and resistance phenotypes. *Curr. Opin. Microbiol.* 15, 577–582. doi: 10.1016/j.mib.2012.07.004

D'Costa, V. M., King, C. E., Kalan, L., Morar, M., Sung, W. W., Schwarz, C., et al. (2011). Antibiotic resistance is ancient. *Nature* 477, 457–461. doi: 10.1038/nature10388

D'Costa, V. M., Mcgrann, K. M., Hughes, D. W., and Wright, G. D. (2006). Sampling the antibiotic resistome. *Science* 311, 374–377. doi: 10.1126/science.1120800

Domingues, S., Harms, K., Fricke, W. F., Johnsen, P. J., Da Silva, G. J., and Nielsen, K. M. (2012). Natural transformation facilitates transfer of transposons, integrons and gene cassettes between bacterial species. *PLoS Pathog.* 8:e1002837. doi: 10.1371/journal.ppat.1002837

Drudge, C. N., Elliott, A. V., Plach, J. M., Ejim, L. J., Wright, G. D., Droppo, I. G., et al. (2012). Diversity of integron- and culture-associated antibiotic resistance genes in freshwater floc. *Appl. Environ. Microbiol.* 78, 4367–4372. doi: 10.1128/AEM.00405-12

Forsberg, K. J., Reyes, A., Wang, B., Selleck, E. M., Sommer, M. O., and Dantas, G. (2012). The shared antibiotic resistome of soil bacteria and human pathogens. *Science* 337, 1107–1111. doi: 10.1126/science.1220761

Franke, A. E., and Clewell, D. B. (1981). Evidence for a chromosome-borne resistance transposon (Tn916) in *Streptococcus faecalis* that is capable of "conjugal" transfer in the absence of a conjugative plasmid. *J. Bacteriol.* 145, 494–502.

Ghinet, M. G., Bordeleau, E., Beaudin, J., Brzezinski, R., Roy, S., and Burrus, V. (2011). Uncovering the prevalence and diversity of integrating conjugative elements in actinobacteria. *PLoS ONE* 6:e27846. doi: 10.1371/journal.pone.0027846

Ghosh, D., Roy, K., Williamson, K. E., White, D. C., Wommack, K. E., Sublette, K. L., et al. (2008). Prevalence of lysogeny among soil bacteria and presence of 16S rRNA and trzN genes in viral-community DNA. *Appl. Environ. Microbiol.* 74, 495–502. doi: 10.1128/AEM.01435-07

Griffith, F. (1928). The significance of pneumococcal types. *J. Hyg. (Lond.)* 27, 113–159. doi: 10.1017/S0022172400031879

Guiral, S., Henard, V., Granadel, C., Martin, B., and Claverys, J. P. (2006). Inhibition of competence development in *Streptococcus pneumoniae* by increased basal-level expression of the ComDE two-component regulatory system. *Microbiology* 152, 323–331. doi: 10.1099/mic.0.28425-0

Heuer, H., Kopmann, C., Binh, C. T., Top, E. M., and Smalla, K. (2009). Spreading antibiotic resistance through spread manure: characteristics of a novel plasmid type with low %G+C content. *Environ. Microbiol.* 11, 937–949. doi: 10.1111/j.1462-2920.2008.01819.x

Horvath, P., and Barrangou, R. (2010). CRISPR/Cas, the immune system of bacteria and archaea. *Science* 327, 167–170. doi: 10.1126/science.1179555

Howard, A., O'donoghue, M., Feeney, A., and Sleator, R. D. (2012). *Acinetobacter baumannii*: an emerging opportunistic pathogen. *Virulence* 3, 243–250. doi: 10.4161/viru.19700

Hughes, V. M., and Datta, N. (1983). Conjugative plasmids in bacteria of the 'pre-antibiotic' era. *Nature* 302, 725–726. doi: 10.1038/302725a0

Humeniuk, C., Arlet, G., Gautier, V., Grimont, P., Labia, R., and Philippon, A. (2002). Beta-lactamases of *Kluyvera ascorbata*, probable progenitors of some plasmid-encoded CTX-M types. *Antimicrob. Agents Chemother.* 46, 3045–3049. doi: 10.1128/AAC.46.9.3045-3049.2002

Johnsborg, O., Eldholm, V., and Havarstein, L. S. (2007). Natural genetic transformation: prevalence, mechanisms and function. *Res. Microbiol.* 158, 767–778. doi: 10.1016/j.resmic.2007.09.004

Knapp, C. W., Dolfing, J., Ehlert, P. A., and Graham, D. W. (2010). Evidence of increasing antibiotic resistance gene abundances in archived soils since 1940. *Environ. Sci. Technol.* 44, 580–587. doi: 10.1021/es901221x

Martinez, J. L. (2008). Antibiotics and antibiotic resistance genes in natural environments. *Science* 321, 365–367. doi: 10.1126/science.1159483

Martinez, J. L. (2012). Bottlenecks in the transferability of antibiotic resistance from natural ecosystems to human bacterial pathogens. *Front. Microbiol.* 2:265. doi: 10.3389/fmicb.2011.00265

Molbak, L., Molin, S., and Kroer, N. (2007). Root growth and exudate production define the frequency of horizontal plasmid transfer in the Rhizosphere. *FEMS Microbiol. Ecol.* 59, 167–176. doi: 10.1111/j.1574-6941.2006.00229.x

Ochman, H., Lawrence, J. G., and Groisman, E. A. (2000). Lateral gene transfer and the nature of bacterial innovation. *Nature* 405, 299–304. doi: 10.1038/35012500

Parsley, L. C., Consuegra, E. J., Kakirde, K. S., Land, A. M., Harper, W. F. Jr., and Liles, M. R. (2010). Identification of diverse antimicrobial resistance determinants carried on bacterial, plasmid, or viral metagenomes from an activated sludge microbial assemblage. *Appl. Environ. Microbiol.* 76, 3753–3757. doi: 10.1128/AEM.03080-09

Perry, J. A., Jones, M. B., Peterson, S. N., Cvitkovitch, D. G., and Levesque, C. M. (2009). Peptide alarmone signalling triggers an auto-active bacteriocin necessary for genetic competence. *Mol. Microbiol.* 72, 905–917. doi: 10.1111/j.1365-2958.2009.06693.x

Petrova, M., Gorlenko, Z., and Mindlin, S. (2011). Tn5045, a novel integron-containing antibiotic and chromate resistance transposon isolated from a permafrost bacterium. *Res. Microbiol.* 162, 337–345. doi: 10.1016/j.resmic.2011.01.003

Piddock, L. J. (2006a). Clinically relevant chromosomally encoded multidrug resistance efflux pumps in bacteria. *Clin. Microbiol. Rev.* 19, 382–402. doi: 10.1128/CMR.19.2.382-402.2006

Piddock, L. J. (2006b). Multidrug-resistance efflux pumps – not just for resistance. *Nat. Rev. Microbiol.* 4, 629–636. doi: 10.1038/nrmicro1464

Poirel, L., Liard, A., Rodriguez-Martinez, J. M., and Nordmann, P. (2005a). Vibrionaceae as a possible source of Qnr-like quinolone resistance determinants. *J. Antimicrob. Chemother.* 56, 1118–1121. doi: 10.1093/jac/dki371

Poirel, L., Rodriguez-Martinez, J. M., Mammeri, H., Liard, A., and Nordmann, P. (2005b). Origin of plasmid-mediated quinolone resistance determinant QnrA. *Antimicrob. Agents Chemother.* 49, 3523–3525. doi: 10.1128/AAC.49.8.3523-3525.2005

Popowska, M., and Krawczyk-Balska, A. (2013). Broad-host-range IncP-1 plasmids and their resistance potential. *Front. Microbiol.* 4:44. doi: 10.3389/fmicb.2013.00044

Seitz, P., and Blokesch, M. (2012). Cues and regulatory pathways involved in natural competence and transformation in pathogenic and environmental Gram-negative bacteria. *FEMS Microbiol. Rev.* 37, 336–363. doi: 10.1111/j.1574-6976.2012.00353.x

Shintani, M., Takahashi, Y., Yamane, H., and Nojiri, H. (2010a). The behavior and significance of degradative plasmids belonging to Inc groups in *Pseudomonas* within natural environments and microcosms. *Microbes Environ.* 25, 253–265. doi: 10.1264/jsme2.ME10155

Shintani, M., Yamane, H., and Nojiri, H. (2010b). Behavior of various hosts of the IncP-7 carbazole-degradative plasmid pCAR1 in artificial microcosms. *Biosci. Biotechnol. Biochem.* 74, 343–349. doi: 10.1271/bbb.90675

Sommer, M. O., Dantas, G., and Church, G. M. (2009). Functional characterization of the antibiotic resistance reservoir in the human microflora. *Science* 325, 1128–1131. doi: 10.1126/science.1176950

Stalder, T., Barraud, O., Casellas, M., Dagot, C., and Ploy, M. C. (2012). Integron involvement in environmental spread of antibiotic resistance. *Front. Microbiol.* 3:119. doi: 10.3389/fmicb.2012.00119

Szczepanowski, R., Linke, B., Krahn, I., Gartemann, K. H., Gutzkow, T., Eichler, W., et al. (2009). Detection of 140 clinically relevant antibiotic-resistance genes in the plasmid metagenome of wastewater treatment plant bacteria showing reduced susceptibility to selected antibiotics. *Microbiology* 155, 2306–2319. doi: 10.1099/mic.0.028233-0

Thomas, C. M., and Nielsen, K. M. (2005). Mechanisms of, and barriers to, horizontal gene transfer between bacteria. *Nat. Rev. Microbiol.* 3, 711–721. doi: 10.1038/nrmicro1234

Trieu-Cuot, P., and Courvalin, P. (1986). Evolution and transfer of aminoglycoside resistance genes under natural conditions. *J. Antimicrob. Chemother.* 18(Suppl. C), 93–102.

Ubeda, C., Maiques, E., Knecht, E., Lasa, I., Novick, R. P., and Penades, J. R. (2005). Antibiotic-induced SOS response promotes horizontal dissemination of pathogenicity island-encoded virulence factors in staphylococci. *Mol. Microbiol.* 56, 836–844. doi: 10.1111/j.1365-2958.2005.04584.x

van Elsas, J. D., and Bailey, M. J. (2002). The ecology of transfer of mobile genetic elements. *FEMS Microbiol. Ecol.* 42, 187–197. doi: 10.1111/j.1574-6941.2002. tb01008.x

Verdet, C., Arlet, G., Barnaud, G., Lagrange, P. H., and Philippon, A. (2000). A novel integron in *Salmonella enterica* serovar Enteritidis, carrying the bla(DHA-1) gene and its regulator gene ampR, originated from *Morganella morganii. Antimicrob. Agents Chemother.* 44, 222–225. doi: 10.1128/AAC.44.1.222-225.2000

Vo, A. T., Van Duijkeren, E., Gaastra, W., and Fluit, A. C. (2010). Antimicrobial resistance, class 1 integrons, and genomic island 1 in *Salmonella* isolates from Vietnam. *PLoS ONE* 5:e9440. doi: 10.1371/journal.pone.0009440

Vos, M., Birkett, P. J., Birch, E., Griffiths, R. I., and Buckling, A. (2009). Local adaptation of bacteriophages to their bacterial hosts in soil. *Science* 325, 833. doi: 10.1126/science.1174173

Wiedenbeck, J., and Cohan, F. M. (2011). Origins of bacterial diversity through horizontal genetic transfer and adaptation to new ecological niches. *FEMS Microbiol. Rev.* 35, 957–976. doi: 10.1111/j.1574-6976.2011.00292.x

Wozniak, R. A., and Waldor, M. K. (2010). Integrative and conjugative elements: mosaic mobile genetic elements enabling dynamic lateral gene flow. *Nat. Rev. Microbiol.* 8, 552–563. doi: 10.1038/nrmicro2382

Wright, G. D. (2007). The antibiotic resistome: the nexus of chemical and genetic diversity. *Nat. Rev. Microbiol.* 5, 175–186. doi: 10.1038/nrmicro1614

Wright, G. D. (2010). Antibiotic resistance in the environment: a link to the clinic? *Curr. Opin. Microbiol.* 13, 589–594. doi: 10.1016/j.mib.2010.08.005

Zhang, X., Mcdaniel, A. D., Wolf, L. E., Keusch, G. T., Waldor, M. K., and Acheson, D. W. (2000). Quinolone antibiotics induce Shiga toxin-encoding bacteriophages, toxin production, and death in mice. *J. Infect. Dis.* 181, 664–670. doi: 10.1086/315239

Mutation in ribosomal protein S5 leads to spectinomycin resistance in *Neisseria gonorrhoeae*

Elena N. Ilina*, Maya V. Malakhova, Ivan N. Bodoev, Nina Y. Oparina, Alla V. Filimonova and Vadim M. Govorun

Research Institute of Physico-Chemical Medicine, Moscow, Russia

Edited by:
Kunihiko Nishino, Osaka University, Japan

Reviewed by:
Lilia Macovei, Harvard Medical School, USA
Petr V. Sergiev, Lomonosov Moscow State University, Russia

****Correspondence:***
Elena N. Ilina, Research Institute of Physico-Chemical Medicine, Malaya Pirogovskaya st., 1a, 119435, Moscow, Russia
e-mail: ilinaen@gmail.com

Spectinomycin remains a useful reserve option for therapy of gonorrhea. The emergence of multidrug-resistant *Neisseria gonorrhoeae* strains with decreased susceptibility to cefixime and to ceftriaxone makes it the only medicine still effective for treatment of gonorrhea infection in analogous cases. However, adoption of spectinomycin as a routinely used drug of choice was soon followed by reports of spectinomycin resistance. The main molecular mechanism of spectinomycin resistance in *N. gonorrhoeae* was C1192T substitution in 16S rRNA genes. Here we reported a Thr-24→Pro mutation in ribosomal protein S5 (RPS5) found in spectinomycin resistant clinical *N. gonorrhoeae* strain, which carried no changes in 16S rRNA. In a series of experiments, the transfer of *rpsE* gene allele encoding the mutant RPS5 to the recipient *N. gonorrhoeae* strains was analyzed. The relatively high rate of transformation [ca. 10^{-5} colony-forming units (CFUs)] indicates the possibility of spread of spectinonycin resistance within gonococcal population due to the horizontal gene transfer (HGT).

Keywords: spectinomycin resistance, spot-transformation, horizontal gene transfer, ribosomal proteins, mutations

INTRODUCTION

Neisseria gonorrhoeae is an obligate pathogen causing gonorrhea, one of the most abundant sexually transmitted diseases. The expansion of drug resistant *N. gonorrhoeae* strains is one of the global contemporary problems. The emergence and spreading of multidrug resistant (MDR) strains, which are resistant to penicillin, tetracycline, and ciprofloxacin, are reported throughout the world. In some countries, including Russia, about 50% of clinical *N. gonorrhoeae* strains identified as MDR (Kubanova et al., 2010; Allen et al., 2011). Until recently, all these strains remain susceptible to spectinomycin and to extended-spectrum cephalosporins (ceftriaxone and cefixime). Recently, *N. gonorrhoeae* strains displayed reduced susceptibility to the extended-spectrum cephalosporins. Moreover, several cases of clinical failures during the cefixime treatment have been reported (Wang et al., 2003; Heymans et al., 2012; Unemo et al., 2012). The spectinomycin remains the only antibiotic still effective in analogous cases. However, adoption of spectinomycin as the routinely used drug of choice was soon followed by reports of spectinomycin resistance (Boslego et al., 1987). The treatment of gonorrhea infection caused by extremely drug resistant (XDR) *N. gonorrhoeae* strains is very difficult, and the extended knowledge of molecular mechanisms of drug resistance is required for development of new tests needed to for routine diagnose in clinical practice.

In general, these are several mechanisms occurring in the bacteria which confer them antibiotic resistance. The most common are known to be drug inactivation, efflux-pumping of the drug out of the cell, and target modification due to single nucleotide change polymorphisms (SNPs) mainly (Davies and Davies, 2010). A bacterial strain can acquire resistance either by mutation of its own genes or by the uptake of exogenous genes by horizontal transfer from other microbes. Within bacterial population horizontal gene transfer (HGT) occurs via conjugation, transformation and transduction. With regards to neisseria genus these bacteria are naturally transformable and are capable to exchange their genetic material with high frequency (Koomey, 1998). This property leads to the rapid dissemination of antibiotic resistance markers and to the panmictic structure of the gonococcal and meningococcal populations.

Spectinomycin belongs to an aminocyclitol antibiotic class which blocks biosynthesis of bacterial proteins. After entering the bacterial cells, spectinomycin binds a ribosome beneath the 34 helix of 16S rRNA and interrupts elongation of the polypeptide during protein synthesis apparently preventing the translocation of the peptidyl tRNA from the A-site to the P-site (Carter et al., 2000; Borovinskaya et al., 2007).

Various bacteria demonstrate spectinomycin resistance, which results from three different mechanisms. The most frequent mechanism is the drug inactivation by adenylylation. Until now a diverse number of adenyltransferases, which exhibit the spectinomycin resistant (Spt-R) phenotype, was described (Shaw et al., 1993). One group of enzymes referred as AAD(3″)(9) [or ANT(3″)(9)] confers combined resistance to spectinomycin and streptomycin. These enzymes were found in a variety of gram-negative bacteria (Yamada et al., 1968; Hollingshead and Vapnek, 1985; Kehrenberg et al., 2005) and also in gram-positive bacteria (Clark et al., 1999). The other group of adenyltransferase referred as AAD(9) [or ANT(9)] confers the Spt-R phenotype only (LeBlanc et al., 1991).

On the other hand, the spectinomycin resistance can result from alteration of 30S subunit of bacterial ribosome due to mutations in chromosomal genes encoding ribosomal RNAs or proteins. Thus, mutations in the spectinomycin binding region of helix 34 of 16S rRNA encompassing the cross-linked positions from 1063 to 1066 and from 1190 to 1193 (in *Escherichia coli* numbering) lead to high level resistance to spectinomycin (Sigmund et al., 1984; Brink et al., 1994). These mutations were discovered for various bacteria such as *Chlamydia psittaci, Borrelia burgdorferi, E. coli, Pasteurella multocida* (Johanson and Hughes, 1995; Binet and Maurelli, 2005; Criswell et al., 2006; Kehrenberg and Schwarz, 2007) including *N. gonorrhoeae* and *N. meningitidis* (Maness et al., 1974; Galimand et al., 2000). Although ribosomal protein S5 (RPS5) is not involved in spectinomycin binding, it is located very close to the antibiotic binding site (within 5 A°) (Wirmer and Westhof, 2006). Accordingly, it has been found that mutations in RPS5 can lead to spectinomycin resistance in *E. coli* (Funatsu et al., 1972; Bilgin et al., 1990) and in *P. multocida* (Kehrenberg and Schwarz, 2007).

Until recently, the only 16S rRNA substitutions were found in Spt-R bacteria from *Neisseria* genus (Maness et al., 1974; Galimand et al., 2000). In this study, we reported the discovery of isolated mutation in RPS5 in Spt-R clinical *N. gonorrhoeae* strain, confirmed by Unemo et al. (2013), and estimate the potential of Spt-R horizontal spread. We established that the 10^{-5} colony-forming units (CFU) from transformation experiments represents a high risk of spectinomycin resistance spread within gonococcal population.

MATERIALS AND METHODS

BACTERIAL STRAINS

N. gonorrhoeae clinical isolates were collected as a part of previous study (Ilina et al., 2008) and stored at a temperature of −80°C. The studied *N. gonorrhoeae* clinical isolates and strains are shown in **Table 1**.

For any manipulations, gonococci were cultivated on the BBL™ GC agar base (Becton Dickinson & Co, USA) supplemented with 1% BBL™ IsoVitaleX™ Enrichment (Becton Dickinson & Co, USA) at 37°C in a humid atmosphere with 5% CO_2 during 20–24 h.

PHENOTYPIC CHARACTERIZATION

Susceptibility testing to penicillin G, tetracycline, ciprofloxacin, spectinomycin and ceftriaxone was performed by agar dilution method in accordance with CLSI recommendations (CLSI document M100-S17, 2007). All antibiotics were manufactured by Sigma, USA. *N. gonorrhoeae* strain ATCC 49226 was used as a control.

GONOCOCCAL TRANSFORMATION

Spot-transformation of gonococci was performed as described (Dillard, 2011). Briefly, 200 ng of amplified DNA fragments in a 10 µl volume were placed into spots (diameter approximately 1.5 cm) on a pre-warmed (37°C) GC base agar plate. The spot was allowed to soak into the plate. Then piliated colonies of *N. gonorrhoeae* recipient strains were streaked across the plate through the DNA spots. After overnight incubation at 37°C in a humid atmosphere with 5% CO_2, colonies were swabbed from the spot with a Dacron swab and re-suspended in 100 µl of storage medium (50% BBL™ Brain Heart Infusion, Becton Dickinson & Co, USA, 30% Fetal Bovine Serum, Gibco, USA, 20% glycerin, Sigma, USA). This suspension of cells was then diluted and plated on both GC base agar alone, and GC base agar supplemented with 64 mg/L of spectinomycin. These plates were incubated at 37°C in a humid atmosphere with 5% CO_2 for one to two days, and individual transformants were picked up from spectinomycin supplemented plate. Selected colonies were cultivated once again on spectinomycin supplemented plates; the obtained

Table 1 | Characteristics of gonococci involved into current investigation.

Name	Description	MICs (mg/L) for					Serotype	NG-MAST sequence type
		PEN	TET	CIP	SPT	CRO		
e03.04	Clinical isolate	0.015	< 0.03	0.001	32–64	< 0.002	P1B3	5187
NG3	Clinical strain derived from e03.04 isolate	0.015–0.03	0.03–0.06	0.001–0.002	4–8	0.0005–0.001	P1B3	5187
NG3.1	Clinical strain derived from e03.04 isolate	< 0.015	0.03–0.06	0.0005–0.001	64–128	0.0005–0.001	P1B3	5187
NG3.2	Clinical strain derived from e03.04 isolate	0.03–0.06	0.03–0.06	0.0005–0.001	64–128	0.001–0.002	P1B3	5187
NG7	Clinical strain, using as a recipient for spot-transformation	0.12–0.25	0.015	0.001	16–32	0.002	P1B3	8633
NG94	Clinical strain, using as a recipient for spot-transformation	0.015–0.03	< 0.03	0.001	16–32	< 0.002	P1B3	8401

PEN, penicillin; TET, tetracycline; CIP, ciprofloxacin; SPT, spectinomycin; CRO, ceftriaxone.

N. gonorrhoeae strains were stored at −80°C. Transformation frequency was calculated as the number of spectinomycin-resistant colony-forming units (SPT^r CFU/ml) per total CFU (CFU/ml).

GENOTYPIC CHARACTERIZATION USES FEW METHODS: PCR AND SEQUENCING AND MALDI-TOF MS

Total genomic DNA from tested *N. gonorrhoeae* strains was isolated by "DNA express" kit (Lytech Ltd, Russia). When necessary, the prepared DNA samples were stored at a temperature of −20°C.

Conventional PCR was done using the genomic DNA as a template and oligonucleotide primers described in **Table 2**. All primers were newly designed using the Oligo_6.31 software (Molecular Biology Insights Inc., USA) and sequences of *N. gonorrhoeae* strain FA1090 (GenBank accession number is NC_002946). Amplification was carried out in 10 μl of 66 mM Tris-HCl pH 9.0; 16.6 mM $(NH_4)_2SO_4$; 2.5 mM $MgCl_2$; 0.2 mM of each dNTP; 5 pmol of each primer (**Table 2**) and 1 unit of TaqPolymerase (Fermentas, Lithuania) under the following conditions: 94°C for 20 s, 60°C for 20 s, and 72°C for 15 s, in 35 cycles. A programmed thermocycler TETRAD DNA ENGINE (MJ Research Inc.) was used. The amplification products were analyzed by electrophoresis in 2% agarose gel.

For further sequencing analysis dephosphorylation of the 5′-end phosphate groups of dNTPs and cleavage of primers in the post-amplification reaction mixture was done by incubation with 0.5 U of shrimp alkaline phosphatase and 0.1 U of exonuclease I (both enzymes from Fermentas, Lithuania) for 20 min at 37°C, followed with inactivation by heating at 85°C for 10 min. Sequence analysis of 16S rRNA genes as well as genes cording the ribosomal proteins S5, S4, and S8 was performed with dedicated primers (**Table 2**) by the modified Sanger method using the ABI Prism™ BigDye® Terminator v. 3.1 Cycle Sequencing Kit and 3730xl DNA Analyzer (Applied Biosystems, USA) according to the manufacturer's instruction. Analysis of the nucleotide sequences as well as deduced amino acid sequences was done using the Vector NTI Advance v. 9.0 software (Infomarks Incorporation, USA).

N. gonorrhoeae multi-antigen typing (NG–MAST) was performed as originally described (Martin et al., 2004). Sequence types were identified via NG-MAST (http://www.ng-mast.net) websites.

The rapid identification of A70C nucleotide substitution in *rpsE* gene, leading to Thr-24→Pro amino acid mutation in RPS5, was done by primer extension reaction followed by MALDI ToF mass spectrometry. For this, PCR was performed as mentioned above with primers form **Table 2**. The dephosphorylation of the 5′-end phosphate groups of dNTPs in the post-amplification reaction mixture was carried out by incubation with 0.5 U of shrimp alkaline phosphatase (Fermentas, Lithuania) for 20 min at 37°C, followed by inactivation of the enzyme by heating for 10 min at 85°C. After that amplicon was used as template in thermocyclic primer extension reaction, carried out in 20 μL of the mixture of 66 mM Tris-HCl pH 9.0; 16.6 mM $(NH_4)_2SO_4$; 2.5 mM $MgCl_2$;

Table 2 | List of primers selected for PCR and sequencing of *N. gonorrhoeae* genes encoding 16S rRNAs, and ribosomal proteins S4, S5, and S8.

Genetic characterization of selected *N. gonorrhoeae* strains

Target	Primers for PCR, 5′-3′ sequence(amplicon length)	Primers for sequencing, 5′-3′ sequence
1st copy of 16S rRNA	aaccgatgaccccctgcttg; gaaaaatgcatggcaggccg (2194 bp)	aaccgatgaccccctgcttg
2nd copy of 16S rRNA	aaccgatgaccccctgcttg; accgtaaccgaatgccccctg (2409 bp)	tgacgtgtgaagccctggtcataa
3rd copy of 16S rRNA	aaccgatgaccccctgcttg; gcaaacccatgacatttacc (2435 bp)	acgctaccaagcaatcaagttgcc
4th copy of 16S rRNA	aaccgatgaccccctgcttg; acgggatcgggaacgaaaac (2432 bp)	tcatcggccgccgatattggcaac
RPS4 (rpsD gene)	tattaaaggtccaggtccaggtcg; catggatgacagtaagatacggcg (954 bp)	as for PCR
RPS5 (rpsE gene)	cgtgcacatgcacgatgagattca; tgagaaggctaaagcagcaggtgt (727 bp)	as for PCR
RPS8 (rpsH gene)	tcaatccattcctcgtaatgcggc; tttacttctacaccagcgggaacc (637 bp)	as for PCR
Genomic DNA fragment for spot transformation	tcaaagcaactgtaggtcgg; tgcgttctggtgctaaaggc (12931 bp)	

Identification of RPS5 Thr-24→Pro mutant strains

Target	Primers for PCR, 5′-3′ sequence (amplicon length)	Primer for primer extension (minisequencing) reaction, 5′-3′ sequence, molecular weight	Composition of dNTP and ddNTP mix	Predicted molecular weight of primer extension reaction products for wild type	Predicted molecular weight of primer extension reaction products for mutant type
A70C mutation in *rpsE* gene	cgtgcacatgcacgatgagattca; tgagaaggc-taaagcagcaggtgt (727 bp)	gacgacctttaactactttgg (6397 Da)	dG, ddT	6685 Da (primer + ddT)	7014 Da (primer + dG +ddT)

The scheme of identification of A70C mutation in rpsE gene by primer extension reaction followed by mass spectrometry measuring is also presented.

0.2 mM of each dGTP and ddTTP, 10 pmol of internal primer (see **Table 2**) and 2 units of TermiPol DNA Polymerase (Solis Biodyne, Estonia) according to the followed profiling: 94°C for 20 s, 58°C for 20 s, and 72°C for 15 s, in 70 cycles.

The products from primer extension reaction were purified using the SpectroCLEAN Kit (Sequenom, USA) according to the manufacturer's instruction.

An aliquote (0.2–1 μL) of purified products from primer extension reaction was spotted onto a matrix, which was preliminarily dried on the MALDI target AnchorChip™ with 400 μm diameter of anchor sports (Bruker Daltonics, Germany). The matrix employed was a saturated solution of 3-hydroxypicolinic acid (Fluka, Germany) in a 1:1 acetonitrile/water mixture (Merck, Germany) mixed with 0.4 M dibasic ammonium citrate (Fluka, Germany) in 9:1 vol. ratio. All solvents were of quality suitable for mass spectrometry. Mass spectra were collected on a Microflex LT MALDI ToF mass spectrometer (Bruker Daltonics, Germany) that was operated in the positive linear mode. A 337 nm nitrogen laser with the 9 Hz pulse frequency was used. Mass spectrometer parameters were optimized for the range of m/z values from 1000 to 10,000, using a peptide standards set for calibration. Each mass spectrum was collected at 30 laser pulses at constant laser power and constant threshold value, in order to enhance the resolution.

ACCESSION NUMBERS

DNA sequences of *rspE* gene alleles of *N. gonorrhoeae* strains NG3, NG3.1, and NG3.2 were deposited into GenBank [accession numbers KF021591, KF021592, and KF021593, respectively].

RESULTS AND DISCUSSION

In this study we identified a molecular mechanism responsible for spectinomycin resistance in gonococci. As a part of unrelated experiment, *N. gonorrhoeae* strains with Spt-R phenotype were occasionally isolated. They were derived from clinical isolate e03.04 belonged to Por1B3 serotype. Collected in 2004 it was identified as susceptible to penicillin, tetracycline, ciprofloxacin, and ceftriaxon. Spectinomycin MIC was defined as 32-64 mg/L, which corresponded to intermediate resistant (Spt-I) phenotype. When the susceptibility profile of this isolate was retested in 2008 two colonies emerged on the plate supplemented with 64 mg/L of spectinomycin. Each colony was seeded once again on plates with the same antibiotic concentration, and then on the plates with 128 mg/L of spectinomycin. It was a poor growth on plates with 128 mg/L of spectinomycin, so two clones grown well under the 64 mg/L of spectinomycin were stored.

It should be noted that neither one of other *N. gonorrhoeae* isolates tested in this experiment nor the same e03.04 clinical isolate examined in repeats revealed any additional colonies survived under 64 mg/L of spectinomycin. Thus we have considered two occasionally isolated Spt-R clones as a small fraction of heterogeneous e03.04 clinical isolate. The collected strains were designated as NG3.1 and NG3.2. Gonococci derived from e03.04 isolate susceptible to spectinomycin treatment were also collected and stored as NG3 *N. gonorrhoeae* clinical strain.

Susceptibility testing data for clinical e03.04 isolate as well as for selected *N. gonorrhoeae* strains is presented in **Table 1**. In accordance with NG-MAST scheme all of them belonged to the same 5187 sequence type that supported the assumption of a common origin of the strains studied. Since, the only previously reported mechanism for Spt-R gonococci was C1192T mutation in 16S rRNA gene (Maness et al., 1974; Galimand et al., 2000), we have sequenced all four copies of 16S rRNA genes located in *N. gonorrhoeae* genomic DNA (for the number of rRNA genes copies see rrnDB database, http://ribosome.mmg.msu.edu/rrndb/index.php). For each tested strain, all four copies of 16S rRNA genes were found identical. Indeed, the 1192 position as well as a locus encoding for the 34 helix of 16S rRNA, which forms the spectinomycin-binding site of ribosome (Carter et al., 2000; Wirmer and Westhof, 2006) possessed the wild-type sequence in NG3 strain as well as in NG3.1 and NG3.2 ones. So, we have proposed that other molecules located close by to the ribosomal spectinomycin-binding site could be involved in formation of Spt-R phenotype.

The crystal structure of the 30S subunit of bacterial ribosome from *E. coli* in complex with spectinomycin (Carter et al., 2000) was taken into account and the ribosomal proteins S4, S5, and S8 were picked up for further examination due to their vicinity to a spectinomycin-binding site. Accordingly, *rpsD*, *rpsE*, and *rpsH* genes were amplified and sequenced. No differences were found between *rpsD*, and *rpsH* genes. However, both Spt-R *N. gonorrhoeae* strains (NG3.1 and NG3.2) carried the same A70C mutation in *rpsE* genes, leading to Thr-24→Pro amino acid substitution at RPS5, which mapped to Ser-22 residue of RPS5 from *E. coli* (**Figure 1**).

The 19–33 loop of RPS5 is known to be RNA binding site, and is the most frequent zone for location of mutations related

```
             1                                                50
ATCC49226    MAKHEIEERG DGLIEKMVAV NRVTKVVKGG RIMAFSALTV VGDGDGRIGM
   FA1090    MAKHEIEERG DGLIEKMVAV NRVTKVVKGG RIMAFSALTV VGDGDGRIGM
      NG3    MAKHEIEERG DGLIEKMVAV NRVTKVVKGG RIMAFSALTV VGDGDGRIGM
    NG3.1    MAKHEIEERG DGLIEKMVAV NRVPKVVKGG RIMAFSALTV VGDGDGRIGM
    NG3.2    MAKHEIEERG DGLIEKMVAV NRVPKVVKGG RIMAFSALTV VGDGDGRIGM
  NM_MC58    MAKHEIEERG DGLIEKMVAV NRVTKVVKGG RIMAFSALTV VGDGDGRIGM
   EC_K12    MA-H-IEKQA GELQEKLIAV NRVSKTVKGG RIFSFTALTV VGDGNGRVGF
  PM_1398    MA-N-IEKQA GELQEKLIAV NRVSKTVKGG RIMSFTALTV VGDGNGRVGF
```

FIGURE 1 | Multiple alignment of RPS5 sequences of NG3, NG3.1, and NG3.2 strains. The Thr-24→Pro mutation is bolded. Deduced amino acid sequences of RPS5 of wild-type *N. gonorrhoeae* (ATCC49226, FA1090), *N. meningitidis* (NM_MC58), *E. coli* (EC_K12), and *P. multocida* (PM_1398) are also presented. Regions involved in formation of resistance to spectinomycin are underlined [according to Davies et al. (1998); Kehrenberg and Schwarz (2007)].

to spectinomycin resistance (Funatsu et al., 1972; Wirmer and Westhof, 2006; Kehrenberg and Schwarz, 2007). Mostly, RPS5 mutations associated with Spt-R phenotype occur simultaneously with 16S rRNA changes. However, the isolated Ser-22→Pro RPS5 mutation in resistant to spectinomycine *E. coli* strain was also described (Wilcox et al., 2001). Basing on this knowledge, we have suggested that the Thr-24→Pro substitution found in RPS5 from NG3.1 and NG3.2 *N. gonorrhoeae* strains confer the Spt-R phenotype.

As an argument, that the single Thr-24→Pro mutation in RPS5 can support a Spt-R phenotype alone, we performed a transformation of spectinomycin sensitive *N. gonorrhoeae* strains by the exogenic DNA fragment contained mutant *rpsE* gene. Furthermore, the experiments described below demonstrated a potential role of HGT in spread of spectinomycin resistance.

The 12931 bp fragments of *N. gonorrhoeae* chromosomal DNA, which include whole *rpsE* gene and the nearest DNA uptake sequences (DUS12, 5′ atgccgtctgaa 3′) on their ends were amplified with primers indicated in **Table 2**. It was done using the NG3 (wild type) and NG3.1 (mutant) genomic DNAs as templates. The presence of DUS12 is known to be necessary for DNA recognition and uptake and therefore, mediates an increase in transformation efficiency (Duffin and Seifert, 2010).

Two different *N. gonorrhoeae* strains—NG7, and NG94, susceptible to spectinomycin were chosen as recipients. For each recipient, the spot transformation by purified amplified DNA fragment contained mutant (or wild) variant of *rpsE* gene was carried out. The principal scheme of an experiment is represented in **Figure 2**. The transformation of recipients by a DNA fragment carried a wild variant of *rpsE* gene was used as a negative control. Each experiment was repeated in triplicate.

As a result, 74.7 ± 5.7 and 15.6 ± 2.5 colonies emerged on GC agar plates supplemented with 64 mg/L of spectinomycin and derived from NG7 and NG94 bacterial cells transformed by mutant *rpsE* gene, respectively (**Table 3**). Bacterial cells transformed by DNA fragment carried wild type of *rpsE* gene formed no colonies on spectinomycin supplemented GC agar plates. Transformation frequency calculated as the number of SPT^r CFU per total CFU was found $2.2 \pm 0.4 \times 10^{-5}$ and $1.7 \pm 0.2 \times 10^{-5}$ for NG7 and NG94 *N. gonorrhoeae* strains, respectively.

Each transformant survived after a re-cultivation on spectinomycin supplemented (64 mg/L) agar plates was tested by sequencing. All tested strains carried A70C mutation in *rpsE* gene identical to NG3.1 and NG3.2 *N. gonorrhoeae* strains and leading to Thr-24→Pro amino acid substitution in RPS5. Otherwise, in accordance with NG MAST, they belonged to the same sequence types as the recipient strains from which they originated.

The spectinomycin MICs were measured for the transformants derived both from NG7 and NG94 *N. gonorrhoeae* recipient strains. In all cases, spectinomycin MICs increased fourfold (from 16–32 mg/L to 64–128 mg/L) and became identical to the ones of NG3.1 and NG3.2 *N. gonorrhoeae* strains.

Described experiments verified that single Thr-24→Pro amino acid substitution in RPS5 confers the Spc-R phenotype of *N. gonorrhoeae* strains.

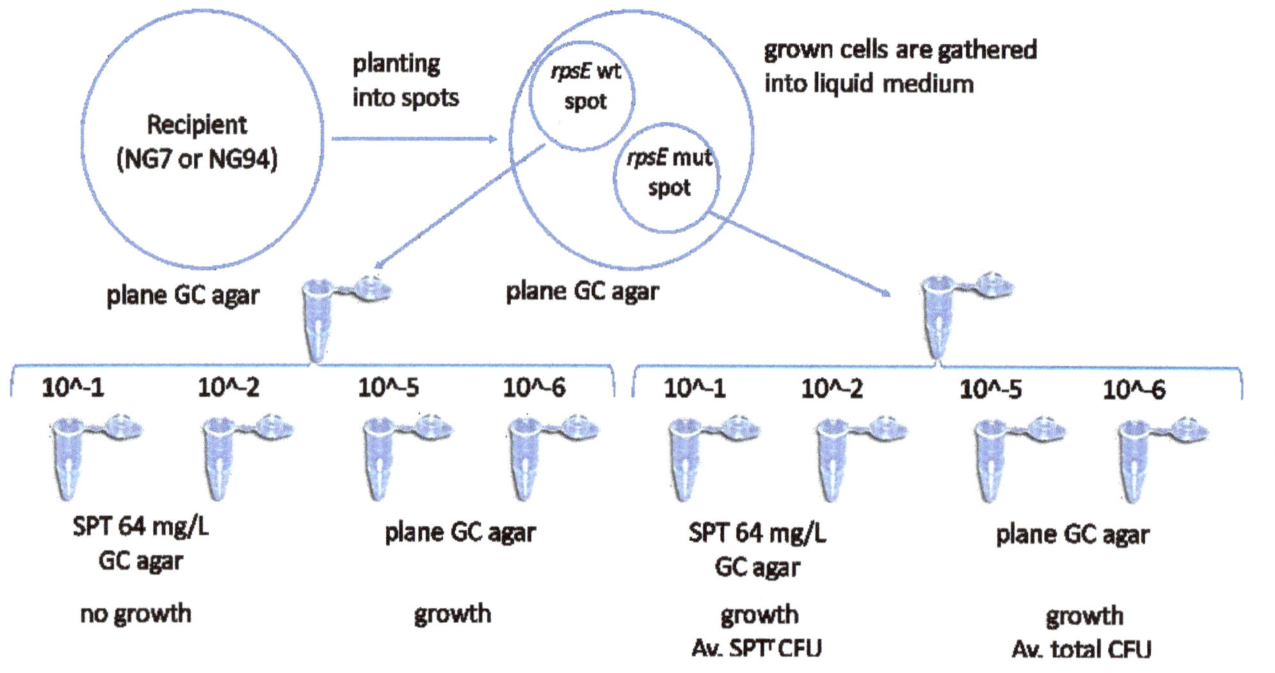

FIGURE 2 | The principal scheme of sport transformation. Amplified DNA fragments carried mutant (mut) and wild type (wt) of *rpsE* gene cording the ribosomal protein S5 (RPS5) were placed in spots on a GC base agar plate. Then piliated colonies of recipient strains (NG7 and NG94) were streaked across the plate through the DNA spots. After overnight incubation, bacterial cells were swabbed from the spots into a liquid medium, diluted and plated on both GC base agar alone, and GC base agar supplemented with 64 mg/L of spectinomycin (SPT). The individual transformants emerged on SPT-supplemented plates were picked up for further examination. Colony-forming units (CFUs) were counted on each plate.

Table 3 | The calculated results of transformation experiments.

Recipient	Av. SPT^r CFUs	Av. SPT^r CFU/ml	Av total CFU/ml	Transformation efficiency
NG7	74.7 ± 5.7	$3.5 \pm 0.4 \times 10^4$	$1.6 \pm 0.5 \times 10^9$	$2.2 \pm 0.4 \times 10^{-5}$
NG94	15.6 ± 2.5	$0.8 \pm 0.2 \times 10^4$	$4.7 \pm 0.2 \times 10^8$	$1.7 \pm 0.2 \times 10^{-5}$

An average data from three replicas is presented.

Furthermore, the transformation efficiency was found relatively high (ca. 10^{-5}) and was not statistically different between both recipient strains. This finding supports the statement that the HGT through the natural transformation permits movement of mutant allele of *rpsE* gene and increases the opportunity for the spread of spectinonycin resistance within gonococcal population.

The RPS5 mutation we verified here appeared to be the same that was described for *N. gonorrhoeae* WHO A strain (Unemo et al., 2013). This mutation results in low-level spectinomycin resistance in gonococci that agrees with our conclusion.

The main issue is that in this study, conducted independently the mutant allele of *rpsE* gene was found in clinical *N. gonorrhoeae* strain isolated in Russia. This emphasizes that the described molecular mechanism of Spt-R phenotype formation is a universal one and spreads worldwide.

To extend the knowledge of frequency of RPS5 Thr-24→Pro mutants the entire laboratory collection of *N. gonorrhoeae* genomic DNA ($n = 1131$) acquired since 2002–2008 years was analyzed. The majority of them ($n = 1113$) were susceptible to spectinomycin, and the 18 strains revealed the Spt-I phenotype (MICs = 32–64 mg/L). Keeping in mind that NG3.1 and NG3.2 strains possessed Thr-24→Pro mutation in RPS5 were found occasionally as a small fraction of a wild population, we did not exclude susceptible to spectinomycin gonococci from the examination.

No more mutant *N. gonorrhoeae* strains have been found. It seems the tested Thr-24→Pro substitution in RPS5 is very rare among gonococci. This may reflect the uncommon use of spectinomycin in therapy of gonorrhea. On the other hand, we cannot deny that gonococci with mutation in ribosomal protein could be somehow defective in their survival and population spreading. Undoubtedly, fitness cost due to such mutation requires further careful investigation.

Nevertheless, our study is an additional evidence of the existing of clinical *N. gonorrhoeae* strains with moderate spectinomycin resistance due to isolated mutations in RPS5. It is very important in terms of the surveillance and the therapy of gonococcal infection. The extended knowledge of the potential mutations responsible for resistant phenotypes is essential in the development of new tests suitable in clinical setting, which aim to establish the correct antimicrobial therapy.

ACKNOWLEDGMENTS

We sincerely thank V. A. Karpov for the oligonucleotide primers synthesis; and M. M. Chukin for the assistance with the sequence instrumentation. We also declare that current investigation was first presented during the 18th International Pathogenic Neisseria Conference, Würzburg, Germany, 2012.

TRANSPARENCY DECLARATION

This research work received financial support from the Ministry of Health of the Russian Federation (Development Contract No 06/311 from 30/05/2008).

REFERENCES

Allen, V. G., Farrell, D. J., Rebbapragada, A., Tan, J., Tijet, N., Perusini, S. J., et al. (2011). Molecular analysis of antimicrobial resistance mechanisms in *Neisseria gonorrhoeae* isolates from Ontario, Canada. *Antimicrob. Agents Chemother.* 55, 703–712. doi: 10.1128/AAC.00788-10

Bilgin, N., Richter, A. A., Ehrenberg, M., Dahlberg, A. E., and Kurland,C. G. (1990). Ribosomal RNA and protein mutants resistant to spectinomycin. *EMBO J.* 9, 735–739.

Binet, R., and Maurelli, A. T. (2005). Fitness cost due to mutations in the 16S rRNA associated with spectinomycin resistance in *Chlamydia psittaci 6BC. Antimicrob. Agents. Chemother.* 49, 4455–4464. doi: 10.1128/AAC.49.11.4455-4464.2005

Borovinskaya, M. A., Shoji, S., Holton, J. M., Fredrick, K., and Cate, J. H. D. (2007). A steric block in translation caused by the antibiotic spectinomycin. *ACS Chem. Biol.* 2, 545–552. doi: 10.1021/cb700100n

Boslego, J. W., Tramont, E. C., Takafuji, E. T., Diniega, B. M., Mitchell, B. S., Small, J. W., et al. (1987). Effect of spectinomycin use on the prevalence of spectinomycin-resistant and of penicillinase-producing *Neisseria gonorrhoeae. N. Engl. J. Med.* 317, 272–278. doi: 10.1056/NEJM198707303170504

Brink, M. F., Brink, G., Verbeet, M. P., and de Boer, H. A. (1994). Spectinomycin interacts specifically with the residues G1064 and C1192 in 16S rRNA, thereby potentially freezing this molecule into an inactive conformation. *Nucleic Acids Res.* 22, 325–331.

Carter, A. P., Clemons, W. M., Brodersen, D. E., Morgan-Warren, R. J., Wimberly, B. T., and Ramakrishnan, V. (2000). Functional insights from the structure of the 30S ribosomal subunit and its interactions with antibiotics. *Nature* 407, 340–348. doi: 10.1038/35030019

Clark, N. C., Olsvik, Ø., Swenson, J. M., Spiegel, C. A., and Tenover, F. C. (1999). Detection of a streptomycin/spectinomycin adenylyltransferase gene (aadA) in *Enterococcus faecalis. Antimicrob. Agents Chemother.* 43, 157–160.

CLSI document M100-S17. (2007). Performance standards for antimicrobialsusceptibilitytesting; seventeenth informational supplement. *Clin. Lab. Stand. Inst.* 27, 1–182.

Criswell, D., Tobiason, V. L., Lodmell, J. S., and Samuels, D. S. (2006). Mutations conferring aminoglycoside and spectinomycin resistance in *Borrelia burgdorferi. Antimicrob. Agents Chemother.* 50, 445–452. doi: 10.1128/AAC.50.2.445-452.2006

Davies, C., Bussiere, D. E., Golden, B. L., Porter, S. J., Ramakrishnan,V., and White, S. W. (1998). Ribosomal proteins S5 and L6: high-resolution crystal structures and roles in protein synthesis and antibiotic resistance. *J. Mol. Biol.* 279, 873–888. doi: 10.1006/jmbi.1998.1780

Davies, J., and Davies, D. (2010). Origins and evolution of antibiotic resistance. *Microbiol. Mol. Biol. Rev.* 74, 417–433. doi: 10.1128/MMBR.00016-10

Dillard, J. P. (2011). "Genetic Manipulation of *Neisseria gonorrhoeae*," in *Current Protocols in Microbiology*, (Wiley Online Library). Available online at: wileyonlinelibrary.com

Duffin, P. M., and Seifert, H. S. (2010). DNA uptake sequence-mediated enhancement of transformation in *Neisseria gonorrhoeae* is strain dependent. *J. Bacteriol.* 192, 4436–4444. doi: 10.1128/JB.00442-10

Funatsu, G., Schiltz, E., and Wittmann, H. G. (1972). Ribosomal proteins. XXVII. Localization of the amino acid exchanges in protein S5 from two *Escherichia coli* mutants resistant to spectinomycin. *Mol. Gen. Genet.* 114, 106–111. doi: 10.1007/BF00332781

Galimand, M., Gerbaud, G., and Courvalin, P. (2000). Spectinomycin resistance in *Neisseria spp.* due to mutations in 16S rRNA. *Antimicrob. Agents Chemother.* 44, 1365–1366. doi: 10.1128/AAC.44.5.1365-1366.2000

Heymans, R., Bruisten, S. M., Golparian, D., Unemo, M., de Vries, H. J., and van Dam, A.P. (2012). Clonally related *Neisseria gonorrhoeae* isolates with decreased susceptibility to the extended-spectrum cephalosporin cefotaxime in Amsterdam, the Netherlands. *Antimicrob. Agents Chemother.* 56, 1516–1522. doi: 10.1128/AAC.05481-11

Hollingshead, S., and Vapnek, D. (1985). Nucleotide sequence analysis of a gene encoding a streptomycin/spectinomycin adenyltransferase. *Plasmid* 13, 17–30.

Ilina, E. N., Vereshchagin, V. A., Borovskaya, A. D., Malakhova, M. V., Sidorenko, S. V., Al Khafaji, N. C., et al. (2008). Relation between genetic markers of drug resistance and susceptibility profile of clinical Neisseria gonorrhoeae strains. *Antimicrob. Agents Chemother.* 52, 2175–2182. doi: 10.1128/AAC.01420-07

Johanson, U., and Hughes, D. (1995). A new mutation in 16S rRNA of *Escherichia coli* conferring spectinomycin resistance. *Nucleic Acids Res.* 23, 464–466. doi: 10.1093/nar/23.3.464

Kehrenberg, C., Catry, B., Haesebrouck, F., de Kruif, A., and Schwarz, S. (2005). Novel Spectinomycin/Streptomycin Resistance Gene, aadA14, from Pasteurella multocida, *Antimicrob. Agents Chemother.* 49, 3046–3049. doi: 10.1128/AAC.49.7.3046-3049.2005

Kehrenberg, C., and Schwarz, S. (2007). Mutations in 16S rRNA and ribosomal protein S5 associated with high-level spectinomycin resistance in *Pasteurella multocida*. *Antimicrob. Agents Chemother.* 51, 2244–2246. doi: 10.1128/AAC.00229-07

Koomey, M. (1998). Competence for natural transformation in *Neisseria gonorrhoeae*: a model system for studies of horizontal gene transfer. *APMIS Suppl.* 84, 56–61.

Kubanova, A., Frigo, N., Kubanov, A., Sidorenko, S., Lesnaya, I., Polevshikova, S., et al. (2010). The Russian gonococcal antimicrobial susceptibility programme (RU-GASP)-national resistance prevalence in 2007 and 2008, and trends during 2005–2008. *Euro Surveill.* 15, pii: 19533.

LeBlanc, D. J., Lee, L. N., and Inamine, J. M. (1991). Cloning and nucleotide base sequence analysis of a spectinomycin adenyltransferase AAD (9) determinant from *Enterococcus faecalis*. *Antimicrob. Agents Chemother.* 35, 1804–1810. doi: 10.1128/AAC.35.9.1804

Maness, M. J., Foster, G. C., and Sparling, P. F. (1974). Ribosomal resistance to streptomycin and spectinomycin in *Neisseria gonorrhoeae*. *J. Bacteriol.* 120, 1293–1299.

Martin, I. M. C., Ison, C. A., Aanensen, D. M., Fenton, K. A., and Spratt, B. G. (2004). Rapid sequence-based identification of gonococcal transmission clusters in a large metropolitan area. *J. Infect. Dis.* 189, 1497–1505. doi: 10.1086/383047

Shaw, K. J., Rather, P. N., Hare, R. S., and Miller, G. H. (1993). Molecular genetics of aminoglycoside resistance genes and familial relationships of the aminoglycoside-modifying enzymes. *Microbiol. Rev.* 57, 138–163.

Sigmund, C. D., Ettayebi, M., and Morgan, E. A. (1984). Antibiotic resistance mutations in 16S and 23S ribosomal RNA genes of Escherichia coli. *Nucleic Acids Res.* 12, 4653–4663. doi: 10.1093/nar/12.11.4653

Unemo, M., Golparian, D., Nicholas, R., Ohnishi, M., Gallay, A., and Sednaoui, P. (2012). High-level cefixime- and ceftriaxone-resistant *Neisseria gonorrhoeae* in France: novel *penA* mosaic allele in a successful international clone causes treatment failure. *Antimicrob. Agents Chemother.* 56, 1273–1280. doi: 10.1128/AAC.05760-11

Unemo, M., Golparian, D., Skogen, V., Olsen, A. O., Moi, H., Syversen, G., et al. (2013). *Neisseria gonorrhoeae* strain with high-level resistance to spectinomycin due to a novel resistance mechanism (mutated ribosomal protein S5) verified in Norway. *Antimicrob. Agents Chemother.* 57, 1057–1061. doi: 10.1128/AAC.01775-12

Wang, S. A., Lee, M. V., O'Connor, N., Iverson, C. J., Ohye, R. G., Whiticar, P. M., et al. (2003). Multidrug-resistant *N. gonorrhoeae* with decreased susceptibility to cefixime—Hawaii, 2001. *Clin. Infect. Dis.* 15, 849–852. doi: 10.1086/377500

Wilcox, S. K., Cavey, G. S., and Pearson, J. D. (2001). Single ribosomal protein mutations in antibiotic-resistant bacteria analyzed by mass spectrometry. *Antimicrob. Agents Chemother.* 45, 3046–3055. doi: 10.1128/AAC.45.11.3046-3055.2001

Wirmer, J., and Westhof, E. (2006). Molecular contacts between antibiotics and the 30S ribosomal particle. *Methods Enzymol.* 415, 180–202. doi: 10.1016/S0076-6879(06)15012-0

Yamada, D., Tipper, D., and Davies, J. (1968). Enzymatic inactivation of streptomycin by R-factor resistant *Escherichia coli*. *Nature* 219, 288–291. doi: 10.1038/219288a0

18

Effect of subtherapeutic vs. therapeutic administration of macrolides on antimicrobial resistance in *Mannheimia haemolytica* and enterococci isolated from beef cattle

Rahat Zaheer[1], Shaun R. Cook[1], Cassidy L. Klima[1], Kim Stanford[2], Trevor Alexander[1], Edward Topp[3], Ron R. Read[4] and Tim A. McAllister[1]*

[1] *Lethbridge Research Centre, Agriculture and Agri-Food Canada, Lethbridge, AB, Canada*
[2] *Alberta Agriculture and Rural Development, Lethbridge, AB, Canada*
[3] *Southern Crop Protection and Food Research Centre, Agriculture and Agri-Food Canada, London, ON, Canada*
[4] *Faculty of Medicine, University of Calgary, Calgary, AB, Canada*

Edited by:
Marilyn C. Roberts, University of Washington, USA

Reviewed by:
Marilyn C. Roberts, University of Washington, USA
Henk Aarts, National Institute for Public Health and the Environment, Netherlands
Michael T. Sweeney, Zoetis, USA

****Correspondence:***
Tim A. McAllister, Lethbridge Research Center, Agriculture and Agri-Food Canada, 5403-1st Ave. South, Lethbridge, AB T1J 4B1, Canada.
e-mail: tim.mcallister@agr.gc.ca

Macrolides are the first-line treatment against bovine respiratory disease (BRD), and are also used to treat infections in humans. The macrolide, tylosin phosphate, is often included in the diet of cattle as a preventative for liver abscesses in many regions of the world outside of Europe. This study investigated the effects of administering macrolides to beef cattle either systemically through a single subcutaneous injection (therapeutic) or continuously in-feed (subtherapeutic), on the prevalence and antimicrobial resistance of *Mannheimia haemolytica* and *Enterococcus* spp. isolated from the nasopharynx and faeces, respectively. Nasopharyngeal and faecal samples were collected weekly over 28 days from untreated beef steers and from steers injected once with tilmicosin or tulathromycin or continuously fed tylosin phosphate at dosages recommended by manufacturers. Tilmicosin and tulathromycin were effective in lowering ($P < 0.05$) the prevalence of *M. haemolytica*, whereas subtherapeutic tylosin had no effect. *M. haemolytica* isolated from control- and macrolide-treated animals were susceptible to macrolides as well as to other antibiotics. Major bacteria co-isolated with *M. haemolytica* from the nasopharynx included *Pasteurella multocida*, *Staphylococcus* spp., *Acinetobacter* spp., *Escherichia coli* and *Bacillus* spp. With the exception of *M. haemolytica* and *P. multocida*, erythromycin resistance was frequently found in other isolated species. Both methods of macrolide administration increased ($P < 0.05$) the proportion of erythromycin resistant enterococci within the population, which was comprised almost exclusively of *Enterococcus hirae*. Injectable macrolides impacted both respiratory and enteric microbes, whereas orally administered macrolides only influenced enteric bacteria.

Keywords: macrolides, antimicrobial resistance, *Mannheimia haemolytica*, enterococci, beef cattle

INTRODUCTION

Bovine respiratory disease (BRD), commonly known as shipping fever continues to be one of the most economically significant health issues in feedlot cattle. The pathogenesis of BRD is multifactorial, being influenced by stress, immune status as well as viral/bacterial interactions within the respiratory tract. Regardless of what initiates the disease, *Mannheimia haemolytica* is considered to be the predominant bacterial pathogen associated with BRD (Confer, 2009).

To reduce or treat BRD, antibiotics are commonly administered to cattle upon arrival in North American feedlots. The use of antimicrobial therapy to control BRD increases in high-density feedlots where conditions are favorable for the introduction and transmission of infectious microbes. The macrolides, tilmicosin and tulathromycin are frequently administered subcutaneously to high-risk cattle, either prophylactically, metaphylactically, or therapeutically to cattle suffering from the disease. In North America, the macrolide tylosin phosphate is also included in beef cattle diets as a growth promoter and to prevent liver abscesses, a practice banned in Europe. After ionophores and tetracycline, macrolides are the most frequently used antimicrobials in cattle production in Canada (CIPARS, 2013). In the United States, a survey of 84% of the US feedlots revealed that about 42% of cattle received tylosin in feed for 138–145 days whereas over two-thirds of the cattle received injectable macrolides (USDA, 1999).

Macrolides belonging to the antimicrobial drug superfamily MLS_B (macrolide–lincosamide–streptogramin B) are classified as category II antimicrobials by the WHO and Health Canada (http://hc-sc.gc.ca/dhp-mps/vet/antimicrob/amr_ram_hum-med-rev-eng.php) emphasizing their importance in treating infections in humans. As reviewed by Gow (2005), as a proportion of total DDDs (Defined Daily Dose) for humans, after penicillins (27%), macrolides (20%) constitute the second most common systemic antibacterial class dispensed by retail pharmacies in Canada, followed by tetracyclines (14%), fluoroquinolones (12%), first- and second-generation cephalosporins (10%).

Although tilmicosin, tulathromycin and tylosin are exclusively used in food animals, they belong to the same category II MLS_B superfamily as erythromycin, which is used in both humans, food and companion animals. Despite having slight structural differences these drugs cross-select for resistance to all drugs of this superfamily, including several drugs used to treat infections in humans such as erythromycin and its derivatives azithromycin and clarithromycin (Roberts, 2008; Desmolaize et al., 2011). Consequently, use of macrolides in livestock could affect the efficacy of these antibiotics in controlling infections in humans through selection for resistance. Macrolide resistance can be conferred by discrete point mutations at nucleotide A2058 and its neighbours in the 23S rRNA, altering the main anchoring point for these antibiotics (Schlünzen et al., 2001) or by methylation of the A2058 at the N6 position as catalyzed by the Erm family of methyltransferases (Skinner et al., 1983). Drug efflux systems have also been shown to result in macrolide resistance (Roberts et al., 1999).

Enterococci are common members of the normal gut flora of both livestock and humans (Yost et al., 2011), but they can also be important human pathogens as *Enterococcus faecalis* and *Enterococcus faecium* are often implicated in nosocomial infections. Macrolide resistant enterococci have been isolated from cattle and depending on the species, could potentially colonize the intestinal tract of humans if they enter the food chain (Giraffa, 2002; Jensen et al., 2002).

The present study investigated and compared the response of respiratory and digestive tract bacteria in feedlot cattle to no antibiotic treatment or treatment with macrolide antibiotics at subtherapeutic (in-feed) or therapeutic (via injection) levels. Our specific objective was to evaluate the effects of administering macrolides to beef cattle either systemically through a single subcutaneous injection (tilmicosin and tulathromycin) or continuously in-feed (tylosin phosphate), on the prevalence and the antimicrobial resistance profiles of faecal *Enterococcus* spp., and *M. haemolytica* from the nasopharynx.

MATERIALS AND METHODS

EXPERIMENTAL DESIGN

The study was conducted at the individual feeding barn facility at the Lethbridge Research Centre (Lethbridge, Alberta, Canada) using 40–eleven month old beef steers (394 ± 37 kg). All steers originated from the same ranch and had not received antibiotics during their lifetime prior to their arrival at the Lethbridge Research Centre. Steers were housed in individual pens with 10 replicate animals for each of the four treatments (1) control, no antibiotics; (2) tilmicosin (Micotil® Elanco Animal Health) single subcutaneous injection at 10 mg/kg bodyweight (BW) on day 1; (3) tulathromycin (Draxxin® Pfizer Animal Health, www.pfizer.ca) single subcutaneous injection at 2.5 mg/kg BW on day 1; (4) tylosin phosphate (Tylan®, Elanco Animal Health, www.elanco.ca) at 11 ppm in feed for the entire 28 day experimental period (**Figure 1**). Adjacent pens within the same treatment group shared a common water trough and cattle within each treatment were housed in separate, but otherwise identical wings of the barn. Throughout the study, care of the steers was in accordance with the guidelines set by the Canadian Council on Animal Care (http://www.ccac.ca/).

DIET AND FEEDING

Steers were housed in individual pens and fed a typical forage-based growing diet consisting of 70% barley silage, 25% barley grain, and 5% supplement (Addah et al., 2011) on a dry matter (DM) basis, for the entire experimental period (**Figure 1**). Steers were fed once daily in a manner that ensured that all feed that was allotted was consumed. To avoid cross contamination of feed, tylosin was mixed with 5 kg of supplement and manually spread over the surface of feed within each of the appropriate pens during the morning feeding. All cattle were provided feed at the same time each day with no feed remaining in the bunk prior to the next feeding. Cattle assigned to the control treatment had no access to medicated feed throughout the entire experiment and were not injected with any antibiotics.

SAMPLING AND SAMPLE PROCESSING

Rectal faecal and nasopharyngeal swab samples were taken from all 40 animals on arrival (day 0) at the facility, and then weekly thereafter for 4 weeks and processed as follows:

Faecal samples

Rectal grab faecal samples were taken and used for subsequent determination of antimicrobial resistant and total numbers of enterococci bacteria. For the isolation of *Enterococcus* species faecal samples (1 g) were diluted 1:5 in phosphate buffered saline, from which serial dilutions were made up to 10^{-5} and 100 μL of each dilution was spread-plated, in duplicate, onto Bile-Esculin-Azide (BEA) agar plates. Dilutions 10^{-1} and 10^{-2} were also spread-plated onto BEA agar containing erythromycin at a concentration of 8 μg/mL of media (BEA+Ery) to isolate macrolide-resistant enterococci. Plates were incubated at 37°C for 24 h and colonies from both BEA and BEA+Ery plates were enumerated. Three to five presumptive *Enterococcus* colonies per sample per media type were isolated and streak-purified onto BEA or BEA+Ery plates accordingly. Purified isolates were stored in glycerol stocks at −80°C until further characterized.

Nasopharyngeal swab samples

Nasopharyngeal swab samples were collected using a commercially available deep, double guarded culture swab (Jorgensen Laboratories, Inc., Loveland, CO, USA) from all 40 steers on arrival at the beef-barn facility prior to administration of antibiotics, and then weekly thereafter for 4 weeks following antibiotic treatment. Swab samples were transported to the lab on ice and immediately suspended in 0.7 mL of Brain Heart Infusion (BHI) broth. Aliquots (100 μL) were cultured at 37°C for 16 h onto BAC-agar plates (tryptic soy agar plates containing 5% sheep blood and 15 μg/mL of bacitracin; Dalynn Biologicals, Inc., Calgary, AB, Canada) with and without the addition of erythromycin (Ery) 8 μg/mL at 37°C for 16 h. Colonies (1–5) indicative of *Mannheimia*, were selected and tested for catalase and oxidase activity as described previously (Klima et al., 2011). Isolates that exhibited typical *M. haemolytica*

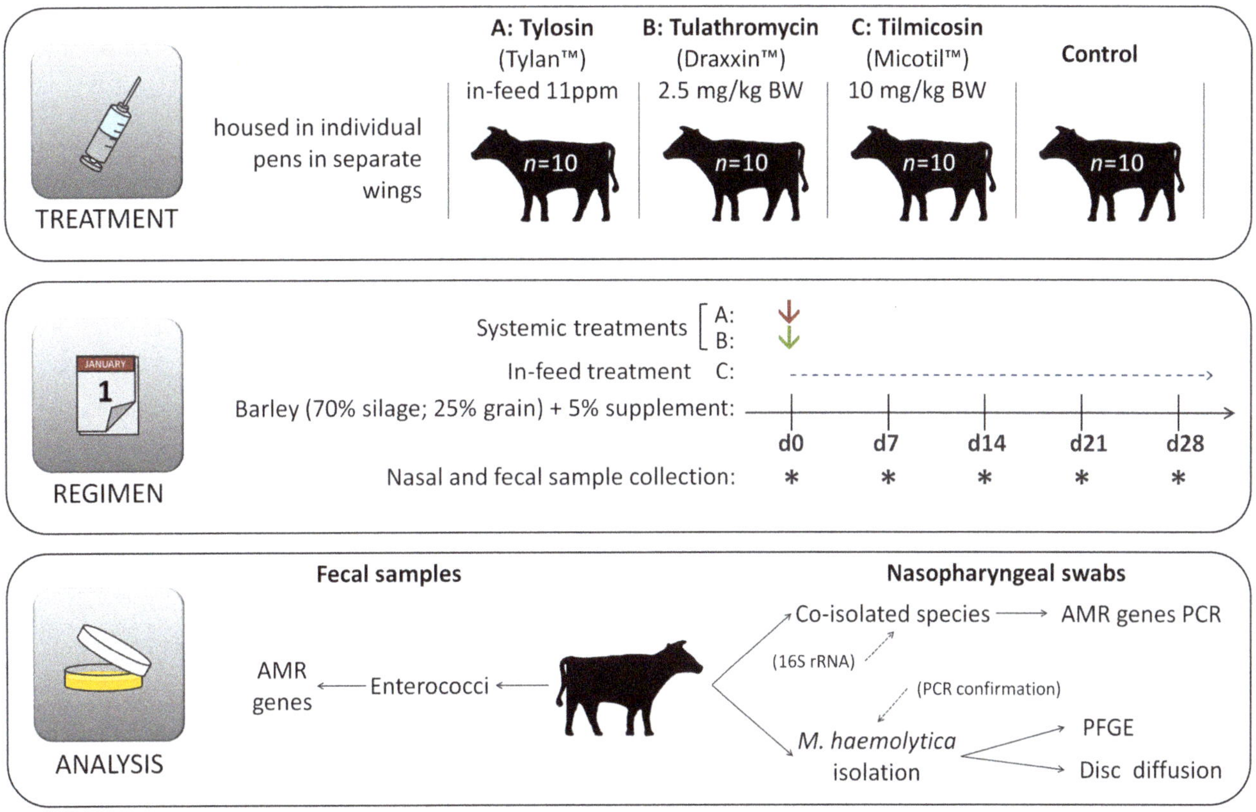

FIGURE 1 | Experimental design. Immediately after first sample collection on day 0 (d0) animals were administered appropriate treatments and hence the same day is also referred as day 1, denoting the beginning of the experimental period. Cattle had no prior direct exposure to antibiotics prior to initiation of the experiment.

colony morphology and were both catalase and oxidase positive were subsequently confirmed using a multiplex PCR assay (Alexander et al., 2008). Confirmed *M. haemolytica* isolates were stored at −80°C in BHI broth containing 20% glycerol for further characterization. Colonies that did not exhibit morphology indicative of *Mannheimia* on BAC or BAC+Ery agar plates were identified and 1–2 colonies representing each morphotype were selected and stored at −80°C in BHI broth containing 20% glycerol until further characterized. Bacitracin in BAC media inhibited the growth of the majority of gram positive bacteria, thereby improving the likelihood of isolating *M. haemolytica.* Although bacitracin resistant gram positive bacteria were co-isolated with *Mannheimia,* these isolates were subsequently identified using 16S rRNA profiling as described below.

CHARACTERIZATION OF *Mannheimia haemolytica* AND CO-ISOLATED NASOPHARYNGEAL BACTERIA

Confirmed *M. haemolytica* isolates were serotyped as previously described (Klima et al., 2011) with antisera prepared in rabbits against formalin-killed whole cells of *M. haemolytica* reference strains UGCC G1 (serotype 1), UGCC G2 (serotype 2), ATCC 29697 (serotype 6), ATCC 29698 (serotype 7), and ATCC 29700 (serotype 9). Isolates were subject to pulsed field gel electrophoresis (PFGE) profiling using *Sal*I restriction enzyme as previously described (Klima et al., 2011). The 16S rRNA genes were PCR amplified from bacteria co-isolated with *M. haemolytica* using universal bacterial 16S rRNA gene primers 27F (5′-AGAGTTTGATCCTGGCTCAG-3′) and 1492R (5′-GGTTACCTTGTTACGACTT-3′) and subject to DNA sequencing (Eurofins MWG Operon, Huntsville, Alabama, USA) using one (27F) or both (27F and 1492R) primers.

ANTIBIOGRAMS

Disk susceptibility tests were conducted for *Mannheimia* in accordance with the Clinical and Laboratory Standards Institute documents M31-A3 and M45-A (CLSI, 2008a,b). The antimicrobials tested, suppliers and resistance breakpoints applied are listed in **Table 1**. Reference strains *Escherichia coli* ATCC 35218, *Staphylococcus aureus* ATCC 25923, *Streptococcus pneumoniae* ATCC 49619, and *M. haemolytica* ATCC 33396 were used as quality controls. Briefly, cultures grown on Muller–Hinton agar supplemented with 5% defibrinated sheep blood (MHB; 16–18 h at 37°C) were suspended into Muller–Hinton broth to an absorbance reading between 0.125 and 0.145 at 625 nm. Using sterile swabs, the prepared inocula were swabbed onto MHB followed by the dispensation of the antibiotic containing disks onto the plate surface. The plates were incubated at 37°C in ambient air, with the exception of *S. pneumoniae* ATCC 49619 which required cultivation in a 5% CO_2 atmosphere for 24 h.

Table 1 | Antimicrobial agents, suppliers, disk contents, and interpretative criteria used for disk susceptibility testing.

Antimicrobial	Supplier	Supplier code	Disk content (μg)	Zone diameter (mm) breakpoints[c]		
				S	I	R
Amoxicillin/clavulanic Acid[a]	BD	AMC-30	20/10	≥27	n/a	≤26
Ampicillin[a]	BD	AM-10	10	≥27	n/a	n/a
Ceftiofur[b]	BD	XNL-30	30	≥21	18–20	≤17
Danofloxacin[b]	Pfizer	DNO	5	≥22	n/a	n/a
Erythromycin[a]	BD	E-15	15	≥27	25–26	≤24
Florfenicol[b]	BD	FF-30	30	≥19	15–18	≤14
Gentamicin[b]	BD	GM-10	10	≥15	13–14	≤12
Oxytetracycline[a]	BD	T-30	30	≥23	n/a	n/a
Spectinomycin[b]	BD	SPT-100	100	≥14	11–13	≤10
Sulfamethoxazole[a]/trimethoprim	BD	SXT	23.75/1.25	≤24	n/a	n/a
Tilmicosin[b]	BD	TIL-15	15	≥14	11–13	≤10
Tulathromycin[b]	Pfizer	TUL	30	≥18	15–17	≤14

[a]*M45-A: Methods for antimicrobial dilution and disk susceptibility testing of infrequently isolated or fastidious bacteria; approved guideline (CLSI, 2008b). Due to the unavailability MIC breakpoints for Mannheimia spp., guidelines for Pasteurella spp. were followed.*

[b]*M31-A3: Performance standard for antimicrobial disk and dilution susceptibility tests for bacteria isolated from animals; approved standard—third edition (CLSI, 2008a).*

[c]*Zone diameter value used to indicate susceptible (S), intermediate (I) and resistant (R), n/a, not available.*

The resulting zones of inhibition were read using the BioMic V3 imaging system (Giles Scientific, Inc., Santa Barbara, CA, USA).

CHARACTERIZATION OF ENTEROCOCCI

The enterococci isolated from faecal samples were confirmed to be *Enterococcus* spp. by PCR using primers Ent-ES-211-233-F (5′-GHACAGAAGTRAAATAYGAAGG-3′) and Ent-EL-74-95-R (5′-GGNCCTAABGTHACTTTNACTG-3′) and 130 select isolates representing both erythromycin susceptible and resistant categories were further analyzed for species identification by pyrosequencing as described by Zaheer et al. (2012). Thirty six select isolates were subject to PFGE profiling using *Sma*I restriction enzyme using an adaptation of the procedure of Turabelidze et al. (2000). Briefly, bacteria from overnight brain-heart infusion-agar (BHI-agar) cultures were harvested using sterile swabs and suspended in cell suspension buffer [100 mM Tris-HCl (pH 8.0) and 100 mM EDTA], to an optical density (OD) of 1.2–1.3 at 610 nm (1-cm light path). Aliquots (1 ml each) of the suspensions were centrifuged (10,000 × g) for 2 min. in a microcentrifuge and 2/3rd of the supernatant was removed from the tube. The bacterial pellet was resuspended in the remaining supernatant, concentrating the cell suspension to an OD_{610} of 3.6–4.0 (ca. 2.5×10^9 CFU/ml). An aliquot (100 μL) of cell suspension was added to an equal volume of lysis buffer (50 mM Tris-HCl (pH 8), 50 mM EDTA, 625 U/ml mutanolysin, 2.5 mg/ml lysozyme, 1.5 mg/ml proteinase K, 20 μg/ml RNase), mixed gently and incubated at 37°C for 10 min. An equal volume of 1.2% molten SeaKem Gold agarose (FMC BioProducts, Rockland, Maine) containing 1% sodium dodecyl sulfate was added, the mixtures were poured in duplicate into 2-cm by 1-cm by 1.5-mm reusable plug molds (Bio-Rad Laboratories, Hercules, CA) and allowed to solidify at room temperature for 10 min. The duplicate plugs were added to a tube containing 1.8 mL of proteolysis solution [0.44 M EDTA (pH 8.0), 1% sarcosyl, 400 μg/ml of proteinase K] and incubated with constant agitation at 300 rpm for 2 h at 55°C. Plugs were washed 3 times for 10 min each in H_2O (1.8 mL), followed by 3 times for 10 min in TE (1.8 mL) in a thermomixer set at 50°C and 300 rpm. One plug was cut in three equal slices latitudinally and two of the gel slices were pre-incubated in 200 μL of 1X restriction enzyme buffer for 15 min at 30°C. DNA in the plugs was restricted with 50 units of *Sma*I in a 200 μL reaction mixture for 3 h at 25°C. As a reference standard *Xba*I digested *Salmonella* serotype Braenderup (H9812) plugs were prepared as previously described (Klima et al., 2011).

The digested plugs were embedded in 1% SeaKem Gold low-melting temperature agarose (Lonza Canada, Inc., Shawinigan, QC) that was dissolved in 0.5 × TBE (45 mM Tris, 45 mM boric acid, 1 mM EDTA, pH 8.0). Prior to incorporation into the gel, digested plugs were incubated with 200 μl of 0.5 × TBE at room temperature for 20 min. The digested DNA were separated by PFGE using a CHEF DRII device (Bio-Rad Laboratories Ltd., Mississauga, ON, Canada), at 12°C. The voltage was maintained at 6 V/cm for a total of 21 h with switch times of 4–40 s for initial 12.5 h followed by switch times of 1.5–6 for 8.5 h. The gels were run in 0.5 × TBE buffer containing 0.45 mM thiourea. After electrophoresis, gels were stained with ethidium bromide (1 μg/ml) in distilled water for 20 min followed by three 20 min washes with distilled water. Gels were photographed with an AlphaImager gel documentation system (Alpha Innotech Corp., St. Leandro, CA). Fragment analysis was performed with BioNumerics V5.1 software (Applied Maths Inc., Austin, TX).

IDENTIFICATION OF MACROLIDE RESISTANCE DETERMINANTS

Erythromycin-resistant isolates were evaluated for the presence of the commonly found macrolide resistance determinants *erm*(A), *erm*(B), *erm*(C), *erm*(F), *erm*(T), *erm*(X), *mef*(A) (http://faculty.washington.edu/marilynr/) by PCR analyses. For generating PCR template, a single bacterial colony was suspended in 50 μL of TE (10 mM Tris.HCl pH 8.0, 1 mM EDTA pH 8.0) and incubated at 95°C for 5 min followed by centrifugation at 10,000 × g for 5 min. Supernatant (2 μL) was used as template in a 20 μL volume PCR reaction mixture using PCR primers and reaction conditions as described elsewhere (Chen et al., 2007; Szczepanowski et al., 2009). The commercially available HotStarTaq Plus Master Mix Kit (Qiagen Canada, Inc., Mississauga, ON, Canada) was used according to manufacturer's instructions. Plasmids containing corresponding gene fragments previously cloned in our laboratory were used as positive controls. Select PCR fragments amplified from erythromycin resistant isolates originating from the present study were verified by DNA sequencing.

STATISTICAL ANALYSIS

Data were analyzed using commercially available statistical analysis software (SAS System for Windows, release 9.1.3, SAS Institute, Cary, NC). Prevalence of *M. haemolytica* and erythromycin resistance in enterococci were analyzed using logistic methodology within the GLIMMIX procedure of SAS, with treatment in the model and day of sampling treated as a repeated measure. Model adjusted means (LS means back-transformed to original scale) and standard errors were reported and used to estimate the efficacy of the antibiotic treatments for controlling *M. haemolytica*. For all tests, the level of significance was set at $P < 0.05$.

ETHICS STATEMENT

Experiments with beef steers were conducted according to the Canadian Council on Animal Care (CCAC) guidelines. The studies were approved by the institutional Animal Care Committee (ACC), Lethbridge Research Centre, Agriculture and Agri-Food Canada, under protocol number 1111. Antibiotics were administered or fed at levels approved by the Canadian Bureau of Veterinary Drugs and recommended by the manufacturer and used in accordance with industry practices.

RESULTS

Mannheimia haemolytica CHARACTERIZATION

A total of 274 suspect *M. haemolytica* isolates were obtained over the duration of the study of which 260 were confirmed by multiplex PCR assay (Alexander et al., 2008). Isolates were obtained from 29 out of the 40 steers used in the experiment. All of the confirmed *M. haemolytica* isolates were serotyped and 160 (1–3 isolates per *Mannheimia* positive animal per sampling event) were tested for antimicrobial susceptibility using the disk diffusion assay, and 65 (one isolate belonging to each of the *M. haemolytica* positive animals for each sampling event) were subjected to PFGE.

Serotyping revealed that 89% (232/260) of the *M. haemolytica* isolates that originated from 93% (27/29) of the positive animals were serotype 1, whereas 8.4% (22/260) of the isolates, all of which originated from a single steer were serotype 2. Two percent (5/260) of the isolates were identified as serotype 6, all of which were obtained from a single steer on the 28th day post treatment. Two main clusters were identified by PFGE analysis, cluster A consisted primarily of serotype 1 isolates with only a single serotype 6 isolate, whereas cluster B was comprised of serotype 2 isolates (**Figure 2**). Two sub-clusters, A1 and A2 were observed within cluster A; A1 solely comprising serotype 1 isolates and A2 consisting of a mixture of serotype 1 and 6 (**Figure 2**).

The prevalence of *M. haemolytica* dropped substantially from steers that were injected with tilmicosin or tulathromycin as compared to levels prior to treatment (**Figure 3A**). Compared to the control, the number of steers harboring *M. haemolytica* was reduced ($P < 0.05$) by systemic treatment with either tilmicosin or tulathromycin over the post treatment sampling period (days 7–28). Compared to the in-feed tylosin, tilmicosin and tulathromycin also resulted in a reduction ($P < 0.05$) in number of cattle positive for *M. haemolytica* (64 and 42%, respectively) (**Figure 3B**). In disk diffusion assays, *M. haemolytica* isolates cultured without erythromycin on primary isolation were all sensitive to amoxicillin/clavulanic acid, ampicillin, ceftiofur, danofloxacin, erythromycin, florfenicol, gentamicin, oxytetracycline, spectinomycin, trimethoprim/sulfamethoxazole, tilmicosin, and tulathromycin.

CHARACTERIZATION OF BACTERIA CO-ISOLATED WITH *M. haemolytica*

The non-*Mannheimia* bacterial colonies originating from nasopharyngeal samples cultured on BAC or BAC+Ery agar plates were divided into 11 morphological groups (**Table 2**). The 16S rRNA gene sequences from 165 select isolates with 5–15 isolates representing each morphology group were subsequently analyzed for genus/species identification through alignments using "seqmatch" (http://rdp.cme.msu.edu/index.jsp) or BLAST (http://blast.ncbi.nlm.nih.gov/). The morphotypes were found to be very consistent with 16S rDNA sequence based bacterial identification and therefore were used to define the identity of collected isolates. One representative of each morphotype per sampling event was used to determine bacterial prevalence. Along with *M. haemolytica* (13%), other bacteria found in abundance included *Pasteurella multocida* (25%), *Staphylococcus* spp. (25%), *Acinetobacter* spp. (9%), *E. coli/Shigella* group (8%), and *Bacillus licheniformis* (7%) (**Figure 4**). Among the *Staphylococcus* spp., *S. epidermidis*, *S. pasteuri*, and *S. cohnii* were abundant and collectively constituted 20% of isolated nasopharyngeal bacterial species, with *S. sciuri* only occasionally isolated. These *Staphylococcus* species had indistinguishable colony morphologies and thus collectively constituted one morphological group (**Table 2**). *Staphylococcus chromogenes* was placed in a separate morphological group due to its distinct yellow color and it constituted 5% of isolated nasopharyngeal bacterial species. Other species such as streptococci, *Macrococcus casseolyticus* and *Bacillus* spp. including *B. clausii* and *B. pumilus* were less abundant (**Figure 4**). However, collectively and irrespective of morphotypes, *Bacillus* spp. constituted ~14% of isolated bacteria.

Erythromycin resistance was found in all isolated bacterial species except *M. haemolytica*, *P. multocida* and other less frequently isolated bacteria (**Table 2**). Of the seven macrolide resistance genes tested by PCR, the *erm*(C) was predominantly found in *Staphylococcus* spp. (**Table 2**). With regard to

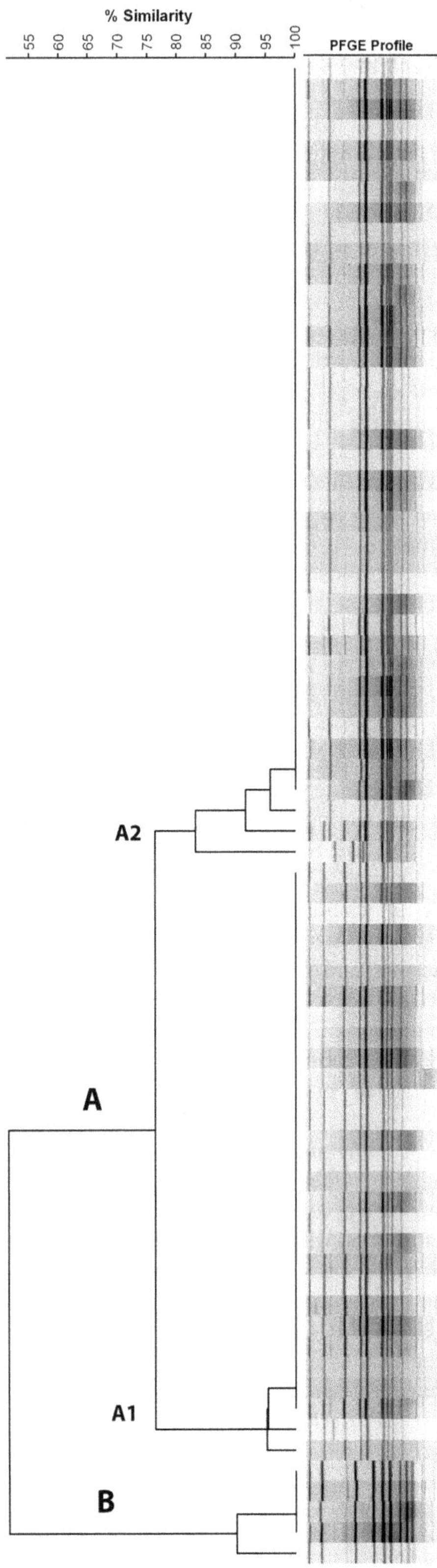

Sample ID	Serotype	Treatment	Day Post-Treatment
151-1-1	1	control	0
151-3-1	1	control	14
151-5-1	1	control	28
152-2-1	1	control	7
152-3-1	1	control	14
153-1-7	1	control	0
153-4-1	1	control	21
156-5-1	1	control	28
157-2-1	1	control	7
157-1-6	1	control	0
160-3-1	1	control	14
160-5-1	1	control	28
161-4-1	1	tilmicosin	21
162-3-1	1	tilmicosin	14
162-5-1	1	tilmicosin	28
166-1-8	1	tilmicosin	0
169-1-6	1	tilmicosin	0
170-1-6	1	tilmicosin	0
171-4-1	1	tulathromycin	21
172-1-6	1	tulathromycin	0
172-4-1	1	tulathromycin	21
172-5-1	1	tulathromycin	28
174-1-7	1	tulathromycin	0
174-1-6	1	tulathromycin	0
175-1-6	1	tulathromycin	0
179-1-9	1	tulathromycin	0
179-5-1	1	tulathromycin	28
182-2-1	1	tylosin phosphate	7
182-3-1	1	tylosin phosphate	14
183-5-1	1	tylosin phosphate	28
184-4-1	1	tylosin phosphate	21
184-5-1	1	tylosin phosphate	28
185-2-1	1	tylosin phosphate	7
188-5-1	1	tylosin phosphate	28
190-3-1	1	tylosin phosphate	14
190-4-1	1	tylosin phosphate	21
153-2-1	1	control	7
188-2-1	1	tylosin phosphate	7
163-5-1	6	tilmicosin	28
151-2-1	1	control	7
151-4-1	1	control	21
152-1-4	1	control	0
153-5-1	1	control	28
156-2-1	1	control	7
156-1-6	1	control	0
156-3-1	1	control	14
157-4-1	1	control	21
158-4-1	1	control	21
158-5-1	1	control	28
160-4-1	1	control	21
162-1-8	1	tilmicosin	0
163-1-6	1	tilmicosin	0
163-4-1	1	tilmicosin	21
167-1-8	1	tilmicosin	0
175-1-7	1	tulathromycin	0
175-5-1	1	tulathromycin	28
176-1-6	1	tulathromycin	0
177-5-1	1	tulathromycin	28
178-3-1	1	tulathromycin	14
179-2-1	1	tulathromycin	7
179-3-1	1	tulathromycin	14
179-4-1	1	tulathromycin	21
183-3-1	1	tylosin phosphate	14
188-1-7	1	tylosin phosphate	0
188-1-6	1	tylosin phosphate	0
190-2-1	1	tylosin phosphate	7
154-1-6	1	control	0
188-1-8	1	tylosin phosphate	0
186-2-1	2	tylosin phosphate	7
186-3-1	2	tylosin phosphate	14
186-4-1	2	tylosin phosphate	21
186-5-1	2	tylosin phosphate	28
186-1-6	2	tylosin phosphate	0

FIGURE 2 | Dendrogram of PFGE *SalI* profiles from representative *M. haemolytica* isolates collected weekly. As an example, sample ID 151-3-1 represents isolate #1 from 3rd sampling event (day 14 post treatment) from animal #151. (Control: animal IDs 151–160; tilmicosin: animal IDs 161–170; tulathromycin: animal IDs 171–180; tylosin: animal IDs 181–190).

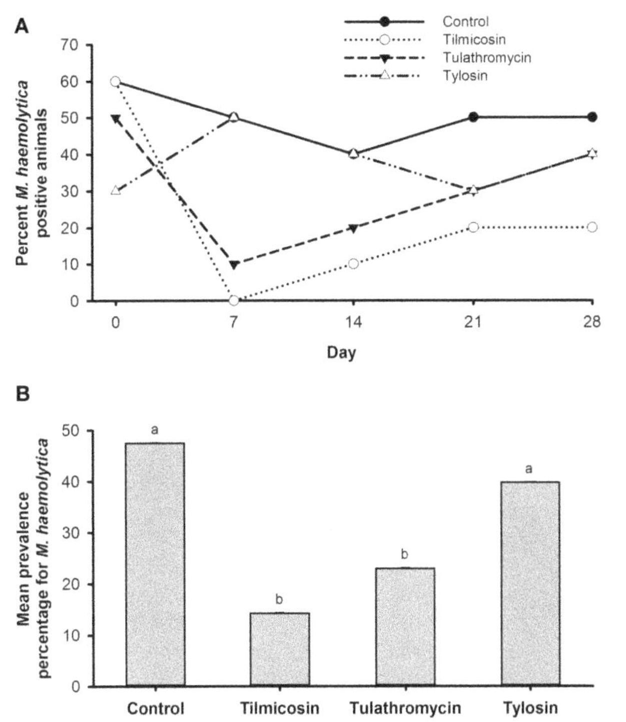

FIGURE 3 | (A) Percentage of animals positive for *M. haemolytica* for each of the five sampling events over 28 days study period. **(B)** Mean percentage of *M. haemolytica* prevalence in animals over the entire study period. Means with different superscripts differ ($P < 0.05$).

other erythromycin-resistant isolates, no resistance determinants matching any of the seven PCR primer pairs were amplified and therefore were considered as "not detected".

EVALUATION OF ENTEROCOCCI PRE- AND POST-MACROLIDE-TREATMENT

Enterococci were isolated from all 40 animals (control and treatment groups) on arrival (day 0), and weekly thereafter for 4 weeks (day 7, 14, 21, and 28). Enterococci colonies obtained on BEA and BEA+Ery plates were enumerated and the proportion of erythromycin resistant colonies was calculated for each sample (**Figure 5**). Compared to the control group, antibiotic treatment groups were 76 times more likely ($P < 0.02$) to have erythromycin resistant enterococci over the study period (days 7–28). Similarly, for all treatment groups, post-treatment samples from the entire study period were 66 times more likely to have erythromycin resistant enterococci ($P < 0.001$) when compared to pre-treatment (day 0) samples. No significant differences in the incidence of erythromycin resistance were observed between injectable (tilmicosin and tulathromycin) and in-feed (tylosin) macrolides.

Speciation of 130 of the enterococci isolates collected from day 0, 7, or 28 revealed that all were *Enterococcus hirae* with the exception of two which were *Enterococcus casseliflavus*. Fifty select isolates of erythromycin resistant enterococci from day 0 and day 7 sampling events were used for the identification of erythromycin resistance determinants. Of the seven macrolide resistance genes investigated via PCR only the *erm*(B) gene was identified in enterococci isolates.

Table 2 | Bacteria co-isolated with *M. haemolytica*.

Morphotypes	Morphology on BAC-agar plates	Species identification based on 16S rDNA sequencing	Ery resistance	Resistance determinant(s)
Mh	Small, glossy, grey, beta-haemolytic	*Mannheimia haemolytica*[a]	–	–
1	Small/small-medium, round, glossy, white	*S. epidermidis, S. cohnii, S. pasteuri, S. saprophyticus, S. sciuri*	+	*erm*(C), *erm*(C), *erm*(C), ND, ND
2	Large, mucoid, semi-transparent, grey-white	*Pasteurella multocida*	–	–
3	Very small, dense, brown/pale, alpha-haemolytic	*Streptococcus/Bacillus*	+	ND
4	Medium/large, wrinkly, crusty, fluid-filled, beta-haemolytic	*Bacillus licheniformis*	+	ND
5	Medium/large, glossy, grey-white, mostly beta-haemolytic	*Escherichia coli/Shigella*	+	–
6	Medium/large, rough edges, flat, granular	*Bacillus clausii/Bacillus spp.*	+	ND
7	Small, glossy, grey/cream	*Acinetobacter lwoffii, Acinetobacter spp.*	+	ND
8	Small/medium, glossy, pale-yellow	*Staphylococcus chromogenes*	NA	ND
9	Small/medium, pale-yellow, concentric with concave center	*Macrococcus caseolyticus*	NA	ND
10	Medium, yellowish, concentric circles, very haemolytic, greenish	*Bacillus pumilus*	NA	ND
U	Unique morphologies found occasionally	*Klebsiella, Neisseria* spp., *Paenibacillus* spp., uncultured bacteria	NA	ND

[a] *Also confirmed by multiplex PCR assay (Alexander et al., 2008); NA, not available, as those morphology groups were less commonly found on BAC plates and not found on BAC+Ery plates; ND, not determined (no positives detected in PCRs with any of the tested macrolide primer sets, see Materials and Methods).*

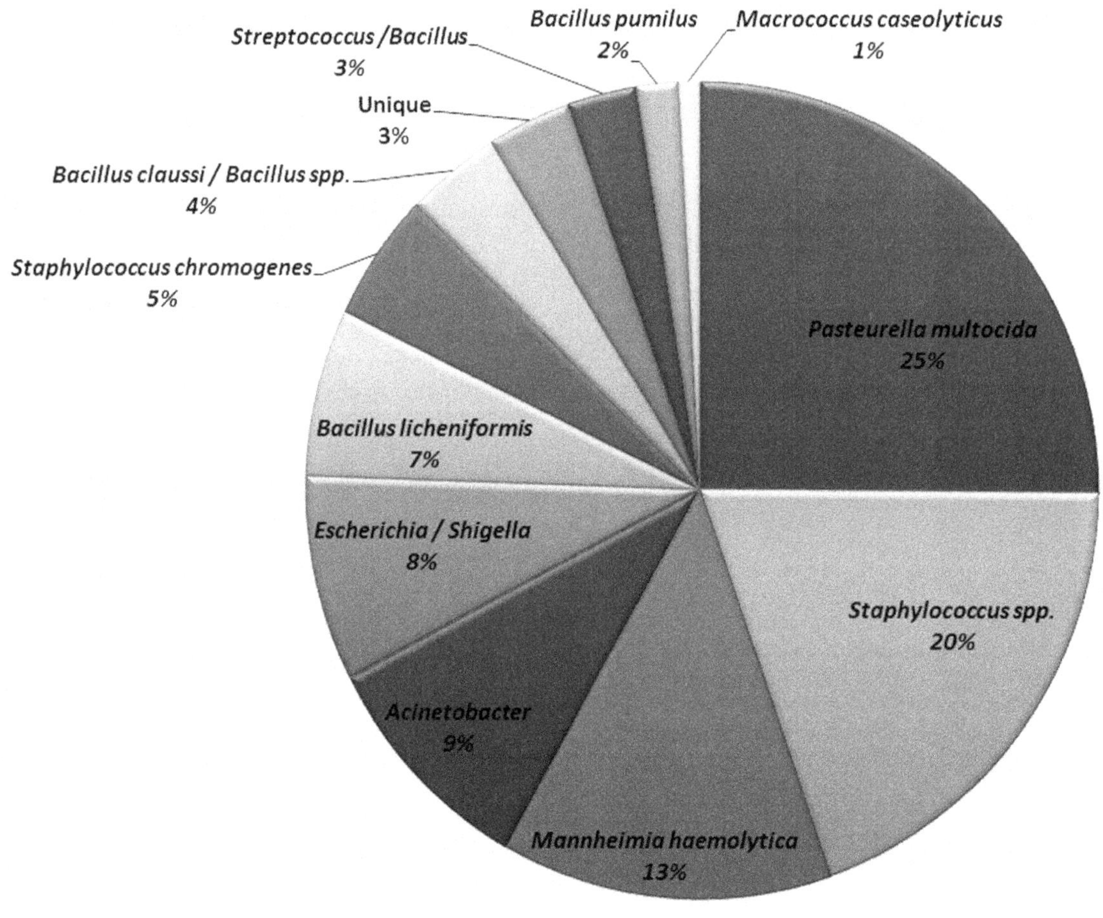

FIGURE 4 | Relative abundance of bacitracin resistant bacterial species isolated from nasopharynx over 28-days sampling period. One representative of each morphology per animal per sampling event were used to determine bacterial species prevalence ($n = 466$).

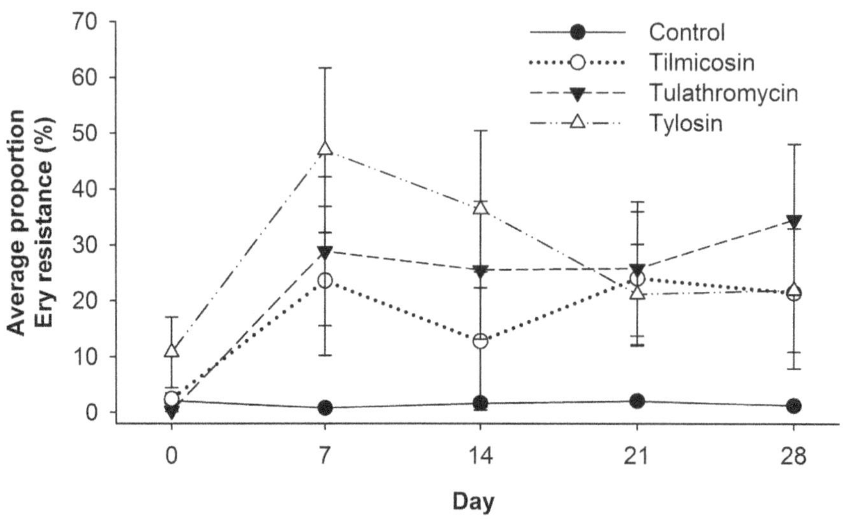

FIGURE 5 | Proportion of erythromycin-resistant faecal enterococci isolates for each of the five sampling events over 28 days study period, with day 0 samples collected prior to antibiotic treatment. From day 7 onward, Control isolates had less resistance detected ($P < 0.05$) than antibiotic treated groups, while resistance noted with injectable macrolides (tilimicosin and tulathormycin) did not differ from that cattle fed tylosin.

A representative 36 erythromycin resistant enterococci from 12 select animals from three sampling events (day 0, 7, and 28) were subject to PFGE and produced three closely related clusters (>85% similarity) (**Figure 6**). In eight of the twelve animals the PFGE profiles from the three sampling events had >90% similarity indicating that erythromycin resistant enterococci likely consisted of a persistent clonal population.

DISCUSSION

The objective of this study was to evaluate and compare the effect of in-feed subtherapeutic and injectable therapeutic administration of macrolides on antimicrobial susceptibility of indicator bacteria from the digestive and respiratory tract of feedlot cattle. For this purpose we selected faecal enterococci and *M. haemolytica* as our indicator bacteria for the digestive and respiratory tract, respectively. Injectable macrolide antimicrobials such as tilmicosin and tulathromycin are commonly used at therapeutic levels in beef cattle production to prevent and treat BRD. The macrolide, tylosin is frequently administered in-feed at subtherapeutic doses for improving feed efficiency and for the reduction of liver abscesses caused by *Fusobacterium necrophorum* and *Actinomyces pyogenes* (www.merckvetmanual.com). The subtherapeutic administration of antibiotics has been hypothesized to promote resistance development as bacteria are exposed to sublethal concentrations of antibiotic for prolonged periods of time. Consequently, the subtherapeutic administration of antibiotics in animal feeds for growth promotion has been proposed as a serious public health concern (Aarestrup and Wegener, 1999; Wegener et al., 1999; McEwen and Fedorka-Cray, 2002). Over the last 6–10 years the minimum inhibitory concentrations (MICs) of tilmicosin and tulathromycin towards *M. haemolytica* have markedly increased (Portis et al., 2012), questioning the continued effectiveness of these antibiotics against the etiological agents of BRD. Furthermore, *M. haemolytica* could serve as a reservoir of macrolide resistance genes, potentially disseminating them to other respiratory pathogens.

Deep nasopharyngeal swabs were taken to isolate *M. haemolytica* as this procedure is quick, simple and relatively non-invasive. In our study, a single systemic administration of therapeutic levels of either tilmicosin or tulathromycin was effective in lowering *M. haemolytica* in the nasopharynx of steers (**Figures 3A,B**). According to the manufacturer, (ELANCO Animal Health, Guelph, On, Canada, www.elanco.ca) injecting cattle with 10 mg of tilmicosin /kg of body weight results in lung concentrations exceeding the MIC(3.12 μg/mL) for *M. haemolytica* for at least 3 days, eliminating it from the respiratory tract for up to 6 days (Frank et al., 2000). Tulathromycin is believed to accumulate in neutrophils and alveolar macrophages (Siegel et al., 2004; Cox et al., 2010), with peak lung levels of 4.1 μg/mL occurring in cattle 24 h after a single injection and concentrations remaining above the MIC for *M. haemolytica* (2.0 μg/mL) for 10 days (www.pfizer.ca). Our data demonstrated that 7 days post-injection, *M. haemolytica* was detected in only one steer treated with tulathromycin and none of the steers treated with tilimicosin, whereas 60% of steers were positive for this bacterium upon arrival (day 0). This suggests that *M. haemolytica* in newly arrived cattle were not macrolide resistant, an observation supported by our inability to isolate erythromycin resistant *M. haemolytica* and likely a reflection of the fact that these cattle had no previous exposure to macrolides.

In contrast to injectable macrolides, tylosin had no effect on the number of *M. haemolytica* in steers administered this antibiotic in feed as compared to cattle that received no antibiotics (**Figures 3A,B**). This observation likely reflects differences in the method and concentration of the antibiotic administered and the sensitivity of *M. haemolytica* to tylosin. Tylosin is not effective at penetrating the outer membrane of Gram-negative bacteria and as a result its MIC (64 μg/mL) against *M. haemolytica* is much higher than either tilimicosin or tulathromycin (Andersen et al., 2012). Tylosin is known to be widely distributed in body fluids and tissues, but comparative pharmacokinetics of its distribution in the digestive tract relative to the respiratory tract when it is administered in feed are poorly characterized (Lewicki, 2006).

Mannheimia haemolytica isolated from animals belonging to control and all three macrolide treatment groups throughout the course of study were found to be susceptible to all tested macrolides indicating that both therapeutic and subtherapeutic administration did not contribute to macrolide resistance in *M. haemolytica* during the study. *Mannheimia haemolytica* isolated in the present study were also susceptible to all other antibiotics tested (**Table 2**). While tilmicosin and tulathromycin are generally effective against *M. haemolytica*, a few isolates originating from Germany, Japan and United States have shown resistance to these antibiotics (Katsuda et al., 2009; Watts and Sweeney, 2010; Michael et al., 2012). An integrative conjugative element (ICE) has been identified in *P. multocida* that exhibits high similarity to ICEs in *P. multocida* 36950, *Histophilus somni* 23364 and an ICE fragment within the incomplete *M. haemolytica* PHL23 genome (Michael et al., 2012). This is a matter of concern as *P. multocida*, *M. haemolytica*, and *H. somni* often share the same ecological niche in the bovine respiratory tract and exchange of this ICE element could lead to macrolide resistance in these BRD pathogens as transfer of this element among *P. multocida*, *M. haemolytica*, and *E. coli* has been demonstrated in the laboratory (Dabo et al., 2007; Watts and Sweeney, 2010).

The majority of *M. haemolytica* isolates collected from asymptomatic animals in this study were serotype 1 (**Figure 2**). The PFGE profiles of serotype 1 and 6 isolates clustered together with a ~83% relatedness, a relationship observed previously for these serotypes (Klima et al., 2011). The predominance of a single serotype in the majority of steers is likely a reflection of sourcing them from the same isolated ranch in southern Alberta and transporting them directly to the Lethbridge Research Centre. This arrangement was necessary to ensure that steers had no exposure to antibiotics prior to arrival. Serotype 1 has frequently been linked to clinical disease and both serotypes 1 and 6 are often isolated from cattle with BRD (Zecchinon et al., 2005). However, none of the steers in the present study exhibited clinical BRD. The BRD complex consists of a bacteria (*M. haemolytica, Pasteurella multocida, Histophulus somni, Mycoplasma bovis*) and viruses (Bovine Viral Diarrhea, Infectious Bovine Rhinotracheltis, Bovine Respiratory Synctial Virus, Parainfluenza Type-3 Virus) which together supress innate immune responses and cause lung damage (Fulton, 2009; Pardon

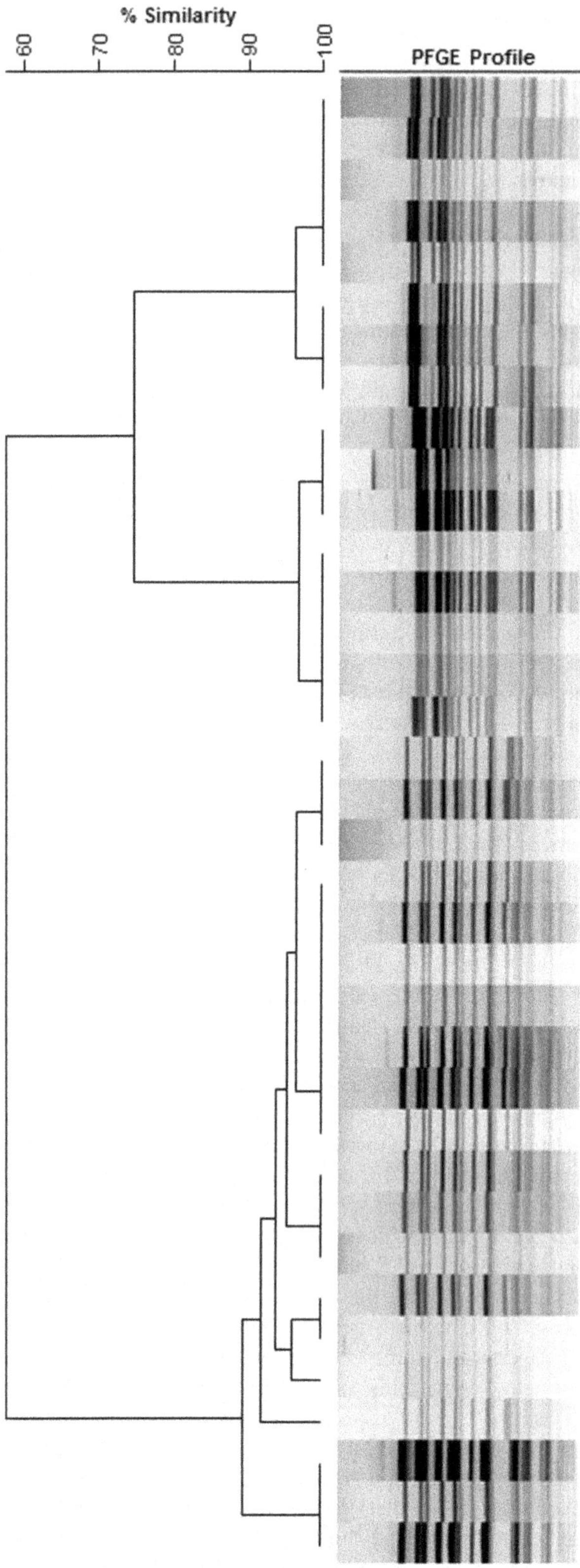

Sample ID	Treatment	Day Post-Treatment
162-ERY-5-1	tilmicosin	28
167-ERY-2-1	tilmicosin	7
167-ERY-5-1	tilmicosin	28
170-ERY-2-1	tilmicosin	7
170-ERY-5-1	tilmicosin	28
162-ERY-1-2	tilmicosin	0
162-ERY-2-1	tilmicosin	7
167-ERY-1-1	tilmicosin	0
173-ERY-2-1	tulathromycin	7
173-ERY-5-1	tulathromycin	28
176-ERY-5-1	tulathromycin	28
172-ERY-1-1	tulathromycin	0
172-ERY-5-1	tulathromycin	28
173-ERY-1-1	tulathromycin	0
176-ERY-1-1	tulathromycin	0
176-ERY-2-1	tulathromycin	7
161-ERY-1-1	tilmicosin	0
161-ERY-2-1	tilmicosin	7
161-ERY-5-1	tilmicosin	28
153-ERY-1-1	control	0
153-ERY-2-1	control	7
153-ERY-5-1	control	28
181-ERY-1-1	tylosin phosphate	0
188-ERY-1-1	tylosin phosphate	0
188-ERY-2-1	tylosin phosphate	7
188-ERY-5-1	tylosin phosphate	28
160-ERY-1-1	control	0
160-ERY-2-1	control	7
160-ERY-5-1	control	28
181-ERY-2-2	tylosin phosphate	7
181-ERY-5-1	tylosin phosphate	28
174-ERY-5-1	tulathromycin	28
170-ERY-1-1	tilmicosin	0
172-ERY-2-1	tulathromycin	7
174-ERY-1-1	tulathromycin	0
174-ERY-2-1	tulathromycin	7

FIGURE 6 | Dendrogram of PFGE *Sma*I profiles from representative erythromycin resistant enterococci from day 0, 7, and 28. As an example, sample ID 153-ERY-5-1 represents isolate #1 collected from BEA+ERY plates on 5th sampling event (day 28) from animal #153. (Control: animal IDs 151–160; tilmicosin: animal IDs 161–170; tulathromycin: animal IDs 171–180; tylosin: animal IDs 181–190.

et al., 2011). It seems likely that in this study the steers lacked the infectious complex necessary for the development of BRD.

Pasturella multocida was the most ubiquitous bacterium isolated from the nasopharynx of steers and in contrast to *M. haemolytica*, prevalence of this bacterium was similar in pre- and post-treatment groups. However, none of the isolated *P. multocida* exhibited resistance to erythromycin. As *P. multocida* were not enumerated, it is possible that macrolides reduced the population of this bacterium. After *P. multocida*, *Staphylococcus* spp. was most abundant with a relative abundances of *S. epidermidis* > *S. pasteuri* > *S. cohnii* > *S. sciuri* > *S. saprophyticus*. Staphylococci are ubiquitous Gram-positive bacteria and are common in the microflora of skin and mucosal surfaces. Currently, there are 31 species recognized in the genus *Staphylococcus* and about half of these are indigenous to humans (Kloos and Bannerman, 1994). The role of some species, such as *S. epidermidis*, *S. saprophyticus*, *S. Pasteuri* and *S. cohni* in human disease has been well documented (Piette and Verschraegen, 2008; Savini et al., 2009). Consistent with previous studies (Aarestrup et al., 2000a; Simeoni et al., 2008), the majority of the erythromycin resistant *Staphylococcus* spp. harbored *erm*(C).

Thirteen percent of the isolated nasopharyngeal bacteria were *M. haemolytica* followed by *Acinetobacter*, Enterobacteriaceae (*Esherichia spp., Shigella spp.)* and *Bacillus* spp. including *B. licheniformis* and *B. clausii*. Most of these bacteria are recognized as part of normal flora of the skin, oropharynx and perineum of healthy individuals. While erythromycin resistance was found in the majority of isolated nasopharyngeal bacteria, macrolide determinants could only be detected in the *Staphylococcus* group. The primers we used to detect seven macrolide resistance genes would not be expected to capture all of the genes potentially conferring resistance. For example, primers for erythromycin resistance genes *erm*(D) and *erm*(34) previously characterized from *B. licheniformis* and *B. clausii*, respectively (Israeli-Reches et al., 1984; Bozdogan et al., 2004) were not included in our panel. Although we observed no increase in the diversity of erythromycin resistant nasopharyngeal bacteria in our study, determinants in those bacteria that possessed them could be disseminated into the broader environment.

Escherichia coli are commonly used as faecal indicator bacteria to assess AMR, but we chose enterococci as *E. coli* are intrinsically resistant to macrolides (Mao and Putterman, 1968). Enterococci are common inhabitants of the normal gut flora of both livestock and humans (Yost et al., 2011). Outside of their normal habitat, enterococci are viewed as pathogens and may present a public health concern as they can be transmitted to humans from other hosts or by ingestion of contaminated food or water (Heuer et al., 2006; Marshall and Levy, 2011). Enterococci, in particular *E. faecalis* and *E. faecium* are recognized as prevalent nosocomial pathogens (Fisher and Phillips, 2009; van Schaik and Willems, 2010) with many isolates being resistant to multiple antibiotics and capable of exchanging DNA with other bacteria (SchjØrring and Krogfelt, 2011). In the present study we did not isolate either *E. faecalis* or *E. faecium*, with *E. hirae* being the predominant species isolated from cattle, a species infrequently associated with hospital infections.

The present study revealed a significant increase in the proportion of erythromycin resistant enterococci following macrolide treatment regardless of the method of administration (**Figure 5**). Oral administration of tylosin was expected to have a direct impact on the enterococci population of the gut, but the occurrence of erythromycin resistant enterococci in cattle administered injectable macrolides was equally marked. Studies submitted to the Food and Drug Administration's Center for Veterinary Medicine (FDA/CVM) showed that with a single subcutaneous dose of tilmicosin to cattle, 24% was recovered in the urine and 68% in the feces, whereas with tulathromycin, 50% was recovered in the feces with 90% of this being in its original form. It has been proposed that tulathromycin losses activity at pH $\leq$ 7.0, (Food and Drug Administration's Center for Veterinary, 2013), but considering that the pH in intestinal digesta and in feces is usually neutral or acidic (Allison et al., 1979; Canh et al., 1997), our results would suggest that this antibiotic selected for resistant enterococci within the intestinal tract. It is possible that the forage rich diet used in our study resulted in intestinal contents having, a pH above 7.0, allowing the concentration of tulathromycin in digesta to exceed the MIC of enterococci. High forage diets in cattle are known to increase colonic pH to ranges between 7.4 and 8.0 (Scott et al., 2000; Loy et al., 2001), but results could be quite different on high grain diets where the pH of digesta is considerably lower.

Similar PFGE profiles were observed for erythromycin resistant enterococci from both pre- and post-treatment samples (**Figure 6**), suggesting that regardless of the method of administration, macrolides selected for erythromycin resistant enterococci that were already in the digestive tract. Selection for resistant enterococci combined with a reduction in susceptible enterococci significantly increased the presence of erythromycin resistant *Enterococcus* spp. within the digestive tract. This observation is of interest considering that the cattle used in this study originated from a very isolated ranch and never had prior direct exposure to macrolides. It would be interesting to examine the persistence of this resistant population for a prolonged period of time to understand population dynamics and to investigate if the metabolic burden/cost of antibiotic resistance genes in the absence of macrolides leads to a decline in resistance within the enterococci population over time. As is typical in industry, cattle in this study were treated with injectable macrolides early in the feeding period. Considering that they would have been fed for an additional 200 days prior to slaughter, loss of resistant enterococci from the intestinal tract at later points in the feeding period is a distinct possibility. However, resistant enterococci may persist in cattle fed tylosin as this antibiotic is often administered for a longer duration of the feeding period.

All of the isolated erythromycin resistant enterococci contained *erm*(B), a gene coding for rRNA adenine N-6-methyltransferase, which methylates the A2058 position of 23S rRNA. Macrolide resistance in enterococci isolates from humans and animal sources in Europe has been well documented (Jensen et al., 1999; Aarestrup et al., 2001). Occurrence of macrolide resistance in enterococci originating from swine is thought to stem from the subtherapeutic use of tylosin (Jackson et al., 2004). The co-existence of macrolide resistance genes with other antibiotic resistance genes has also been observed, most notably a link between resistance to macrolides and vancomycin (Aarestrup et al., 2000b), attributable to *erm*(B) and the *vanA* gene occurring in close proximity on the same plasmid. The increased occurrence of both *erm* and *tet* (tetracycline resistance) genes in faecal microbial communities from beef cattle fed subtherapeutic levels of tylosin has also been identified (Chen et al., 2008). Linkage of determinants for MLS_B and chloramphenicol resistance has also been found on a single conjugative plasmid in *E. faecium* and dissemination of this cluster among streptogramin-resistant enterococci occurs (Werner et al., 2000). Resistance to MLS_B antibiotics in Gram-positive cocci colonizing humans is now recognized to be a serious problem, negatively affecting clinical outcomes (Lim et al., 2002; DiPersio and DiPersio, 2006).

Regardless of the hypothesized prospects of subtherapeutic administration of antimicrobials contributing towards AMR development, there is limited and conflicting data as to the extent that subtherapeutic vs. therapeutic drug administration contributes to livestock mediated antimicrobial resistance. Studies have shown that subtherapeutic administration of tylosin had no impact on the prevalence of erythromycin resistant *Campylobacter* in feedlot cattle (Inglis et al., 2005), whereas with broiler chickens the frequency of macrolide resistant *Campylobacter* in cecal contents was increased with subtherapeutic vs. therapeutic doses of tylosin (Ladely et al., 2007). These discrepancies may reflect species-specific (cattle vs. chicken) differences in gastrointestinal physiology and diet. Others have found that short-term therapeutic use of chlortetracycline in the diet was no less likely to select for resistant *Salmonella* populations than long-term subtherapeutic use (Kobland et al., 1987). In-feed and subcutaneous administration of oxytetracycline were also equally responsible for increasing the proportion of feedlot cattle excreting tetracycline resistant *E. coli* in faeces (Checkley et al., 2010).

The present study offers a comparison of subtherapeutic and therapeutic drug administration with regards to the prevalence of resistance among bacteria from two independent locations in cattle. In conclusion, the injectable macrolides had impact on both respiratory and enteric microbes whereas orally administered macrolides only influenced enteric bacteria. Therapeutic levels of tilmicosin and tulathromycin were effective in lowering nasopharyngeal *M. haemolytica*, whereas the in-feed levels of tylosin had no effect on the prevalence of this bacterium. *M. haemolytica* isolates from control and macrolide treated animals were found to be susceptible to macrolides as well as other antibiotics tested. The lack of AMR in *M. haemolytica* may be attributed to the possible absence of AMR determinants in *Mannheimia* as well as other closely related bacteria such as *P. multocida*. Erythromycin resistance was detected in nasopharyngeal bacteria co-isolated with *M. haemolytica*, regardless of the treatment group. All three macrolides increased the occurrence of erythromycin resistance *Enterococcus* spp. within the intestinal tract of cattle, but the species identified were not those most frequently linked to nosocomial infections in humans. To our knowledge this is the first report on increased occurrence of macrolide resistance in enterococci after systemic macrolide usage in cattle. It would be interesting to monitor the post-treatment AMR resistance over a period of weeks to months beyond treatment to determine if these macrolide-resistant enterococci continue to persist within the faecal bacterial populations of cattle.

ACKNOWLEDGMENTS

This study was conducted with funding from SAGES program of Agriculture and Agri-Food Canada in partnership with the University of Calgary. We thank Ruth Barbieri, Lorna Selinger, Shea Brennan, Wendi Smart, and animal handling staff for their technical assistance.

REFERENCES

Aarestrup, F. M., Agersł, Y., Ahrens, P., Jłrgensen, J. C., Madsen, M., and Jensen, L. B. (2000a). Antimicrobial susceptibility and presence of resistance genes in staphylococci from poultry. *Vet. Microbiol.* 74, 353–364.

Aarestrup, F. M., Kruse, H., Tast, E., Hammerum, A. M., and Jensen, L. B. (2000b). Associations between the use of antimicrobial agents for growth promotion and the occurrence of resistance among *Enterococcus faecium* from broilers and pigs in Denmark, Finland, and Norway. *Microb. Drug Resist.* 6, 63–70.

Aarestrup, F. M., and Wegener, H. C. (1999). The effects of antibiotic usage in food animals on the development of antimicrobial resistance of importance for humans in *Campylobacter* and *Escherichia coli*. *Microbes. Infect.* 1, 639–644.

Aarestrup, F. M. A., Seyfarth, M., Emborg, H. D., Pedersen, K., Hendriksen, R. S., and Bager, F. (2001). Effect of abolishment of the use of antimicrobial agents for growth promotion on occurrence of antimicrobial resistance in fecal enterococci from food animals in Denmark. *Antimicrob. Agents Chemother.* 45, 2054–2059.

Addah, W., Baah, J., Groenewegen, P., Okine, E. K., and McAllister, T. A. (2011). Comparison of the fermentation characteristics, aerobic stability and nutritive value of barley and corn silages ensiled with or without a mixed bacterial inoculant. *Can. J. Anim. Sci.* 91, 133–146.

Alexander, T. W., Cook, S. R., Yanke, L. J., Booker, C. W., Morley, P. S., Read, R. R., et al. (2008). A multiplex polymerase chain reaction assay for the identification of *Mannheimia haemolytica*, *Mannheimia glucosida* and *Mannheimia ruminalis*. *Vet. Microbiol.* 130, 165–175.

Allison, M. J., Robinson, I. M., Bucklin, J. A., and Booth, G. D. (1979). Comparison of bacterial populations of the pig cecum and colon based upon enumeration with specific energy sources. *Appl. Environ. Microbiol.* 37, 1142–1151.

Andersen, N. M., Poehlsgaard, J., Warrass, R., and Douthwaite, S. (2012). Inhibition of protein synthesis on the ribosome comparing tildipirosin with other veterinary macrolides. *Antimicrob. Agents Chemother.* 56, 6033–6036.

Bozdogan, B., Galopin, S., and Leclercq, R. (2004). Characterization of a new erm-related macrolide resistance gene present in probiotic strains of *Bacillus clausii*. *Appl. Environ. Microbiol.* 70, 280–284.

Canh, T. T., Verstegen, M. W. A., Aarnink, A. J. A., and Schrama, J. W. (1997). Influence of dietary factors on nitrogen partitioning and composition of urine and feces of fattening pigs. *J. Anim. Sci.* 75, 700–706.

Checkley, S. L., Campbell, J. R., Chirino-Trejo, M., Janzen, E. D., and Waldner, C. L. (2010). Associations between antimicrobial use and the prevalence of antimicrobial resistance in fecal *Escherichia coli* from feedlot cattle in western Canada. *Can. Vet. J.* 51, 853–861.

Chen, J., Fluharty, F. L., St-Pierre, N., Morrison, M., and Yu, Z. (2008). Technical note: occurrence in fecal microbiota of genes conferring resistance to both macrolide-lincosamide-streptogramin B and tetracyclines concomitant with feeding of beef cattle with tylosin. *J. Anim. Sci.* 86, 2385–2391.

Chen, J., Yu, Z., Michel F. C. Jr., Wittum, T., and Morrison, M. (2007). Development and application of real-time PCR assays for quantification of *erm* genes conferring resistance to macrolides-lincosamides-streptogramin B in livestock manure and manure management systems. *Appl. Environ. Microbiol.* 73, 4407–4416.

CIPARS. (2013). Canadian Integrated Program for Antimicrobial Resistance Surveillance Report. Available online at: http://www.phac-aspc.gc.ca/cipars-ca/cipars-picra/pubs-eng.php#ar (last accessed date: 8 March 2013).

Clinical and Laboratory Standards Institute (2008a). *Performance Standards for Antimicrobial Disk and Dilution Susceptibility Tests for Bacteria Isolated from Animals; Approved Standard - 3rd Edn. Document M31-A3.* Wayne, PA: Clinical and Laboratory Standards Institute.

Clinical and Laboratory Standards Institute (2008b). *Methods for Antimicrobial Dilution and Disk Susceptibility Testing of Infrequently Isolated or Fastidious Bacteria; Approved Guideline. Document M45-A.* Wayne, PA: Clinical and Laboratory Standards Institute.

Confer, A. W. (2009). Update on bacterial pathogenesis in BRD. *Anim. Health Res. Rev.* 10, 145–148.

Cox, S. R., McLaughlin, C., Fielder, A. E., Yancey, M. F., Bowersock, T. L., Garcia-Tapia, D., et al. (2010). Rapid and prolonged distribution of tulathromycin into lung homogenate and pulmonary epithelial lining fluid of Holstein calves following a single subcutaneous administration of 2.5 mg/kg body weight. *Int. J. Appl. Res. Vet. Med.* 8, 129–137.

Dabo, S. M., Taylor, J. D., and Confer, A. W. (2007). *Pasteurella multocida* and bovine respiratory disease. *Anim. Health Res. Rev.* 8, 129–150.

Desmolaize, B., Rose, S., Warrass, R., and Douthwaite, S. (2011). A novel *Erm* monomethyltransferase in antibiotic-resistant isolates of *Mannheimia haemolytica* and *Pasteurella multocida*. *Mol. Microbiol.* 80, 184–194.

DiPersio, L. P., and DiPersio, J. R. (2006). High rates of erythromycin and clindamycin resistance among OBGYN isolates of group B *Streptococcus*. *Diagn. Microbiol. Infect. Dis.* 54, 79–82.

Fisher, K., and Phillips, C. (2009). The ecology, epidemiology and virulence of *Enterococcus*. *Microbiol.* 55, 1749–1757.

Food and Drug Administration's Center for Veterinary Medicine (FDA/CVM). (2013). Tulathromycin solution for parenteral injection for treatment of bovine and swine respiratory diseases: microbiological effects on bacteria of human health concern, a qualitative risk estimation. Available online at: www.fda.gov/downloads/AdvisoryCommittees/CommitteesMeetingMaterials/VeterinaryMedicineAdvisoryCommittee/UCM127196.pdf (last accessed date: 8 March 2013).

Frank, G. H., Briggs, R. E., Loan, R. W., Purdy, C. W., and Zehr, E. S. (2000). Effect of tilmicosin treatment on *Pasteurella haemolytica* organisms in nasal secretion specimens of calves with respiratory tract disease. *Am. J.Vet. Res.* 61, 525–529.

Fulton, R. W. (2009). Bovine respiratory disease research (1983–2009). *Anim. Health Res. Rev.* 10, 131–139.

Giraffa, G. (2002). Enterococci from foods. *FEMS Microbiol. Rev.* 26, 163–171.

Gow, S. (2005). Antimicrobial resistance, prudent use, and the Canadian integrated program for antimicrobial resistance surveillance (CIPARS). *Large Anim. Vet Rounds* 5, 1–6.

Heuer, O. E., Hammerum, A. M., Collignon, P., Collignon, P., and Wegener, H. C. (2006). Human health hazard from antimicrobial-resistant enterococci in animals and food. *Clin. Infect. Dis.* 43, 911–916.

Inglis, G. D., McAllister, T. A., Busz, H. W., Yanke, L. J., Morck, D. W., Olson, M. E., et al. (2005). Effects of subtherapeutic administration of antimicrobial agents to beef cattle on the prevalence of antimicrobial resistance in *Campylobacter jejuni* and *Campylobacter hyointestinalis*. *Appl. Environ. Microbiol.* 71, 3872–3881.

Israeli-Reches, M., Weinrauch, Y., and Dubnau, D. (1984). Evolutionary relationships of the *Bacillus licheniformis* macrolide-lincosamide-streptogramin B resistance elements. *Mol. Gen. Genet.* 194, 362–367.

Jackson, C. R., Fedorka-Cray, P. J., Barrett, J. B., and Ladely, S. R. (2004). Effects of tylosin use on erythromycin resistance in enterococci isolated from swine. *Appl. Environ. Microbiol.* 70, 4205–4210.

Jensen, L. B., Frimodt-Moller, N., and Aarestrup, F. M. (1999). Presence of *erm* gene classes in gram-positive bacteria of animal and human origin in Denmark. *FEMS Microbiol. Lett.* 170, 151–158.

Jensen, L. B., Hammerum, A. M., Bager, F., and Aarestrup, F. M. (2002). Streptogramin resistance among *Enterococcus faecium* isolated from production animals in Denmark in 1997. *Microb. Drug Resist.* 8, 369–374.

Katsuda, K., Kohmoto, M., Mikami, O., and Uchida, I. (2009). Antimicrobial resistance and genetic characterization of fluoroquinolone-resistant *Mannheimia haemolytica* isolates from cattle with bovine pneumonia. *Vet. Microbiol.* 139, 74–79.

Klima, C. L., Alexander, T. W., Read, R. R., Gow, S. P., Booker, C. W., Hannon, S., et al. (2011). Genetic characterization and antimicrobial susceptibility of *Mannheimia haemolytica* isolated from the nasopharynx of feedlot cattle. *Vet. Microbiol.* 149, 390–398.

Kloos, W., and Bannerman, T. L. (1994). Update on clinical significance of coagulase-negative staphylococci. *Clin. Microbiol. Rev.* 7, 117–140.

Kobland, J. D., Gale, G. O., Gustafson, R. H., and Simkins, K. L. (1987). Comparison of therapeutic versus subtherapeutic levels of chlortetracycline in the diet for selection of resistant *salmonella* in experimentally challenged chickens. *Poult. Sci.* 66, 1129–1137.

Ladely, S. R., Harrison, M. A., Fedorka-Cray, P. J., Berrang, M. E., Englen, M. D., and Meinersmann, R. J. (2007). Development of macrolide-resistant Campylobacter in broilers administered subtherapeutic or therapeutic concentrations of tylosin. *J. Food Prot.* 70, 1945–1951.

Lewicki, J. (2006). Tylosin. A review of pharmacokinetics, residues in food animals and analytical methods. FAO website: ftp://ftp.fao.org/ag/agn/food/tylosin2006.pdf (last accessed date: 8 March 2013).

Lim, J. A., Kwon, A. R., Kim, S. K., Chong, Y., Lee, K., and Choi, E. C. (2002). Prevalence of resistance to macrolide, lincosamide and streptogramin antibiotics in Gram-positive cocci isolated in a Korean hospital. *J. Antimicrob. Chemother.* 49, 489–495.

Loy, T., Wilson, C., Bailey, D., Klopfenstein, T. J., and Moxley, R. A. (2001). Influence of restricted intake and reduced dietary starch on colonic pH and *E. coli* prevalence. *Nebraska Beef Report* MP76-A, 86–88.

Marshall, B. M., and Levy, S. B. (2011). Food animals and antimicrobials: impacts on human health. *Clin. Microbiol. Rev.* 24, 718–733.

Mao, J. C., and Putterman, M. (1968). Accumulation in gram-postive and gram-negative bacteria as a mechanism of resistance to erythromycin. *J. Bacteriol.* 95, 1111–1117.

McEwen, S. A., and Fedorka-Cray, P. J. (2002). Antimicrobial use and resistance in animals. *Clin. Infect. Dis.* 34, S93–S106.

Michael, G. B., Kadlec, K., Sweeney, M. T., Brzuszkiewicz, E., Liesegang, H., Daniel, R., et al. (2012). ICEPmu1, an integrative conjugative element (ICE) of *Pasteurella multocida*: analysis of the regions that comprise 12 antimicrobial resistance genes. *J. Antimicrob. Chemother.* 67, 84–90.

Pardon, B., De Bleecker, K., Dewulf, J., Callens, J., Boyen, F., Catry, B., et al. (2011). Prevalence of respiratory pathogens in diseased, non-vaccinated, routinely medicated veal calves. *Vet. Rec.* 169, 278.

Piette, A., and Verschraegen, G. (2008). Role of coagulase-negative staphylococci in human disease. *Vet. Microbiol.* 134, 45–54.

Portis, E., Lindeman, C., Johansen, L., and Stoltman, G. (2012). A ten-year (2000–2009) study of antimicrobial susceptibility of bacteria that cause bovine respiratory disease complex–*Mannheimia haemolytica*, *Pasteurella multocida*, and *Histophilus somni*–in the United States and Canada. *J. Vet. Diagn. Invest.* 24, 932–944.

Roberts, M. C. (2008). Update on macrolide-lincosamide-streptogramin, ketolide, and oxazolidinone resistance genes. *FEMS Microbiol. Lett.* 282, 147-159

Roberts, M. C., Sutcliffe, J., Courvalin, P., Jensen, L. B., Rood, J., and Seppala, H. (1999). Nomenclature for macrolide and macrolide-lincosamide-streptogramin B resistance determinants. *Antimicrob. Agents Chemother.* 43, 2823–2830.

Savini, V., Catavitello, C., Carlino, D., Bianco, A., Pompilio, A., Balbinot, A., et al. (2009). *Staphylococcus pasteuri* bacteraemia in a patient with leukaemia. *J. Clin.Pathol.* 62, 957–958.

SchjØrring, S., and Krogfelt, K. A. (2011). Assessment of bacterial antibiotic resistance transfer in the gut. *Int. J. Microbiol.* 2011:ID 312956. doi: 10.1155/2011/312956

Schlünzen, F., Zarivach, R., Harms, J., Bashan, A., Tocilj, A., Albrecht, R., et al. (2001). Structural basis for the interaction of antibiotics with the peptidyl transferase centre in eubacteria. *Nature* 413, 814–821.

Scott, T., Wilson, C., Bailey, D., Klopfendtein, T. J., and Milton, T. (2000). Influence of diet on total and acid resistant *E. coli* and colonic pH. *Nebraska Beef Report* MP73-A, 39–43.

Siegel, T. W., Earley, D. L., Smothers, C. D., Sun, F., and Ricketts, A. P. (2004). Cellular uptake of the triamilide tulathromycin by bovine and porcine phagocytic cells *in vitro*. *J. Anim. Sci.* 82, 186.

Simeoni, D., Rizzotti, L., Cocconcelli, P., Gazzola, S., Dellaglio, F., and Torriani, S. (2008). Antibiotic resistance genes and identification of staphylococci collected from the production chain of swine meat commodities. *Food Microbiol.* 25, 196–201.

Skinner, R., Cundliffe, E., and Schmidt, F. J. (1983). Site of action of a ribosomal RNA methylase responsible for resistance to erythromycin and other antibiotics. *J. Biol. Chem.* 258, 12702–12706.

Szczepanowski, R., Linke, B., Krahn, I., Gartemann, K. H., Gützkow, T., Eichler, W., et al. (2009). Detection of 140 clinically relevant antibiotic-resistance genes in the plasmid metagenome of wastewater treatment plant bacteria showing reduced susceptibility to selected antibiotics. *Microbiol.* 155, 2306–2319.

Turabelidze, D., Kotetishvili, M., Kreger, A., Morris, J. G. Jr., and Sulakvelidze, A. (2000). Improved pulsed-field gel electrophoresis for typing vancomycin-resistant enterococci. *J. Clin. Microbiol.* 38, 4242–4245.

USDA. (1999). Report part III: health management and biosecurity in U.S. feedlots 1999. Available online at: http://www.aphis.usda.gov/animal_health/nahms/feedlot/downloads/feedlot99/Feedlot99_dr_PartIII.pdf (last accessed date: 8 March 2013).

van Schaik, W., and Willems, R. J. (2010). Genome-based insights into the evolution of enterococci. *Clin. Microbiol. Infect.* 16, 527–532.

Watts, J. L., and Sweeney, M. T. (2010). Antimicrobial resistance in bovine respiratory disease pathogens: measures, trends, and impact on efficacy. *Vet. Clin. North Am. Food Anim. Pract.* 26, 79–88.

Wegener, H. C., Aarestrup, F. M., Jensen, L. B., Hammerum, A. M., and Bager, F. (1999). Use of antimicrobial growth promoters in food animals and *Enterococcus faecium* resistance to therapeutic antimicrobial drugs in Europe. *Emerg. Infect. Dis.* 5, 329–335.

Werner, G., Hildebrandt, B., Klare, I., and Witte, W. (2000). Linkage of determinants for streptogramin A, macrolide-lincosamide-streptogramin B, and chloramphenicol resistance on a conjugative plasmid in *Enterococcus faecium* and dissemination of this cluster among streptogramin-resistant enterococci. *Int. J. Med. Microbiol.* 290, 543–548.

Yost, C. K., Diarra, M. S., and Topp, E. (2011). "Animals and humans as sources of fecal indicator bacteria," in *The Fecal Bacteria*, eds M. J. Sadowsky and R. L. Whitman (Washington DC: ASM Press), 67–91.

Zaheer, R., Yanke, L. J., Church, D., Topp, E., Read, R. R., and McAllister, T. A. (2012). High-throughput species identification of enterococci using pyrosequencing. *J. Microbiol. Methods* 89, 174–178.

Zecchinon, L., Fett, T., and Desmecht, D. (2005). How *Mannheimia haemolytica* defeats host defence through a kiss of death mechanism. *Vet. Res.* 36, 133–156.

Characterization of fluoroquinolone resistance and *qnr* diversity in *Enterobacteriaceae* from municipal biosolids

Ella Kaplan[1,2], Maya Ofek[1,2], Edouard Jurkevitch[2] and Eddie Cytryn[1]*

[1] Department of Soil Chemistry, Plant Nutrition and Microbiology, Institute of Soil, Water and Environmental Sciences, The Volcani Center, Agricultural Research Organization, Beit Dagan, Israel
[2] Department of Agroecology and Plant Health, The Robert H. Smith Faculty of Agriculture, Food and Environment, The Hebrew University of Jerusalem, Jerusalem, Israel

Edited by:
Marilyn C. Roberts, University of Washington, USA

Reviewed by:
Charles W. Knapp, University of Strathclyde, UK
Carlos F. Amábile-Cuevas, Fundación Lusara, Mexico

***Correspondence:**
Eddie Cytryn, Department of Soil Chemistry, Plant Nutrition and Microbiology, Institute of Soil, Water and Environmental Sciences, The Volcani Center, Agricultural Research Organization, P.O. Box 6, Beit Dagan 50250, Israel
e-mail: eddie@volcani.agri.gov.il

Municipal biosolids produced during activated sludge treatment applied in wastewater treatment plants, are significant reservoirs of antibiotic resistance, since they assemble both natural and fecal microbiota, as well as residual concentrations of antibiotic compounds. This raises major concerns regarding the environmental and epidemiological consequences of using them as fertilizers for crops. The second generation fluoroquinolone ciprofloxacin is probably the most abundant antibiotic compound detected in municipal biosolids due to its widespread use and sorption properties. Although fluoroquinolone resistance was originally thought to result from mutations in bacterial gyrase and topoisomerase IV genes, it is becoming apparent that it is also attributed to plasmid-associated resistance factors, which may propagate environmental antibiotic resistance. The objective of this study was to assess the impact of the activated sludge process on fluoroquinolone resistance. The scope of resistances and mobile genetic mechanisms associated with fluoroquinolone resistance were evaluated by screening large collections of ciprofloxacin-resistant *Enterobacteriaceae* strains from sludge ($n = 112$) and from raw sewage ($n = 89$). Plasmid-mediated quinolone resistance determinants (*qnrA*, *B*, and *S*) were readily detected in isolates from both environments, the most dominant being *qnr*S. Interestingly, all *qnr* variants were significantly more abundant in sludge isolates than in the isolates from raw sewage. Almost all ciprofloxacin-resistant isolates were resistant to multiple antibiotic compounds. The sludge isolates were on the whole resistant to a broader range of antibiotic compounds than the raw sewage isolates; however, this difference was not statistically significant. Collectively, this study indicates that the activated sludge harbors multi-resistant bacterial strains, and that mobile quinolone-resistance elements may have a selective advantage in the activated sludge.

Keywords: activated sludge, biosolids, fluoroquinolone, ciprofloxacin, antibiotic resistance, *qnr*, integron

INTRODUCTION

Municipal biosolids produced during the activated sludge process in secondary wastewater treatment are often utilized as fertilizers for a wide array of crops, due to their availability and high nutrient content (Dröge et al., 2000; Golet et al., 2003). However, despite the obvious advantages of this practice, sludge application may have highly negative ecological and epidemiological ramifications. Wastewater treatment plants (WWTPs) represent an endless pool of commensal human and farm animal bacteria (Dröge et al., 2000; Zhang et al., 2009), which are constantly exposed to a wide range of anthropogenic compounds, such as antibiotics. These compounds can select for resistant strains of both pathogenic and non-pathogenic bacteria, by means of both vertical and horizontal gene transfer (Pellegrini et al., 2011).

The application of municipal biosolids to soil may not only result in transfer of resistant bacterial strains, but also in dissemination of antibiotic resistance genes (ARGs) that can enhance environmental antibiotic resistance reservoirs. Indeed, there is growing perception that ARGs are emerging contaminants with the ability to spread from anthropogenic sources, such as WWTPs, into natural environments (LaPara et al., 2011; Li et al., 2012; Pruden et al., 2012). Although municipal biosolids are generally stabilized before application to soils, a recent study detected significant levels of ARGs in biosolids subsequent to different stabilization methods (Ma et al., 2011; Munir and Xagoraraki, 2011), and elevated levels of these genes were even observed in soil samples after land application of biosolids (Munir and Xagoraraki, 2011).

Fluoroquinolones are fully synthetic broad-spectrum antibacterial agents that are becoming increasingly popular in the treatment of clinical infections. The mechanism by which fluoroquinolones inhibit cell proliferation was well elaborated by Jacoby (2005) and by Strahilevitz et al. (2009).

Ciprofloxacin is a second generation fluoroquinolone and is the fifth most commonly prescribed antibacterial with over 20 million outpatient prescriptions written in the US alone in 2010.

The metabolism of ciprofloxacin in the human body is only partial and so it is excreted in both urine (45–62%) and feces (15–25%), and transported to WWTPs through municipal sewage systems (Golet et al., 2003). During wastewater treatment, a large fraction of ciprofloxacin is removed from the aqueous phase and absorbed into the sludge, thereby accumulating in dewatered sludge, where concentrations of up to 50 mg/kg dry weight have been detected (Golet et al., 2002; McClellan and Halden, 2010).Field experiments have demonstrated that sorption of fluoroquinolones to municipal sludge results in long-term persistence, which continues even after application to agricultural soils (Golet et al., 2003).

When fluoroquinolones were first introduced for clinical use in the mid 1980s the likelihood for the emergence of resistance was considered to be negligible, because bacteria would have to spontaneously acquire two or more non-fatal mutations in the catalytic sites of the gyrase/topoisomerase IV enzymes to evade the antibiotic effect (Robicsek et al., 2006). Nonetheless, shortly after fluoroquinolones became one of the top antibiotic compounds in nosocomial use, resistance became a common global phenomenon (Robicsek et al., 2006; Strahilevitz et al., 2007). Originally, fluoroquinolone resistance was attributed to mutations in specific areas of DNA gyrase genes (*gyrA*, *parC*, and *parE*), known as quinolone resistance-determining regions. However, in the late 1990s emerging evidence indicated acquisition of fluoroquinolone resistance in a non-clonal manner (Robicsek et al., 2006), with the detection of a plasmid-mediated-quinolone-resistance mechanism by Martinez-Martinez et al. (1998). This plasmid encoded a pentapeptide-repeat protein termed QnrA (for quinolone resistance) that increased quinolone resistance levels between 8- and 64-fold in *Escherichia coli*. Although the resistance of these isolates was approximately 10-fold lower than traditional mutation-associated minimal inhibitory concentration (MIC), they were found to have increased probabilities for acquisition of additional resistance mechanisms (Tran and Jacoby, 2002). Experiments conducted with a purified, His6 QnrA determined that it eliminated the quinolone action by directly binding to gyrase and preventing the antibiotic from binding to the DNA, thus being trapped in the lethal gyrase–DNA–quinolone cleavage complex (Tran and Jacoby, 2002; Tran et al., 2005; Strahilevitz et al., 2009).

The worldwide expansion of *qnr* was rapid. In a study conducted in Alabama in 1994 by Martinez-Martinez et al. (1998), the newly defined *qnr*A variant was identified in only one host-associated *Klebsiella pneumoniae* isolate, and was not detected among any other of 350 Gram-negative isolates that were screened over 6 months. Ten years later, the prevalence of *qnr*A among ciprofloxacin-resistant *K. pneumoniae* isolates rose to 11% (in a 3-year survey done in six US states; Wang et al., 2004). During this period of time, *qnr*A-like determinants were also found in 7.7% of ciprofloxacin-resistant *E. coli* isolates in Shanghai, China (Wang et al., 2003). In light of these, and many other studies, it may be suggested that the increase in fluoroquinolone resistance was driven by the increase in *qnr* prevalence, which is horizontally transferred and confers a selective advantage to plasmid bearing bacteria (Martinez-Martinez et al., 1998; Nordmann and Poirel, 2005; Strahilevitz et al., 2007).

Several other variants of the Qnr protein have been discovered to date, including QnrB, QnrS, and the rarer QnrC and QnrD. All Qnr proteins involve a similar mechanism of protecting the bacterial gyrase/topoisomerase IV from the quinolone, and vary in size from 214 to 221 amino acids (Strahilevitz et al., 2009). Other studies show that although originating in different bacterial hosts, *qnr* genes are mostly found adjacent to sulfonamide resistance genes – *sul-I* and *sul-II*, and are often carried on class-1 integrons, in proximity to the integrase (*intl-1*) gene, which are prevalent in a wide range of ecological habitats (Tran and Jacoby, 2002; Strahilevitz et al., 2009; Pellegrini et al., 2011).

The objective of this study was to assess the phenotypic and genotypic scope of quinolone resistance in raw sewage and in WWTP sludge and to determine whether quinolone resistant bacteria, and specifically if plasmid-associated quinolone-resistance genes are enriched in WWTPs during sewage treatment. We isolated a large collection of ciprofloxacin-resistant *Enterobacteriaceae* from both the raw sewage entering the WWTP, and from dewatered sludge, and these isolates were screened for *qnrA*, *B*, and *S* variants, and for class-1 integron-associated integrase (*intl-1*) genes. Ciprofloxacin-resistant isolates were also screened against 1 μg/ml ciprofloxacin and six other antibiotic compounds to assess levels of multi-resistance in these environments. The initial isolation of the analyzed *Enterobacteriaceae* was conducted on 0.4 μg/ml ciprofloxacin, which corresponds to intermediate ciprofloxacin (IC) resistance that is a characteristic of *qnr*-harboring isolates. This is approximately 2.5-fold below MIC values associated with gyrase/topoisomerase IV mutant strains (Hopkins et al., 2005; Nordmann and Poirel, 2005; Gosling et al., 2012).

MATERIALS AND METHODS

SITE DESCRIPTION AND SAMPLING PROTOCOL

The Dan Region Wastewater Treatment and Reclamation Project (termed Shafdan), is the largest and most complex wastewater treatment facility in Israel. It treats approximately 340,000 m^3 of sewage daily from the entire metropolitan Tel Aviv area including five major hospitals. Secondary treatment is conducted in 12 activated sludge reservoirs with retention times ranging from 12–14 h. Approximately 15,000 m^3 of sludge are produced daily (1% dry weight).

Triplicate dewatered sludge and raw sewage samples were taken from the Shafdan WWTP in three individual sampling profiles (April 2012, May 2012, and October 2012). Dewatered sludge (18% water content) was sampled in sterile 100 ml test tubes, and the raw sewage was collected from WWTP influent in 1 l bottles. Samples were transferred to the lab on ice within 1 h, and raw sewage samples were concentrated by centrifuging for 10 min at 1000 *g*.

ENTEROBACTERIACEAE ISOLATION AND CHARACTERIZATION

Five grams of dewatered activated sludge or raw sewage samples were suspended in 40 ml of sterile 0.1 M ammonium phosphate buffer [$(NH_4)_2HPO_4$], shaken laterally at 350 rpm for 45 min, at room temperature, and centrifuged twice for 10 min at 500 rpm; each time supernatant was transferred into new 50 ml sterile tubes and pellet was discarded. Supernatant was then centrifuged for 10 min at 8,000 rpm, and the pellet was resuspended in 20 ml sterile saline solution. Samples were serially diluted and filtered onto 25 mm, 0.45 μm pore size polycarbonate membranes (GE Healthcare, Chalfont St. Giles, UK). Filters were aseptically placed on 45 mm Petri dishes containing modified membrane thermotolerant *Escherichia coli* (mTEC) agar, which selects for *Enterobacteriaceae*. The modified mTEC method www.epa.gov/nerlcwww/documents/1603sp02.pdf uses the chromogen 5-bromo-6-chloro-3-indolyl-β-D-glucuronide (Magenta Gluc) as the differential agent (Francy and Darner, 2000).

Serial dilutions were platted on media with or without IC concentrations (0.4 μg/ml). This sub-MIC value was selected, because, as mentioned above, it is believed to be a ciprofloxacin concentration which will allow us to screen for *Enterobacteriaceae* that harbor plasmid-mediated fluoroquinolone resistance (Hopkins et al., 2005; Gosling et al., 2012). Plates were incubated for 2 h at 37°C and then for 20–22 h at 45°C as previously described (Francy and Darner, 2000).

The taxonomic affiliation of the isolates was determined by plating on CHROMagar Orientation medium agar plates (CHROMagar Microbiology, Paris, France). CHROMagar typing indicated that all of the *Enterobacteriaceae* isolates from both the raw sewage and the sludge biosolids were affiliated with either the *E. coli* (16.1% of sludge isolates and 11.2% of raw sewage isolates) or *Klebsiella* (78.6% of sludge isolates and 70.8% of raw sewage isolates) genera.

There was no statistical difference in the ration of *E. coli* to *Klebsiella* genera in the sludge relative to the raw sewage.

All of the non-*Enterobacteriaceae* isolates were not used for further analysis. The taxonomic affiliation of 20 of the isolates was further assessed by phylogenetic analysis of partial 16S rRNA gene fragments. Standard Sanger sequencing was conducted at HyLabs (Rehovot, Israel) and the taxonomic affiliation of the sequences was determined by basic local alignment search tool (BLAST). In total, 201 sub-MIC *Enterobacteriaceae* isolates were obtained (112 from the activated sludge, and 89 from the raw sewage), and further analyzed as described below.

RESISTANCE PHENOTYPING

Ninety activated sludge and 87 raw sewage, sub-MIC ciprofloxacin-resistant isolates were screened for resistance to other antibiotic compounds as follows: isolates were transferred aseptically to Müller-Hinton (MH)-agar containing one of the eight different antibiotics at European Committee on Antibiotic Susceptibility Testing (EUCAST) clinical MIC breakpoint concentrations according to standard procedures (http://www.eucast.org/clinical_breakpoints): ciprofloxacin (1 μg/ml), ampicillin (8 μg/ml), ceftriaxone (2 μg/ml), chloramphenicol (8 μg/ml), and gentamicin (4 μg/ml). In addition, isolates were also screened against nalidixic acid (32 μg/ml) and tetracycline (30 μg/ml). Plates were incubated at 37°C overnight, and colony formation was assessed.

DNA EXTRACTION FROM ISOLATES

DNA was extracted from all samples using a modified bead-beating method. Bacteria cells were grown overnight in 5 ml Luria-Bertani (LB) broth containing ciprofloxacin (0.4 μg/μl). After harvest, cells were lysed in extraction buffer [100 mM Tris–HCl, pH 8.0; 100 mM potassium phosphate buffer pH 8.0; 1% cetyltrimethylammonium bromide (CTAB); and 2% sodium dodecyl sulfate (SDS)] followed by bead-beating (in the Fast Prep FP 120, Bio101, Savant Instruments Inc., Holbrook, NY, USA). The crude extracts were mixed with KCl to a final concentration of 0.5 M, incubated for 5 min, and centrifuged. DNA present in the supernatant was bound to glassmilk (0.5–10 μm silica particles, Sigma Chemical Co., St. Louis, MO, USA) with 6 M NaI. The silica was then resuspended in an ethanol-based wash buffer solution (Boyle and Lew, 1995) and transferred to a centrifuge tube filter (0.22 μm cut-off nylon filter, Costar, Corning Inc., Corning, NY, USA) that bound the DNA to the silica and retained it on the filter until eluted with 60°C Tris–EDTA (TE) into a sterile tube. Extracted DNA samples were stored at −20°C until use.

PCR DETECTION OF *qnr* VARIANTS AND *intI-1* GENES

Detection of the *qnr* variants was accomplished by means of a modified multiplex, touchdown PCR protocol based on a previously described method and primers (Cattoir et al., 2007). Briefly, the protocol involved 20 initial cycles: 5 min 94°C, 30 s 94°C, 30 s 60–50°C (each cycles reducing 0.5°C), 20 s 72°C, repeating the latter three steps; 15 additional cycles: 30 s 94°C, 30 s 50°C, 20 s 72°C; and a final cool down step for 10 min, at 72°C followed by a slow descent to 10°C.

For detection of the *intI-1* gene, the following PCR protocol was conducted, using previously reported primers (Gaze et al., 2011): 25 cycles: 3 min 95°C, 1 min 95°C, 30 s 58°C, 10 s 72°C repeating the latter three steps, 10 min 72°C and a slow descent to 10°C. Both PCR programs were executed in a final volume of 12.5 μl containing: 8 ng of purified DNA, 5 U Dream-Taq polymerase (MBI Fermentas, Lithuania), 1× Dream-Taq Buffer, 1.5 mM $MgCl_2$, 200 μM dNTPs, 0.4 μM primers.

STATISTICAL ANALYSES

Statistical analyses were conducted using the Statistica software application (StatSoft, Inc., Tulsa, OK, USA). Multiple statistical comparisons were conducted using the Tukey's HSD (honestly significant difference) test, in which mean values that do not share any letters are considered significantly different. Pairwise comparisons were conducted using the Fisher's exact test. Compared values were considered statistically significant when p values were less than 0.05.

RESULTS

ESTIMATION OF CIPROFLOXACIN-RESISTANT *ENTEROBACTERIACEAE*

Enterobacteriaceae levels in both raw sewage and dewatered, activated sludge ranged between 10^7 and 5×10^8 CFU/mg. Resistance to IC concentrations (0.4 μg/ml) reduced the number of colony forming units in both sample types by approximately two orders of magnitude (**Figure 1**), with no significant differences in the relative abundances of IC-resistant isolates in the sludge in comparison to the sewage isolates.

SCREENING FOR MULTI-RESISTANCE

The raw sewage and activated sludge *Enterobacteriaceae* isolates were highly resistant to EUCAST clinical MIC breakpoint

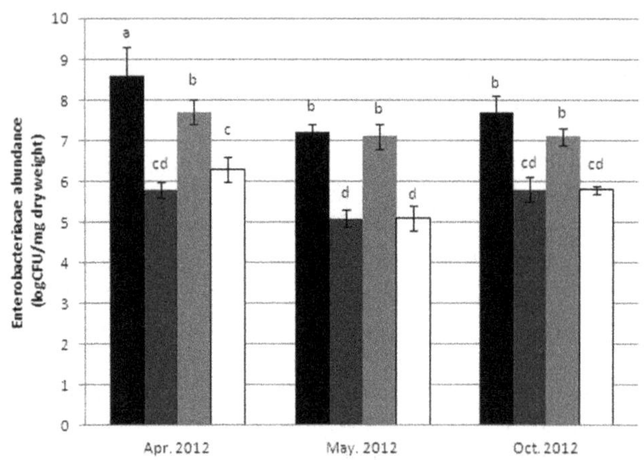

FIGURE 1 | Abundance of *Enterobacteriaceae* in dewatered sludge: non-selective media (black bars) and 0.4 µg/ml ciprofloxacin-amended media (dark gray bars); and in raw sewage: non-selective media (light gray bars), and 0.4 µg/ml ciprofloxacin-amended media (white bars). Error bars indicate standard deviation. Mean values that do not share any letters are considered significantly different (Tukey's HSD $p < 0.05$).

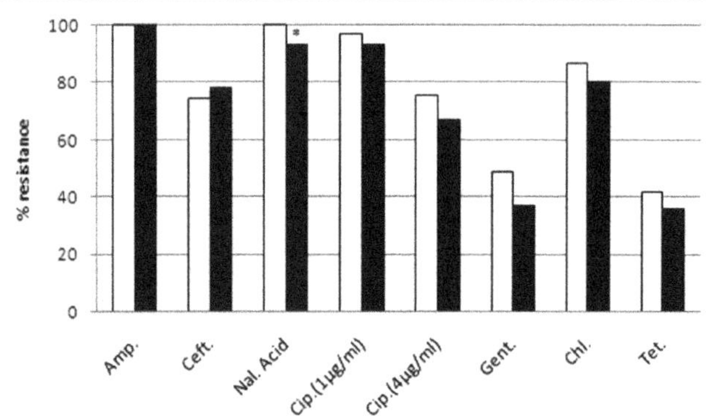

FIGURE 2 | Resistance of sludge (white bars) and raw sewage (gray bars) intermediate ciprofloxacin-resistant isolates to additional antibiotic compounds at MIC concentrations. Asterisk indicates statistically significant (Fisher's exact test $p < 0.05$) differences between sampling locations.

concentrations (**Figure 2**). With the exception of ceftriaxone, the ratio of IC isolates resistant to additional antibiotic compounds (at MIC concentrations) was generally higher in the dewatered sludge than in the raw sewage; however, this was only statistically significant for nalidixic acid. The efficacy of different antibiotics against the sewage and sludge isolates was highly similar for all of the antibiotics tested, as shown in **Figure 2.** Additional discrepancies were observed in the resistance profiles of the two environments when examining the scope of multi-resistance of the IC isolates. The sludge IC isolates were generally resistant to a larger range of antibiotic compounds; however, this was not statistically significant (**Figure 3**).

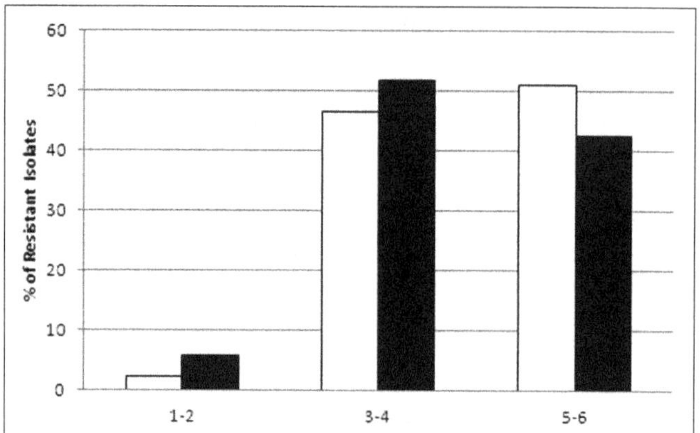

FIGURE 3 | Level of multi-resistance in intermediate ciprofloxacin-resistant isolates from sludge (white bars) and raw sewage (gray bars). The *x*-axis shows the abundance of the strains resistant to 1–2, 3–4, and 5–6 additional antibiotic compounds.

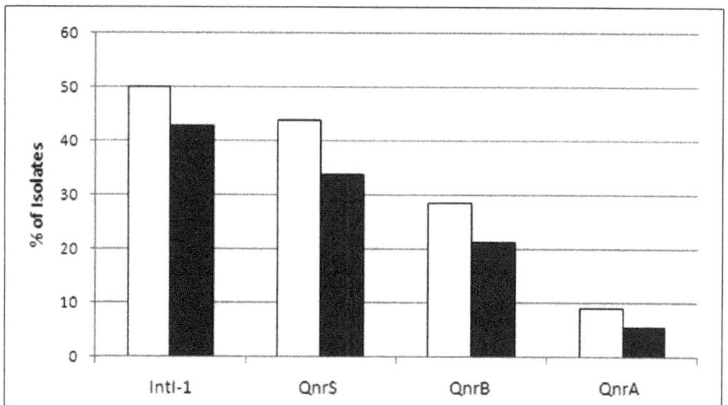

FIGURE 4 | The abundance of the different variants of *qnr* and of the *intl-1* genes in sludge (white bars) and raw sewage (gray bars) intermediate ciprofloxacin-resistant isolates.

DETECTION OF *qnr* VARIANTS AND PRESENCE OF CLASS-1 INTEGRONS

In total, 75% of the sludge IC isolates and 59.6% of the raw sewage IC isolates were found to harbor at least one *qnr* variant. This suggests a possible enrichment of plasmid-mediated quinolone resistance in the activated sludge ($p < 0.05$). The *qnrS* variant was the most abundant, detected in 43.8 and 33.7% of the sludge and raw sewage IC isolates, respectively; the *qnrB* variant accounted for 28.5 and 21.3%, respectively; and *qnrA* was detected in 9 and 5.6%, respectively (**Figure 4**).

The *intl-1* gene was found in 50 and 42.7% of sludge and raw sewage IC isolates, respectively (**Figure 4**). Although *qnr*S was the most prevalent variant detected in both sludge and raw sewage, *qnr*B was found to have the strongest association with *intl-1* (**Figure 5**).

Contingency tests were conducted on the question whether specific populations of bacteria (*E. coli* and *Klebsiella*) are more or less prone to carry the different *qnr* variants or the *intl-1* gene. No such correlation was found.

Several studies have found that *qnr* genes are associated with class-1 integrons. Therefore, the linkage between *qnr* and *intl-1* genes was more comprehensively explored. Approximately 81.5% of the raw sewage *intl-1*-positive IC isolates were *qnr* positive (I^+Q^+), whereas only 29.4% of the *intl-1*-negative IC isolates harbored *qnr* (I^-Q^+). This stands in complete contrast to the

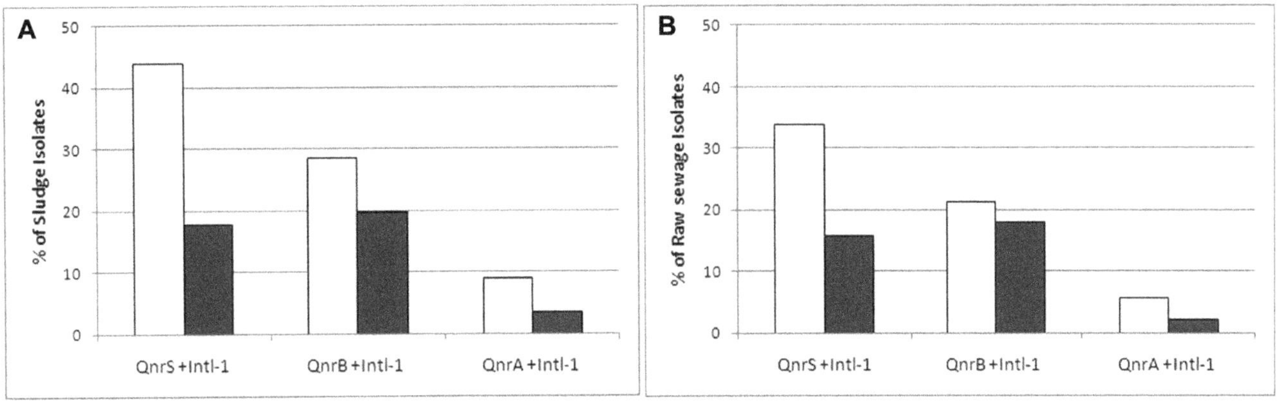

FIGURE 5 | *White bars*: the relative abundance of intermediate ciprofloxacin-resistant isolates carrying *qnr* variants (A, B, S) from the sludge (A), and raw sewage (B); *Gray bars*: the abundance of *intI-1* positive isolates among those *qnr*-positive isolates.

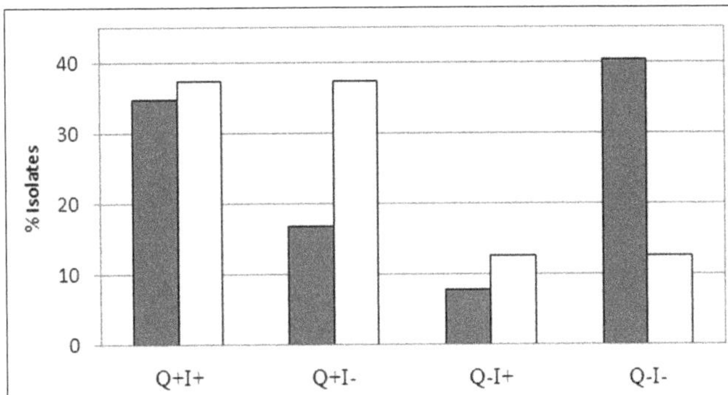

FIGURE 6 | Correlation between *qnr* and *intI-1* presence: isolates exhibited a negative correlation between *qnr* (Q) and their *intI-1* (I) content in sludge (white bars) and raw sewage (gray bars).

activated sludge, where 75% of both the I^+ and I^- IC isolates contained *qnr* genes (**Figure 6**).

DISCUSSION

Wastewater treatment plants are man-made ecological niches that assemble high concentrations of fecal and environmental bacteria. These giant "chemostats" have the potential to serve as hotspots for horizontal gene transfer. Horizontal transfer of ARGs in activated sludge is an actual concern, due to the potential evolution of multi-resistance strains, which are later discharged into agricultural environments when municipal biosolids are used as fertilizer. These ARGs can readily enter water supplies and the food chain, and henceforth may have significant epidemiological ramifications. Bacterial pathogens from municipal biosolids are generally not considered as high risk factors for disease propagation, since the sludge is generally stabilized by anaerobic digestion or compostation prior to application as fertilizer. However, a fraction of sludge bacteria, and more notably, horizontally transferable genetic entities harboring ARGs can survive sludge stabilization processes and this gene pool may be disseminated into the soil microbiome following municipal sludge application.

In this study we focused on plasmid-mediated quinolone resistance (Qnr) determinants. Although these determinants have been found to occur on chromosomal DNA in certain environmental bacteria (Poirel et al., 2005), they are considered to be almost exclusively plasmid-borne in *Enterobacteriaceae* (Rodriguez-Martinez et al., 2011). This characteristic is especially concerning due to the clinical importance of fluoroquinolones and the rapid spread of plasmid-associated resistance. We isolated a large group of *Enterobacteriaceae* resistant to IC concentrations from both raw sewage ($n = 89$) and activated sludge ($n = 112$, in order to assess the potential influence of the activated sludge process on (a) the relative abundance of IC resistance; (b) the scope of resistance to other antibiotics; and (c) the abundance of selected mobile genetic elements.

Interestingly, although no significant increase in the level of IC-resistant isolates was observed when comparing the sludge to the raw sewage, the sludge IC isolates were characterized by a significantly higher ratio of *qnr*-positive variants, indicating that these plasmid-associated elements enhance the fitness of the *Enterobacteriaceae* isolates in the activated sludge. This may be due to the *qnr* genes themselves, or alternatively to additional genes that are carried on mobile genetic elements that also harbor the *qnr* genes. The acquisition of plasmids carrying *qnr* genes increases the MIC of ciprofloxacin for wild-type *E. coli* J53 from 0.016 to 0.25 μg/ml (Robicsek et al., 2006) and therefore, it may be assumed that *qnr* confers a selective advantage to bacteria residing in the sludge, where ciprofloxacin concentrations of up to 0.05 μg/mg have been detected (Golet et al., 2002; McClellan and Halden, 2010).

We discovered that although the activated sludge process did not appear to select for a specific resistance, there appeared to be an increase in the degree of multi-resistance of the sludge IC isolates relative to the raw sewage isolates. However, with the exception of nalidixic acid, the increase of IC sludge vs. raw sewage isolates resistant to additional antibiotics was not statistically significant, and therefore a larger pool of isolates will need to be screened before this hypothesis can be established.

Typically, plasmid-mediated quinolone resistance was thought to be associated with class-1 integrons (Robicsek et al., 2006; Lapierre et al., 2008). However, the increased abundance of *qnr* elements observed in the sludge isolates relative to the raw sewage appears to stem from *qnr* elements that were not *intl-1* positive (**Figure 6**), suggesting that the *qnr* genes that proliferate in the sludge IC isolates are not associated with class-1 integrons. In total, raw sewage IC isolates that harbored the *intl-1* gene had a probability of 81.5% to carry a *qnr* gene, whereas only 75% of the *intl-1* positive sludge IC isolates carried a *qnr* gene (I^+Q^+). If the integron was indeed the genetic platform on which *qnr* resides, one would expect to see a correlated decrease between *qnr* and *intl-1* in class-1 integron negative isolates in both raw sewage and sludge. In reality, while only 29% of *intl-1* negative raw sewage isolates harbored a *qnr* gene, 75% of *intl-1* negative sludge isolates were. In contrast, 67% of the *qnr*-positive raw sewage isolates were also positive for *intl-1*, whereas only 50% of the sludge isolates did. Furthermore, only 16% of the *qnr*-negative raw sewage IC isolates carried the *intl-1* gene, whereas 50% of the *qnr*-negative sludge isolates did. This strongly suggests that *qnr* genes are not essentially associated with type-1 integrons, and that the dynamics of *qnr* in sludge may differ from that in raw sewage. A few studies have shown that the association between qnr and class-1 integrons is not mandatory. For example, Richter et al. (2010) identified an association between a *qnr* gene and a Tn2012 transposon. This novel transposon was comprised of a transposase gene (ISEcp1C) and a *qnr*B19 gene that were inserted into a Tn1721 transposon, a non-conjugative transposon from the Tn3 family. This genetic structure allows the *in vitro* dissemination of the *qnr*B19 gene into conjugative strains (Cattoir et al., 2008).

In conclusion, as depicted from our data, the presence of *qnr* (both with and without corresponding *intl-1* genes) is favored in the WWTP process irrespective of class-1 integron presence, thereby eliminating the suggested linkage between class-1 integrons and plasmid-associated quinolone resistance. This is of particular interest since it was previously described that qnr tend to be found in correlation to the class-1 integrons, and could suggest a different, negative correlation between those two genetic entities. Future research will need to screen the flanking regions of these *qnrs* in order to determine which mobile genetic elements the *qnrs* are located on, and if there are ubiquitous flanking genes that potentially bestow a selective advantage in the activated sludge environment.

ACKNOWLEDGMENTS

We would like to thank Dr. Zohar Pasternak for statistical assistance and Dr. Pinchas Fine and Mr. Lior Aboksis for technical assistance. This study was funded by the Israeli Ministry of Environmental Protection (grant #103-1-3).

REFERENCES

Boyle, J. S., and Lew, A. M. (1995). An inexpensive alternative to glassmilk for DNA purification. *Trends Genet.* 11, 8. doi: 10.1016/S0168-9525(00)88977-5

Cattoir, V., Nordmann, P., Silva-Sanchez, J., Espinal, P., and Poirel, L. (2008). ISEcp1-mediated transposition of qnrB-like gene in *Escherichia coli*. *J. Antimicrob. Chemother.* 52, 2929–2932. doi: 10.1128/AAC.00349-08

Cattoir, V., Poirel, L., Rotimi, V., Soussy, C. J., and Nordmann, P. (2007). Multiplex PCR for detection of plasmid-mediated quinolone resistance qnr genes in ESBL-producing enterobacterial isolates. *J. Antimicrob. Chemother.* 60, 394–397. doi: 10.1093/jac/dkm204

Dröge, M., Pühler, A., and Selbitschka, W. (2000). Phenotypic and molecular characterization of conjugative antibiotic resistance plasmids isolated from bacterial communities of activated sludge. *Mol. Gen. Genet.* 263, 471–482. doi: 10.1007/s004380051191

Francy, D. S., and Darner, R. A. (2000). Comparison of methods for determining *Escherichia coli* concentrations in recreational waters. *Water Res.* 34, 2770–2778. doi: 10.1016/S0043-1354(00)00031-2

Gaze, W. H., Zhang, L., Abdouslam, N. A., Hawkey, P. M., Calvo-Bado, L., Royle, J., et al. (2011). Impacts of anthropogenic activity on the ecology of class 1 integrons and integron-associated genes in the environment. *ISME J.* 5, 1253–1261. doi: 10.1038/ismej.2011.15

Golet, E. M., Alder, A. C., and Giger, W. (2002). Environmental exposure and risk assessment of fluoroquinolone antibacterial agents in wastewater and river water of the Glatt Valley Watershed, Switzerland. *Environ. Sci. Technol.* 36, 3645–3651. doi: 10.1021/es0256212

Golet, E. M., Xifra, I., Siegrist, H., Alder, A. C., and Giger, W. (2003). Environmental exposure assessment of fluoroquinolone antibacterial agents from sewage to soil. *Environ. Sci. Technol.* 37, 3243–3249. doi: 10.1021/es0264448

Gosling, R. J., Clouting, C. S., Randall, L. P., Horton, R. A., and Davies, R. H. (2012). Ciprofloxacin resistance in *E. coli* isolated from turkeys in Great Britain. *Avian Pathol.* 41, 83–89. doi: 10.1080/03079457.2011.640659

Hopkins, K. L., Davies, R. H., and Threlfall, E. J. (2005). Mechanisms of quinolone resistance in *Escherichia coli* and *Salmonella*: recent developments. *Int. J. Antimicrob. Agents* 25, 358–373. doi: 10.1016/j.ijantimicag.2005.02.006

Jacoby, G. A. (2005). Mechanisms of resistance to quinolones. *Clin. Infect. Dis* 41, S120–S126. doi: 10.1086/428052

LaPara, T. M., Burch, T. R., McNamara, P. J., Tan, D. T., Yan, M., and Eichmiller, J. J. (2011). Tertiary-treated municipal wastewater is a significant point source of antibiotic resistance genes into Duluth-Superior Harbor. *Environ. Sci. Technol.* 45, 9543–9549. doi: 10.1021/es202775r

Lapierre, L., Cornejo, J., Borie, C., Toro, C., and San Martín, B. (2008). Genetic characterization of antibiotic resistance genes linked to class 1 and class 2 integrons in commensal strains of *Escherichia coli* isolated from poultry and swine. *Microb. Drug Resist.* 14, 265–272. doi: 10.1089/mdr.2008.0810

Li, J., Wang, T., Shao, B., Shen, J., Wang, S., and Wu, Y. (2012). Plasmid-mediated quinolone resistance genes and antibiotic residues in wastewater and soil adjacent to swine feedlots: potential transfer to agricultural lands. *Environ. Health Perspect.* 120, 1144–1149. doi: 10.1289/ehp.1104776

Ma, Y., Wilson, C. A., Novak, J. T., Riffat, R., Aynur, S., Murthy, S., et al. (2011). Effect of various sludge digestion conditions on sulfonamide, macrolide, and tetracycline resistance genes and class I integrons. *Environ. Sci. Technol.* 45, 7855–7861. doi: 10.1021/es200827t

Martinez-Martinez, L., Pascual, A., and Jacoby, G. A. (1998). Quinolone resistance from a transferable plasmid. *Lancet* 351, 797–799. doi: 10.1016/S0140-6736(97)07322-4

McClellan, K., and Halden, R. U. (2010). Pharmaceuticals and personal care products in archived U.S. biosolids from the 2001 EPA national sewage sludge survey. *Water Res.* 44, 658–668. doi: 10.1016/j.watres.2009.12.032

Munir, M., and Xagoraraki, I. (2011). Levels of antibiotic resistance genes in manure, biosolids, and fertilized soil. *J. Environ. Qual.* 40, 248–255. doi: 10.2134/jeq2010.0209

Nordmann, P., and Poirel, L. (2005). Emergence of plasmid-mediated resistance to quinolones in Enterobacteriaceae. *J. Antimicrob. Chemother.* 56, 463–469. doi: 10.1093/jac/dki245

Pellegrini, C., Celenza, G., Segatore, B., Bellio, P., Setacci, D., Amicosante, G., et al. (2011). Occurrence of class 1 and 2 integrons in resistant Enterobacteriaceae collected from a urban wastewater treatment plant: first report from central Italy. *Microb. Drug Resist.* 17,229-234 doi: 10.1089/mdr.2010.0117

Poirel, L., Rodriguez-Martinez, J. M., Mammeri, H., Liard, A., and Nordmann, P. (2005). Origin of plasmid-mediated quinolone resistance determinant QnrA. *J.*

Antimicrob. Chemother. 49, 3523–3525. doi: 10.1128/AAC.49.8.3523-3525.2005

Pruden, A., Arabi, M., and Storte, H. N. (2012). Correlation between upstream human activities and riverine antibiotic resistance genes. *Environ. Sci. Technol.* 46, 11541–11549. doi: 10.1021/es302657r

Richter, S. N., Frassona, I., Bergob, C., Manganellia, R., Cavallarob, A., and Palù, G. (2010). Characterisation of qnr plasmid-mediated quinolone resistance in Enterobacteriaceae from Italy: association of the qnrB19 allele with the integron element ISCR1 in *Escherichia coli. Int. J. Antimicrob. Agents* 35, 578–583. doi: 10.1016/j.ijantimicag.2010.02.015

Robicsek, A., Jacoby, G. A., and Hooper, D. C. (2006). The worldwide emergence of plasmid-mediated quinolone resistance. *Lancet Infect. Dis.* 6, 629–640. doi: 10.1016/S1473-3099(06)70599-0

Rodriguez-Martinez, J. M., Cano, M. E., Velasco, C., Martinez-Martinez, L., and Pascual, A. (2011). Plasmid-mediated quinolone resistance: an update. *J. Infect. Chemother.* 17, 149–182. doi: 10.1007/s10156-010-0120-2

Strahilevitz, J., Engelstein, D., Adler, A., Temper, V., Moses, A. E., Block, C., et al. (2007). Changes in qnr prevalence and Fluoroquinolone resistance in clinical isolates of *Klebsiella pneumoniae* and *Enterobacter* spp. collected from 1990 to 2005. *J. Antimicrob. Chemother.* 51, 3001–3003. doi: 10.1128/AAC.00256-07

Strahilevitz, J., Jacoby, G. A., Hooper, D. C., and Robicsek, A. (2009). Plasmid-mediated quinolone resistance: a multifaceted threat. *Clin. Microbiol. Rev.* 22, 664–689. doi: 10.1128/CMR.00016-09

Tran, J. H., and Jacoby, G. A. (2002). Mechanism of plasmid-mediated quinolone resistance. *Proc. Natl. Acad. Sci. U.S.A.* 99, 5638–5642. doi: 10.1073/pnas.082092899

Tran, J. H., Jacoby, G. A., and Hooper, D. C. (2005). Interaction of the plasmid-encoded quinolone resistance protein qnr with *Escherichia coli* DNA gyrase. *J. Antimicrob. Chemother.* 49, 118–125. doi: 10.1128/AAC.49.1.118-125.2005

Wang, M., Sahm, D. F., Jacoby, G. A., and Hooper, D. C. (2004). Emerging plasmid-mediated quinolone resistance associated with the qnr gene in *Klebsiella pneumoniae* clinical isolates in the United States. *J. Antimicrob. Chemother.* 48, 1295–1299. doi: 10.1128/AAC.48.4.1295-1299.2004

Wang, M., Tran, J. H., Jacoby, G. A., Zhang, Y., Wang, F., and Hooper, D. C. (2003). Plasmid-mediated quinolone resistance in clinical isolates of *Escherichia coli* from Shanghai, China. *J. Antimicrob. Chemother.* 47, 2242–2248. doi: 10.1128/AAC.47.7.2242-2248.2003

Zhang, Y., Marrs, C. F., Simon, C., and Xi, C. (2009). Wastewater treatment contributes to selective increase of antibiotic resistance among *Acinetobacter* spp. *Sci. Total Environ.* 407, 3702–3706. doi: 10.1016/j.scitotenv.2009.02.013

20

Mechanisms of antimicrobial resistance in finfish aquaculture environments

Claudio D. Miranda[1], Alfredo Tello[2] and Patricia L. Keen[3]*

[1] Department of Aquaculture, Universidad Católica del Norte, Coquimbo, Chile
[2] Instituto Tecnológico del Salmón, INTESAL de SalmonChile, Puerto Montt, Chile
[3] Department of Civil Engineering, University of British Columbia, Vancouver, BC, Canada

Edited by:
Marilyn C. Roberts, University of Washington, USA
Reviewed by:
Lisa Nonaka, Dokkyo Medical University, Japan
Henning Sørum, Norwegian School of Veterinary Science, Norway
***Correspondence:**
Patricia L. Keen, Department of Civil Engineering, University of British Columbia, 2002 - 6250 Applied Science Lane, Vancouver, BC V6T 1Z4, Canada
e-mail: patricia.keen@civil.ubc.ca

Consumer demand for affordable fish drives the ever-growing global aquaculture industry. The intensification and expansion of culture conditions in the production of several finfish species has been coupled with an increase in bacterial fish disease and the need for treatment with antimicrobials. Understanding the molecular mechanisms of antimicrobial resistance prevalent in aquaculture environments is important to design effective disease treatment strategies, to prioritize the use and registration of antimicrobials for aquaculture use, and to assess and minimize potential risks to public health. In this brief article we provide an overview of the molecular mechanisms of antimicrobial resistance in genes found in finfish aquaculture environments and highlight specific research that should provide the basis of sound, science-based policies for the use of antimicrobials in aquaculture.

Keywords: antimicrobials, antimicrobial resistance, fish, aquaculture

INTRODUCTION

Through a continuous process of expansion, intensification, and diversification, aquaculture has become the fastest-growing food industry in the world (Bostock et al., 2010). With production of new species and the expansion of the production of current species to new geographical locations, the risk of disease and need for treatment continues to increase. This risk is compounded by the uncertainties introduced by global climate change, which may affect the emergence and dynamics of new and existing pathogens (Tirado et al., 2010), and consequently the use of antimicrobials and the prevalence of antimicrobial resistance.

The major concern surrounding the use of antimicrobials in aquaculture is considered to be the potential to favor the development of a reservoir of antimicrobial resistance genes (ARGs) that may be eventually transferred to clinically relevant bacteria (FAO/OIE/WHO, 2006). So far, lack of data, methodological constraints, and the complexity of characterizing exposure pathways have prevented the derivation of quantitative estimates of the risk that this may pose to public health. Nevertheless, there is consensus in the scientific community and international organizations concerned with human health, animal health, and food security that steps should be taken to minimize it (FAO/OIE/WHO, 2006; Smith, 2008; Heuer et al., 2009; WHO, 2011). On a global scale, several of the major classes of antimicrobials are being used or have been used in aquaculture. Among these are sulphonamides, penicillins, macrolides, quinolones, phenicols, and tetracyclines (Sapkota et al., 2008), all of which are listed as critically or highly important antimicrobials in human medicine (WHO, 2011). However, the judicious use of antimicrobials in global aquaculture is important to effectively treat bacterial fish diseases and maintain fish health and welfare.

The molecular mechanism, genomic context, and prevalence of genes conferring resistance to antimicrobials determine their clinical relevance (i.e., whether they confer low- vs. high-level clinical resistance, their ability to be mobilized by lateral gene transfer, and their frequency of occurrence). Thus, knowledge of ARGs from aquaculture environments is important to design and prioritize monitoring programs that may generate data that eventually becomes relevant for performing quantitative risk assessments and develop sound treatment strategies to control fish disease. Within this general scope, we provide this article as an overview of the molecular mechanisms, genomic context, and prevalence of quinolone, tetracycline, and phenicol resistance genes that have been reported to occur in aquaculture environments.

ANTIMICROBIAL RESISTANCE GENES IN AQUACULTURE ENVIRONMENTS

Quinolones (i.e., oxolinic acid, flumequine, and enrofloxacin), tetracyclines [i.e., oxytetracycline (OTC)], and phenicols (i.e., florfenicol) are among the most widely used antimicrobial compounds in aquaculture, and they have been used extensively to control bacterial fish disease in salmon farming [SERNAPESCA (Chile), 2009; Burridge et al., 2010; Rico et al., 2012]. Although the use of quinolones in salmon farming currently accounts for less than 1% of the overall use of antimicrobials, they continue to be used in aquaculture production in several Asian countries [SERNAPESCA (Chile), 2009; Burridge et al., 2010; Rico et al., 2012]. Quinolones, tetracyclines, and phenicols have been reported to be selective for a variety of ARGs and tend to occur in mobile genetic elements that favor their dissemination (i.e., transposons, plasmids, and integrons; Cloeckaert et al., 2000; Chopra and Roberts, 2001; Kümmerer, 2004; Schwarz et al., 2004; Roberts, 2005).

QUINOLONE RESISTANCE

The protein targets of quinolones are the bacterial enzymes, DNA gyrase and topoisomerase IV. DNA gyrase is a tetrameric enzyme encoded by the *gyrA* and *gyrB* genes, and its main activity is to catalyze the negative supercoiling of bacterial DNA. Topoisomerase IV is also a tetrameric enzyme and it is encoded by the *parC* and *parE* genes; its function is to decatenate and relax the activity of daughter replicons following DNA replication (Anderson et al., 1998; Hawkey, 2003).

The acquisition of quinolone resistance is primarily due to chromosomal mutations in topoisomerases genes (i.e., *gyrA*, *gyrB*, *parC*, and *parE*) and mutations that reduce drug accumulation by decreasing uptake or increasing efflux (Drlica and Zhao, 1997; Ruiz, 2003). Additionally, at least three mechanisms of quinolone resistance are known to be plasmid encoded: (1) Qnr proteins; (2) AAC(6)-Ib-cr aminoglycoside acetyltransferases; and (3) QepA and OqxAB efflux pumps. Qnr proteins protect DNA gyrase and type IV topoisomerase from quinolone inhibition (Tran and Jacoby, 2002; Jacoby, 2005) and the AAC(6)-Ib-cr determinant acetylates several fluoroquinolones. Plasmid-encoded QepA and OqxAB are active efflux pumps that may extrude hydrophilic fluoroquinolones such as enrofloxacin (Li, 2005; Poirel et al., 2008, 2012; Cattoir and Nordmann, 2009; Rodríguez-Martínez et al., 2011).

Various point mutations in the quinolone resistance-determining regions of the *gyrA* and/or *parC* genes have been detected in quinolone-resistant strains of the fish pathogens *Aeromonas hydrophila*, *Vibrio anguillarum*, and *V. parahaemolyticus* (Okuda et al., 1999; Rodkhum et al., 2008; Lukkana et al., 2012). Levels of quinolone resistance in Gram-negative bacteria are suggested to be high when associated with point mutations in both the *gyrA* and *parC* genes, whereas only an intermediate level of resistance is associated with point mutations in the *gyrA* gene only. However, high-level resistance to oxolinic acid associated with a single mutation in the *gyrA* gene has been reported for strains of the fish pathogens *Aeromonas salmonicida*, *Edwardsiella tarda*, and *Photobacterium damselae* (Oppegaard and Sørum, 1994; Goñi-Urriza et al., 2002; Kim et al., 2005, 2011; Ozanne et al., 2005). The extensive administration of quinolones in fish farming has been linked to increased mutations in DNA gyrase and topoisomerase IV in quinolone-resistant fish pathogens such as *Yersinia ruckeri*, *Flavobacterium psychrophilum*, and *V. anguillarum* (Gibello et al., 2004; Izumi and Aranishi, 2004; Colquhoun et al., 2007; Izumi et al., 2007; Shah et al., 2012).

Plasmid-mediated quinolone resistance in bacteria associated with fish farms has been detected in several countries. Ishida et al. (2010) detected the *qnr* and *aac(6′)-Ib-cr* resistance determinants in bacterial strains isolated from fish farm water samples in Egypt. Recently, Buschmann et al. (2012) reported the occurrence of topoisomerase protection genes *qnrA*, *qnrB*, and *qnrS*, the putative enzymatic inactivation gene *aac(69)-Ib-cr* and the efflux pump gene *oqxA* among strains isolated from un-polluted and fish farm-impacted marine sediments in Chile. Jiang et al. (2012) found a high prevalence of *qnrB* and *qnrS* genes in *Escherichia coli* strains recovered from Chinese farmed fish while *qnrD* and *aac(6′)-Ib-cr* genes occurred less frequently. Han et al. (2012) found 17 strains encoding chromosomal mutations in *gyrA*, 11 strains encoding mutations in *parC*, and a few strains carrying the *qnrS1*-like and *qnrS2* genes among 33 *Aeromonas* spp. isolated from diseased fish and from water samples. The identification of QnrS determinants in *Aeromonas* spp. suggests that they may act as an environmental reservoir of *qnrS* genes, as already described for *tet* genes (Rhodes et al., 2000; Schmidt et al., 2001a). Some *qnr* genes have also been described in the Vibrionaceae family and it is suggested that water-borne Vibrionaceae may constitute a natural reservoir for Qnr-like quinolone-resistance determinants (Poirel et al., 2005; Cattoir et al., 2007; Cattoir and Nordmann, 2009). Evidence suggests that *qnr*-plasmids are most commonly integron associated and carry multiple resistance determinants, providing resistance to several classes of antimicrobials, including beta-lactams and aminoglycosides (Li, 2005).

TETRACYCLINE RESISTANCE

Oxytetracycline is a broad-spectrum bacteriostatic antimicrobial, active against a wide variety of Gram-positive and Gram-negative bacteria, which is extensively used in fish farming. Tetracyclines bind reversibly to the 70S ribosome of prokaryotes and block protein synthesis (Chopra, 1985; Roberts, 1996).

Mechanisms of tetracycline resistance include active efflux, ribosomal protection, ribosomal RNA mutations, and tetracycline inactivation (Speer and Salyers, 1989; Salyers et al., 1990; Burdett, 1991; Levy, 1992; Speer et al., 1992; Taylor and Chau, 1996). Tetracycline resistance in fish farm-associated bacteria has been found to be mainly mediated by one or more of the Tet family of proton-dependent efflux pumps or via ribosomal protection by cytoplasmic proteins found widely in Gram-negative bacteria (Roberts, 2005; Roberts et al., 2012).

Several *tet* determinants have been identified in fish farm bacteria from a number of geographical locations and fish species (DePaola et al., 1988; Adams et al., 1998; Rhodes et al., 2000; Schmidt et al., 2001a; Furushita et al., 2003; Miranda et al., 2003; Akinbowale et al., 2007; Seyfried et al., 2010; Gao et al., 2012). The genes *tet*(A), *tet*(B), *tet*(E), *tet*(H), *tet*(L), *tet*(34), and *tet*(35) were found in tetracycline-resistant bacteria isolated from Chilean salmon farms (Miranda et al., 2003). Recently, Seyfried et al. (2010) detected the presence of *tet*(A), *tet*(B), *tet*(D), *tet*(E), *tet*(G), *tet*(M), *tet*(O), *tet*(Q), *tet*(S), and *tet*(W) genes in medicated and non-medicated feed samples and water samples from non-commercial fish farms in the United States. Similarly, Jun et al. (2004) found a high prevalence of *tet*(A) and *tet*(D) genes associated with mobile plasmids and *tet*(B) and *tet*(G) genes associated with non-mobile elements in *Edwardsiella tarda* strains isolated from fish farms in Korea. Nonaka et al. (2007) found a high incidence of *tet*(M)-carrying *Vibrio* strains in fish farms and Agersø et al. (2007) detected *tet*(E) in *Aeromonas* strains from Danish fish farms associated with large plasmids capable of horizontal transfer to *Escherichia coli*. Nawaz et al. (2009) found a high prevalence of *tet*(B) and, to a lesser extent, *tet*(A), *tet*(C) and the co-occurrence of *tet*(A) and *tet*(B) in *Escherichia coli* isolated from farm-raised catfish. Kim et al. (2004) reported the occurrence of *tet*(M) and *tet*(S) in tetracycline-resistant bacteria from fish farms in Korea and Nonaka and Suzuki (2002) found the novel OTC-resistance determinant *tet*(34) in a *Vibrio* strain isolated from cultured yellowtail (*Seriola quinqueradiata*).

The spread of *tet* genes is often facilitated by their location on mobile genetic elements, such as plasmids and transposons (Roberts, 1994; DePaola and Roberts, 1995; Chopra and Roberts,

2001). Tn1721 and Tn1721-like elements, for example, are known to play a significant role in the global dissemination of the *tet*(A) gene (Rhodes et al., 2000; Sørum et al., 2003; Chenia and Vietze, 2012). Miranda et al. (2003) found the *tet*(H) gene as part of the transposon Tn5706 in *Moraxella* and *Acinetobacter* strains isolated from salmon farms. In addition, they were able to transfer *tet*(B) and *tet*(34) genes from strains of *Serratia liquefaciens*, *Pseudomonas pseudoalcaligenes*, and *Brevundimonas vesicularis*. Similarly, Furushita et al. (2003) transferred *tet*(B), *tet*(D), and *tet*(Y) genes from bacterial isolates from different Japanese fish farms by conjugation and Adams et al. (1998) reported that various OTC-resistant isolates of *Aeromonas salmonicida* transferred R-plasmids carrying the *tet*(A) gene to environmental and clinical isolates of *Aeromonas* spp. Class 1 integrons harboring different combinations of the resistance gene cassettes *ant(3'')Ia*, *aac(6'')Ia*, *dhfr1*, *oxa2a*, and/or *pse1* and *tet* genes were also detected in a large number of plasmid bearing *Aeromonas* spp. strains isolated from tilapia, trout, and koi cultures in South Africa (Jacobs and Chenia, 2007). In *Edwardsiella ictaluri* strains isolated from diseased freshwater catfish in Vietnam, Dung et al. (2009) found the *tet*(A) gene associated with a high-molecular weight plasmid belonging to the Inc*K* group. In addition, all strains were able to transfer their *tet*(A)-carrying plasmids to *Escherichia coli* recipients.

Several studies have also reported the co-occurrence of tetracycline and sulphonamide resistances genes. Agersø and Petersen (2007) showed that *tet*(39) and *sul2* genes located on plasmids of different sizes to be common among clonally distinct *Acinetobacter* spp. from fish farms in Thailand. Su et al. (2011) detected the genes *tet*(A), *tet*(C), and the sulphonamide-resistance gene, *sul2*, in more than 50% of the strains of Enterobacteriaceae they isolated from fish farms in China. Gao et al. (2012) recently reported the co-occurrence of tetracycline- and sulphonamide-resistance genes in *Bacillus* species isolated from aquaculture farms in China.

PHENICOL RESISTANCE

Florfenicol is a synthetic fluorinated analog of chloramphenicol whose bacteriostatic activity is based on a reversible binding to the 50S subunit of 70S bacterial ribosomes that prevents peptide elongation (Schwarz et al., 2004). The replacement of a hydroxyl group with a fluorine atom protects florfenicol from inactivation by chloramphenicol acetyltransferases (CATs), a common mechanism of bacterial resistance to chloramphenicol (Shaw and Leslie, 1991; Schwarz et al., 2004). The effectiveness of florfenicol against a number of relevant fish pathogens makes it a very valuable drug for the fish farming industry (Fukui et al., 1987; Nordmo et al., 1994; Samuelsen et al., 1998, 2003; Bruun et al., 2000; Gaunt et al., 2003; McGinnis et al., 2003; Michel et al., 2003; Samuelsen and Bergh, 2004).

Mechanisms of resistance to florfenicol include specific and non-specific drug transporters, RNA methyltransferases, and specific hydrolases (Paulsen et al., 1996; Schwarz et al., 2004; Poole, 2005; Long et al., 2006; Tao et al., 2012). Genes *floR* and *fexA* belong to the major facilitator superfamily and code for efflux proteins that export florfenicol out of the cell (Schwarz et al., 2004). The gene *cfr*, which has been shown to be an RNA methyltransferase that belongs to the recently discovered radical *S*-adenosylmethionine (SAM) superfamily of proteins (Sofia et al., 2001), inhibits ribose methylation and thereby causes resistance to florfenicol, chloramphenicol, and clindamycin (Long et al., 2006).

Most studies of florfenicol resistance in fish farming have reported the occurrence of the *floR* gene. Dang et al. (2007) detected the *floR* gene in tetracycline-resistant bacteria isolated from aquaculture sites in China, and Ishida et al. (2010) detected the *floR* gene in four strains of Gram-negative bacteria isolated from fish farms in Africa. In North America, McIntosh et al. (2008) reported the occurrence of *Aeromonas salmonicida* strains carrying a conjugative IncA/C plasmid harboring *floR*, *sul2*, and *tetA* genes that were transferable to *Aeromonas hydrophila* and *Edwardsiella tarda*. Welch et al. (2009) detected IncA/C plasmid-mediated florfenicol resistance in the catfish pathogen *Edwardsiella ictaluri*, and Gordon et al. (2008) reported a multiresistant *Aeromonas bestiarum* strain carrying a plasmid harboring the *floR*, *tetY*, *sul2*, and *strA–strB* resistance genes. A relatively recent study showed that many florfenicol-resistant bacterial strains isolated from Chilean salmon farms carried the *floR* gene, whereas others possessed non-specific efflux pumps that conferred florfenicol resistance (Fernández-Alarcón et al., 2010). In fish farm impacted marine sediments, Buschmann et al. (2012) recently reported the occurrence of several strains containing plasmid-borne *floR*, *tet*, and *qnr* genes.

PRIORITIZING RESEARCH AND POLICY NEEDS

The studies discussed in the previous sections support the hypothesis that fish farms represent a reservoir of diverse ARGs, many of which may be readily mobilized by lateral gene transfer. Given the extent of global aquaculture and its fast-paced growth, it is imperative that research needs with regards to the use of antimicrobials and the emergence and potential spread of antimicrobial resistance are prioritized. This research should form the basis of sound, science-based policies that contribute to the sustainability of the aquaculture industry and minimize risks to public health. Further studies are needed to explore the prevalence of antimicrobial resistance in zoonotic fish pathogens such as *Aeromonas hydrophila*, *Edwardsiella tarda*, *Mycobacterium fortuitum*, *Mycobacterium marinum*, *Photobacterium damselae*, *Pseudomonas fluorescens*, and *Streptococcus iniae* (Austin and Austin, 2012). Moreover, there are important knowledge gaps regarding the co-occurrence of antimicrobial-resistant bacteria from aquaculture environments with human pathogens throughout production cycles and across a range of aquaculture environments, the transfer rate of resistance genes between aquaculture and clinically relevant bacteria under field or semi-field conditions, and the epidemiology of antimicrobial resistance in areas of intense aquaculture activity.

Good management strategies can make a significant contribution to minimize the use of antimicrobials in fish and the emergence and spread of antimicrobial resistance in aquaculture environments. Among these precautionary practices are the use of "good quality" fish stocks, reducing stocking densities, maintaining overall good environmental conditions (e.g., dissolved O_2 levels), the implementation of proper biosecurity measures, the development of effective vaccines and vaccination programs, and the rotation of antimicrobial compounds in the treatment of fish disease. Although the use of antimicrobials in human medicine places constraints on the type of antimicrobials that may be used in veterinary medicine, the rotation of antimicrobials in aquaculture may play an important role in reducing the chances of selection, co-selection, and dissemination of antimicrobial resistance. In this context, it is also important that efforts are directed toward creating incentives for the development and registration of antimicrobials for aquaculture use in addition to implementation of antimicrobial stewardship practices.

REFERENCES

Adams, C. A., Austin, B., Meaden, P. G., and McIntosh, D. (1998). Molecular characterization of plasmid-mediated oxytetracycline resistance in *Aeromonas salmonicida*. *Appl. Environ. Microbiol.* 64, 4194–4201.

Agersø, Y., Bruun, M. S., Dalsgaard, I., and Larsen, J. L. (2007). The tetracycline resistance gene tet(E) is frequently occurring and present on large horizontally transferable plasmids in *Aeromonas* spp. from fish farms. *Aquaculture* 266, 47–52. doi: 10.1016/j.aquaculture.2007.01.012

Agersø, Y., and Petersen, A. (2007). The tetracycline resistance determinant Tet 39 and the sulphonamide resistance gene sulII are common among resistant *Acinetobacter* spp. isolated from integrated fish farms in Thailand. *J. Antimicrob. Chemother.* 59, 23–27. doi: 10.1093/jac/dkl419

Akinbowale, O. L., Peng, H., and Barton, M. D. (2007). Diversity of tetracycline resistance genes in bacteria from aquaculture sources in Australia. *J. Appl. Microbiol.* 103, 2016–2025. doi: 10.1111/j.1365-2672.2007.03445.x

Anderson, V. E., Gootz, T. D., and Osheroff, N. (1998). Topoisomerase IV catalysis and the mechanism of quinolone action. *J. Biol. Chem.* 273, 17879–17885. doi: 10.1074/jbc.273.28.17879

Austin, B., and Austin, D. (2012). *Bacterial Fish Pathogens: Disease of Farmed and Wild Fish.* Dordrecht: Springer Science + Business Media.

Bostock, J., McAndrew, B., Richards, R., Jauncey, K., Telfer, T., Lorenzen, K., et al. (2010). Aquaculture: global status and trends. *Philos. Trans. R. Soc. Lond. B Biol. Sci.* 365, 2897–2912. doi: 10.1098/rstb.2010.0170

Bruun, M. S., Schmidt, A. S., Lone Madsen, L., and Dalsgaard, I. (2000). Antimicrobial resistance patterns in Danish isolates of *Flavobacterium psychrophilum*. *Aquaculture* 187, 201–212. doi: 10.1016/S0044-8486(00)00310-0

Burdett, V. (1991). Purification and characterization of tet(M), a protein that renders ribosomes resistant to tetracycline. *J. Biol. Chem.* 266, 2872 2877.

Burridge, L., Weis, J. S., Cabello, F., Pizarro, J., and Bostick, K. (2010). Chemical use in salmon aquaculture: a review of current practices and possible environmental effects. *Aquaculture* 306, 7–23. doi: 10.1016/j.aquaculture.2010.05.020

Buschmann, A. H., Tomova, A., López, A., Maldonado, M. A., Henríquez, L. A., Ivanova, L., et al. (2012). Salmon aquaculture and antimicrobial resistance in the marine environment. *PLoS ONE* 7:e42724. doi: 10.1371/journal.pone.0042724

Cattoir, V., and Nordmann, P. (2009). Plasmid-mediated quinolone resistance in Gram-negative bacterial species: an update. *Curr. Med. Chem.* 16, 1028–1046. doi: 10.2174/092986709787581879

Cattoir, V., Poirel, L., Mazel, D., Soussy, C. J., and Nordmann, P. (2007). *Vibrio splendidus* as the source of plasmid-mediated QnrS-like quinolone resistance determinants. *Antimicrob. Agents Chemother.* 51, 2650–2651. doi: 10.1128/AAC.00070-07

Chenia, H. Y., and Vietze, C. (2012). Tetracycline resistance determinants of heterotrophic bacteria isolated from a South African tilapia aquaculture system. *Afr. J. Microbiol. Res.* 6, 6761–6768. doi: 10.5897/AJMR10.840

Chopra, I. (1985). "Mode of action of the tetracyclines and the nature of bacterial resistance to them," in *The Tetracyclines. Handbook of Experimental Pharmacology*, Vol. 78, eds J. J. Hlavka and J. H. Boothe (Berlin: Springer-Verlag KG), 317–392.

Chopra, I., and Roberts, M. C. (2001). Tetracycline antibiotics: mode of action, applications, molecular biology, and epidemiology of bacterial resistance. *Microbiol. Mol. Biol. Rev.* 65, 232–260. doi: 10.1128/MMBR.65.2.232-260.2001

Cloeckaert, A., Baucheron, S., and Chaslus-Dancla, E. (2001). Nonenzymatic chloramphenicol resistance mediated by IncC plasmid R55 is encoded by a *flo*R gene variant. *Antimicrob. Agents Chemother.* 45, 2381–2382. doi: 10.1128/AAC.45.8.2381-2382.2001

Cloeckaert, A., Baucheron, S., Flaujac, S., Schwarz, S., Kehrenberg, C., Martel, J., et al. (2000). Plasmid-mediated florfenicol resistance encoded by the *flo*R gene in *Escherichia coli* isolated from cattle. *Antimicrob. Agents Chemother.* 44, 2858–2860. doi: 10.1128/AAC.44.10.2858-2860.2000

Colquhoun, D. J., Aarflot, L., and Melvold, C. F. (2007). *gyr*A and *par*C mutations and associated quinolone resistance in *Vibrio anguillarum* serotype O2b strains isolated from farmed Atlantic cod (*Gadus morhua*) in Norway. *Antimicrob. Agents Chemother.* 51, 2597–2599. doi: 10.1128/AAC.00315-07

Dang, H., Zhang, X., Song, L., Chang, Y., and Yang, G. (2007). Molecular determination of oxytetracycline-resistant bacteria and their resistance genes from mariculture environments of China. *J. Appl. Microbiol.* 103, 2580–2592. doi: 10.1111/j.1365-2672.2007.03494.x

DePaola, A., Flynn, P. A., McPhearson, R. M., and Levy, S. B. (1988). Phenotypic and genotypic characterization of tetracycline- and oxytetracycline resistant *Aeromonas hydrophila* from cultured channel catfish (*Ictalurus punctatus*) and their environments. *Appl. Environ. Microbiol.* 54, 1861–1863.

DePaola, A., and Roberts, M. C. (1995). Class D and E tetracycline resistance determinants in Gram-negative catfish pond bacteria. *Mol. Cell. Probes* 9, 311–313. doi: 10.1016/S0890-8508(95)91572-9

Drlica, K., and Zhao, X. L. (1997). DNA gyrase, topoisomerase IV, and the 4-quinolones. *Microbiol. Rev.* 61, 377–392.

Dung, T. T., Haesebrouck, F., Sorgeloos, P., Tuan, N. A., Pasmans, F., Smet, A., et al. (2009). IncK plasmid-mediated tetracycline resistance in *Edwarsiella ictaluri* isolates from diseased freshwater catfish in Vietnam. *Aquaculture* 295, 157–159. doi: 10.1016/j.aquaculture.2009.07.010

FAO/OIE/WHO. (2006). *Report of a Joint FAO/OIE/WHO Expert Consultation on Antimicrobial Use in Aquaculture and Antimicrobial Resistance: Seoul, Republic of Korea, June 13–16, 2006.* Seoul: WHO.

Fernández-Alarcón, C., Miranda, C. D., Singer, R. S., López, Y., Rojas, R., Bello, H., et al. (2010). Detection of the *flo*R gene in a diversity of florfenicol resistant Gram-negative bacilli from freshwater salmon farms in Chile. *Zoonoses Public Health* 57, 181–188. doi: 10.1111/j.1863-2378.2009.01243.x

Fukui, H., Fujihara, Y., and Kano, T. (1987). In vitro and in vivo antibacterial activities of florfenicol, a new fluorinated analog of thiamphenicol, against fish pathogens. *Fish Pathol.* 22, 201–207. doi: 10.3147/jsfp.22.201

Furushita, M., Shiba, T., Maeda, T., Yhata, M., Kaneoka, A., Takahashi, Y., et al. (2003). Similarity of tetracycline resistance genes isolated from fish farm bacteria to those from clinical isolates. *Appl. Environ. Microbiol.* 69, 5336–5342. doi: 10.1128/AEM.69.9.5336-5342.2003

Gao, P., Mao, D., Luo, Y., Wang, L., Xu, B., and Xu, L. (2012). Occurrence of sulphonamide and tetracycline-resistant bacteria and resistance genes in aquaculture environment. *Water Res.* 46, 2355–2364. doi: 10.1016/j.watres.2012.02.004

Gaunt, P., Endris, R., Khoo, L., Leard, T., Jack, S., Santucci, T., et al. (2003). Preliminary assessment of the tolerance and efficacy of florfenicol against *Edwardsiella ictaluri* administered in feed to channel catfish. *J. Aquat. Anim. Health* 15, 239–247. doi: 10.1577/H03-022

Gibello, A., Porrero, M. C., Blanco, M. M., Vela, A. I., Liébana, P., Moreno, M. A., et al. (2004). Analysis of the gyrA gene of clinical *Yersinia ruckeri* isolates with reduced susceptibility to quinolones. *Appl. Environ. Microbiol.* 70, 599–602. doi: 10.1128/AEM.70.1.599-602.2004

Goñi-Urriza, M., Arpin, C., Capdepuy, M., Dubois, V., Caumette, P., and Quentin, C. (2002). Type II topoisomerase quinolone resistance-determining regions of *Aeromonas caviae*, *A. hydrophila* and *A. sobria* complexes and mutations associated with quinolone resistance. *Antimicrob. Agents Chemother.* 46, 350–359. doi: 10.1128/AAC.46.2.350-359.2002 PMCid:PMC127024

Gordon L, Cloeckaert A, Doublet, B., Schwarz, S., Agnès Bouju-Albert, A., Ganière, J. P., et al. (2008). Complete sequence of the *flo*R-carrying multiresistance plasmid pAB5S9 from freshwater *Aeromonas bestiarum*. *J. Antimicrob. Chemother.* 62, 65–71. doi: 10.1093/jac/dkn166

Han, J. E., Kim, J. H., Cheresca, C. H., Shin, S. P., Jun, J. W., Chai, J. Y., et al. (2012). First description of the qnrS-like (qnrS5) gene and analysis of quinolone resistance-determining regions in motile *Aeromonas* spp. from diseased fish and water. *Res. Microbiol.* 163, 73–79. doi: 10.1016/j.resmic.2011.09.001

Hawkey, P. M. (2003). Mechanisms of quinolone action and microbial response. *J. Antimicrob. Chemother.* 51, S1, 29–35. doi: 10.1093/jac/dkg207

Heuer, O. E., Kruse, H., Grave, K., Collignon, P., Karunasagar, I., and Angulo, F. J. (2009). Human health consequences of use of antimicrobial agents in aquaculture. *Clin. Infect. Dis.* 49, 1248–1253. doi: 10.1086/605667

Ishida, Y., Ahmed, A. M., Mahfouz, N. B., Kimura, T., El-Khodery, S. A., Moawad, A. A., et al. (2010). Molecular analysis of antimicrobial resistance in Gram-negative bacteria isolated from fish farms in Egypt. *J. Vet. Med. Sci.* 72, 727–734. doi: 10.1292/jvms.09-0538

Izumi, S., and Aranishi, F. (2004). Relationship between *gyr*A mutations and quinolone resistance in *Flavobacterium psychrophilum* isolates. *Appl. Environ. Microbiol.* 70, 3968–3972. doi: 10.1128/AEM.70.7.3968-3972.2004

Izumi, S., Ouchi, S., Kuge, T., Arai, H., Mito, T., Fujii, H., et al. (2007). PCR–RFLP genotypes associated with quinolone resistance in isolates of *Flavobacterium psychrophilum*. *J. Fish Dis.* 30, 141–147. doi: 10.1111/j.1365-2761.2007.00797.x

Jacobs, L., and Chenia, H. Y. (2007). Characterization of integrons and tetracycline resistance determinants in *Aeromonas* spp. isolated from South African aquaculture systems. *Int. J. Food Microbiol.* 114, 295–306. doi: 10.1016/j.ijfoodmicro.2006.09.030

Jacoby, G. A. (2005). Mechanisms of resistance to quinolones. *Clin. Infect. Dis.* 41, S120–S126. doi: 10.1086/428052

Jiang, H. X., Tang, D., Liu, Y. H., Zhang, X. H., Zeng, Z. L., Xu, L., et al. (2012). Prevalence and characteristics of β-lactamase and plasmid-mediated quinolone resistance genes in *Escherichia coli* isolated from farmed fish in China. *J. Antimicrob. Chemother.* 67, 2350–2353. doi: 10.1093/jac/dks250

Jun, L. J., Jeong, J. B., Huh, M. D., Chung, J. K., Choi, D. L., Lee, C. H., et al. (2004). Detection of tetracycline-resistance determinants by multiplex polymerase chain reaction in *Edwardsiella tarda* isolated from fish farms in Korea. *Aquaculture* 240, 89–100. doi: 10.1016/j.aquaculture.2004.07.025

Kim, J. H., Hwang, S. Y., Son, J. S., Han, J. E., Jun, J. W., Shin, S. P., et al. (2011). Molecular characterization of tetracycline- and quinolone-resistant *Aeromonas salmonicida* isolated in Korea. *J. Vet. Sci.* 12, 41–48. doi: 10.4142/jvs.2011.12.1.41

Kim, M. J., Hirono, I., and Aoki, T. (2005). Detection of quinolone-resistant genes in *Photobacterium damselae* subsp. piscicida strains by targeting-induced local lesions in genomes. *J. Fish Dis.* 28, 463–471. doi: 10.1111/j.1365-2761.2005.00652.x

Kim, S. R., Nonaka, L., and Suzuki, S. (2004). Occurrence of tetracycline resistance genes tet(M) and tet(S) in bacteria from marine aquaculture sites. *FEMS Microbiol. Lett.* 237, 147–156. doi: 10.1111/j.1574-6968.2004.tb09690.x

Kümmerer, K. (2004). Resistance in the environment. *J. Antimicrob. Chemother.* 54, 311–320. doi: 10.1093/jac/dkh325

Levy, S. B. (1992). Active efflux mechanisms for antimicrobial resistance. *Antimicrob. Agents Chemother.* 36, 695–703. doi: 10.1128/AAC.36.4.695

Li, X. Z. (2005). Quinolone resistance in bacteria: emphasis on plasmid-mediated mechanisms. *Int. J. Antimicrob. Agents* 25, 453–463. doi: 10.1016/j.ijantimicag.2005.04.002

Long, K. S., Poehlsgaard, J., Kehrenberg, C., Schwarz, S., and Vester, B. (2006). The Cfr rRNA methyltransferase confers resistance to phenicols, lincosamides, oxazolidinones, pleuromutilins, and streptogramin A antibiotics. *Antimicrob. Agents Chemother.* 50, 2500–2505. doi: 10.1128/AAC.00131-06

Lukkana, M., Wongtavatchai, J., and Chuanchuen, R. (2012). Class 1 integrons in *Aeromonas hydrophila* isolates from farmed Nile tilapia (*Oreochromis nilotica*). *J. Vet. Med. Sci.* 74, 435–440. doi: 10.1292/jvms.11-0441

McGinnis, A., Gaunt, P., Santucci, T., Simmons, R., and Endris, R. (2003). In vitro evaluation of the susceptibility of *Edwardsiella ictaluri*, etiological agent of enteric septicemia in channel catfish, *Ictalurus punctatus* (Rafinesque), to florfenicol. *J. Vet. Diagn. Invest.* 15, 576–579. doi: 10.1177/104063870301500612

McIntosh, D., Cunningham, D., Ji, B., Fekete, F. A., Parry, E. M., Clark, S. E., et al. (2008). Transferable, multiple antibiotic and mercury resistance in Atlantic Canadian isolates of *Aeromonas salmonicida* subsp. *Salmonicida* is associated with carriage of an IncA/C plasmid similar to the *Salmonella enterica* plasmid pSN254. *J. Antimicrob. Chemother.* 61, 1221–1228. doi: 10.1093/jac/dkn123

Michel, C., Kerouault, B., and Martin, C. (2003). Chloramphenicol and florfenicol susceptibility of fish-pathogenic bacteria isolated in France: comparison of minimum inhibitory concentration, using recommended provisory standards for fish bacteria. *J. Appl. Microbiol.* 95, 1008–1015. doi: 10.1046/j.1365-2672.2003.02093.x

Miranda, C. D., Kehrenberg, C., Ulep, C., Schwarz, S., and Roberts, M. C. (2003). Diversity of tetracycline resistance genes in bacteria from Chilean salmon farms. *Antimicrob. Agents Chemother.* 47, 883–888. doi: 10.1128/AAC.47.3.883-888.2003

Nawaz, M., Khan, A. A., Khan, S., Sung, K., Kerdahi, K., and Steele, R. (2009). Molecular characterization of tetracycline-resistant genes and integrons from avirulent strains of *Escherichia coli* isolated from catfish. *Foodborne Pathog. Dis.* 6, 553–559. doi: 10.1089/fpd.2008.0204

Nonaka, L., Ikeno, K., and Suzuki, S. (2007). Distribution of tetracycline resistance gene, *tet*(M), in Gram-positive and Gram-negative bacteria isolated from sediment and seawater at a coastal aquaculture site in Japan. *Microbes Environ.* 22, 355–364. doi: 10.1264/jsme2.22.355

Nonaka, L., and Suzuki, S. (2002). New $Mg2^{+}$-dependent oxytetracycline resistance determinant Tet 34 in *Vibrio* isolates from marine fish intestinal contents. *Antimicrob. Agents Chemother.* 46, 1550–1552. doi: 10.1128/AAC.46.5.1550-1552.2002

Nordmo, R., Varma, K. J., Sutherland, I. H., and Brokken, E. S. (1994). Florfenicol in Atlantic salmon, *Salmo salar* L.: field evaluation of efficacy against furunculosis in Norway. *J. Fish Dis.* 17, 239–244. doi: 10.1111/j.1365-2761.1994.tb00219.x

Okuda, J., Hayakawa, E., Nishibuchi, M., and Nishino, T. (1999). Sequence analysis of the *gyr*A and *par*C homologues of a wild type strain of *Vibrio parahaemolyticus* and its fluoroquinolone-resistant mutants. *Antimicrob. Agents. Chemother.* 43, 1156–1162.

Oppegaard, H., and Sørum, H. (1994). *gyr*A mutations in quinolone-resistant isolates of the fish pathogen *Aeromonas salmonicida*. *Antimicrob. Agents Chemother.* 38, 2460–2464. doi: 10.1128/AAC.38.10.2460

Ozanne, B., Benveniste, R., Tipper, D., and Davies, J. (2005). Molecular cloning of the *gyr*A gene and characterization of its mutation in clinical isolates of quinolone-resistant *Edwarsiella tarda*. *Dis. Aquat. Org.* 67, 259–266. doi: 10.3354/dao067259

Paulsen, I. T., Brown, M., and Skurray, R. (1996). Proton-dependent multidrug efflux systems. *Microbiol. Rev.* 60, 575–608.

Poirel, L., Cattoir, V., and Nordmann, P. (2008). Is plasmid-mediated quinolone resistance a clinically significant problem? Clin. *Microbiol. Infect.* 14, 295–297. doi: 10.1111/j.1469-0691.2007.01930.x

Poirel, L., Cattoir, V., and Nordmann, P. (2012). Plasmid-mediated quinolone resistance: interactions between human, animal, and environmental ecologies. *Front. Microbiol.* 3:24. doi: 10.3389/fmicb.2012.00024

Poirel, L., Liard, A., Rodriguez-Martinez, J. M., and Nordmann, P. J. (2005). *Vibrionaceae* as a possible source of Qnr-like quinolone resistance determinants. *J. Antimicrob. Chemother.* 56, 1118–1121. doi: 10.1093/jac/dki371

Poole, K. (2005). Efflux-mediated antimicrobial resistance. *J. Antimicrob. Chemother.* 56, 20–51. doi: 10.1093/jac/dki171

Rhodes, G., Huys, G., Swings, J., McGann, P., Hiney, M., Smith, P., et al. (2000). Distribution of oxytetracycline resistance plasmids between aeromonads in hospital and aquaculture environments: implication of Tn1721 in dissemination of the tetracycline resistance determinant Tet A. *Appl. Environ. Microbiol.* 66, 3883–3890. doi: 10.1128/AEM.66.9.3883-3890.2000

Rico, A., Satapornvanit, K., Haque, M. M., Min, J., Nguyen, P. T., Telfer, T. C., et al. (2012). Use of chemicals and biological products in Asian aquaculture and their potential environmental risks: a critical review. *Rev. Aquac.* 4, 75–93. doi: 10.1111/j.1753-5131.2012.01062.x

Roberts, M. C. (1994). Epidemiology of tetracycline-resistance determinants. *Trends Microbiol.* 2, 353–357. doi: 10.1016/0966-842X(94)90610-6

Roberts, M. C. (1996). Tetracycline resistance determinants: mechanisms of action, regulation of expression, genetic mobility, and distribution. *FEMS Microbiol. Rev.* 19, 1–24. doi: 10.1111/j.1574-6976.1996.tb00251.x

Roberts, M. C. (2005). Update on acquired tetracycline resistance genes. *FEMS Microbiol. Lett.* 245, 195–203. doi: 10.1016/j.femsle.2005.02.034

Roberts, M. C., Schwarz, S., and Aarts, H. J. M. (2012). Erratum: acquired antibiotic resistance genes: an overview. *Front. Microbiol.* 3:384. doi: 10.3389/fmicb.2012.00384

Rodkhum, C., Maki, T., Hirono, I., and Aoki, T. (2008). *gyrA* and *parC* associated with quinolone resistance in *Vibrio anguillarum*. *J. Fish Dis.* 31, 395–399. doi: 10.1111/j.1365-2761.2007.00843.x

Rodríguez-Martínez, J. M., Cano, M. E., Velasco, C., Martínez-Martínez, L., and Pascual, A. (2011). Plasmid-mediated quinolone resistance: an update. *J. Infect. Chemother.* 17, 149–182. doi: 10.1007/s10156-010-0120-2

Ruiz, J. (2003). Mechanisms of resistance to quinolones: target alterations, decreased accumulation and DNA gyrase protection. *J. Antimicrob. Chemother.* 51, 1109–1117. doi: 10.1093/jac/dkg222

Salyers, A. A., Speer, B. S., and Shoemaker, N. B. (1990). New perspectives in tetracycline resistance. *Mol. Microbiol.* 4, 151–156. doi: 10.1111/j.1365-2958.1990.tb02025.x

Samuelsen, O. B., and Bergh, Ø. (2004). Efficacy of orally administered florfenicol and oxolinic acid in the treatment of vibriosis in cod (*Gadus morhua* L.). *Aquaculture* 235, 27–35. doi: 10.1016/S0044-8486(03)00446-0

Samuelsen, O. B., Bergh, Ø., and Ervik, A. (2003). A single-dose pharmacokinetic study of florfenicol in cod (*Gadus morhua* L.) held in seawater at 8°C and in vitro antibacterial activity against some *Vibrio anguillarum* strains isolated from diseased cod. *Dis. Aquat. Org.* 56, 127–133. doi: 10.3354/dao056127

Samuelsen, O. B., Hjeltnes, B., and Glette, J. (1998). Efficacy of orally administered florfenicol in the treatment of furunculosis in Atlantic salmon. *J. Aquat. Anim. Health.* 10, 56–61. doi: 10.1577/1548-8667(1998)010<0056:EOOAFI>2.0.CO;2

Sapkota, A., Sapkota, A. R., Kucharski, M., Burke, J., McKenzie, S., Walker, P., et al. (2008). Aquaculture practices and potential human health risks: current knowledge and future priorities. *Environ. Int.* 34, 1215–1226. doi: 10.1016/j.envint.2008.04.009

Schmidt, A. S., Bruun, M. S., Dalsgaard, I., and Larsen, J. L. (2001a). Incidence, distribution, and spread of tetracycline resistance determinants and integron-associated antibiotic resistance genes among motile aeromonads from a fish farming environment. *Appl. Environ. Microbiol.* 67, 5675–5682. doi: 10.1128/AEM.67.12.5675-5682.2001

Schmidt, A. S., Bruun, M. S., Larsen, J. L., and Dalsgaard, I. (2001b). Characterization of class 1 integrons associated with R-plasmids in clinical *Aeromonas salmonicida* isolates from various geographical areas. *J. Antimicrob. Chemother.* 47, 735–743. doi: 10.1093/jac/47.6.735

Schwarz, S., Kehrenberg, C., Doublet, B., and Cloeckaert, A. (2004). Molecular basis of bacterial resistance to chloramphenicol and florfenicol. *FEMS Microbiol. Rev.* 28, 519–542. doi: 10.1016/j.femsre.2004.04.001

SERNAPESCA (Chile). (2009). *Informe De Uso De Antimicrobianos 2005–2009.* Report available at: http://www.sernapesca.cl/index.php?option=com_remository&Itemid=246&func=select&id=35&orderby=2&page=2.

Seyfried, E. E., Newton, R. J., Rubert, K. F., Pedersen, J. A., and McMahon, K. D. (2010). Occurrence of tetracycline resistance genes in aquaculture facilities with varying use of oxytetracycline. *Microb. Ecol.* 59, 799–807. doi: 10.1007/s00248-009-9624-7

Shah, S. Q., Nilsen, H., Bottolfsen, K., Colquhoun, D. J., and Sørum, H. (2012). DNA gyrase and topoisomerase IV mutations in quinolone-resistant *Flavobacterium psychrophilum* isolated from diseased salmonids in Norway. *Microb. Drug Resist.* 18, 207–214. doi: 10.1089/mdr.2011.0142

Shaw, W. V., and Leslie, A. G. (1991). Chloramphenicol acetyltransferase. *Annu. Rev. Biophys. Biophys. Chem.* 20, 363–386. doi: 10.1146/annurev.bb.20.060191.002051

Smith, P. (2008). Aquaculture and florfenicol resistance in *Salmonella enterica* Typhimurium DT104 (letter). *Emerg. Infect. Dis.* 14, 1327–1328. doi: 10.3201/eid1408.080329

Sofia, H. J., Chen, G., Hetzler, B. G., Reyes-Spindola, J. F., and Miller, N. E. (2001). Radical SAM, a novel protein superfamily linking unresolved steps in familiar biosynthetic pathways with radical mechanisms: functional characterization using new analysis and information visualization methods. *Nucleic Acids Res.* 29, 1097–1106. doi: 10.1093/nar/29.5.1097

Sørum, H., L'Abee-Lund, T. M., Solberg, A., and Wold, A. (2003). Integron-containing incU R plasmid pRAS1 and pAr-32 from the fish pathogen *Aeromonas salmonicida*. *Antimicrob. Agents Chemother.* 47, 1285–1290. doi: 10.1128/AAC.47.4.1285-1290.2003

Speer, B. S., and Salyers, A. A. (1989). Novel aerobic tetracycline resistance gene that chemically modifies tetracycline. *J. Bacteriol.* 171, 148–153.

Speer, B. S., Shoemaker, N. B., and Salyers, A. A. (1992). Bacterial resistance to tetracycline: mechanisms, transfer, and clinical significance. *Clin. Microbiol. Rev.* 5, 387–399.

Su, H. C., Ying, G. G., Tao, R., Zhang, R. Q., Fogarty, L. R., and Kolpin, D. W. (2011). Occurrence of antibiotic resistance and characterization of resistance genes and integrons in Enterobacteriaceae isolated from integrated fish farms in South China. *J. Environ. Monit.* 13, 3229–3236. doi: 10.1039/c1em10634a

Tao, W., Lee, M. H., Wu, J., Kim, N. H., Kim, J.-C., Chung, E., et al. (2012). Inactivation of chloramphenicol and florfenicol by a novel chloramphenicol hydrolase. *Appl. Environ. Microbiol.* 78, 6295–6301. doi: 10.1128/AEM.01154-12

Taylor, D. E., and Chau, A. (1996). Tetracycline resistance mediated by ribosomal protection. *Antimicrob. Agents Chemother.* 40, 1–5.

Tirado, M. C., Clarke, R., Jaykus, L. A., McQuatters-Gollop, A., and Frank, J. M. (2010). Climate change and food safety: a review. *Food Res. Int.* 43, 1745–1765. doi: 10.1016/j.foodres.2010.07.003

Tran, J. H., and Jacoby, G. A. (2002). Mechanism of plasmid-mediated quinolone resistance. *Proc. Natl. Acad. Sci. U.S.A.* 99, 5638–5642. doi: 10.1073/pnas.082092899

Welch, T. J., Evenhuis, J., White, D. G., McDermott, P. F., Harbottle, H., Miller, R. A., et al. (2009). IncA/C plasmid-mediated florfenicol resistance in the catfish pathogen *Edwardsiella ictaluri*. *Antimicrob. Agents Chemother.* 53, 845–846. doi: 10.1128/AAC.01312-08

WHO. (2011). *Critically Important Antimicrobials for Human Medicine,* 3rd Revision. Available at: http://apps.who.int/iris/bitstream/10665/77376/1/9789241504485_eng.pdf.

21

Beta-lactamase induction and cell wall metabolism in Gram-negative bacteria

Ximin Zeng and Jun Lin*

Department of Animal Science, The University of Tennessee, Knoxville, TN, USA

Edited by:
Lixin Zhang, Institute of Microbiology, Chinese Academy of Sciences, China

Reviewed by:
Sabeel Padinhara Valappil, The University of Liverpool, UK
Yixin Shi, Arizona State University, USA

****Correspondence:***
Jun Lin, Department of Animal Science, The University of Tennessee, 2506 River Drive, Knoxville, TN 37996-4574, USA.
e-mail: jlin6@utk.edu

Production of beta-lactamases, the enzymes that degrade beta-lactam antibiotics, is the most widespread and threatening mechanism of antibiotic resistance. In the past, extensive research has focused on the structure, function, and ecology of beta-lactamases while limited efforts were placed on the regulatory mechanisms of beta-lactamases. Recently, increasing evidence demonstrate a direct link between beta-lactamase induction and cell wall metabolism in Gram-negative bacteria. Specifically, expression of beta-lactamase could be induced by the liberated murein fragments, such as muropeptides. This article summarizes current knowledge on cell wall metabolism, beta-lactam antibiotics, and beta-lactamases. In particular, we comprehensively reviewed recent studies on the beta-lactamase induction by muropeptides via two major molecular mechanisms (the AmpG–AmpR–AmpC pathway and BlrAB-like two-component regulatory system) in Gram-negative bacteria. The signaling pathways for beta-lactamase induction offer a broad array of promising targets for the discovery of new antibacterial drugs used for combination therapies. Therefore, to develop effective mitigation strategies against the widespread beta-lactam resistance, examination of the molecular basis of beta-lactamase induction by cell wall fragment is highly warranted.

Keywords: beta-lactamase, regulation, peptidoglycan

INTRODUCTION

Bacteria should continuously maintain and shape their envelopes to adapt enormous stresses they encounter in different niches and to meet physiological needs, such as growth and multiplication. Bacterial envelope is highly organized as a layer structure including cell wall, membrane(s), and the possible space between them. The structure of cell envelope varies in prokaryotes. In general, Gram-positive bacteria contain a thick layer of cell wall as well as a layer of cytoplasmic membrane. However, Gram-negative bacteria (e.g., *Escherichia coli*) typically contain an outer membrane, an intervening periplasmic space where a thin layer of cell wall resides, and a layer of cytoplasmic membrane.

The bacterial cell wall is unique to bacteria and plays a critical role in maintaining cell integrity. In addition, the conserved cell wall components, such as monomeric disaccharide tetrapeptide, could serve as a signal to trigger host immunologic or pathologic responses (Goldman et al., 1982; Melly et al., 1984; Viala et al., 2004; Watanabe et al., 2004; Dziarski and Gupta, 2005; Cloud-Hansen et al., 2006; Strober et al., 2006). Thus, given its significant role in bacterial pathophysiology, cell wall has been an effective target for developing various antimicrobials with different mode of actions, such as beta-lactam and glycopeptide antibiotics. Of these, beta-lactam antibiotics are the most commercially available antibiotics in the market. Until 2010, beta-lactam antibiotics account for sales of approximately 53% of the total antibiotic market worldwide (42 billion US dollars; Hamad, 2010). Beta-lactam antibiotics inhibit bacterial cell wall biosynthesis, consequently leading to cell lysis and death. Specifically, beta-lactam antibiotics bind and acylate active site of penicillin-binding protein (PBP), the enzyme essential for the biosynthesis of bacteria cell wall.

To counteract bactericidal effect of beta-lactams, bacteria have quickly evolved defense systems in which production of beta-lactamase is a major beta-lactam resistance mechanism. Bacterial resistance to beta-lactam antibiotics has become a worldwide health care problem, as exemplified by the recent emergence of broad-range beta-lactam resistant NDM-1 (New Delhi metallo-beta-lactamase 1) strains (Kumarasamy et al., 2010). Beta-lactamase is an enzyme that could hydrolyze beta-lactam ring, consequently deactivating beta-lactam antibiotics. In Gram-negative bacteria, the beta-lactamase was usually produced at very high concentration constitutively or by induction via direct interaction of beta-lactam antibiotic with regulatory system (e.g., MecR1/MecI in *Staphylococcus aureus*; Kogut et al., 1956; Richmond, 1963, 1965; Pollock, 1965; Zhu et al., 1992; Fuda et al., 2005; Safo et al., 2005). In Gram-negative bacteria, the expression level of beta-lactamase is usually low; however, it has been observed that production of beta-lactamase was inducible but molecular basis for this phenomenon was not clear (Ambler, 1980; Jacobs et al., 1997).

In the past, extensive research has focused on the structure, function, and ecology of beta-lactamases while limited efforts were placed on the regulatory mechanisms of beta-lactamases. In 1990s, the induction of beta-lactamase AmpC was observed to be correlated to the recycling process of cell wall in Gram-negative

---

Abbreviations: GlcNAc, *N*-acetylglucosamine; LT, lytic transglycosylase; MurNAc, *N*-acetylmuramic acid; PBP, penicillin-binding protein; PG, peptidoglycan; TCRS, two-component regulatory system.

bacteria, which shed light on the molecular basis of beta-lactamase induction (Jacobs et al., 1994). In the past two decades, accumulating evidence have shown the relationship between muropeptide release and beta-lactamase induction in Gram-negative bacteria (Holtje et al., 1994; Jacobs et al., 1994, 1997; Korsak et al., 2005). However, in Gram-positive bacteria, there is little evidence showing the induction of beta-lactamases by liberated murein fragments. Recently, Amoroso et al. (2012) observed that a cell wall fragment could re-enter in the cytoplasm of *Bacillus licheniformis* and function as a signal to induce the expression of beta-lactamase. However, whether this cell wall fragment is the major signal for beta-lactamase induction in this Gram-positive bacterium still needs to be determined in the future. Given the lack of information on the relationship between beta-lactamase induction and cell wall metabolism in Gram-positive bacteria, in this review, we only summarize the relevant background information and recent research on the mechanisms of beta-lactamase induction by cell wall fragments in Gram-negative bacteria. In addition, we also discuss potential strategies to mitigate beta-lactam resistance by targeting beta-lactamase induction pathways.

PEPTIDOGLYCAN BIOSYNTHESIS AND RECYCLING

In Gram-negative bacteria, peptidoglycan (PG), also called murein, is a mesh structure with units of continuous biopolymer residing on the intervening space between the outer and inner (cytoplasmic) membrane. Specifically, PG is a polysaccharide composed of repeating β-(1,4)-GlcNAc-β-(1,4)-MurNAc disaccharide interconnected by oligopeptide stems via covalent bond (Glauner et al., 1988; **Figure 1**). The PG maintains cell integrity by sustaining internal osmotic pressure and keeps the regular bacterial shape. The glycan strand in *E. coli* is averagely composed of 29 disaccharide-peptide units (Glauner, 1988).

The PG biosynthesis involves multi-stage enzymatic activities. First, the PG monomer unit (disaccharide with oligopeptide stem) is attached to a lipid in the cytoplasmic leaf of inner membrane (van Heijenoort, 2001b; Barreteau et al., 2008; Bouhss et al., 2008). Second, the PG monomer-lipid intermediate is flipped into periplasm and catalyzed into the end of extending glycan chain by glycosyltransferases (Goffin and Ghuysen, 1998; van Heijenoort, 2001a; Sauvage et al., 2008). Finally, the stem oligopeptides [L-Ala-γ-D-Glu-meso-A2pm-(L)-D-Ala-D-Ala pentapeptide in *E. coli*, **Figure 1**] that is linked to MurNAc are cross-linked to the adjacent stem oligopeptides from other glycan chains by transpeptidases (Goffin and Ghuysen, 2002; Sauvage et al., 2008). These transpeptidases are the target of beta-lactam antibiotics and also called PBPs (including PBP1a, PBP1b, PBP1c, PBP2, and PBP3; Goffin and Ghuysen, 1998; Sauvage et al., 2008). Thus, PBPs are involved in the final stage of PG synthesis. Each bacterial cell may produce different PBPs, leading to various types of cross-linkage, such as D-Ala → (D)-meso-A2pm, (L)-meso-A2pm → (D)-meso-A2pm, and so on (van Heijenoort, 2011), for making a rigid mesh structure of PG.

Notably, PG is not a static biological structure. The structural units of PG changes dynamically during bacterial growth and doubling, with old units degraded and new materials added. Instead of starting over the complete *de novo* synthesis as described above, large quantities of the new materials added are recycled from the degraded PG units. It's estimated that up to 60% of the parental cell wall is made of the recycled PG units during active bacterial growth (de Pedro et al., 2001; Park and Uehara, 2008).

The PG recycling also involves multi-stage enzymatic activities. First, the lytic transglycosylase (LT) cleaves the glycan strand between the MurNAc and GlcNAc, and forms the 1,6-anhydro bond at the newly exposed MurNAc end in the mean time. With the aid of the endopeptidases (e.g., PBP4) that could break the cross-linkage between stem oligopeptides, anhydro muropeptide monomers (GlcNAc-anhydro-MurNAc-peptides) are liberated from PG. The main muropeptides are GlcNAc-anhMurNAc-L-Ala-γ-D-Glu-meso-A2pm-D-Ala (GlcNAc-anhydroMurNAc-tetrapeptide), with small amount of tri-, pentapeptides (Glauner, 1988). Second, these muropeptides are transported into cytoplasm through the inner membrane transporter AmpG (Park and Uehara, 2008). Subsequently, in cytoplasm, the GlcNAc sugar residue is removed by the glycoside hydrolase NagZ (Cheng et al., 2000; Votsch and Templin, 2000). The resulting population of 1,6-anhydroMurNAc-oligopeptides are further transformed to UDP-MurNAc-pentapeptide (Park and Uehara, 2008), a PG precursor that can be reincorporated into the PG biosynthesis pathway (Park and Uehara, 2008). The muropeptides also could serve as a signal to induce the production of beta-lactamase, which will be discussed below in Section "Mechanisms of Beta-lactamase Induction."

BETA-LACTAM ANTIBIOTICS AND BETA-LACTAMASE

In 1928, Alexander Fleming observed the bactericidal effect of *Penicillium notatum*, leading to the identification of the first beta-lactam antibiotic, penicillin (Fleming, 1929). Since then, a variety of beta-lactam antibiotics with different antimicrobial profiles have been discovered or synthesized, such as penicillin derivatives (penams), cephalosporins (cephems), monobactams, and carbapenems. All beta-lactam antibiotics share a common core containing a four-member beta-lactam ring (**Figure 2**). This beta-lactam ring displays phenomenal structural mimicry with the backbone of the D-alanyl-D-alanine, the substrate of PBP (**Figure 2**). Therefore, penicillin has been proposed to act as a substrate analog and binds to the active site of transpeptidases for inhibition of synthesis of the cross-linked PG (Tipper and Strominger, 1965). This hypothesis was later supported by the evidence that transpeptidases could bind radioactive-labeled penicillin; thus, transpeptidases were also called as PBPs (Cooper et al., 1949; Maass and Johnson, 1949a,b; Cooper, 1955; Schepartz and Johnson, 1956; Markov et al., 1960; Spratt and Pardee, 1975).

Beta-lactam antibiotics have been a primary choice for physicians to treat bacterial infections due to their high specificity and potent killing effect. Clinical introduction of beta-lactam antibiotics has ever claimed to be a historical victory against bacterial infection; the mortality rate due to bacterial infections in the USA was drastically dropped from 797 to 36 per 100,000 individuals between 1900 and 1980 (Armstrong et al., 1999). The emergence of antibiotic resistant bacteria quickly becomes the ghost of modern medicine (Cohen, 2000). In fact, even during the ground-breaking discovery of penicillin, Alexander Fleming has already isolated the *E. coli*, *Salmonella enterica* serovar Typhi, and *Haemophilus influenza* strains that were resistant to penicillin (Fleming, 1929).

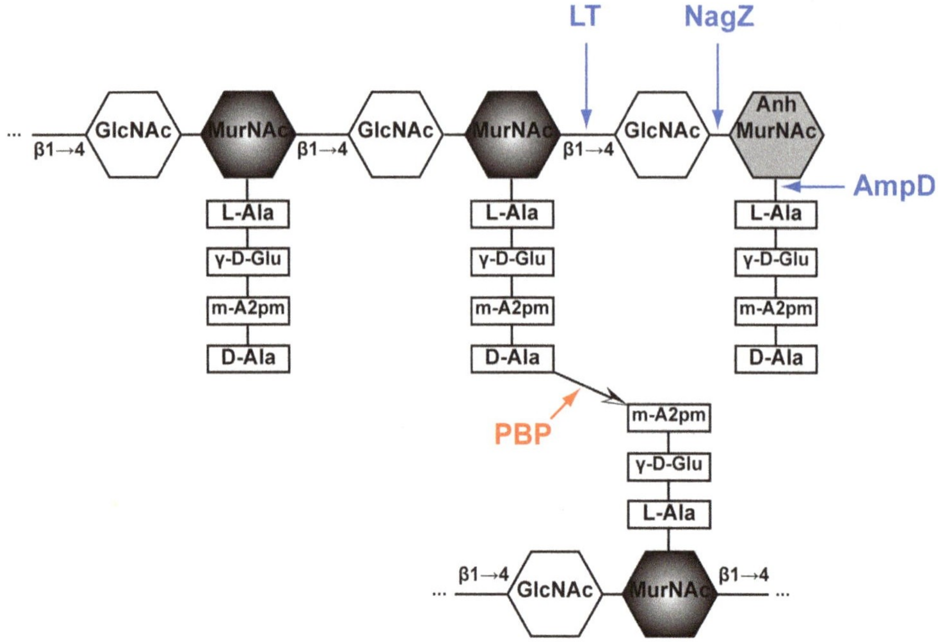

FIGURE 1 | Schematic structure of PG and target sites of different enzymes (pointed by color arrows). The synthetic enzyme (PBP) is highlighted in red while the lytic enzymes (NagZ, AmpD, and LT) are highlighted in blue. Notably, NagZ and AmpD catalyze the liberated muropeptides instead of intact PG. Hexagons denote sugars while rectangles denote stem amino acids. The cross-linkage (⟶) between the top and bottom glycan strands is D-Ala → meso-A2pm. LT, lytic transglycosylase; PBP, penicillin-binding protein, m-A2pm, meso-diaminopimelic acid; AnhMurNAc, 1,6-anhydro-MurNAc; β1 → 4, β-(1,4)-glycosidic bond.

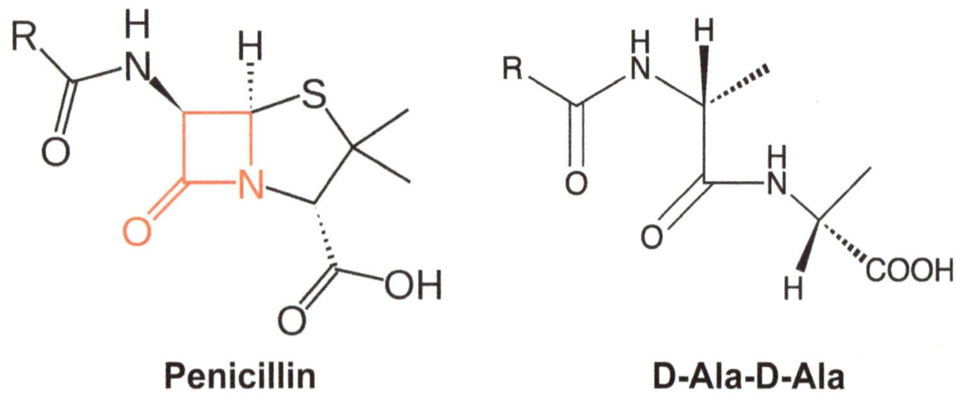

FIGURE 2 | The mimicry of beta-lactam antibiotics to D-alanyl-D-alanine (D-Ala-D-Ala). The four-member lactam ring in penicillin was highlighted in red.

Although numerous efforts have been placed on the discovery new generation of beta-lactam antibiotics to further improve their clinical efficacy, bacteria have been evolving with an unbeatable pace to fail those new beta-lactams (Culotta, 1994). To address this serious public health issue, it is imperative to study the molecular basis of beta-lactam resistance so that we can overcome beta-lactam resistance by targeting resistance mechanisms.

The molecular mechanisms of beta-lactam resistance have been widely studied (Ogawara, 1981; Fuda et al., 2004; Jovetic et al., 2010; Harris and Ferguson, 2012). To evade the bactericidal effects of beta-lactam antibiotics, Gram-negative bacteria have evolved multiple strategies, such as production of beta-lactamases (Korfmann and Wiedemann, 1988; Jacoby, 2009), production of novel PBPs with reduced affinity to beta-lactam antibiotics (Fuda et al., 2004), reducing beta-lactam antibiotics entry through mutations in porins, and expelling beta-lactam antibiotics out of cells using multi-drug efflux pumps (Kohler et al., 1999). Of these mechanisms, producing beta-lactamases, the enzymes that could hydrolyze beta-lactam ring, is still the most efficient strategy (Abraham and Chain, 1940; Jacoby and Munoz-Price, 2005). It has been proposed that beta-lactamases and the PBPs may share a common ancestor due to the presence of certain sequence homology (Massova and Mobashery, 1998). Recently, Fernandez et al. (2012) observed that overexpression beta-lactamases changed the

PG composition and affected bacterial fitness, likely due to the residual transpeptidase activity of the beta-lactamases.

Given the tight link between beta-lactam resistance and the beta-lactamase activity, it is not surprising that past studies were primarily focused on the structure, function, and ecology of beta-lactamases. Particularly, many epidemiological, clinical, and ecological studies are focused on the detection and characterization of specific beta-lactamase genes with little attention on the regulatory mechanism of beta-lactamases. The first "cryptic" beta-lactamase, AmpC (originally named AmpA), was identified in beta-lactam sensitive *E. coli* K-12 by stepwise selection on beta-lactam antibiotics containing medium (Eriksson-Grennberg et al., 1965; Eriksson-Grennberg, 1968). The beta-lactam resistant derivatives constitutively produced high-level of beta-lactamases, suggesting the presence of an inducible beta-lactamase gene in *E. coli* K-12 (Linstrom et al., 1970). Later, the AmpC gene was cloned and characterized as a beta-lactamase (Jaurin and Grundstrom, 1981). The expression of *ampC* normally is maintained at low level and dependent on growth rate (Jaurin et al., 1981). However, a single nucleotide mutation in the promoter region (likely an attenuator) of *ampC* led to overexpression of beta-lactamase, indicating that the *ampC* was subjected to regulation (Jaurin et al., 1981). Then the *ampC* was observed to be widely distributed in different enterobacterial species, such as *Salmonella enterica* serovar Typhimurium, *Pseudomonas aeruginosa*, *Serratia marcescens*, and *Klebsiella pneumonia*; interestingly, the *ampC* was inducible under treatment of beta-lactam antibiotics (Bergstrom et al., 1982). However, the expression of *ampC* in *E. coli* was not induced by beta-lactam antibiotics due to the lack of a regulator gene *ampR* adjacent to the *ampC* in the chromosome (Honore et al., 1986). Complementation of *E. coli* with a plasmid containing the *ampR–ampC* operon from *Enterobacter cloacae* restored the phenotype of beta-lactamase induction (Kraft et al., 1999).

The induction of beta-lactamase is of great clinical importance. For example, prolonged administration of beta-lactam antibiotics could lead to emergence of *P. aeruginosa* mutants resistance to multiple beta-lactam antibiotics, eventually leading to treatment failure and patient death (Livermore, 1987; Sanders, 1987; Giwercman et al., 1990; Juan et al., 2005). Therefore, significant progresses have been made on the molecular basis of the beta-lactamase induction in Gram-negative bacteria in the past two decades.

MECHANISMS OF BETA-LACTAMASE INDUCTION

Understanding the molecular basis of beta-lactamase induction would facilitate us to develop effective combination therapy strategy by inhibiting the induction of beta-lactamase. Gram-negative bacteria have evolved two major mechanisms for beta-lactamase induction, the AmpG–AmpR–AmpC pathway and the two-component regulatory system (TCRS; **Figure 3**). Recent progresses in this significant research area are summarized below.

THE AmpG–AmpR–AmpC PATHWAY

As mentioned above, in many bacteria belonging to Enterobacteriaceae family, AmpC expression is induced by beta-lactam antibiotics. Since beta-lactam antibiotics treatment can trigger the release of large amount of muropeptides in periplasm, which could be subjected to cell wall recycling process, the relationship between cell wall recycling and beta-lactamase induction has been examined and confirmed in recent studies. Briefly, in the AmpG–AmpR–AmpC pathway, beta-lactam antibiotics treatment breaks the balance of PG biosynthesis (e.g., due to the inhibited PBP and the functional LT), consequently liberating GlcNAc-anhydro-MurNAc-oligopeptides in periplasm (Templin et al., 1992). The GlcNAc-anhydro-MurNAc-oligopeptides are further transported into cytoplasm through AmpG transporter (Park and Uehara, 2008). The GlcNAc moiety is removed by enzyme NagZ, leading the accumulated PG products (mainly anhydro-MurNAc-tetrapeptides). In cytoplasm, anhydro-MurNAc-oligopeptide are the inducer of beta-lactamase expression through the interaction with AmpR (Lindquist et al., 1989; Jacobs et al., 1997).

AmpR is a LysR type transcriptional regulator and is encoded immediately upstream of *ampC* with opposite direction (Lindquist et al., 1989; Jacobs et al., 1997). AmpR was demonstrated as an activator for *ampC* using *in vitro* transcription assay (Jacobs et al., 1997). However, production of *ampC* was still repressed even if bacterial host contains functional AmpR, unless exogenous beta-lactam antibiotic was added (Honore et al., 1986; Lindquist et al., 1989; Lodge et al., 1990; Jacobs et al., 1997). Therefore, it has been hypothesized that the activator function of AmpR was inhibited by certain cellular metabolite, which was demonstrated as the cell wall synthesis precursor, UDP-MurNAc-pentapeptide (Jacobs et al., 1997). This inhibition was abolished in the mutant with point mutation in AmpR (G102E; Bartowsky and Normark, 1991), indicating the role of the residue G for the association of UDP-MurNAc-pentapeptide. Upon the treatment of beta-lactam antibiotics, the accumulated intracellular anhydro-MurNAc-oligopeptides could displace the AmpR-associated UDP-MurNAc-pentapeptide, triggering conformational change of AmpR, and subsequently activating the transcription of *ampC* (Jacobs et al., 1997). The DNase I-protection assay showed the binding site of AmpR was in a 39-bp region upstream of the *ampC* transcription start site (−40 to −88; Jacobs et al., 1997). Interestingly, AmpR in *P. aeruginosa* is a global transcriptional factor whose regulon includes beta-lactamases, proteases, quorum sensing, and other virulence factors (Kong et al., 2005; Balasubramanian et al., 2012).

Among the PG cycling process, there is a negative effector to fine-tune the expression of AmpC. A cytoplasmic *N*-acetylmuramoyl-L-alanine amidase, named AmpD (Holtje et al., 1994), could dissociate stem peptides from the anhydro-MurNAc or GlcNAc-anhydro-MurNAc, therefore, reducing concentrations of the inducing muropeptides and mitigating the overexpression of AmpC (Jacobs et al., 1994).

Consistent with these observations on the relationship between PG cycling and beta-lactamase induction, perturbation of PG recycling also affected AmpC induction, suggesting potential pharmaceutical targets. For example, overproduction of the LT MltB stimulated beta-lactamase induction whereas specific inhibition of LT Slt70 by bulgecin repressed AmpC expression (Kraft et al., 1999). In addition, mutation of all six LT enzymes (Slt70, MltA, MltB, MltC, MltD, and EmtA) in *E. coli* decreased the beta-lactamase activities (Korsak et al., 2005).

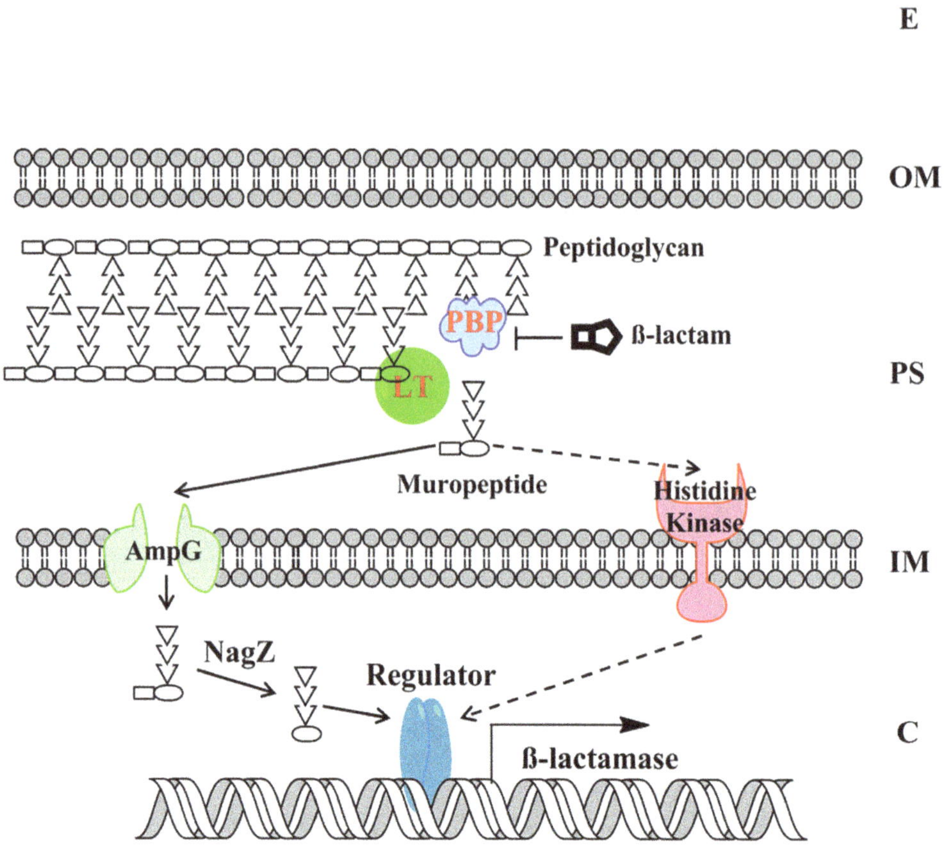

FIGURE 3 | The model of beta-lactamase induction in Gram-negative bacteria. The beta-lactamase induction by muropeptides via two major molecular mechanisms, the AmpG–AmpR–AmpC pathway and the BlrAB-like two-component regulatory system, are presented. The signaling pathway via two-component regulatory system is only supported by limited studies to date and is shown in dashed arrows. The "Regulator" denotes AmpR-like regulator or two-component response regulator. The "beta-lactamase" denotes the beta-lactamase that is subjected to induction. E, extracellular environment; OM, outer membrane; PS, periplasmic space; IM, inner membrane; C, cytoplasm.

Different versions of AmpG–AmpR–AmpC regulatory pathways exist in bacteria. For example, *E. coli* and *Shigella* spp. lacks an *ampR* gene (Bergstrom et al., 1982; Honore et al., 1986), leading to the low level, non-inducible expression of AmpC. The AmpC gene in *E. coli* was primarily regulated by an attenuator sequence in promoter region (Jaurin et al., 1981). The overexpression of AmpC can be achieved either by mutating attenuator (Jaurin et al., 1981) or by introducing an AmpR regulator (Kraft et al., 1999); the similar pathway was also observed in *Acinetobacter baumannii* (Bou and Martinez-Beltran, 2000). In *Salmonella*, the chromosomal AmpC–AmpR is usually absent, which may be due to unbearable production cost of AmpC (Morosini et al., 2000). However, clinical *Salmonella* strains can acquire AmpC–AmpR through horizontally transferred mobile elements (Barnaud et al., 1998). In *Serratia marcescens*, besides AmpR regulation, the post-transcriptional regulation also influences the expression of AmpC. Specifically, the half-life of *ampC* transcript could be affected by a 126-bp, non-encoding region that forms a stem-loop structure (Mahlen et al., 2003). In *P. aeruginosa* PAO1, interestingly, there are three copies of *ampD* genes, which contributed to the stepwise up-regulation of AmpC with the discrete mutation of each copy of *ampD* (Juan et al., 2006).

THE BlrAB-LIKE TWO-COMPONENT REGULATORY SYSTEM

The TCRS, which involves sensing specific environmental stimuli (Capra and Laub, 2012), was also observed to be involved in the induction of beta-lactamase. In *Aeromonas* spp., the AmpC and two other chromosomally encoded beta-lactamases were regulated by the response regulator BlrA of a TCRS instead of an AmpR-type regulator (Alksne and Rasmussen, 1997). Complementation study demonstrated that overexpression of BlrA in *E. coli* enhanced the expression of the *Aeromonas*-derived beta-lactamase in *E. coli* MC1061 while the beta-lactamase was expressed at low level in the absence of BlrA (Alksne and Rasmussen, 1997).

The closest TCRS homolog of BlrAB in *E. coli* is CreBC (Amemura et al., 1986; Wanner and Wilmes-Riesenberg, 1992). Interestingly, the beta-lactamases from *Aeromonas hydrophila* could be regulated by the CreBC TCRS system in the Cre$^+$ *E. coli* strain such as DH5α (Avison et al., 2000, 2001). The "*cre*/*blr*-tag" signature, which is the "TTCACnnnnnnTTCAC" motif located in the promoter of Cre-regulon, was identified in *E. coli* (Avison et al., 2001). These "cre/blr-tag" also reside in promoters of *Aeromonas*-derivative beta-lactamases (Niumsup et al., 2003), and the induction of those beta-lactamases by overexpressed BlrA was dependent on the presence of "*cre/blr*-tag" (Avison et al., 2004).

In *P. aeruginosa*, inactivation of a non-essential PBP was shown to trigger overproduction of a chromosomal AmpC gene and this overproduction is dependent on CreBC TCRS (Moya et al., 2009). Interestingly, among the 32 tested *E. coli* TCRS response regulators, overexpression of FimZ conferred increased level of beta-lactam resistance through the action of AmpC in *E. coli* (Hirakawa et al., 2003).

Despite above evidence showing that TCRS is also involved in the induction of beta-lactamase, the identity of the corresponding cues to which the TCRS respond for beta-lactamase induction is still unknown. We speculate that specific degraded PG components may serve as a signal for the response regulator to induce the production of beta-lactamase. This hypothesis needs to be examined in the future.

OTHER MECHANISMS

Another novel beta-lactamase induction pathway was discovered in *Ralstonia pickettii* (Girlich et al., 2006). The chromosomally encoded beta-lactamases (OXA-22 and OXA-60) were regulated by ORF-RP3 (short for RP3), a gene located at 192-bp upstream of the ATG codon of *oxa-60*. Inactivation of RP3 resulted in the abolishment of induction of the both beta-lactamases; complementation of the RP3 restored the inducible expression of OXA-22 and OXA-60 (Girlich et al., 2006). DNase I footprinting showed that RP3 specifically bound to tandem repeats upstream at the transcriptional start sites of OXA-22 and OXA-60 genes, suggesting RP3 is a novel positive-regulator for beta-lactamase induction (Girlich et al., 2009).

PHARMACEUTICAL IMPLICATIONS OF BETA-LACTAMASE INDUCTION MECHANISM

Discovery of beta-lactamase inhibitors is a promising strategy to combat the prevalent beta-lactam resistance (Bush and Macielag, 2010; Harris and Ferguson, 2012). However, this approach is challenged by the variable affinity of the inhibitors to different beta-lactamases and by the overwhelming quantity of the beta-lactamases produced in resistant cells. Based on the information reviewed here, we propose that the signaling pathways of beta-lactamase induction offer a broad array of promising targets for the discovery of new antibacterial drugs used for combination therapies. The inhibitors targeting beta-lactamase induction pathway may prevent the emergence of beta-lactam resistance and enhance the efficacy of clinical beta-lactam antibiotics, as what we have observed for the efflux pump inhibitors (Lomovskaya and Bostian, 2006). In supporting this hypothesis, the frequency of emergence of ceftazidime resistance in *blrAB* mutant in *P. aeruginosa* was below the detection limit ($<1 \times 10^{-11}$), which is far below that for the wild-type parent strain (3×10^{-8}; Moya et al., 2009).

The potential targets in the beta-lactamase induction pathway as well as the known inhibitors are summarized in **Table 1**. Several inhibitors have been identified for LTs that play a critical role in the initializing the PG cycling. The LT inhibitor bulgecin could induce cell lysis and morphology changes in the presence of beta-lactam antibiotics although bulgecin alone did not show any antibacterial activity against *E. coli* (Imada et al., 1982; Nakao et al., 1986; Bonis et al., 2012). The major molecular target of bulgecin was the soluble LT Slt70 (Templin et al., 1992). In a 2.8-Å resolution crystallographic structure of Slt70-bulgecin complex, one single bulgecin molecule was found to be located in the active site of Slt70, indicating that bulgecin may act as an analog of an oxocarbenium ion intermediate in the reaction catalyzed by Slt70 (Thunnissen et al., 1995). The beta-hexosaminidase inhibitor *N*-acetylglucosamine thiazoline (NAG-thiazoline) was also found to inhibit the LT sMltB from *P. aeruginosa* (Reid et al., 2004a,b). Another inhibitor, hexa-*N*-acetylchitohexaose, can inhibit the LT from bacteriophage lambda (Leung et al., 2001). Interestingly, a proteinaceous inhibitor of vertebrate lysozymes (Ivy), which has conserved CKPHDC motif, was also found to control the autolytic activity of bacterial LTs (Clarke et al., 2010).

Regarding other targets in beta-lactamase induction pathway, PUGNAc and modified EtBuPUG can inhibit the function of NagZ by the mimicry of the oxocarbenium ion-like transition state (Stubbs et al., 2007). Unlike PUGNAc that is also a potent inhibitor against human *O*-GlcNAcase and beta-hexosaminidase, EtBuPUG displayed 100-fold selectivity toward to NagZ. The function of inner membrane permease AmpG in laboratory strains of *P. aeruginosa* can be inhibited by carbonyl cyanide *m*-chlorophenylhydrazone (CCCP), a general inhibitor of proton motive force, consequently leading to an increased susceptibility to beta-lactam antibiotics (Cheng and Park, 2002; Zhang et al., 2010). However, it is important to mention that CCCP also targets other energy-dependent systems, such as drug efflux pump; thus, the linkage between reduced beta-lactam resistance and AmpG inhibition was not clearly demonstrated in these studies.

Although a panel of inhibitors that target the PG recycling pathway have been identified (**Table 1**), it is still largely unknown if these inhibitors repress the inducible beta-lactam resistance effectively in Gram-negative bacteria, consequently enhancing the

Table 1 | The inhibitors targeting the beta-lactamase induction pathway.

Target	Function	Inhibitor
LT	Non-hydrolytic cleave PG with the concomitant formation of 1,6-anhydro-MurNAc	Bulgecin A (Templin et al., 1992); NAG-thiazoline (Reid et al., 2004a,b); hexa-*N*-acetylchitohexaose (Leung et al., 2001); Ivy (Clarke et al., 2010)[a]
NagZ	Cleave disaccharide oligopeptides to release 1,6-anhydro-MurNAc-peptide	PUGNAc, EtBuPUG (Stubbs et al., 2007)
AmpG	Inner membrane permease of the 1,6-GlcNAc-anhydro-MurNAc-peptides	CCCP (Zhang et al., 2010)
AmpR	Binary regulator of AmpC	UDP-*N*-acetylmuramic acid peptides (Jacobs et al., 1997)

[a] *Proteinaceous inhibitor, also the inhibitor of vertebrate lysozymes.*

to beta-lactam antibiotics. *Microbiol. Rev.* 45, 591–619.

Park, J. T., and Uehara, T. (2008). How bacteria consume their own exoskeletons (turnover and recycling of cell wall peptidoglycan). *Microbiol. Mol. Biol. Rev.* 72, 211–227; table of contents.

Pollock, M. R. (1965). Purification and properties of penicillinases from two strains of Bacillus licheniformis: a chemical, physicochemical and physiological comparison. *Biochem. J.* 94, 666–675.

Reid, C. W., Blackburn, N. T., and Clarke, A. J. (2004a). The effect of NAG-thiazoline on morphology and surface hydrophobicity of *Escherichia coli. FEMS Microbiol. Lett.* 234, 343–348.

Reid, C. W., Blackburn, N. T., Legaree, B. A., Auzanneau, F. I., and Clarke, A. J. (2004b). Inhibition of membrane-bound lytic transglycosylase B by NAG-thiazoline. *FEBS Lett.* 574, 73–79.

Richmond, M. H. (1963). Purification and properties of the exopenicillinase from *Staphylococcus aureus. Biochem. J.* 88, 452–459.

Richmond, M. H. (1965). Wild-type variants of exopenicillinase from *Staphylococcus aureus. Biochem. J.* 94, 584–593.

Safo, M. K., Zhao, Q., Ko, T. P., Musayev, F. N., Robinson, H., Scarsdale, N., et al. (2005). Crystal structures of the BlaI repressor from *Staphylococcus aureus* and its complex with DNA: insights into transcriptional regulation of the bla and mec operons. *J. Bacteriol.* 187, 1833–1844.

Sanders, C. C. (1987). Chromosomal cephalosporinases responsible for multiple resistance to newer beta-lactam antibiotics. *Annu. Rev. Microbiol.* 41, 573–593.

Sauvage, E., Kerff, F., Terrak, M., Ayala, J. A., and Charlier, P. (2008). The penicillin-binding proteins: structure and role in peptidoglycan biosynthesis. *FEMS Microbiol. Rev.* 32, 234–258.

Schepartz, S. A., and Johnson, M. J. (1956). The nature of the binding of penicillin by bacterial cells. *J. Bacteriol.* 71, 84–90.

Spratt, B. G., and Pardee, A. B. (1975). Penicillin-binding proteins and cell shape in *E. coli. Nature* 254, 516–517.

Strober, W., Murray, P. J., Kitani, A., and Watanabe, T. (2006). Signalling pathways and molecular interactions of NOD1 and NOD2. *Nat. Rev. Immunol.* 6, 9–20.

Stubbs, K. A., Balcewich, M., Mark, B. L., and Vocadlo, D. J. (2007). Small molecule inhibitors of a glycoside hydrolase attenuate inducible AmpC-mediated beta-lactam resistance. *J. Biol. Chem.* 282, 21382–21391.

Templin, M. F., Edwards, D. H., and Holtje, J. V. (1992). A murein hydrolase is the specific target of bulgecin in *Escherichia coli. J. Biol. Chem.* 267, 20039–20043.

Thunnissen, A. M., Rozeboom, H. J., Kalk, K. H., and Dijkstra, B. W. (1995). Structure of the 70-kDa soluble lytic transglycosylase complexed with bulgecin A. Implications for the enzymatic mechanism. *Biochemistry* 34, 12729–12737.

Tipper, D. J., and Strominger, J. L. (1965). Mechanism of action of penicillins: a proposal based on their structural similarity to acyl-D-alanyl-D-alanine. *Proc. Natl. Acad. Sci. U.S.A.* 54, 1133–1141.

van Heijenoort, J. (2001a). Formation of the glycan chains in the synthesis of bacterial peptidoglycan. *Glycobiology* 11, 25R–36R.

van Heijenoort, J. (2001b). Recent advances in the formation of the bacterial peptidoglycan monomer unit. *Nat. Prod. Rep.* 18, 503–519.

van Heijenoort, J. (2011). Peptidoglycan hydrolases of *Escherichia coli. Microbiol. Mol. Biol. Rev.* 75, 636–663.

Viala, J., Chaput, C., Boneca, I. G., Cardona, A., Girardin, S. E., Moran, A. P., et al. (2004). Nod1 responds to peptidoglycan delivered by the *Helicobacter pylori* cag pathogenicity island. *Nat. Immunol.* 5, 1166–1174.

Votsch, W., and Templin, M. F. (2000). Characterization of a beta-*N*-acetylglucosaminidase of *Escherichia coli* and elucidation of its role in muropeptide recycling and beta-lactamase induction. *J. Biol. Chem.* 275, 39032–39038.

Wanner, B. L., and Wilmes-Riesenberg, M. R. (1992). Involvement of phosphotransacetylase, acetate kinase, and acetyl phosphate synthesis in control of the phosphate regulon in *Escherichia coli. J. Bacteriol.* 174, 2124–2130.

Watanabe, T., Kitani, A., Murray, P. J., and Strober, W. (2004). NOD2 is a negative regulator of Toll-like receptor 2-mediated T helper type 1 responses. *Nat. Immunol.* 5, 800–808.

Zhang, Y., Bao, Q., Gagnon, L. A., Huletsky, A., Oliver, A., Jin, S., et al. (2010). ampG gene of *Pseudomonas aeruginosa* and its role in beta-lactamase expression. *Antimicrob. Agents Chemother.* 54, 4772–4779.

Zhu, Y., Englebert, S., Joris, B., Ghuysen, J. M., Kobayashi, T., and Lampen, J. O. (1992). Structure, function, and fate of the BlaR signal transducer involved in induction of beta-lactamase in *Bacillus licheniformis. J. Bacteriol.* 174, 6171–6178.

22

The intrinsic resistome of bacterial pathogens

Jorge Olivares, Alejandra Bernardini, Guillermo Garcia-Leon, Fernando Corona, Maria B. Sanchez and Jose L. Martinez*

Centro Nacional de Biotecnología, Consejo Superior de Investigaciones Científicas, Madrid, Spain

Edited by:
Marcelo Tolmasky, California state University Fullerton, USA

Reviewed by:
Morten Otto Alexander Sommer, Technical University of Denmark, Denmark
Alfonso J. Soler-Bistue, Institut Pasteur, France

****Correspondence:***
Jose L. Martinez, Centro Nacional de Biotecnología, Consejo Superior de Investigaciones Científicas, Darwin 3, 28049 Madrid, Spain.
e-mail: jlmtnez@cnb.csic.es

Intrinsically resistant bacteria have emerged as a relevant health problem in the last years. Those bacterial species, several of them with an environmental origin, present naturally low-level susceptibility to several drugs. It has been proposed that intrinsic resistance is mainly the consequence of the impermeability of cellular envelopes, the activity of multidrug efflux pumps or the lack of appropriate targets for a given family of drugs. However, recently published articles indicate that the characteristic phenotype of susceptibility to antibiotics of a given bacterial species depends on the concerted activity of several elements, what has been named as intrinsic resistome. These determinants comprise not just classical resistance genes. Other elements, several of them involved in basic bacterial metabolic processes, are of relevance for the intrinsic resistance of bacterial pathogens. In the present review we analyze recent publications on the intrinsic resistomes of *Escherichia coli* and *Pseudomonas aeruginosa*. We present as well information on the role that global regulators of bacterial metabolism, as Crc from *P. aeruginosa*, may have on modulating bacterial susceptibility to antibiotics. Finally, we discuss the possibility of searching inhibitors of the intrinsic resistome in the aim of improving the activity of drugs currently in use for clinical practice.

Keywords: intrinsic resistance, MDR efflux pump, biofilms, swarming, phenotypic resistance, persistence

Clinical definition of antibiotic resistance is mainly based on the bacterial response to treatment. One microorganism is considered as resistant if there exists a high likelihood of therapeutic failure upon antibiotic treatment. Consequently, resistance has been operationally defined in the basis of breakpoints of the minimal inhibitory concentrations (MICs). More recently, an ecological definition of antibiotic resistance is emerging, which is based in the MIC value identifying the upper limit of the wild-type population (Turnidge et al., 2006). This is defined as the ecological cut off (ECOFF) value and all strains presenting MICs above ECOFF are considered resistant from an ecological point of view, even if they are classified as susceptible in the basis of clinical breakpoints. When defining the intrinsic resistome, we are facing the same situation. Bacteria are classically considered intrinsically resistant in the basis of the clinical definition, in other words, if their infections cannot be treated with a given antibiotic. Three are the most relevant causes of this intrinsic resistance: lack of the target, activity of chromosomally encoded antibiotic-inactivating enzymes and reduced uptake of the antibiotic, the later includes reduced permeability of the cellular envelopes and activity of efflux pumps (Nikaido, 1989, 1994; Li et al., 1994; Fernandez and Hancock, 2012). More recently, in the same line of the ecological definition of resistance, the "intrinsic resistome" has been defined as the set of elements that contributes directly or indirectly to antibiotic resistance, and whose presence is independent of previous antibiotic exposure and is not due to horizontal gene transfer (HGT; Fajardo et al., 2008; Wright, 2010).

This definition encompasses all the chromosomally encoded elements that have not been recently acquired as the consequence of the recent human use of antibiotics for therapy and farming purposes. Consequently, for any bacterial species an intrinsic resistome can be defined, irrespective on whether or not this species is classified as intrinsically resistant in the basis of clinical breakpoints. From the studies on the intrinsic resistome, two categories of genes have emerged (Fajardo et al., 2008). Those which inactivation make bacteria more resistant to antibiotics and those which inactivation make bacteria more susceptible. The first ones define elements that are relevant for the acquisition of resistance. For instance, the mutation in a transcriptional repressor of a multidrug (MDR) efflux pump turns the microorganism more resistant to antibiotics (Alonso and Martinez, 1997, 2000, 2001). Mapping these elements is important to define the capability of an organism to evolve toward resistance by mutation (Martinez and Baquero, 2000) and is thus relevant for predicting the evolution of resistance (Martinez et al., 2007, 2011a). The other group of elements define the determinants that contribute to the natural phenotype of susceptibility to antibiotics of a given species, and constitute the *bona fide* intrinsic resistome. Inactivation of these elements make bacteria more susceptible to antibiotics, which may be useful for improving efficacy of current drugs (Martinez, 2012). This has been the situation of inhibitors of plasmid-encoded β-lactamases, which have been demonstrated to be efficient drugs to be used in combination with β-lactams (Reading and Cole, 1977). Similarly, the inhibition of a MDR efflux pump (or another mechanism of intrinsic resistance) might also improve the efficacy of antibiotics currently in use or allow the utilization of others (Lomovskaya et al., 1999; Renau et al., 1999; Lomovskaya and Watkins, 2001). For instance, macrolides are not used for treatment of Gram-negative infections because these organisms are intrinsically resistant to this family of antibiotics. However, the major *Escherichia coli* efflux pump AcrAB extrudes macrolides and its inactivation might increase the susceptibility of *Escherichia coli* to these antibiotics (Chollet et al., 2004). This evidence indicates that macrolides might be useful for treating Gram-negative infections if they are used in combination with an inhibitor of MDR efflux pumps.

As stated above, the main causes of intrinsic resistance from a clinical viewpoint are lack of the target and the inactivation, low uptake and efflux of the antibiotic. However, all bacterial species harbor in their genomes genes encoding MDR efflux pumps, and several present also chromosomally encoded antibiotic-inactivating enzymes, even though they are not classified as intrinsically resistant from the clinical point of view (Saier et al., 1998; Webber and Piddock, 2003; Piddock, 2006; Poole, 2007; Vila and Martinez, 2008; Nikaido, 2009). The study of the intrinsic resistome of bacterial pathogens has shown that in addition to these elements, several others contribute to the phenotype of resistance. Among them, there are the aforementioned classical resistance genes, but there exist also several other elements belonging to all functional categories, including elements of the bacterial general metabolism (Fajardo et al., 2008). These results indicate that the specific phenotype of susceptibility to antibiotics of a given bacterial species is an emergent property consequence of the concerted action of several elements (Girgis et al., 2009). The large functional diversity of the elements of the intrinsic resistome indicates this has not evolved to specifically counteract the activity of the antibiotics. Together with the proposal that antibiotics might be molecular signals at the low concentrations they are likely present in natural ecosystems (Davies, 2006; Linares et al., 2006; Yim et al., 2006, 2007; Fajardo and Martinez, 2008), this situation allows a complementary view to the traditional weapons/shields roles that antibiotics and their resistance genes may have at natural ecosystems (Martinez, 2008; Aminov, 2009, 2010; Fajardo et al., 2009; Martinez et al., 2009a; Allen et al., 2010; Davies and Davies, 2010; Sengupta et al., 2013).

Studying the intrinsic resistome is of relevance for predicting evolution of resistance (Martinez et al., 2007, 2011a), for understanding the linkage between resistance and other bacterial processes as virulence (Martinez and Baquero, 2002; Martinez et al., 2009a,b) or metabolism (Martinez and Rojo, 2011), and for defining novel targets which inactivation make bacteria more susceptible to antibiotics (Martinez et al., 2011b; Martinez, 2012). In this article we present information of those organisms (*Escherichia coli* and *Pseudomonas aeruginosa*) for which more information on their intrinsic resistome is available. We discuss as well some issues concerning transient phenotypic resistance, which also depends on the intrinsic capabilities of the bacteria for evading antibiotics action (**Figure 1**). Finally, we present updated information on studies on the development of inhibitors of resistance.

METHODS FOR ANALYZING THE INTRINSIC RESISTOME

Genome-wide analysis of the intrinsic resistome of a given microorganism requires using high-throughput technologies. Among them, the use of insertion or deletion libraries, allows determining the contribution of each single gene to the

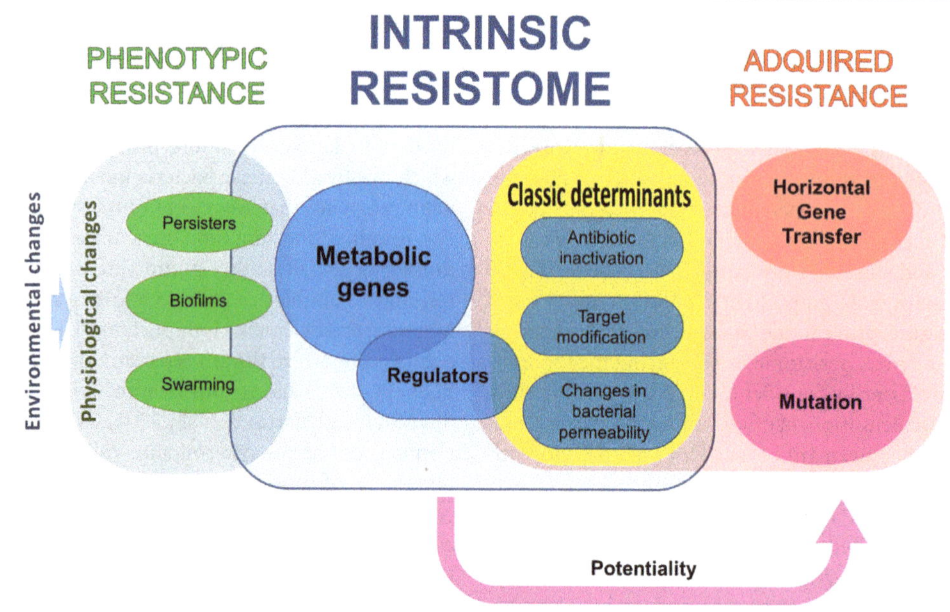

FIGURE 1 | The different elements in bacterial resistance to antibiotics. All bacteria have a repertoire of elements that contribute to their characteristic phenotype of susceptibility to antibiotics, what has been dubbed as intrinsic resistome. Some of the elements of this resistome are classical resistance elements, as antibiotic-inactivating enzymes, whereas others belong to all functional categories. The mutation of some of these elements makes bacteria more susceptible to antibiotics, whereas for some others increased resistance is acquired. Nevertheless, acquisition of a phenotype of increased resistance to antibiotics not always implies a genetic change, either because of mutation or as the consequence of the acquisition of a resistance gene by horizontal gene transfer. Phenotypic, non-inheritable resistance can be achieved by different processes that include, among others, growth in biofilms, swarming adaptation, and development of persistence.

characteristic phenotype of a given bacteria (Liu et al., 2010). This method is the best suited to determine if the inactivation of a gene changes bacterial susceptibility. However, it does not allow analyzing the effect of mutations that do not fully inactivate a given determinant but changes its activity. Alternatively, the use of plasmid libraries containing each open reading frame of a given genome allows to establish the contribution to resistance of each gene when is overexpressed or when it is transferred to a heterologous host (Soo et al., 2011; Spindler et al., 2013). This method is only useful for analyzing acquired resistance, but not for studying genes which inactivation alters the bacterial susceptibility to antimicrobials. The use of high-throughput sequencing and microarray technologies is also useful for studying intrinsic resistance. These methodologies can be used for comparing populations grown in the absence and in the presence of antibiotics. These populations can be formed by the type of libraries above mentioned (transposon-tagged of expression libraries), in which case the enrichment of mutants or clones in the presence of antibiotics allow defining genes contributing to resistance (Girgis et al., 2009; Zhang et al., 2012; Spindler et al., 2013). While these methods are faster and cheaper than methods based in analyzing the susceptibility of each single mutant/clone, their main drawback is that among all potential determinants that contribute to resistance, only those with lower fitness costs will be enriched and several of the elements that may be detected by classical susceptibility tests would not be detected using enrichment-based technologies. This drawback may be a benefit when the analysis is not made on a library, but using a wild-type strain. In these circumstances, sequencing the evolving population allows in a single step defining the mutations that produce resistance and present the smallest fitness costs among those analyzed, as well as to determine potential compensatory mutations (Gullberg et al., 2011; Toprak et al., 2012). These mutations are the most likely found in clinical isolates (Martinez et al., 2007, 2011a; Shcherbakov et al., 2010).

THE *Escherichia coli* INTRINSIC RESISTOME

Although *Escherichia coli* is traditionally considered a susceptible organism, acquired resistance to antibiotics was first detected in enteric bacteria, *Escherichia coli*, *Shigella*, and *Salmonella*, in the late 1950s to early 1960s (Watanabe, 1963). Nowadays, *Escherichia coli* accounts for 17.3% of clinical infections requiring hospitalization and is the second most common cause of infection behind *Staphylococcus aureus* (18.8%). Among outpatient infections, *Escherichia coli* is the most common organism (38.6%).

The antibiotic intrinsic resistome of *Escherichia coli* has been studied by testing the susceptibility to several antibiotics of mutants from gene knockout collections (Tamae et al., 2008; Liu et al., 2010) or transposon-tagged mutant libraries (Girgis et al., 2009). The results from these screenings showed that several genes participate in the phenotype of susceptibility to antibiotics in this species. Among them, some are classical resistance genes. Indeed, this bacterium has different known resistance mechanisms; such as the AmpC β-lactamase and MDR efflux systems like AcrAB–TolC (Lindberg and Normark, 1986; Ma et al., 1993; Lubelski et al., 2007; Jacoby, 2009). In addition, *Escherichia coli* harbors several genes that might be of relevance for its susceptibility to antibiotics as those involved in the repair of DNA damage or cell membrane synthesis and integrity. In addition to these comprehensive analysis, other studies based on the whole-genome sequence of strains evolving in the presence of antibiotics (Toprak et al., 2012) or on the enrichment of specific mutants of transposon-tagged libraries grown with antibiotics have been used to track genes relevant for the development of resistance (Zhang et al., 2012). However, in this type of analysis, mutants are competing one to each other and only those with the highest fitness will be selected.

Escherichia coli as a Gram-negative bacterium presents two cell membranes, and both are non-specific barriers preventing drug influx into the cell. The lipopolysaccharide (LPS) of the outer membrane protects the cell against hydrophobic antibiotics and polycationic compounds such as aminoglycosides and polymyxins. LPS presents anionic groups and it is the first barrier where some antibiotics bind (Hancock, 1984). Because of this, changes in the LPS can alter the susceptibility to antibiotics. For instance, the loss of *rffA*, a gene encoding an enzyme implicated in the LPS synthesis, increases susceptibility to gentamicin (Tamae et al., 2008). The *Enterobacteriaceae* common antigen (ECA) is also an intrinsic resistance element that provides protection against organic acids (Barua et al., 2002). In a similar way as happens with the LPS, changes in ECA may alter the susceptibility to antibiotics. In line with this reasoning is the finding that inactivation of the ECA biosynthesis protein WzxE increases *Escherichia coli* susceptibility to nalidixic acid and amikacin (Girgis et al., 2009). Mechanisms that control the negative charge of the outer membrane, as the Yrb system and the Pmr regulon, modulate the bacterial susceptibility to neutral or negatively charged compounds, such as nalidixic acid, lomefloxacin, and doxycycline (Girgis et al., 2009).

The gates of entry of several nutrients through the outer membrane are the porins, which are also used by antibiotics for entering into the cell (Nikaido, 1994). Many *Escherichia coli* strains have developed resistance to antibiotics as β-lactams and quinolones by mutations in the genes that encode porins or regulate their expression (Hirai et al., 1986; Adler et al., 2013). In addition, transient down-regulation of the expression of the porins can also trigger phenotypic resistance (Fernandez and Hancock, 2012). A general mechanism that prevents the cellular accumulation of drugs is their active extrusion from the cell or from the cytoplasmic membrane through MDR efflux pumps (Nikaido, 1998a,b). The AcrAB–TolC system of *Escherichia coli* is one of the best-characterized MDR transporters (Ma et al., 1995). This system consists of AcrA, a membrane fusion protein; AcrB, a transporter of the RND family; and TolC, an outer membrane protein. AcrAB–TolC is a major determinant for drug intrinsic resistance in *Escherichia coli* (Sulavik et al., 2001). Furthermore, its expression is increased in the presence of bile salts, which are present in the habitat of *Escherichia coli*, the gut (Thanassi et al., 1997; Rosenberg et al., 2003). This means that *Escherichia coli* might present a lower susceptibility to antibiotics when is growing inside its host as the consequence of the overexpression of the MDR efflux pump AcrAB–TolC. Several other MDR transporters pro vide resistance to a narrow range of compounds. *Escherichia coli* contains five putative ABC-type MDR-like transporters. However, none of these systems provides an appreciable drug resistance to *Escherichia coli*, excepting YbjYZ (macrolide-specific ABC-type efflux carrier), which confers resistance to macrolides composed of 14- and 15-membered lactones, as erythromycin (Kobayashi et al., 2001; Nishino and Yamaguchi, 2001). The EmrAB is another MDR pump that protects the cell from several chemically unrelated antimicrobial agents, e.g., the protonophores carbonyl cyanide *m*-chlorophenylhydrazone and tetrachlorosalicyl anilide and the antibiotics nalidixic acid and thiolactomycin (Lomovskaya et al., 1995).

In addition to MDR efflux pumps, *Escherichia coli* harbors antibiotic-inactivating enzymes. It is worth mentioning that whilst MDR efflux pumps usually confer low-level resistance to a wide range of compounds, antibiotic-inactivating enzymes confer frequently high-level resistance to antibiotics belonging to a single structural family. All *Escherichia coli* strains have the chromosomally encoded β-lactamase AmpC. Although it contributes to resistance to antibiotics, it is difficult to assume that this is its original functional role if we take into consideration that the natural habitat of *Escherichia coli* is the gut, which microbiota does not include β-lactam producers. AmpC β-lactamases hydrolyze broad and extended-spectrum cephalosporins but are not inhibited by β-lactamases inhibitors such as clavulanic acid (Jacoby, 2009). Considering that β-lactams inhibit peptidoglycan transpeptidation, determinants involved in this process might be important for the susceptibility to these antibiotics. This is the case for *mltB* and *slt*, which encode membrane-bound lytic murein transglycosylases (von Rechenberg et al., 1996) and of *ampG*, which encodes a transporter involved in the recycling of murein (Jacobs et al., 1994). These genes are not only relevant for β-lactam susceptibility. They are also important for the regular physiology of *Escherichia coli*, since the loss of *mltB*, *slt*, *ampG*, and *ampC* is deleterious (Girgis et al., 2009).

Among those determinants involved in the intrinsic resistance of *Escherichia coli*, some deal with the general response to stress, including the repair of damaged DNA. It is known that quinolones produce DNA damage and induce the SOS repair system (Howard et al., 1993). However, other antibiotics with a different mechanism of action as nitrofurantoin and metronidazol can also damage DNA, and the RecF pathway of DNA repair of single-strand breaks and gaps (*recF*, *recO*, *recR*, *recQ*, and *recJ*; Amundsen and Smith, 2003) is important to prevent damages caused by these drugs. It has been reported that the generation of hydroxyl radicals leading to double-strands breaks contributes to cell death caused by bactericidal antibiotics (Kohanski et al., 2008). In this sense DNA repair mechanisms involved in the maintenance of DNA integrity as the RecBCD system or genes involved in the response of the cell to damaging agents (*dinG*, *xseA*, *xseB*, and *gshB*) constitute a valuable battery of defense mechanisms against antibiotics (Liu et al., 2010). A similar response to stress might be in the basis of the role of ribosomal proteins on intrinsic resistance. Indeed, several genes that encode ribosomal proteins (*rplA*, *rpmE*, *rpmJ*) or proteins involved in their modification (*rimK*) have a role in the susceptibility to a set of antibiotics belonging to different structural families (Liu et al., 2010).

Resistance is also provided by some genes that encode elements that are involved in the regulation of gene expression (*dksA*, *fur*, *hfq*, *hns*, *mfd*, *nusB*, *rseA*, *xapR*, *yciT*; Liu et al., 2010). These genes act in different ways, some of them involved in the stress response. For instance the DksA transcription factor regulates genes involved in double-strand break repair (Meddows et al., 2005). However, other determinants are global regulators of basic processes of the bacterial physiology. This is the case of Fur, that is the master regulator in the response to iron availability (Bagg and Neilands, 1987), an environmental cue with relevance for infection (de Lorenzo and Martinez, 1988; Martinez et al., 1990). This indicates that bacterial physiology and the bacterial response to environmental inputs are cornerstones for the phenotype of susceptibility to antibiotics. In addition to genes with known functions, there are several other determinants of the *Escherichia coli* intrinsic resistome which functional role is not known. This is the case of *yecR* and *yfgC*. Removal of *yfgC* decreases the MIC of vancomycin, rifampicin, and ampicillin (Tamae et al., 2008). *yfgC* has homology to peptidases, and apparently it is located in the bacterial inner membrane (Gardy et al., 2005). The existence of elements of unknown function conferring resistance to several antibiotics bear witness regarding the complexity and the variety of intrinsic resistance mechanisms encoded in the *Escherichia coli* genome.

THE INTRINSIC RESISTOME OF *Pseudomonas aeruginosa*

Pseudomonas aeruginosa is one of the most metabolically versatile bacteria described so far (Lister et al., 2009). This particular feature allows it to colonize multiple environments, being isolated from seawater (Levin and Cabelli, 1972), soil (Green et al., 1974), interacting mutualistically with plant roots (Green et al., 1974; Walker et al., 2004), as a plant pathogen (Walker et al., 2004; Records, 2011) and infecting animals (Petersen et al., 2002), including humans (Stover et al., 2000). In addition of its role in infections, *P. aeruginosa* has been isolated at hospitals in different inorganic surfaces, from ventilation and intubation equipments, contact lens and even in hydrotherapy pools (Morales et al., 2012). This versatility and ability to survive on minimum nutritional requirements (Favero et al., 1971) have made this bacterium one of the most successful nosocomial opportunistic pathogens (Lister et al., 2009).

Not only is this ability to survive anywhere the cause of the ecological success of this organism. This bacterium also shows high levels of antibiotic resistance which often makes impossible its eradication. Evolutionary forces have built its high resistance, and countless elements contribute to intrinsic and acquired resistance of this bacterium, considered a model organism to study mechanisms of resistance (Poole et al., 1993).

Although the recent acquisition of antibiotic resistance genes has been extensively described in *P. aeruginosa* (Woodford et al., 2011), these acquired elements are not the unique cause of antibiotic resistance in *P. aeruginosa*; multiple elements contribute substantially to the resistance of this bacterium. Many works have been performed in order to unravel the intrinsic resistome of *P. aeruginosa*. Transposon-tagged libraries have demonstrated that the inactivation of several genes cause changes in antibiotic susceptibility. The majority of these genes are not related with the cell envelope or efflux pumps and many of them are involved in bacterial metabolism (Breidenstein et al., 2008; Fajardo et al., 2008; Schurek et al., 2008; Alvarez-Ortega et al., 2010; Fernandez et al.,

2013). Mutants with changes in susceptibility to ciprofloxacin, aminoglycosides, β-lactams, and polymyxin B have been identified using this method.

Ciprofloxacin is a broad-spectrum fluoroquinolone that target the bacterial enzymes DNA gyrase and topoisomerase IV (Drlica and Zhao, 1997). Thirty-five and 79 mutants with increased and decreased susceptibilities to this antibiotic, respectively (Breidenstein et al., 2008), were identified in a screening of a PA14 mutant transposon library (Liberati et al., 2006). The majority of these mutants demonstrated only twofold changes in susceptibility compared with the respective isogenic strain; just the mutant in *ftsK* was eightfold more susceptible. Mutants in four genes involved in DNA replication and repair (Holliday junction helicase *ruvA*, the ATP-dependent RNA helicase *recG*, recombinase *xerD*, and the site specific recombinase *sss*) present increased susceptibility to ciprofloxacin. Additionally, *ruvA*, *xerD*, and *fstK* grow slower compared with the wild-type. On the contrary, mutants in genes *nuoBDGHIJLN* that encode a dehydrogenase are less susceptible to ciprofloxacin. These mutants in the *nuo* operon present decreased susceptibility to tobramycin also (Schurek et al., 2008) supporting the idea that some of the elements involved in intrinsic resistance have not evolved to counteract the activity of a specific antibiotic (Fajardo et al., 2008; Martinez and Rojo, 2011).

Despite this apparent lack of specificity, there is not a common response to all antibiotics, even for those belonging to the same structural family. In a screening using imipenem, meropenem and ceftazidime just one mutant (PA0908) presented reduced susceptibility to all three antibiotics and two (*glnK* and *ftsK*) showed increased susceptibility to all three antibiotics (Alvarez-Ortega et al., 2010). Even more, the mutant in *ftsK*, which encodes a protein involved in cell division (Lewenza et al., 2005), presents an increased susceptibility to ciprofloxacin too (Breidenstein et al., 2008). In the same way, mutants in many genes that were more susceptible to β-lactams (PA0401, *pyrB* and *pyrD*; Alvarez-Ortega et al., 2010) presented decreased susceptibility to polymyxin B (Fernandez et al., 2013). However, this is not a general trend, since mutants in *galU*, *ampR*, *lptc*, *aroB*, *wapR*, and *ssg* showed decreased susceptibility to β-lactams and they are more susceptible to polymyxin B also (Fernandez et al., 2013). The majority of these genes participate actively in the central metabolism of *P. aeruginosa* (Stover et al., 2000) reinforcing the idea that genes involved in metabolism can play an important role in the intrinsic resistance to antibiotics of the microorganisms.

The cell membrane is considered one of the principal contributors to intrinsic resistance (Nikaido, 1989). In this way mutations in many genes that take part in the LPS synthesis in *P. aeruginosa* produce changes of the susceptibility against β-lactams and tobramycin. A mutant in *wapR*, which encodes a protein involved in the biosynthesis of the LPS core (Poon et al., 2008), is less susceptible to ceftazidime and meropenem; mutations in adjacent genes (PA5001, PA5002, PA5003, and PA5005) which participate in the LPS synthesis also present reduced susceptibility to ceftazidime and some mutants present cross resistance with meropenem (Alvarez-Ortega et al., 2010). A similar effect was observed in mutants of genes involved in the O-antigen synthesis (*wbpZ*, *wbpY*, *wzt*, *wzm*, and *wbpW*). These mutants presented decreased susceptibility to tobramycin, demonstrating the importance of the cellular membrane as a barrier to avoid the entrance of antibiotics inside the cell (Schurek et al., 2008).

Efflux pumps contribute considerably to antibiotic resistance in *P. aeruginosa*. They are involved in the extrusion of toxic substances, including antibacterial compounds, from inside the cell to the external environment (Webber and Piddock, 2003). In this bacterium, 12 different RND-type efflux systems (Blair and Piddock, 2009) that can eventually contribute to antibiotic resistance have been described. However, only MexAB-OprM has shown to play a relevant role on the intrinsic resistance of *P. aeruginosa* to antibiotics (Kohler et al., 1997). Expression of the other efflux pumps under standard growing conditions is too low to achieve resistance, an issue that is also frequently described for other bacteria (Grkovic et al., 2001, 2002). However, MDR efflux pumps can be overexpressed, and hence render resistance, either because of mutations in their regulatory elements or because of the presence of effectors that trigger their expression (Grkovic et al., 2001, 2002; Blair and Piddock, 2009; Hernandez et al., 2009, 2011).

Since intrinsic resistance is a multifactorial phenomenon, it might be modulated by global regulators. This is the case of the *P. aeruginosa* "catabolite repression control" regulator Crc (MacGregor et al., 1991). Crc is a post-transcriptional repressor that regulates the use of preferred carbon sources in nutrient-complex ecosystems (Morales et al., 2004; Moreno et al., 2009). Recent work has shown that inhibition of Crc makes *P. aeruginosa* less virulent and more susceptible to different antibiotics (Linares et al., 2010), the latter being a consequence of increased expression of transporters and changes in the LPS composition. This shows the existence of networks connecting antibiotic resistance, bacterial virulence and metabolism. The hubs of these networks may be good targets in the search of novel antimicrobials targeting simultaneously resistance, virulence, and bacterial physiology.

PHENOTYPIC RESISTANCE

Most studies on antibiotic resistance are based in the analysis of resistant organisms that have acquired the phenotype of resistance as the consequence of genetic, inheritable, changes, which can be mutations (including gene rearrangements) of the acquisition, through HGT, of resistance genes (Walsh, 2000). However, there are other situations, grouped under the name of phenotypic resistance, in which bacteria present a non-inheritable situation of resistance to the antibiotics (Levin, 2004; Levin and Rozen, 2006). Phenotypic resistance is thus defined as a transient situation in which a bacterial population, usually susceptible to antibiotics, is transiently resistant (**Figure 1**). The elements contributing to this phenotype are a part of the intrinsic resistome that are only unveiled under specific growing conditions (Martinez et al., 1994). Below, some examples of phenotypic resistance are described.

PERSISTENCE

Persistence is defined as a situation in which a bacterial subpopulation is not killed by a given antibiotic under conditions in which the bulk of the population is inhibited. Once antibiotic is removed and growth resumes, persistent cells behave as antibiotic susceptible as the original population, which means that persistence is not the consequence of a genetic change. The existence of persister cells into a population is known since 1944, when this phenomenon was first reported for staphylococcal infections treated with penicillin (Bigger, 1944). Currently, persistence has been described for many other bacterial species and antibiotics. As stated, persisters are phenotypic variants that present increased resistance to antibiotics and are genetically identical to the wild-type. The percentage of persisters in a given culture can be as high as 1% of stationary-phase cells for several microorganisms (Kim and Wood, 2010). Establishment of a persistent subpopulation does not require previous antibiotic exposure.

The presence of persister cells in infections increase the chance of survival of the bacteria in the presence of antibiotics, an issue particularly relevant in the case of chronic infections. Because of this, the analysis of the genes and mechanisms responsible for the development of a persister phenotype is of relevance to implement novel therapeutic approaches based on the eradication of antibiotic resistant persistent cells.

The first gene described to be involved in the development of persistence was *hipA* (Moyed and Bertrand, 1983) in *Escherichia coli*. HipA is a toxin that belongs to the *hipBA* toxin/antitoxin system (TA systems; Correia et al., 2006), which overexpression inhibits cell growth and induces antibiotic resistance by persister formation. Other TA systems as MqsRA (Kim and Wood, 2010) or TisAB (Dorr et al., 2010; Lewis, 2010) have been also associated to the formation of persister cells, indicating that a misbalance in the production of toxin and antitoxin may be in the basis of this phenotype.

Toxin/antitoxin systems are highly distributed among different bacterial species. Usually, these systems are formed by two components, a toxin that inhibits cell growth and an antitoxin that impedes the activity of the toxin. At the moment, three general TA systems have been described. The antitoxins of TA types I and III are small RNAs, whereas the toxins of the type II TA systems are inhibited by protein antitoxins (Gerdes et al., 1997, 2005; Blower et al., 2011). Recent work has shown that type II TA systems are highly relevant for developing persistence in *Escherichia coli* and that the simultaneous deletion of 10 TA loci from the chromosome of *Escherichia coli* reduced the fraction of persistent cells by at least 100-fold (Maisonneuve et al., 2011; Gerdes and Maisonneuve, 2012).

In addition to TA systems, other factors modulate the development of persistence. Among them, elements involved in the regular bacterial metabolism have shown to be relevant. This is the case of *phoU*, which encodes a negative global regulator that suppresses the cellular metabolic activity, altering expression of several elements with relevance for bacterial physiology, ranking from flagella-encoding genes to genes encoding energy production enzymes (Li and Zhang, 2007).

In depth analysis on the mechanisms of persistence has shown that there are two types of persistent cells (Balaban et al., 2004), which further supports the idea that there exist different routes toward the development of persistence. Type I persisters constitute a pre-existing population of resting cells that are generated at stationary phase. These cells when are inoculated into fresh medium from stationary phase switch back to growing cells with a characteristic extended time lag. An example of genes involved in this phenotype is *hipA7* (Moyed and Bertrand, 1983). Type II persisters constitute a subpopulation of slowly growing cells. An example of genes involved in this phenotype is *hipQ* (Wolfson et al., 1990).

In agreement with the potential role that both bacterial metabolism and TA systems may have on the establishment of persistence, transcriptomic analysis of persister cells have shown that persistence is associated with the down-regulation of biosynthetic genes and the up-regulation of several TA modules (RelBE, MazEF, DinJYafQ, YgiU; Lewis, 2010), Some of these TA systems are known to affect translation (Christensen et al., 2001; Pedersen et al., 2002), which explains their effect in dormancy and consequently on antibiotic resistance. The SOS response, which up-regulates DNA repair functions, also induces several TA genes in *Escherichia coli*, whose promoters contain a Lex box: *symER, hokE, yafN/yafO*, and *tisAB/istR* (Dorr et al., 2010). This means that TA systems, and hence the formation of persister cells, can be activated by factors that trigger the SOS system. It is known that some antibiotics, such as quinolones, induce the emergence of persister cells (Dorr et al., 2010). Since these antibiotics produce DNA damage and activate the SOS system, it is likely possible that the effect of quinolones on persistence is SOS-dependent. The role of other stresses on persistence has been studied. This is the case of oxidative stress that is important during infection due to the immune response. However, this stress only induces persistence against fluoroquinolones but not for other antibiotics such as kanamycin. Surprisingly, this phenotype is due to the overexpression of the MDR efflux pump AcrAB–TolC (Wu et al., 2012). This indicates that transient expression of classic antibiotic resistance mechanisms forming part of the intrinsic resistome may be of relevance for the establishment of persistence.

One important issue for avoiding persistence would be finding elements which mutation impede the development of persistent cells. However, the analysis of a transposon mutants library of *Escherichia coli* (Hu and Coates, 2005; Hansen et al., 2008) and of the comprehensive Kei collection (Baba et al., 2006), did not allow identifying any gene which mutation fully impede the phenotype of persistence. These data suggest a great degree of redundancy in the elements and pathways involved in the development of persistence. Even though TA systems could be good candidates to decrease the fraction of persister cells in a given population, their high number, with 671 TA systems already identified in 126 prokaryotic genomes (Pandey and Gerdes, 2005) makes difficult developing drugs directed to reduce persistence by targeting these systems.

Another approach for eliminating persisters can be by shifting their metabolic state. A recent report shows that this is feasible by specific metabolic stimuli that allow the recovery of the proton motive force of persistent cells, enabling their killing by aminoglycosides (Allison et al., 2011).

BIOFILM

Biofilm is a structured population of bacteria embedded in a matrix, which is composed by polysaccharides, proteins, and extracellular DNA. It has been shown than cells growing in biofilms are less susceptible to antibiotics than those growing planktonically

(Mah and O'Toole, 2001; Amini et al., 2011). This phenotypic resistance is relevant for the treatment of infections on intubated or catheterized patients, as well as in infections of prosthesis and some chronic infections as those of cystic fibrosis patients that involve the colonization of surfaces (Costerton et al., 1999) in which biofilm formation is frequent. The antibiotic resistance associated with biofilms depends on several causes, some due to the structure of the extracellular matrix, some other to the physiological state of biofilm-growing bacteria; which is different to that of planktonic cells. Even inside the biofilm, bacteria show different metabolic states, because there is a gradient of nutrients and oxygen between the surface of the biofilm and its deeper region.

The extracellular matrix may change the activity of the antibiotics by two different reasons; by diminishing the diffusion of the antibiotic or by sequestering it through its binding to the matrix. This is not a general trend, since in several occasions, slow diffusion of the antibiotic is not the most important element in the phenotypic resistance displayed by biofilms (Walters et al., 2003; Stewart et al., 2009; Singh et al., 2010). Another aspect in which the extracellular matrix may participate in the phenotype of resistance of biofilms is by triggering specific mechanisms of resistance. DNA, a macromolecule capable of chelate cations, is one of the components of the extracellular matrix. Since a reduced concentrations of divalent cations trigger expression of the regulator of resistance to cationic antimicrobials PhoP–PhoQ (Mulcahy et al., 2008), the extracellular matrix trigger itself resistance to these drugs.

When analyzing the role of the metabolic state of bacteria on the phenotypic resistance of biofilms, it has been shown that the degree of resistance depends on the region of the biofilm and on the antibiotic involved. Different regions of the biofilms contain subpopulations in different metabolic stages that mainly depend on the oxygen and nutrients availability (Huang et al., 1995; Sternberg et al., 1999). It has been described than oxygen-rich regions of *P. aeruginosa* biofilms are highly susceptible to quinolones whilst cells in these regions are phenotypically resistant to cationic peptides, and the opposite occurs at regions of the biofilms with low oxygen tension (Rani et al., 2007). Altogether, these results indicate that the phenotypic resistance of bacterial biofilms depend on several factors that operate simultaneously.

SWARMING

Swarming is a specific type of movement of bacterial populations. It is characterized by the formation of hyper-flagellated cells in nutrient-rich environments. It is supposed that this type of motility allows the colonization of such environments. Consequently, swarming is just the most visible phenotype of a complex physiological adaptation process that is dependent on cell–cell signaling [quorum-sensing (QS)] and on nutrients availability (Fraser and Hughes, 1999). The capability of swarm has been described in different microorganisms, including *Escherichia coli, Serratia marcescens, Burkholderia thailandensis, Bacillus subtilis, Salmonella enterica* serovar Typhimurium, and *P. aeruginosa* (Kim et al., 2003; Overhage et al., 2008a; Lai et al., 2009), and it might be of relevance for the colonization of surfaces during infection, as for instance in the lungs of cystic fibrosis patients. A relevant characteristic of swarmer cells consists on their reduced susceptibility to different antibiotics (Kim et al., 2003; Overhage et al., 2008b; Lai et al., 2009).

Transcriptomic analyses of *P. aeruginosa* have shown that several genes change their expression during swarm cell differentiation. Some of these genes encode porins and efflux pumps, such as MexGHI-OpmD. A differential expression of these genes in swarmer cells might be involved in their phenotype of reduced susceptibility to antibiotics (Overhage et al., 2008a). Nevertheless, the reasons for this transient phenotype of antibiotic resistance are still far to be fully understood, since there are other elements that might be involved in the phenotype. For instance, several proteases (Lon, AsrA, PfpI, ClpS, and ClpP) that affect swarming motility are also relevant for the formation of biofilms, and therefore for phenotypic antibiotic resistance (Marr et al., 2007; Kindrachuk et al., 2011; Fernandez and Hancock, 2012).

Quorum-sensing seems to play a key role in swarming differentiation. It has been shown that PvdQ, an acylase that hydrolyzes the QS signal 3-oxo-C12-HSL [*N*-(3-oxo-dodecanoyl)-l-homoserine lactone] is involved in swarming. The analysis of cells either over-expressing or lacking PvdQ showed that PvdQ reduced *P. aeruginosa* outer membrane permeability, thereby elevating antibiotic resistance under swarming conditions, upon which this protein is up-regulated (Wang et al., 2013). A similar effect of reduced permeability has been shown for *Salmonella enterica* swarmer cells. In particular the expression of the porin OmpA, which is used for the entrance of nutrients and some antibiotics is low in swarming cells (Sugawara and Nikaido, 1992; Kim and Surette, 2004), suggesting that changes in the permeability of the cellular envelopes, in response to nutrients' availability, might be in the basis of the antibiotic resistance phenotype displayed by swarmer cells.

There are some common factors that might induce the different situations of phenotypic resistance above described. Changes in the environment as the lack of nutrients or low oxygen levels, which reduce the growth rates, occur in stationary phase and this induces persisters, which are much more abundant in this growth phase. These nutritional cues also take place in some regions of bacterial biofilms, mainly at their deepest zone, and are relevant for their reduced susceptibility to antibiotics. QS signaling is a relevant system in the basis of biofilm formation, which is also involved in triggering the bacterial physiological reprogramming that occurs in swarmer cells. Expression of TA systems occurs in response to external signaling, and is involved in the generation of persister cells, but also are differentially expressed during biofilm formation, directly or *via* QS signaling. Cellular damage produced by toxic compounds, antibiotics included, may induce the SOS response, which triggers expression of reparation systems and usually also reduces metabolic activity, a situation that induces the formation of persister cells and is also foreseen in biofilms.

It thus seems that bacterial populations have developed a battery of mechanisms to respond to stress and these mechanisms are also useful to transiently resist the activity of antibiotics.

INHIBITORS OF RESISTANCE DETERMINANTS

One of the areas under development in the search for novel drugs to fight infections is the study of inhibitors of resistance (Baquero et al., 2011; Martinez et al., 2011b; Martinez, 2012). The use of these drugs in combination with those antibiotics against which the mechanisms of resistance operate, increases bacterial susceptibility to the antimicrobials. The first inhibitors of resistance were developed against mechanisms acquired through HGT, in particular plasmid-encoded β-lactamases (Bush, 1988). However, the definition of intrinsic resistome offers the possibility of developing inhibitors that increase susceptibility to all isolates of a given species (Garcia-Leon et al., 2012). For instance, the inhibition of MDR efflux pumps, which makes Gram-negative bacteria susceptible to macrolides, will allow the use of these compounds for treating infections by Gram-negative microorganisms.

Although clavulanic acid, the first inhibitor of β-lactamases was described more than 40 years ago (Reading and Cole, 1977), few other inhibitors, all of them inhibiting the same type of β-lactamases, are already in the market. Main efforts have focused on the inhibitors of other β-lactamases (Drawz and Bonomo, 2010) and MDR efflux pumps (Lomovskaya and Watkins, 2001). In the case of aminoglycoside-inactivating enzymes, the development of inhibitors is problematic due to the large number and variability of families of these resistance elements.

Based on the Ambler's classification (Ambler et al., 1991), the β-lactamases are divided into four classes: class A, C, and D being serine β-lactamases, and class B being metallo-β-lactamases (MBLs). The commercially available β-lactamase inhibitors (BLIs), clavulanic acid, sulbactam and tazobactam, are only effective against class A β-lactamases. However, their combinations with β-lactam antibiotics are still effective, despite the emergence of resistance, either because of gene-dosage effect (Martinez et al., 1987, 1989; Reguera et al., 1991), either because of mutations that make β-lactamase resilient to inhibition (Blazquez et al., 1993; Canica et al., 1998; Salverda et al., 2010; Frase et al., 2011; Li et al., 2012).

The discovery that carbapenems may inhibit some β-lactamases opened the possibility of finding antibiotics with dual activities, antimicrobial and inhibitor of resistance (Buynak, 2006). However, this can be a difficult task, since antibiotics as cefoxitin may either inhibit or induce expression of β-lactamases depending on their concentration (Tsuey-Ching et al., 2012). Because of this, mathematical models are being implemented to establish reliable dosage regimes (Bhagunde et al., 2012) and novel derivatives are being developed to surpass these problems. Among them, *N*-acyl β-sultams obtained, by sulfonylation of β-lactams and addition of an acyl group, inhibit *Enterobacter cloacae* class C β-lactamase (Page et al., 2003). Penicillin and cephalosporin sulfone derivatives are also part of the pipeline of BLIs. LN-1-255 is a penicillin sulfone that is active against OXA-type β-lactamases and is being used as model for further improvements in this type of inhibitors (Pattanaik et al., 2009; Drawz et al., 2010).

In addition to β-lactams that inhibit β-lactamases, there are also non-β-lactams able to inhibit these enzymes. One of the families receiving more attention is the one formed by boronic acids (Kiener and Waley, 1978), which are potential inhibitors of all types of serine β-lactamases (Tan et al., 2010), and seem to be effective even against penicillin-binding proteins (PBPs) resistant to β-lactams (Zervosen et al., 2012). Nevertheless clinical use of these compounds is compromised because of the toxicity of boron. Another class of non-β-lactam BLIs is formed by the diazabicyclooctanes (DBOs). There are two compounds of this family under clinical trials: MK-7655 and NXL104 (avibactam) (Coleman, 2011). MK-7655 is a potent inhibitor of class A and C β-lactamases, that can be used in combination with imipenem to kill AmpC and KPC (*Klebsiella pneumoniae* carbapenemase) producers (Hirsch et al., 2012). Avibactam is a promising BLI that inhibits class A and C β-lactamases, including BlaC from *Mycobacterium tuberculosis* (Xu et al., 2012). In combination with ceftazidime, avibactam protects β-lactams from hydrolysis in β-lactamase-producing *Enterobacteriaceae* and *P. aeruginosa* (Dubreuil et al., 2012; Levasseur et al., 2012). More recently it has been proposed that a triple combination avibactam, ceftazidime, and metronidazole will be useful for treating complicated intra-abdominal infections, which may present a mixed population of *Enterobacteriaceae* and anaerobes (Dubreuil et al., 2012; Lucasti et al., 2013).

Finding common inhibitors for all MBLs is a difficult task, due to the diversity of class B β-lactamases (Drawz and Bonomo, 2010). However, different structural families of inhibitors are under development, including tetrahydropyrimidine-2-thione and pyrrole derivatives (Hussein et al., 2012), 3-mercapto-1,2,4-triazoles and *N*-acylated thiosemicarbazides (Faridoon et al., 2012), *N*-heterocyclic dicarboxylic acids and pyridylmercaptothiadiazoles (Feng et al., 2012), 2-substituted 4,5-dihydrothiazole-4-carboxylic acids (Chen et al., 2012), or mercaptoacetate (Wachino et al., 2012).

Although most inhibitors of β-lactamases target a specific family of these enzymes, efforts have been made to develop drugs capable to inactivate a large range of β-lactamases. Among them single molecules as mercaptomethylpenicillinates (Buynak et al., 2004) or reverse hydroxamates and oximes (Ganta et al., 2009) are under development as well as combinations of compounds as BAL30376, which is a mixture of BAL19764, a siderophore monobactam active to class B MBLs, BAL29880, a bridged monobactam active to class C β-lactamases, and clavulanate (Livermore et al., 2010; Page et al., 2011).

In addition to traditional methods in searching enzyme's inhibitors, information derived from other studies may help in developing β-lactamases inhibitors. In this regard, the finding of a small protein, produced by the same producer of clavulanic acid, *Streptomyces clavuligerus* (Reading and Cole, 1977; Yuan et al., 2011) and capable to inhibit class A β-lactamases opens the possibility of developing peptides or haptamers capable to inhibit β-lactamases. Similarly, the finding that the active site structures and the catalytic mechanisms of N-terminal nucleophile hydrolase (a component of the bacterial proteasome) and β-lactamases are similar, allows discovering cross-inhibition of both enzymes by compounds as *O*-aryloxycarbonyl hydroxamates (Pelto and Pratt, 2008) or 1,3,4-oxathiazol-2-ones (Adediran et al., 2012). This opens the possibility of testing already known inhibitors of the bacterial proteasome as inhibitors of β-lactamases.

Beta-lactamases inhibitors will be very useful, but only for treating infections by those organisms presenting a β-lactamase. A wider spectrum of activity might have the efflux pumps inhibitors (EPIs). MDR efflux pumps are present in all bacterial species contributing to intrinsic and acquired (when overexpressed) resistance to all family of drugs. Since any single efflux pump can extrude a wide range of antibiotics belonging to different structural families, its inhibition will simultaneously increase the bacterial susceptibility to several antibiotics (Vila and Martinez, 2008). *In vitro* work has shown that inhibition of efflux pumps makes bacteria more susceptible to antibiotics and also reduces the probability of emergence of antibiotic resistant mutants (Lomovskaya et al., 2001). In addition, since some efflux pumps contribute to the virulence of bacterial pathogens, their inhibition will also impair their capability for producing infections (Hirakata et al., 2009), including the formation of biofilms (Baugh et al., 2012).

Theoretically, there are different alternatives for inhibiting MDR determinants (Fernandez and Hancock, 2012). One that could serve for inhibiting all efflux pumps would be the inhibition of energy sources required for pumps activity. Unfortunately activity of MDR efflux pumps is coupled either to the membrane potential, either to ATP, both of which are key element for any eukaryotic of prokaryotic cell. This means that most of these potential inhibitors will be too toxic to be used. There are, however, some elements that are specific for bacteria and could be used as potential targets. This is the case of TonB, a protein involved in the activity of *P. aeruginosa* MDR efflux pumps by coupling the energized state of the membrane to the operation of bacterial transporters (Zhao et al., 1998).

Other ways of inhibiting the activity of efflux pumps include the interference with the pump assembly or the blockage of its activity, for instance using antibodies as has been described for SmrA from *Stenotrophomonas maltophilia* (Al-Hamad et al., 2011), the development of effectors precluding the release of the MDR repressor from its operator DNA, and the competition with antibiotics transported by the efflux pump.

One of the first EPIs with potential therapeutic use is the synthetic dipeptide amide phenylalanine-arginyl-β-naphthylamide, which inhibits several Gram-negative efflux pumps (Lomovskaya et al., 2001; Mahamoud et al., 2006), although not all of them (Sanchez et al., 2003). This molecule is a competitive inhibitor that binds to the same site used by the pump to bind the antibiotic. Some efforts have been made in the optimization of diamide-containing EPIs (Watkins et al., 2003). However, it has been shown that the moieties that are responsible for their unfavorable toxicological properties, are also essential for their activity, a situation that impedes their therapeutic use (Lomovskaya and Bostian, 2006).

Pyridopyrimidines and arylpiperazines have also been assayed as EPIs of MDR pumps and major efforts have been performed for their optimization (Nakayama et al., 2004a,b; Yoshida et al., 2006a,b, 2007). Differing to the previously described dipeptide amides, that only impede the action of the antibiotics they compete, pyridopyrimidines increase the susceptibility to all substrates of the efflux pumps, indicating a different mechanism of action (Lomovskaya and Bostian, 2006).

Although some efforts on the development of EPIs against efflux pumps for Gram-positive organisms, as *Staphylococcus aureus* NorA, have been made (Markham et al., 1999; Holler et al., 2012b; Sabatini et al., 2012), most EPIs so far described inhibit efflux pumps from Gram-negative organisms with some degree of specificity. Among them, pyridopyrimidines inhibit MexAB-OprM of *P. aeruginosa* (Yoshida et al., 2007), 1-(1-naphthylmethyl)-piperazine reversed multidrug resistance in *A. baumannii* but not in *P. aeruginosa* (Pannek et al., 2006), or 13-cyclopentylthio-5-OH tetracycline (13-CPTC), a semisynthetic tetracycline analogue that binds TetB pump of *Escherichia coli* (Nelson and Levy, 1999).

The finding that plant-produced compounds are substrates and inducers of efflux pumps (Matilla et al., 2007) suggests that these compounds may also inhibit MDR determinants. Indeed, it has been shown that plant extracts contain a variety of EPIs (Tegos et al., 2002; Musumeci et al., 2003; Lewis and Ausubel, 2006; Stavri et al., 2007), which may be useful for increasing the susceptibility to antibiotics of different bacterial species (Groblacher et al., 2012a,b; Holler et al., 2012a; Roy et al., 2012; Zhou et al., 2012).

In addition of inhibitors targeting specifically classical resistance elements, the study of the intrinsic resistome opens the possibility of looking for inhibitors of targets that contribute to resistance despite they are not classical resistance determinants. This is the case of the *P. aeruginosa* cyanide-insensitive terminal oxidase. Mutants defective in this gene are hypersusceptible to antibiotics (Tavankar et al., 2003). Consequently, inhibition of this component of the respiratory chain will increase the overall susceptibility of *P. aeruginosa* to antibiotics. Same situation happens with global regulators as the *P. aeruginosa* Crc post-transcriptional repressor (Morales et al., 2004; Moreno et al., 2009). Mutants defective in this gene are hypersusceptible to different antibiotics (Linares et al., 2010); hence its inhibition will increase susceptibility to these antibiotics.

An interesting approach in the search of inhibitors of resistance is the screening of non-antibiotic compounds, which had been already tested for other diseases, and may be used as helper compounds to improve efficacy of antibiotics (Martins et al., 2008). The benefit of using these compounds is that their use has been already approved, so as novel long and costly toxicological trials are not needed. Among them some anesthetics, antihistaminic, and psychotherapeutic compounds have demonstrated to improve the activity of antibiotics (Kristiansen and Amaral, 1997). Within this group of compounds some of them change the permeability of the bacterial membrane (Martins et al., 2008), as the anti-inflammatory drug diclofenac (Dutta et al., 2007) or the anti-psychotic chlorpromazine (Blair and Piddock, 2009), whereas for others, the mechanism of action is not known.

A more recent approach for improving the activity of the antibiotics is by enhancing the cellular responses associated to the antibiotics induced cell death pathway. It has been proposed that bactericidal antibiotics induce a cell pathway that involves the generation of oxygen reactive species (Kohanski et al., 2007, 2010). Understanding this pathway may reveal targets for adjuvants that improve the efficacy of the antibiotics (Farha and Brown, 2013). By using *Escherichia coli* whole-genome metabolic models and further experimental validation of predicted targets, it has been shown that inactivation of some elements increase susceptibility to oxidants and antibiotics (Brynildsen et al., 2013), which opens the possibility of searching a new family of drugs capable to increase the activity of antibiotics.

ACKNOWLEDGMENTS

Work in our laboratory is supported by grants BIO2011-25255 from the Spanish Ministry of Science and Innovation, PROMPT from CAM, REIPI from the Instituto de Salud Carlos III, and HEALTH-F3-2011-282004 (EVOTAR) and HEALTH-F3-2010-241476 (PAR) from the European Union. Guillermo Garcia-Leon is the recipient of a FPI fellowship, Alejandra Bernardini is the recipient of a "La Caixa" fellowship and Fernando Corona is the recipient of a JAE predoctoral fellowship.

REFERENCES

Adediran, S. A., Lin, G., Pelto, R. B., and Pratt, R. F. (2012). Crossover inhibition as an indicator of convergent evolution of enzyme mechanisms: a β-lactamase and a N-terminal nucleophile hydrolase. *FEBS Lett.* 586, 4186–4189.

Adler, M., Anjum, M., Andersson, D. I., and Sandegren, L. (2013). Influence of acquired beta-lactamases on the evolution of spontaneous carbapenem resistance in *Escherichia coli*. *J. Antimicrob. Chemother.* 68, 51–59.

Al-Hamad, A., Burnie, J., and Upton, M. (2011). Enhancement of antibiotic susceptibility of *Stenotrophomonas maltophilia* using a polyclonal antibody developed against an ABC multidrug efflux pump. *Can. J. Microbiol.* 57, 820–828.

Allen, H. K., Donato, J., Wang, H. H., Cloud-Hansen, K. A., Davies, J., and Handelsman, J. (2010). Call of the wild: antibiotic resistance genes in natural environments. *Nat. Rev. Microbiol.* 8, 251–259.

Allison, K. R., Brynildsen, M. P., and Collins, J. J. (2011). Metabolite-enabled eradication of bacterial persisters by aminoglycosides. *Nature* 473, 216–220.

Alonso, A., and Martinez, J. L. (1997). Multiple antibiotic resistance in *Stenotrophomonas maltophilia*. *Antimicrob. Agents Chemother.* 41, 1140–1142.

Alonso, A., and Martinez, J. L. (2000). Cloning and characterization of SmeDEF, a novel multidrug efflux pump from *Stenotrophomonas maltophilia*. *Antimicrob. Agents Chemother.* 44, 3079–3086.

Alonso, A., and Martinez, J. L. (2001). Expression of multidrug efflux pump SmeDEF by clinical isolates of *Stenotrophomonas maltophilia*. *Antimicrob. Agents Chemother.* 45, 1879–1881.

Alvarez-Ortega, C., Wiegand, I., Olivares, J., Hancock, R. E., and Martinez, J. L. (2010). Genetic determinants involved in the susceptibility of *Pseudomonas aeruginosa* to beta-lactam antibiotics. *Antimicrob. Agents Chemother.* 54, 4159–4167.

Ambler, R. P., Coulson, A. F., Frere, J. M., Ghuysen, J. M., Joris, B., Forsman, M., et al. (1991). A standard numbering scheme for the class A beta-lactamases. *Biochem. J.* 276(Pt 1), 269–270.

Amini, S., Hottes, A. K., Smith, L. E., and Tavazoie, S. (2011). Fitness landscape of antibiotic tolerance in *Pseudomonas aeruginosa* biofilms. *PLoS Pathog.* 7:e1002298. doi: 10.1371/journal.ppat.1002298

Aminov, R. I. (2009). The role of antibiotics and antibiotic resistance in nature. *Environ. Microbiol.* 11, 2970–2988.

Aminov, R. I. (2010). A brief history of the antibiotic era: lessons learned and challenges for the future. *Front. Microbiol.* 1:134. doi: 10.3389/fmicb.2010.00134

Amundsen, S. K., and Smith, G. R. (2003). Interchangeable parts of the *Escherichia coli* recombination machinery. *Cell* 112, 741–744.

Baba, T., Ara, T., Hasegawa, M., Takai, Y., Okumura, Y., Baba, M., et al. (2006). Construction of *Escherichia coli* K-12 in-frame, single-gene knockout mutants: the Keio collection. *Mol. Syst. Biol.* 2, 2006.0008.

Bagg, A., and Neilands, J. B. (1987). Ferric uptake regulation protein acts as a repressor, employing iron (II) as a cofactor to bind the operator of an iron transport operon in *Escherichia coli*. *Biochemistry* 26, 5471–5477.

Balaban, N. Q., Merrin, J., Chait, R., Kowalik, L., and Leibler, S. (2004). Bacterial persistence as a phenotypic switch. *Science* 305, 1622–1625.

Baquero, F., Coque, T. M., and De La Cruz, F. (2011). Eco-evo drugs and strategies: the need for novel tools to fight antibiotic resistance. *Antimicrob. Agents Chemother.* 55, 3649–3660.

Barua, S., Yamashino, T., Hasegawa, T., Yokoyama, K., Torii, K., and Ohta, M. (2002). Involvement of surface polysaccharides in the organic acid resistance of Shiga Toxin-producing *Escherichia coli* O157:H7. *Mol. Microbiol.* 43, 629–640.

Baugh, S., Ekanayaka, A. S., Piddock, L. J., and Webber, M. A. (2012). Loss of or inhibition of all multidrug resistance efflux pumps of *Salmonella enterica* serovar Typhimurium results in impaired ability to form a biofilm. *J. Antimicrob. Chemother.* 67, 2409–2417.

Bhagunde, P., Chang, K. T., Hirsch, E. B., Ledesma, K. R., Nikolaou, M., and Tam, V. H. (2012). Novel modeling framework to guide design of optimal dosing strategies for beta-lactamase inhibitors. *Antimicrob. Agents Chemother.* 56, 2237–2240.

Bigger, J. (1944). Treatment of Staphylococcal infections with penicillin by intermittent sterilisation. *Lancet* 244, 497–500.

Blair, J. M., and Piddock, L. J. (2009). Structure, function, and inhibition of RND efflux pumps in Gram-negative bacteria: an update. *Curr. Opin. Microbiol.* 12, 512–519.

Blazquez, J., Baquero, M. R., Canton, R., Alos, I., and Baquero, F. (1993). Characterization of a new TEM-type beta-lactamase resistant to clavulanate, sulbactam, and tazobactam in a clinical isolate of *Escherichia coli*. *Antimicrob. Agents Chemother.* 37, 2059–2063.

Blower, T. R., Salmond, G. P., and Luisi, B. F. (2011). Balancing at survival's edge: the structure and adaptive benefits of prokaryotic toxin–antitoxin partners. *Curr. Opin. Struct. Biol.* 21, 109–118.

Breidenstein, E. B., Khaira, B. K., Wiegand, I., Overhage, J., and Hancock, R. E. (2008). Complex ciprofloxacin resistome revealed by screening a *Pseudomonas aeruginosa* mutant library for altered susceptibility. *Antimicrob. Agents Chemother.* 52, 4486–4491.

Brynildsen, M. P., Winkler, J. A., Spina, C. S., Macdonald, I. C., and Collins, J. J. (2013). Potentiating antibacterial activity by predictably enhancing endogenous microbial ROS production. *Nat. Biotechnol.* 31, 160–165.

Bush, K. (1988). Beta-lactamase inhibitors from laboratory to clinic. *Clin. Microbiol. Rev.* 1, 109–123.

Buynak, J. D. (2006). Understanding the longevity of the beta-lactam antibiotics and of antibiotic/beta-lactamase inhibitor combinations. *Biochem. Pharmacol.* 71, 930–940.

Buynak, J. D., Chen, H., Vogeti, L., Gadhachanda, V. R., Buchanan, C. A., Palzkill, T., et al. (2004). Penicillin-derived inhibitors that simultaneously target both metallo- and serine-beta-lactamases. *Bioorg. Med. Chem. Lett.* 14, 1299–1304.

Canica, M. M., Caroff, N., Barthelemy, M., Labia, R., Krishnamoorthy, R., Paul, G., et al. (1998). Phenotypic study of resistance of beta-lactamase-inhibitor-resistant TEM enzymes which differ by naturally occurring variations and by site-directed substitution at Asp276. *Antimicrob. Agents Chemother.* 42, 1323–1328.

Chen, P., Horton, L. B., Mikulski, R. L., Deng, L., Sundriyal, S., Palzkill, T., et al. (2012). 2-substituted 4,5-dihydrothiazole-4-carboxylic acids are novel inhibitors of metallo-beta-lactamases. *Bioorg. Med. Chem. Lett.* 22, 6229–6232.

Chollet, R., Chevalier, J., Bryskier, A., and Pages, J. M. (2004). The AcrAB-TolC pump is involved in macrolide resistance but not in telithromycin efflux in *Enterobacter aerogenes* and *Escherichia coli*. *Antimicrob. Agents Chemother.* 48, 3621–3624.

Christensen, S. K., Mikkelsen, M., Pedersen, K., and Gerdes, K. (2001). RelE, a global inhibitor of translation, is activated during nutritional stress. *Proc. Natl. Acad. Sci. U.S.A.* 98, 14328–14333.

Coleman, K. (2011). Diazabicyclooctanes (DBOs): a potent new class of non-beta-lactam beta-lactamase inhibitors. *Curr. Opin. Microbiol.* 14, 550–555.

Correia, F. F., D'Onofrio, A., Rejtar, T., Li, L., Karger, B. L., Makarova, K., et al. (2006). Kinase activity of overexpressed HipA is required for growth arrest and multidrug tolerance in *Escherichia coli*. *J. Bacteriol.* 188, 8360–8367.

Costerton, J. W., Stewart, P. S., and Greenberg, E. P. (1999). Bacterial biofilms: a common cause of persistent infections. *Science* 284, 1318–1322.

Davies, J. (2006). Are antibiotics naturally antibiotics? *J. Ind. Microbiol. Biotechnol.* 33, 496–499.

Davies, J., and Davies, D. (2010). Origins and evolution of antibiotic resistance. *Microbiol. Mol. Biol. Rev.* 74, 417–433.

de Lorenzo, V., and Martinez, J. L. (1988). Aerobactin production as a virulence factor: a reevaluation. *Eur. J. Clin. Microbiol. Infect. Dis.* 7, 621–629.

Dorr, T., Vulic, M., and Lewis, K. (2010). Ciprofloxacin causes persister formation by inducing the TisB toxin in *Escherichia coli*. *PLoS Biol.* 8:e1000317. doi: 10.1371/journal.pbio.1000317

Drawz, S. M., Bethel, C. R., Doppalapudi, V. R., Sheri, A., Pagadala, S. R., Hujer, A. M., et al. (2010). Penicillin sulfone inhibitors of class D beta-lactamases. *Antimicrob. Agents Chemother.* 54, 1414–1424.

Drawz, S. M., and Bonomo, R. A. (2010). Three decades of beta-lactamase inhibitors. *Clin. Microbiol. Rev.* 23, 160–201.

Drlica, K., and Zhao, X. (1997). DNA gyrase, topoisomerase IV, and the 4-quinolones. *Microbiol. Mol. Biol. Rev.* 61, 377–392.

Dubreuil, L. J., Mahieux, S., Neut, C., Miossec, C., and Pace, J. (2012). Anti-anaerobic activity of a new beta-lactamase inhibitor NXL104 in combination with beta-lactams and metronidazole. *Int. J. Antimicrob. Agents* 39, 500–504.

Dutta, N. K., Annadurai, S., Mazumdar, K., Dastidar, S. G., Kristiansen, J. E., Molnar, J., et al. (2007). Potential management of resistant microbial infections with a novel non-antibiotic: the anti-inflammatory drug diclofenac sodium. *Int. J. Antimicrob. Agents* 30, 242–249.

Fajardo, A., Linares, J. F., and Martinez, J. L. (2009). Towards an ecological approach to antibiotics and antibiotic resistance genes. *Clin. Microbiol. Infect.* 15(Suppl. 1), 14–16.

Fajardo, A., and Martinez, J. L. (2008). Antibiotics as signals that trigger specific bacterial responses. *Curr. Opin. Microbiol.* 11, 161–167.

Fajardo, A., Martinez-Martin, N., Mercadillo, M., Galan, J. C., Ghysels, B., Matthijs, S., et al. (2008). The neglected intrinsic resistome of bacterial pathogens. *PLoS ONE* 3:e1619. doi: 10.1371/journal.pone.0001619

Farha, M. A., and Brown, E. D. (2013). Discovery of antibiotic adjuvants. *Nat. Biotechnol.* 31, 120–122.

Faridoon, Hussein, W. M., Vella, P., Islam, N. U., Ollis, D. L., Schenk, G., et al. (2012). 3-mercapto-1,2,4-triazoles and N-acylated thiosemicarbazides as metallo-beta-lactamase inhibitors. *Bioorg. Med. Chem. Lett.* 22, 380–386.

Favero, M. S., Carson, L. A., Bond, W. W., and Petersen, N. J. (1971). *Pseudomonas aeruginosa*: growth in distilled water from hospitals. *Science* 173, 836–838.

Feng, L., Yang, K. W., Zhou, L. S., Xiao, J. M., Yang, X., Zhai, L., et al. (2012). N-heterocyclic dicarboxylic acids: broad-spectrum inhibitors of metallo-beta-lactamases with co-antibacterial effect against antibiotic-resistant bacteria. *Bioorg. Med. Chem. Lett.* 22, 5185–5189.

Fernandez, L., Alvarez-Ortega, C., Wiegand, I., Olivares, J., Kocincova, D., Lam, J. S., et al. (2013). Characterization of the polymyxin B resistome of *Pseudomonas aeruginosa. Antimicrob. Agents Chemother.* 57, 110–119.

Fernandez, L., and Hancock, R. E. (2012). Adaptive and mutational resistance: role of porins and efflux pumps in drug resistance. *Clin. Microbiol. Rev.* 25, 661–681.

Frase, H., Toth, M., Champion, M. M., Antunes, N. T., and Vakulenko, S. B. (2011). Importance of position 170 in the inhibition of GES-type beta-lactamases by clavulanic acid. *Antimicrob. Agents Chemother.* 55, 1556–1562.

Fraser, G. M., and Hughes, C. (1999). Swarming motility. *Curr. Opin. Microbiol.* 2, 630–635.

Ganta, S. R., Perumal, S., Pagadala, S. R., Samuelsen, O., Spencer, J., Pratt, R. F., et al. (2009). Approaches to the simultaneous inactivation of metallo- and serine-beta-lactamases. *Bioorg. Med. Chem. Lett.* 19, 1618–1622.

Garcia-Leon, G., Sanchez, M. B., and Martinez, J. L. (2012). The Inactivation of intrinsic antibiotic resistance determinants widens the mutant selection window for quinolones in *Stenotrophomonas maltophilia. Antimicrob. Agents Chemother.* 56, 6397–6399.

Gardy, J. L., Laird, M. R., Chen, F., Rey, S., Walsh, C. J., Ester, M., et al. (2005). PSORTb v.2.0: expanded prediction of bacterial protein subcellular localization and insights gained from comparative proteome analysis. *Bioinformatics* 21, 617–623.

Gerdes, K., Christensen, S. K., and Lobner-Olesen, A. (2005). Prokaryotic toxin–antitoxin stress response loci. *Nat. Rev. Microbiol.* 3, 371–382.

Gerdes, K., Gultyaev, A. P., Franch, T., Pedersen, K., and Mikkelsen, N. D. (1997). Antisense RNA-regulated programmed cell death. *Annu. Rev. Genet.* 31, 1–31.

Gerdes, K., and Maisonneuve, E. (2012). Bacterial persistence and toxin–antitoxin loci. *Annu. Rev. Microbiol.* 66, 103–123.

Girgis, H. S., Hottes, A. K., and Tavazoie, S. (2009). Genetic architecture of intrinsic antibiotic susceptibility. *PLoS ONE* 4:e5629. doi: 10.1371/journal.pone.0005629

Green, S. K., Schroth, M. N., Cho, J. J., Kominos, S. K., and Vitanza-Jack, V. B. (1974). Agricultural plants and soil as a reservoir for *Pseudomonas aeruginosa. Appl. Microbiol.* 28, 987–991.

Grkovic, S., Brown, M. H., and Skurray, R. A. (2001). Transcriptional regulation of multidrug efflux pumps in bacteria. *Semin. Cell Dev. Biol.* 12, 225–237.

Grkovic, S., Brown, M. H., and Skurray, R. A. (2002). Regulation of bacterial drug export systems. *Microbiol. Mol. Biol. Rev.* 66, 671–701.

Groblacher, B., Kunert, O., and Bucar, F. (2012a). Compounds of *Alpinia katsumadai* as potential efflux inhibitors in *Mycobacterium smegmatis. Bioorg. Med. Chem.* 20, 2701–2706.

Groblacher, B., Maier, V., Kunert, O., and Bucar, F. (2012b). Putative mycobacterial efflux inhibitors from the seeds of *Aframomum melegueta. J. Nat. Prod.* 75, 1393–1399.

Gullberg, E., Cao, S., Berg, O. G., Ilback, C., Sandegren, L., Hughes, D., et al. (2011). Selection of resistant bacteria at very low antibiotic concentrations. *PLoS Pathog.* 7:e1002158. doi: 10.1371/journal.ppat.1002158

Hancock, R. E. (1984). Alterations in outer membrane permeability. *Annu. Rev. Microbiol.* 38, 237–264.

Hansen, S., Lewis, K., and Vulic, M. (2008). Role of global regulators and nucleotide metabolism in antibiotic tolerance in *Escherichia coli. Antimicrob. Agents Chemother.* 52, 2718–2726.

Hernandez, A., Mate, M. J., Sanchez-Diaz, P. C., Romero, A., Rojo, F., and Martinez, J. L. (2009). Structural and functional analysis of SmeT, the repressor of the *Stenotrophomonas maltophilia* multidrug efflux pump SmeDEF. *J. Biol. Chem.* 284, 14428–14438.

Hernandez, A., Ruiz, F. M., Romero, A., and Martinez, J. L. (2011). The binding of triclosan to SmeT, the repressor of the multidrug efflux pump SmeDEF, induces antibiotic resistance in *Stenotrophomonas maltophilia. PLoS Pathog.* 7:e1002103. doi: 10.1371/journal.ppat.1002103

Hirai, K., Aoyama, H., Irikura, T., Iyobe, S., and Mitsuhashi, S. (1986). Differences in susceptibility to quinolones of outer membrane mutants of *Salmonella typhimurium* and *Escherichia coli. Antimicrob. Agents Chemother.* 29, 535–538.

Hirakata, Y., Kondo, A., Hoshino, K., Yano, H., Arai, K., Hirotani, A., et al. (2009). Efflux pump inhibitors reduce the invasiveness of *Pseudomonas aeruginosa. Int. J. Antimicrob. Agents* 34, 343–346.

Hirsch, E. B., Ledesma, K. R., Chang, K. T., Schwartz, M. S., Motyl, M. R., and Tam, V. H. (2012). In vitro activity of MK-7655, a novel beta-lactamase inhibitor, in combination with imipenem against carbapenem-resistant Gram-negative bacteria. *Antimicrob. Agents Chemother.* 56, 3753–3757.

Holler, J. G., Christensen, S. B., Slotved, H. C., Rasmussen, H. B., Guzman, A., Olsen, C. E., et al. (2012a). Novel inhibitory activity of the *Staphylococcus aureus* NorA efflux pump by a kaempferol rhamnoside isolated from *Persea lingue* Nees. *J. Antimicrob. Chemother.* 67, 1138–1144.

Holler, J. G., Slotved, H. C., Molgaard, P., Olsen, C. E., and Christensen, S. B. (2012b). Chalcone inhibitors of the NorA efflux pump in *Staphylococcus aureus* whole cells and enriched everted membrane vesicles. *Bioorg. Med. Chem.* 20, 4514–4521.

Howard, B. M., Pinney, R. J., and Smith, J. T. (1993). Function of the SOS process in repair of DNA damage induced by modern 4-quinolones. *J. Pharm. Pharmacol.* 45, 658–662.

Hu, Y., and Coates, A. R. (2005). Transposon mutagenesis identifies genes which control antimicrobial drug tolerance in stationary-phase *Escherichia coli. FEMS Microbiol. Lett.* 243, 117–124.

Huang, C. T., Yu, F. P., Mcfeters, G. A., and Stewart, P. S. (1995). Nonuniform spatial patterns of respiratory activity within biofilms during disinfection. *Appl. Environ. Microbiol.* 61, 2252–2256.

Hussein, W. M., Fatahala, S. S., Mohamed, Z. M., Mcgeary, R. P., Schenk, G., Ollis, D. L., et al. (2012). Synthesis and kinetic testing of tetrahydropyrimidine-2-thione and pyrrole derivatives as inhibitors of the metallo-beta-lactamase from *Klebsiella pneumonia* and *Pseudomonas aeruginosa. Chem. Biol. Drug Des.* 80, 500–515.

Jacobs, C., Huang, L. J., Bartowsky, E., Normark, S., and Park, J. T. (1994). Bacterial cell wall recycling provides cytosolic muropeptides as effectors for beta-lactamase induction. *EMBO J.* 13, 4684–4694.

Jacoby, G. A. (2009). AmpC beta-lactamases. *Clin. Microbiol. Rev.* 22, 161–182.

Kiener, P. A., and Waley, S. G. (1978). Reversible inhibitors of penicillinases. *Biochem. J.* 169, 197–204.

Kim, W., Killam, T., Sood, V., and Surette, M. G. (2003). Swarm-cell differentiation in *Salmonella enterica* serovar typhimurium results in elevated resistance to multiple antibiotics. *J. Bacteriol.* 185, 3111–3117.

Kim, W., and Surette, M. G. (2004). Metabolic differentiation in actively swarming *Salmonella. Mol. Microbiol.* 54, 702–714.

Kim, Y., and Wood, T. K. (2010). Toxins Hha and CspD and small RNA regulator Hfq are involved in persister cell formation through MqsR in *Escherichia coli*. *Biochem. Biophys. Res. Commun.* 391, 209–213.

Kindrachuk, K. N., Fernandez, L., Bains, M., and Hancock, R. E. (2011). Involvement of an ATP-dependent protease, PA0779/AsrA, in inducing heat shock in response to tobramycin in *Pseudomonas aeruginosa*. *Antimicrob. Agents Chemother.* 55, 1874–1882.

Kobayashi, N., Nishino, K., and Yamaguchi, A. (2001). Novel macrolide-specific ABC-type efflux transporter in *Escherichia coli*. *J. Bacteriol.* 183, 5639–5644.

Kohanski, M. A., Dwyer, D. J., and Collins, J. J. (2010). How antibiotics kill bacteria: from targets to networks. *Nat. Rev. Microbiol.* 8, 423–435.

Kohanski, M. A., Dwyer, D. J., Hayete, B., Lawrence, C. A., and Collins, J. J. (2007). A common mechanism of cellular death induced by bactericidal antibiotics. *Cell* 130, 797–810.

Kohanski, M. A., Dwyer, D. J., Wierzbowski, J., Cottarel, G., and Collins, J. J. (2008). Mistranslation of membrane proteins and two-component system activation trigger antibiotic-mediated cell death. *Cell* 135, 679–690.

Kohler, T., Michea-Hamzehpour, M., Henze, U., Gotoh, N., Curty, L. K., and Pechere, J. C. (1997). Characterization of MexE-MexF-OprN, a positively regulated multidrug efflux system of *Pseudomonas aeruginosa*. *Mol. Microbiol.* 23, 345–354.

Kristiansen, J. E., and Amaral, L. (1997). The potential management of resistant infections with non-antibiotics. *J. Antimicrob. Chemother.* 40, 319–327.

Lai, S., Tremblay, J., and Deziel, E. (2009). Swarming motility: a multicellular behaviour conferring antimicrobial resistance. *Environ. Microbiol.* 11, 126–136.

Levasseur, P., Girard, A.-M., Claudon, M., Goossens, H., Black, M. T., Coleman, K., et al. (2012). In vitro antibacterial activity of the ceftazidime–avibactam (NXL104) combination against *Pseudomonas aeruginosa* clinical isolates. *Antimicrob. Agents Chemother.* 56, 1606–1608.

Levin, B. R. (2004). Microbiology. Non-inherited resistance to antibiotics. *Science* 305, 1578–1579.

Levin, B. R., and Rozen, D. E. (2006). Non-inherited antibiotic resistance. *Nat. Rev. Microbiol.* 4, 556–562.

Levin, M. A., and Cabelli, V. J. (1972). Membrane filter technique for enumeration of *Pseudomonas aeruginosa*. *Appl. Microbiol.* 24, 864–870.

Lewenza, S., Gardy, J. L., Brinkman, F. S., and Hancock, R. E. (2005). Genome-wide identification of *Pseudomonas aeruginosa* exported proteins using a consensus computational strategy combined with a laboratory-based PhoA fusion screen. *Genome Res.* 15, 321–329.

Lewis, K. (2010). Persister cells. *Annu. Rev. Microbiol.* 64, 357–372.

Lewis, K., and Ausubel, F. M. (2006). Prospects for plant-derived antibacterials. *Nat. Biotechnol.* 24, 1504–1507.

Li, M., Conklin, B. C., Taracila, M. A., Hutton, R. A., and Skalweit, M. J. (2012). Substitutions at position 105 in SHV family beta-lactamases decrease catalytic efficiency and cause inhibitor resistance. *Antimicrob. Agents Chemother.* 56, 5678–5686.

Li, X. Z., Livermore, D. M., and Nikaido, H. (1994). Role of efflux pump(s) in intrinsic resistance of *Pseudomonas aeruginosa*: resistance to tetracycline, chloramphenicol, and norfloxacin. *Antimicrob. Agents Chemother.* 38, 1732–1741.

Li, Y., and Zhang, Y. (2007). PhoU is a persistence switch involved in persister formation and tolerance to multiple antibiotics and stresses in *Escherichia coli*. *Antimicrob. Agents Chemother.* 51, 2092–2099.

Liberati, N. T., Urbach, J. M., Miyata, S., Lee, D. G., Drenkard, E., Wu, G., et al. (2006). An ordered, nonredundant library of *Pseudomonas aeruginosa* strain PA14 transposon insertion mutants. *Proc. Natl. Acad. Sci. U.S.A.* 103, 2833–2838.

Linares, J. F., Gustafsson, I., Baquero, F., and Martinez, J. L. (2006). Antibiotics as intermicrobial signaling agents instead of weapons. *Proc. Natl. Acad. Sci. U.S.A.* 103, 19484–19489.

Linares, J. F., Moreno, R., Fajardo, A., Martinez-Solano, L., Escalante, R., Rojo, F., et al. (2010). The global regulator Crc modulates metabolism, susceptibility to antibiotics and virulence in *Pseudomonas aeruginosa*. *Environ. Microbiol.* 12, 3196–3212.

Lindberg, F., and Normark, S. (1986). Contribution of chromosomal beta-lactamases to beta-lactam resistance in enterobacteria. *Rev. Infect. Dis.* 8(Suppl. 3), S292–S304.

Lister, P. D., Wolter, D. J., and Hanson, N. D. (2009). Antibacterial-resistant *Pseudomonas aeruginosa*: clinical impact and complex regulation of chromosomally encoded resistance mechanisms. *Clin. Microbiol. Rev.* 22, 582–610.

Liu, A., Tran, L., Becket, E., Lee, K., Chinn, L., Park, E., et al. (2010). Antibiotic sensitivity profiles determined with an *Escherichia coli* gene knockout collection: generating an antibiotic bar code. *Antimicrob. Agents Chemother.* 54, 1393–1403.

Livermore, D. M., Mushtaq, S., and Warner, M. (2010). Activity of BAL30376 (monobactam BAL19764 + BAL29880 + clavulanate) versus Gram-negative bacteria with characterized resistance mechanisms. *J. Antimicrob. Chemother.* 65, 2382–2395.

Lomovskaya, O., and Bostian, K. A. (2006). Practical applications and feasibility of efflux pump inhibitors in the clinic – a vision for applied use. *Biochem. Pharmacol.* 71, 910–918.

Lomovskaya, O., Lee, A., Hoshino, K., Ishida, H., Mistry, A., Warren, M. S., et al. (1999). Use of a genetic approach to evaluate the consequences of inhibition of efflux pumps in *Pseudomonas aeruginosa*. *Antimicrob. Agents Chemother.* 43, 1340–1346.

Lomovskaya, O., Lewis, K., and Matin, A. (1995). EmrR is a negative regulator of the *Escherichia coli* multidrug resistance pump EmrAB. *J. Bacteriol.* 177, 2328–2334.

Lomovskaya, O., Warren, M. S., Lee, A., Galazzo, J., Fronko, R., Lee, M., et al. (2001). Identification and characterization of inhibitors of multidrug resistance efflux pumps in *Pseudomonas aeruginosa*: novel agents for combination therapy. *Antimicrob. Agents Chemother.* 45, 105–116.

Lomovskaya, O., and Watkins, W. (2001). Inhibition of efflux pumps as a novel approach to combat drug resistance in bacteria. *J. Mol. Microbiol. Biotechnol.* 3, 225–236.

Lubelski, J., Konings, W. N., and Driessen, A. J. (2007). Distribution and physiology of ABC-type transporters contributing to multidrug resistance in bacteria. *Microbiol. Mol. Biol. Rev.* 71, 463–476.

Lucasti, C., Popescu, I., Ramesh, M. K., Lipka, J., and Sable, C. (2013). Comparative study of the efficacy and safety of ceftazidime/avibactam plus metronidazole versus meropenem in the treatment of complicated intra-abdominal infections in hospitalized adults: results of a randomized, double-blind, Phase II trial. *J. Antimicrob. Chemother.* 68, 1183–1192.

Ma, D., Cook, D. N., Alberti, M., Pon, N. G., Nikaido, H., and Hearst, J. E. (1993). Molecular cloning and characterization of acrA and acrE genes of *Escherichia coli*. *J. Bacteriol.* 175, 6299–6313.

Ma, D., Cook, D. N., Alberti, M., Pon, N. G., Nikaido, H., and Hearst, J. E. (1995). Genes acrA and acrB encode a stress-induced efflux system of *Escherichia coli*. *Mol. Microbiol.* 16, 45–55.

MacGregor, C. H., Wolff, J. A., Arora, S. K., and Phibbs, P. V. Jr. (1991). Cloning of a catabolite repression control (crc) gene from *Pseudomonas aeruginosa*, expression of the gene in *Escherichia coli*, and identification of the gene product in *Pseudomonas aeruginosa*. *J. Bacteriol.* 173, 7204–7212.

Mah, T. F., and O'Toole, G. A. (2001). Mechanisms of biofilm resistance to antimicrobial agents. *Trends Microbiol.* 9, 34–39.

Mahamoud, A., Chevalier, J., Davin-Regli, A., Barbe, J., and Pages, J. M. (2006). Quinoline derivatives as promising inhibitors of antibiotic efflux pump in multidrug resistant *Enterobacter aerogenes* isolates. *Curr. Drug Targets* 7, 843–847.

Maisonneuve, E., Shakespeare, L. J., Jorgensen, M. G., and Gerdes, K. (2011). Bacterial persistence by RNA endonucleases. *Proc. Natl. Acad. Sci. U.S.A.* 108, 13206–13211.

Markham, P. N., Westhaus, E., Klyachko, K., Johnson, M. E., and Neyfakh, A. A. (1999). Multiple novel inhibitors of the NorA multidrug transporter of *Staphylococcus aureus*. *Antimicrob. Agents Chemother.* 43, 2404–2408.

Marr, A. K., Overhage, J., Bains, M., and Hancock, R. E. (2007). The Lon protease of *Pseudomonas aeruginosa* is induced by aminoglycosides and is involved in biofilm formation and motility. *Microbiology* 153, 474–482.

Martinez, J. L. (2008). Antibiotics and antibiotic resistance genes in natural environments. *Science* 321, 365–367.

Martinez, J. L. (2012). The antibiotic resistome: challenge and opportunity for therapeutic intervention. *Future Med. Chem.* 4, 347–359.

Martinez, J. L., and Baquero, F. (2000). Mutation frequencies and antibiotic resistance. *Antimicrob. Agents Chemother.* 44, 1771–1777.

Martinez, J. L., and Baquero, F. (2002). Interactions among strategies associated with bacterial infection: pathogenicity, epidemicity, and antibiotic resistance. *Clin. Microbiol. Rev.* 15, 647–679.

Martinez, J. L., Baquero, F., and Andersson, D. I. (2007). Predicting antibiotic resistance. *Nat. Rev. Microbiol.* 5, 958–965.

Martinez, J. L., Baquero, F., and Andersson, D. I. (2011a). Beyond serial passages: new methods for predicting the emergence of resistance to novel antibiotics. *Curr. Opin. Pharmacol.* 11, 439–445.

Martinez, J. L., Rojo, F., and Vila, J. (2011b). Are nonlethal targets useful for developing novel antimicrobials? *Future Microbiol.* 6, 605–607.

Martinez, J. L., Blazquez, J., and Baquero, F. (1994). Non-canonical mechanisms of antibiotic resistance. *Eur. J. Clin. Microbiol. Infect. Dis.* 13, 1015–1022.

Martinez, J. L., Cercenado, E., Rodriguez-Creixems, M., Vincente-Perez, M. F., Delgado-Iribarren, A., and Baquero, F. (1987). Resistance to beta-lactam/clavulanate. *Lancet* 2, 1473.

Martinez, J. L., Delgado-Iribarren, A., and Baquero, F. (1990). Mechanisms of iron acquisition and bacterial virulence. *FEMS Microbiol. Rev.* 6, 45–56.

Martinez, J. L., Fajardo, A., Garmendia, L., Hernandez, A., Linares, J. F., Martinez-Solano, L., et al. (2009a). A global view of antibiotic resistance. *FEMS Microbiol. Rev.* 33, 44–65.

Martinez, J. L., Sanchez, M. B., Martinez-Solano, L., Hernandez, A., Garmendia, L., Fajardo, A., et al. (2009b). Functional role of bacterial multidrug efflux pumps in microbial natural ecosystems. *FEMS Microbiol. Rev.* 33, 430–449.

Martinez, J. L., and Rojo, F. (2011). Metabolic regulation of antibiotic resistance. *FEMS Microbiol. Rev.* 35, 768–789.

Martinez, J. L., Vicente, M. F., Delgado-Iribarren, A., Perez-Diaz, J. C., and Baquero, F. (1989). Small plasmids are involved in amoxicillin-clavulanate resistance in *Escherichia coli. Antimicrob. Agents Chemother.* 33, 595.

Martins, M., Dastidar, S. G., Fanning, S., Kristiansen, J. E., Molnar, J., Pages, J. M., et al. (2008). Potential role of non-antibiotics (helper compounds) in the treatment of multidrug-resistant Gram-negative infections: mechanisms for their direct and indirect activities. *Int. J. Antimicrob. Agents* 31, 198–208.

Matilla, M. A., Espinosa-Urgel, M., Rodriguez-Herva, J. J., Ramos, J. L., and Ramos-Gonzalez, M. I. (2007). Genomic analysis reveals the major driving forces of bacterial life in the rhizosphere. *Genome Biol.* 8, R179.

Meddows, T. R., Savory, A. P., Grove, J. I., Moore, T., and Lloyd, R. G. (2005). RecN protein and transcription factor DksA combine to promote faithful recombinational repair of DNA double-strand breaks. *Mol. Microbiol.* 57, 97–110.

Morales, E., Cots, F., Sala, M., Comas, M., Belvis, F., Riu, M., et al. (2012). Hospital costs of nosocomial multi-drug resistant *Pseudomonas aeruginosa* acquisition. *BMC Health Serv. Res.* 12:122. doi: 10.1186/1472-6963-12-122

Morales, G., Linares, J. F., Beloso, A., Albar, J. P., Martinez, J. L., and Rojo, F. (2004). The *Pseudomonas putida* Crc global regulator controls the expression of genes from several chromosomal catabolic pathways for aromatic compounds. *J. Bacteriol.* 186, 1337–1344.

Moreno, R., Marzi, S., Romby, P., and Rojo, F. (2009). The Crc global regulator binds to an unpaired A-rich motif at the *Pseudomonas putida* alkS mRNA coding sequence and inhibits translation initiation. *Nucleic Acids Res.* 37, 7678–7690.

Moyed, H. S., and Bertrand, K. P. (1983). hipA, a newly recognized gene of *Escherichia coli* K-12 that affects frequency of persistence after inhibition of murein synthesis. *J. Bacteriol.* 155, 768–775.

Mulcahy, H., Charron-Mazenod, L., and Lewenza, S. (2008). Extracellular DNA chelates cations and induces antibiotic resistance in *Pseudomonas aeruginosa* biofilms. *PLoS Pathog.* 4:e1000213. doi: 10.1371/journal.ppat.1000213

Musumeci, R., Speciale, A., Costanzo, R., Annino, A., Ragusa, S., Rapisarda, A., et al. (2003). *Berberis aetnensis* C. Presl. extracts: antimicrobial properties and interaction with ciprofloxacin. *Int. J. Antimicrob. Agents* 22, 48–53.

Nakayama, K., Kawato, H., Watanabe, J., Ohtsuka, M., Yoshida, K., Yokomizo, Y., et al. (2004a). MexAB-OprM specific efflux pump inhibitors in *Pseudomonas aeruginosa*. Part 3: optimization of potency in the pyridopyrimidine series through the application of a pharmacophore model. *Bioorg. Med. Chem. Lett.* 14, 475–479.

Nakayama, K., Kuru, N., Ohtsuka, M., Yokomizo, Y., Sakamoto, A., Kawato, H., et al. (2004b). MexAB-OprM specific efflux pump inhibitors in *Pseudomonas aeruginosa*. Part 4: addressing the problem of poor stability due to photoisomerization of an acrylic acid moiety. *Bioorg. Med. Chem. Lett.* 14, 2493–2497.

Nelson, M. L., and Levy, S. B. (1999). Reversal of tetracycline resistance mediated by different bacterial tetracycline resistance determinants by an inhibitor of the Tet(B) antiport protein. *Antimicrob. Agents Chemother.* 43, 1719–1724.

Nikaido, H. (1989). Outer membrane barrier as a mechanism of antimicrobial resistance. *Antimicrob. Agents Chemother.* 33, 1831–1836.

Nikaido, H. (1994). Prevention of drug access to bacterial targets: permeability barriers and active efflux. *Science* 264, 382–388.

Nikaido, H. (1998a). Antibiotic resistance caused by gram-negative multidrug efflux pumps. *Clin. Infect. Dis* 27(Suppl. 1), S32–S41.

Nikaido, H. (1998b). Multiple antibiotic resistance and efflux. *Curr. Opin. Microbiol.* 1, 516–523.

Nikaido, H. (2009). Multidrug resistance in bacteria. *Annu. Rev. Biochem.* 78, 119–146.

Nishino, K., and Yamaguchi, A. (2001). Analysis of a complete library of putative drug transporter genes in *Escherichia coli. J. Bacteriol.* 183, 5803–5812.

Overhage, J., Bains, M., Brazas, M. D., and Hancock, R. E. (2008a). Swarming of *Pseudomonas aeruginosa* is a complex adaptation leading to increased production of virulence factors and antibiotic resistance. *J. Bacteriol.* 190, 2671–2679.

Overhage, J., Bains, M., Brazas, M. D., and Hancock, R. E. W. (2008b). Swarming of *Pseudomonas aeruginosa* is a complex adaptation leading to increased production of virulence factors and antibiotic resistance . *J. Bacteriol.* 190, 2671–2679.

Page, M. G., Dantier, C., Desarbre, E., Gaucher, B., Gebhardt, K., and Schmitt-Hoffmann, A. (2011). In vitro and in vivo properties of BAL30376, a beta-lactam and dual beta-lactamase inhibitor combination with enhanced activity against Gram-negative bacilli that express multiple beta-lactamases. *Antimicrob. Agents Chemother.* 55, 1510–1519.

Page, M. I., Hinchliffe, P. S., Wood, J. M., Harding, L. P., and Laws, A. P. (2003). Novel mechanism of inhibiting beta-lactamases by sulfonylation using beta-sultams. *Bioorg. Med. Chem. Lett.* 13, 4489–4492.

Pandey, D. P., and Gerdes, K. (2005). Toxin-antitoxin loci are highly abundant in free-living but lost from host-associated prokaryotes. *Nucleic Acids Res.* 33, 966–976.

Pannek, S., Higgins, P. G., Steinke, P., Jonas, D., Akova, M., Bohnert, J. A., et al. (2006). Multidrug efflux inhibition in *Acinetobacter baumannii*: comparison between 1-(1-naphthylmethyl)-piperazine and phenyl-arginine-beta-naphthylamide. *J. Antimicrob. Chemother.* 57, 970–974.

Pattanaik, P., Bethel, C., Hujer, A. M., Hujer, K. M., Distler, A. M., Taracila, M., et al. (2009). Strategic design of an effective beta-lactamase inhibitor: LN-1-255, a 6-alkylidene-2′-substituted penicillin sulfone. *J. Biol. Chem.* 284, 945–953.

Pedersen, K., Christensen, S. K., and Gerdes, K. (2002). Rapid induction and reversal of a bacteriostatic condition by controlled expression of toxins and antitoxins. *Mol. Microbiol.* 45, 501–510.

Pelto, R. B., and Pratt, R. F. (2008). Kinetics and mechanism of inhibition of a serine beta-lactamase by O-aryloxycarbonyl hydroxamates. *Biochemistry* 47, 12037–12046.

Petersen, A. D., Walker, R. D., Bowman, M. M., Schott, H. C. II, and Rosser, E. J. Jr. (2002). Frequency of isolation and antimicrobial susceptibility patterns of *Staphylococcus intermedius* and *Pseudomonas aeruginosa* isolates from canine skin and ear samples over a 6-year period (1992-1997). *J. Am. Anim. Hosp. Assoc.* 38, 407–413.

Piddock, L. J. (2006). Clinically relevant chromosomally encoded multidrug resistance efflux pumps in bacteria. *Clin. Microbiol. Rev.* 19, 382–402.

Poole, K. (2007). Efflux pumps as antimicrobial resistance mechanisms. *Ann. Med.* 39, 162–176.

Poole, K., Krebes, K., Mcnally, C., and Neshat, S. (1993). Multiple antibiotic resistance in *Pseudomonas aeruginosa*: evidence for involvement of an efflux operon. *J. Bacteriol.* 175, 7363–7372.

Poon, K. K., Westman, E. L., Vinogradov, E., Jin, S., and Lam, J. S. (2008). Functional characterization of MigA and WapR: putative rhamnosyltransferases involved in outer core oligosaccharide biosynthesis of *Pseudomonas aeruginosa. J. Bacteriol.* 190, 1857–1865.

Rani, S. A., Pitts, B., Beyenal, H., Veluchamy, R. A., Lewandowski, Z., Davison, W. M., et al. (2007). Spatial patterns of DNA replication, protein synthesis, and oxygen concentration within bacterial biofilms reveal diverse physiological states. *J. Bacteriol.* 189, 4223–4233.

Reading, C., and Cole, M. (1977). Clavulanic acid: a beta-lactamase-inhiting beta-lactam from *Streptomyces clavuligerus. Antimicrob. Agents Chemother.* 11, 852–857.

Records, A. R. (2011). The type VI secretion system: a multipurpose delivery system with a phage-like machinery.

Mol. Plant Microbe Interact. 24, 751–757.

Reguera, J. A., Baquero, F., Perez-Diaz, J. C., and Martinez, J. L. (1991). Factors determining resistance to beta-lactam combined with beta-lactamase inhibitors in *Escherichia coli. J. Antimicrob. Chemother.* 27, 569–575.

Renau, T. E., Leger, R., Flamme, E. M., Sangalang, J., She, M. W., Yen, R., et al. (1999). Inhibitors of efflux pumps in *Pseudomonas aeruginosa* potentiate the activity of the fluoroquinolone antibacterial levofloxacin. *J. Med. Chem.* 42, 4928–4931.

Rosenberg, E. Y., Bertenthal, D., Nilles, M. L., Bertrand, K. P., and Nikaido, H. (2003). Bile salts and fatty acids induce the expression of *Escherichia coli* AcrAB multidrug efflux pump through their interaction with Rob regulatory protein. *Mol. Microbiol.* 48, 1609–1619.

Roy, S. K., Pahwa, S., Nandanwar, H., and Jachak, S. M. (2012). Phenylpropanoids of *Alpinia galanga* as efflux pump inhibitors in *Mycobacterium smegmatis* mc(2) 155. *Fitoterapia* 83, 1248–1255.

Sabatini, S., Gosetto, F., Serritella, S., Manfroni, G., Tabarrini, O., Iraci, N., et al. (2012). Pyrazolo[4,3-c][1,2]benzothiazines 5,5-dioxide: a promising new class of *Staphylococcus aureus* NorA efflux pump inhibitors. *J. Med. Chem.* 55, 3568–3572.

Saier, M. H. Jr., Paulsen, I. T., Sliwinski, M. K., Pao, S. S., Skurray, R. A., and Nikaido, H. (1998). Evolutionary origins of multidrug and drug-specific efflux pumps in bacteria. *FASEB J.* 12, 265–274.

Salverda, M. L., De Visser, J. A., and Barlow, M. (2010). Natural evolution of TEM-1 β-lactamase: experimental reconstruction and clinical relevance. *FEMS Microbiol. Rev.* 6, 1015–1036.

Sanchez, P., Le, U., and Martinez, J. L. (2003). The efflux pump inhibitor Phe-Arg-beta-naphthylamide does not abolish the activity of the *Stenotrophomonas maltophilia* SmeDEF multidrug efflux pump. *J. Antimicrob. Chemother.* 51, 1042–1045.

Schurek, K. N., Marr, A. K., Taylor, P. K., Wiegand, I., Semenec, L., Khaira, B. K., et al. (2008). Novel genetic determinants of low-level aminoglycoside resistance in *Pseudomonas aeruginosa. Antimicrob. Agents Chemother.* 52, 4213–4219.

Sengupta, S., Chattopadhyay, M. K., and Grossart, H. P. (2013). The multifaceted roles of antibiotics and antibiotic resistance in nature. *Front. Microbiol.* 4:47. doi: 10.3389/fmicb.2013.00047

Shcherbakov, D., Akbergenov, R., Matt, T., Sander, P., Andersson, D. I., and Bottger, E. C. (2010). Directed mutagenesis of *Mycobacterium smegmatis* 16S rRNA to reconstruct the in-vivo evolution of aminoglycoside resistance in *Mycobacterium tuberculosis. Mol. Microbiol.* 77, 830–840.

Singh, R., Ray, P., Das, A., and Sharma, M. (2010). Penetration of antibiotics through *Staphylococcus aureus* and *Staphylococcus epidermidis* biofilms. *J. Antimicrob. Chemother.* 65, 1955–1958.

Soo, V. W., Hanson-Manful, P., and Patrick, W. M. (2011). Artificial gene amplification reveals an abundance of promiscuous resistance determinants in *Escherichia coli. Proc. Natl. Acad. Sci. U.S.A.* 108, 1484–1489.

Spindler, E. C., Boyle, N. R., Hancock, R. E., and Gill, R. T. (2013). Genome-wide identification of genes conferring energy related resistance to a synthetic antimicrobial Peptide (bac8c). *PLoS ONE* 8:e55052. doi: 10.1371/journal.pone.0055052

Stavri, M., Piddock, L. J., and Gibbons, S. (2007). Bacterial efflux pump inhibitors from natural sources. *J. Antimicrob. Chemother.* 59, 1247–1260.

Sternberg, C., Christensen, B. B., Johansen, T., Toftgaard Nielsen, A., Andersen, J. B., Givskov, M., et al. (1999). Distribution of bacterial growth activity in flow-chamber biofilms. *Appl. Environ. Microbiol.* 65, 4108–4117.

Stewart, P. S., Davison, W. M., and Steenbergen, J. N. (2009). Daptomycin rapidly penetrates a *Staphylococcus epidermidis* biofilm. *Antimicrob. Agents Chemother.* 53, 3505–3507.

Stover, C. K., Pham, X. Q., Erwin, A. L., Mizoguchi, S. D., Warrener, P., Hickey, M. J., et al. (2000). Complete genome sequence of *Pseudomonas aeruginosa* PAO1, an opportunistic pathogen. *Nature* 406, 959–964.

Sugawara, E., and Nikaido, H. (1992). Pore-forming activity of OmpA protein of *Escherichia coli. J. Biol. Chem.* 267, 2507–2511.

Sulavik, M. C., Houseweart, C., Cramer, C., Jiwani, N., Murgolo, N., Greene, J., et al. (2001). Antibiotic susceptibility profiles of *Escherichia coli* strains lacking multidrug efflux pump genes. *Antimicrob. Agents Chemother.* 45, 1126–1136.

Tamae, C., Liu, A., Kim, K., Sitz, D., Hong, J., Becket, E., et al. (2008). Determination of antibiotic hypersensitivity among 4,000 single-gene-knockout mutants of *Escherichia coli. J. Bacteriol.* 190, 5981–5988.

Tan, Q., Ogawa, A. M., Painter, R. E., Park, Y. W., Young, K., and Dininno, F. P. (2010). 4,7-Dichloro benzothien-2-yl sulfonylaminomethyl boronic acid: first boronic acid-derived beta-lactamase inhibitor with class A, C, and D activity. *Bioorg. Med. Chem. Lett.* 20, 2622–2624.

Tavankar, G. R., Mossialos, D., and Williams, H. D. (2003). Mutation or overexpression of a terminal oxidase leads to a cell division defect and multiple antibiotic sensitivity in *Pseudomonas aeruginosa. J. Biol. Chem.* 278, 4524–4530.

Tegos, G., Stermitz, F. R., Lomovskaya, O., and Lewis, K. (2002). Multidrug pump inhibitors uncover remarkable activity of plant antimicrobials. *Antimicrob. Agents Chemother.* 46, 3133–3141.

Thanassi, D. G., Cheng, L. W., and Nikaido, H. (1997). Active efflux of bile salts by *Escherichia coli. J. Bacteriol.* 179, 2512–2518.

Toprak, E., Veres, A., Michel, J. B., Chait, R., Hartl, D. L., and Kishony, R. (2012). Evolutionary paths to antibiotic resistance under dynamically sustained drug selection. *Nat. Genet.* 44, 101–105.

Tsuey-Ching, Y., Hecht, D., Tsai, J. J., and Hu, R. M. (2012). Cefoxitin is both an inhibitor of class A beta-lactamase of *Xanthomonas campestris* pv. *campestris str.* 17 and an inducer of its gene. *Res. Microbiol.* 163, 550–556.

Turnidge, J., Kahlmeter, G., and Kronvall, G. (2006). Statistical characterisation of bacterial wild-type MIC value distributions and the determination of epidemiological cut-off values. *Clin. Microbiol. Infect* 12, 418–425.

Vila, J., and Martinez, J. L. (2008). Clinical impact of the over-expression of efflux pump in nonfermentative gram-negative bacilli, development of efflux pump inhibitors. *Curr. Drug Targets* 9, 797–807.

von Rechenberg, M., Ursinus, A., and Holtje, J. V. (1996). Affinity chromatography as a means to study multienzyme complexes involved in murein synthesis. *Microb. Drug Resist.* 2, 155–157.

Wachino, J. I., Yamaguchi, Y., Mori, S., Kurosaki, H., Arakawa, Y., and Shibayama, K. (2012). Structural insights into the subclass B3 metallo-beta-lactamase, SMB-1, and the mode of inhibition by the common metallo-beta-lactamase inhibitor, mercaptoacetate. *Antimicrob. Agents Chemother.* 57, 101–109.

Walker, T. S., Bais, H. P., Deziel, E., Schweizer, H. P., Rahme, L. G., Fall, R., et al. (2004). *Pseudomonas aeruginosa*-plant root interactions. Pathogenicity, biofilm formation, and root exudation. *Plant Physiol.* 134, 320–331.

Walsh, C. (2000). Molecular mechanisms that confer antibacterial drug resistance. *Nature* 406, 775–781.

Walters, M. C. III, Roe, F., Bugnicourt, A., Franklin, M. J., and Stewart, P. S. (2003). Contributions of antibiotic penetration, oxygen limitation, and low metabolic activity to tolerance of *Pseudomonas aeruginosa* biofilms to ciprofloxacin and tobramycin. *Antimicrob. Agents Chemother.* 47, 317–323.

Wang, L., Zhang, C., Gong, F., Li, H., Xie, X., Xia, C., et al. (2013). Influence of *Pseudomonas aeruginosa* pvdQ gene on altering antibiotic susceptibility under swarming conditions. *Curr. Microbiol.* 66, 152–161.

Watanabe, T. (1963). Infective heredity of multiple drug resistance in bacteria. *Bacteriol. Rev.* 27, 87–115.

Watkins, W. J., Landaverry, Y., Leger, R., Litman, R., Renau, T. E., Williams, N., et al. (2003). The relationship between physicochemical properties, in vitro activity and pharmacokinetic profiles of analogues of diamine-containing efflux pump inhibitors. *Bioorg. Med. Chem. Lett.* 13, 4241–4244.

Webber, M. A., and Piddock, L. J. (2003). The importance of efflux pumps in bacterial antibiotic resistance. *J. Antimicrob. Chemother.* 51, 9–11.

Wolfson, J. S., Hooper, D. C., Mchugh, G. L., Bozza, M. A., and Swartz, M. N. (1990). Mutants of *Escherichia coli* K-12 exhibiting reduced killing by both quinolone and beta-lactam antimicrobial agents. *Antimicrob. Agents Chemother.* 34, 1938–1943.

Woodford, N., Turton, J. F., and Livermore, D. M. (2011). Multiresistant Gram-negative bacteria: the role of high-risk clones in the dissemination of antibiotic resistance. *FEMS Microbiol. Rev.* 35, 736–755.

Wright, G. D. (2010). The antibiotic resistome. *Expert Opin. Drug Discov.* 5, 779–788.

Wu, Y., Vulic, M., Keren, I., and Lewis, K. (2012). Role of oxidative stress in persister tolerance. *Antimicrob. Agents Chemother.* 56, 4922–4926.

Xu, H., Hazra, S., and Blanchard, J. S. (2012). NXL104 irreversibly inhibits the beta-lactamase from *Mycobacterium tuberculosis*. *Biochemistry* 51, 4551–4557.

Yim, G., Wang, H. H., and Davies, J. (2006). The truth about antibiotics. *Int. J. Med. Microbiol.* 296, 163–170.

Yim, G., Wang, H. H., and Davies, J. (2007). Antibiotics as signalling molecules. *Philos. Trans. R. Soc. B Biol. Sci.* 362, 1195–1200.

Yoshida, K., Nakayama, K., Kuru, N., Kobayashi, S., Ohtsuka, M., Takemura, M., et al. (2006a). MexAB-OprM specific efflux pump inhibitors in *Pseudomonas aeruginosa*. Part 5: carbon-substituted analogues at the C-2 position. *Bioorg. Med. Chem.* 14, 1993–2004.

Yoshida, K., Nakayama, K., Yokomizo, Y., Ohtsuka, M., Takemura, M., Hoshino, K., et al. (2006b). MexAB-OprM specific efflux pump inhibitors in *Pseudomonas aeruginosa*. Part 6: exploration of aromatic substituents. *Bioorg. Med. Chem.* 14, 8506–8518.

Yoshida, K., Nakayama, K., Ohtsuka, M., Kuru, N., Yokomizo, Y., Sakamoto, A., et al. (2007). MexAB-OprM specific efflux pump inhibitors in *Pseudomonas aeruginosa*. Part 7: highly soluble and in vivo active quaternary ammonium analogue D13-9001, a potential preclinical candidate. *Bioorg. Med. Chem.* 15, 7087–7097.

Yuan, J., Chow, D. C., Huang, W., and Palzkill, T. (2011). Identification of a beta-lactamase inhibitory protein variant that is a potent inhibitor of *Staphylococcus* PC1 beta-lactamase. *J. Mol. Biol.* 406, 730–744.

Zervosen, A., Bouillez, A., Herman, A., Amoroso, A., Joris, B., Sauvage, E., et al. (2012). Synthesis and evaluation of boronic acids as inhibitors of penicillin binding proteins of classes A, B and C. *Bioorg. Med. Chem.* 20, 3915–3924.

Zhang, X., Paganelli, F. L., Bierschenk, D., Kuipers, A., Bonten, M. J., Willems, R. J., et al. (2012). Genome-wide identification of ampicillin resistance determinants in *Enterococcus faecium*. *PLoS Genet.* 8:e1002804. doi: 10.1371/journal.pgen.1002804

Zhao, Q., Li, X. Z., Mistry, A., Srikumar, R., Zhang, L., Lomovskaya, O., et al. (1998). Influence of the TonB energy-coupling protein on efflux-mediated multidrug resistance in *Pseudomonas aeruginosa*. *Antimicrob. Agents Chemother.* 42, 2225–2231.

Zhou, X., Jia, F., Liu, X., and Wang, Y. (2012). Total alkaloids of *Sophorea alopecuroides*-induced down-regulation of AcrAB-TolC efflux pump reverses susceptibility to Ciprofloxacin in clinical multidrug resistant *Escherichia coli* isolates. *Phytother. Res.* 26, 1637–1643.

23

Lack of efflux mediated quinolone resistance in *Salmonella enterica* serovars Typhi and Paratyphi A

Sylvie Baucheron[1,2]*, Isabelle Monchaux[1,2], Simon Le Hello[3], François-Xavier Weill[3] and Axel Cloeckaert[1,2]*

[1] *UMR1282 Infectiologie et Santé Publique, Institut National de la Recherche Agronomique, Nouzilly, France*
[2] *UMR1282 Infectiologie et Santé Publique, Université François Rabelais de Tours, Tours, France*
[3] *Institut Pasteur, Unité des Bactéries Pathogènes Entériques, Centre National de Référence des Escherichia coli, Shigella et Salmonella, Paris, France*

Edited by:
Kunihiko Nishino, Osaka University, Japan

Reviewed by:
Kunihiko Nishino, Osaka University, Japan
Peter Heisig, University of Hamburg, Germany

****Correspondence:***
Sylvie Baucheron and Axel Cloeckaert, Unité Infectiologie et Santé Publique site 213, Institut National de la Recherche Agronomique, 37380 Nouzilly, France
e-mail: sylvie.baucheron@tours.inra.fr; axel.cloeckaert@tours.inra.fr

Salmonella enterica serovars Typhi and Paratyphi A isolates from human patients in France displaying different levels of resistance to quinolones or fluoroquinolones were studied for resistance mechanisms to these antimicrobial agents. All resistant isolates carried either single or multiple target gene mutations (i.e., in *gyrA*, *gyrB*, or *parC*) correlating with the resistance levels observed. Active efflux, through upregulation of multipartite efflux systems, has also been previously reported as contributing mechanism for other serovars. Therefore, we investigated also the occurrence of non-target gene mutations in regulatory regions affecting efflux pump expression. However, no mutation was detected in these regions in both Typhi and Paratyphi isolates of this study. Besides, no overexpression of the major efflux systems was observed for these isolates. Nevertheless, a large deletion of 2334 bp was identified in the *acrS-acrE* region of all *S.* Typhi strains but which did not affect the resistance phenotype. As being specific to *S.* Typhi, this deletion could be used for specific molecular detection purposes. In conclusion, the different levels of quinolone or FQ resistance in both *S.* Typhi and *S.* Paratyphi A seem to rely only on target modifications.

Keywords: *Salmonella*, ciprofloxacin, transcriptional regulatory genes, *acrS*, efflux pumps

INTRODUCTION

Enteric fever caused by the human-adapted pathogens *Salmonella enterica* serovars Typhi (*S.* Typhi) and Paratyphi A (*S.* Paratyphi A), B, and C, remains a major health problem (Crump and Mintz, 2010). A global epidemiologic study estimated that during the year 2000 typhoid fever caused 21.7 million illnesses and 21,7000 deaths and paratyphoid fever caused 5.4 million illnesses (Crump et al., 2004). During the past decade *S.* Paratyphi A was responsible for a growing proportion of enteric fever in Asia (Ochiai et al., 2005; Crump and Mintz, 2010). Enteric fever being associated with poor sanitation and unsafe food and water, it particularly affects children and adolescents in developing countries of Asia, Africa and Latin America (Crump et al., 2004; Bhan et al., 2005; Crump and Mintz, 2010). In developed countries, patients are most often ill-returned travellers or migrant workers (Bhan et al., 2005; Connor and Schwartz, 2005; Hassing et al., 2013).

To treat these infections, fluoroquinolones (FQ) and third-generation cephalosporins have been considered as first-line drugs, owing to the resistance to ampicillin, chloramphenicol, and trimethoprim/sulfamethoxazole that appeared during the 1980s (Hassing et al., 2011, 2013). Multidrug resistance (MDR) in *S.* Typhi is encoded mainly by resistance genes carried by large conjugative plasmids and has been reported worldwide (Le et al., 2007). As a consequence of a widespread FQ usage, *S.* Typhi and *S.* Paratyphi A isolates resistant to nalidixic acid (NAL^R, minimum inhibitory concentration [MIC] > 16 mg/L) and with decreased susceptibility to ciprofloxacin (CIP^{DS}, MIC 0.125–1.0 mg/L) have also emerged. Such NAL^R-CIP^{DS} *S.* Typhi and *S.* Paratyphi A have been isolated in endemic areas and also in developed countries (Roumagnac et al., 2006; Le et al., 2007; Gaborieau et al., 2010; Accou-Demartin et al., 2011; Hassing et al., 2011, 2013).

Resistance to quinolones in *Salmonella* spp. is mostly attributed to point mutations in the quinolone resistance-determining regions (QRDRs) of the target genes *gyrA*, *gyrB*, *parC*, and *parE* (Cloeckaert and Chaslus-Dancla, 2001; Piddock, 2002; Velge et al., 2005; Giraud et al., 2006). For the *gyrA* gene, coding the A subunit of DNA gyrase, a single mutation resulting in an amino acid substitution at the position 83 (Serine to Phenylalanine or to Tyrosine) or at the position 87 (Aspartic acid to Asparagine or Glycine) has been the most frequently described in NAL^R-CIP^{DS} *S.* Typhi and *S.* Paratyphi A isolates (Bhan et al., 2005; Renuka et al., 2005; Le et al., 2007; Gaborieau et al., 2010; Hassing et al., 2011). A second mutation leading to the amino acid change at the position 80 (Serine to Isoleucine or to Arginine) of the ParC subunit of topoisomerase IV was described to increase the CIP MIC ($\geq$ 0.5 mg/L) in *S.* Typhi and *S.* Paratyphi A human isolates from India (Gaind et al., 2006). Whereas three mutations, i.e., a double mutation in *gyrA* at both codons 83 and 87 and one mutation in *parC*, were shown to confer CIP resistance (MIC >1 mg/L) in *S.* Typhi and *S.* Paratyphi A human isolates from India or from Taiwan (Gaind et al., 2006; Lee et al., 2013).

Moreover, the varying levels of CIP resistance observed in *S.* Typhi and *S.* Paratyphi A isolates with only a single *gyrA* mutation suggest that other mechanisms could be involved in quinolone resistance in this serovar (Renuka et al., 2005).

Resistance to FQ in *S.* Typhimurium has also been attributed to active efflux mechanism, due to overproduction of the AcrAB-TolC efflux system (Giraud et al., 2000, 2006; Cloeckaert and Chaslus-Dancla, 2001; Piddock, 2006). We have previously reported the contribution of the AcrAB-TolC efflux system in resistance to FQ in several MDR epidemic clones of *S.* Typhimurium, such as *S.* Typhimurium of phage types DT204 or DT104 (Baucheron et al., 2002, 2004a,b). Among the chromosomal loci affecting AcrAB-TolC expression, the *ramRA* locus appears to be the most important in *Salmonella* spp. (Abouzeed et al., 2008; Kehrenberg et al., 2009). *ramR* encodes a repressor protein (RamR) belonging to the TetR family of repressor proteins, and has been shown to be the local repressor protein of *ramA* transcription (Abouzeed et al., 2008; Baucheron et al., 2012); while *ramA* encodes a transcriptional activator protein (RamA) belonging to the AraC/XylS family of regulatory proteins (Nikaido et al., 2008; Bailey et al., 2010). The latter is involved in upregulating expression of the AcrAB-TolC system (Nikaido et al., 2008; Bailey et al., 2010). Several mutations in *ramR* or its binding site upstream of *ramA*, affecting expression of this efflux system, have been detected in clinical isolates of serovar Typhimurium or Kentucky and of minor serovars Hadar, Infantis, Livingstone, or Schwarzengrund (Abouzeed et al., 2008; Kehrenberg et al., 2009; Hentschke et al., 2010; Akiyama and Khan, 2012; Baucheron et al., 2013).

In the present study, we have characterized mechanisms involved in resistance to quinolones or fluroquinolones in 21 *S.* Typhi and *S.* Paratyphi A strains displaying different levels of resistance to these drugs and isolated from patients in France during the period 1997–2008. For a subset of strains, with suspected increased efflux activity, we investigated the occurrence of mutations in the global *ram*, *sox* and *mar* regulatory loci of AcrAB-TolC, and in the local *acrR* and *acrS* repressor genes of the AcrAB and AcrEF pumps, respectively (Abouzeed et al., 2008; Kehrenberg et al., 2009).

MATERIALS AND METHODS

BACTERIAL STRAINS

The twenty one strains including 16 *S.* Typhi and 5 *S.* Paratyphi A selected for this study were collected by the French National Reference Center for *Salmonella*, Institut Pasteur, Paris, France. They were isolated in France from travellers or migrants between 1997 and 2008 (**Table 1**). The selection was made to obtain diversity in terms of geographic origin, year of isolation, genetic lineages (haplotype for *S.* Typhi; Roumagnac et al., 2006), and phenotype of resistance to quinolones (**Table 1**).

Table 1 | *Salmonella enterica* serovars Typhi and Paratyphi A strains analyzed in this study.

Strain	Country	Year of isolation	Haplo type	Antimicrobial resistance pattern	MIC (mg/L)		Substitution(s) in the QRDR of:				AcrA production ratio*
					NAL	CIP	GyrA	GyrB	ParC	ParE	
***SALMONELLA* TYPHI**											
06–423	India	2006	ND	Pansusceptible	4	0.015	WT	WT	WT	WT	1
06–426	India	2006	ND	CIP^{DS}	16	0.125	WT	S464Y	WT	WT	1
02–1180	India	2002	H45	NALCIP^{DS}	64	0.125	D87G	WT	WT	WT	1
05–3275	Morocco	2005	H6	NALCIP^{DS}	64	0.125	D87N	WT	WT	WT	1
4(02)MB	Vietnam	1997	H58	ASCSulTmpTeNAL	128	0.03	S83Y	WT	WT	WT	0.5
222(97)MN	Vietnam	1996	ND	ASCSulTmpTeNALCIP^{DS}	128	0.125	S83F	WT	WT	WT	0.5
43(97)MN	Vietnam	1996	H63	ASCSulTmpTeNALCIP^{DS}	128	0.125	S83F	WT	WT	WT	0.5
98–3139	Mexico	1998	H50	NALCIP^{DS}	128	0.125	S83F	WT	WT	WT	0.5
02–7744	India	2002	H52	NALCIP^{DS}	128	0.125	S83F	WT	WT	WT	0.5
226(97)MN	Vietnam	1996	H61	ASCSulTmpTeNALCIP^{DS}	128	0.25	S83F	WT	WT	WT	0.5
97–2307	India	1997	H63	NALCIP^{DS}	256	0.125	S83F	WT	WT	WT	0.5
318(98)MB	Vietnam	1998	H58	ASCSulTmpTeNALCIP^{DS}	512	0.25	S83Y	WT	WT	WT	1
39(98)MN	Vietnam	1998	H58	ASCSulTmpTeNALCIP^{DS}	512	0.25	S83F	WT	WT	WT	1
4(02)MN	Vietnam	2000	H58	ASCSulTmpTeNALCIP^{DS}	1024	0.25	S83F	WT	WT	D420N	1
5(04)MN	Vietnam	2004	ND	NALCIP^{DS}	1024	0.25	S83F	WT	WT	D420N	1
04–2176	India	2004	H58	SSpSulTmpTeNALCIP	1024	8	S83F; D87N	WT	S80I	WT	1
***SALMONELLA* PARATYPHI A**											
08–8903	Senegal	2008		Pansusceptible	8	0.030	WT	WT	WT	WT	2
07–6329	Burkina Faso	2007		CIP^{DS}	16	0.25	WT	S464F	WT	WT	2
05–208	India	2005		NALCIP^{DS}	256	0.50	S83F	WT	WT	WT	2
08–4271	Guinea Bissau	2008		NACIP^{DS}	1024	1	S83F	WT	WT	WT	2
08–2580	India	2008		NALCIP^{DS}	1024	1	S83F	WT	WT	WT	3

**AcrA expression was measured by dot blotting with an anti-AcrA polyclonal antibody.*

ND, not determined.

WT, wild type.

A, amoxicillin; S, streptomycin; Sp, spectinomycin; C, chloramphenicol; Sul, sulfamethoxazole; Tmp, trimethoprim; Te, tetracycline; NAL, nalidixic acid; CIP, ciprofloxacin; CIP^{DS}, decreased susceptibility to ciprofloxacin.

D, aspartic acid; F, phenylalanine; G, glycine; I, isoleucine; N, asparagine; S, serine; Y, tyrosine.

ANTIMICROBIAL SUSCEPTIBILITY TESTING

Antimicrobial susceptibility was investigated by the standard disk diffusion method according to the recommendations of the Antibiogram Committee of the French Society for Microbiology (CA-SFM) (www.sfm-microbiologie.org/). The MICs of NAL and CIP were determined by the standard agar doubling dilution method as described previously (Baucheron et al., 2002). The NAL^R isolates were defined as having a MIC > 16 mg/L. The CIP^R isolates were defined as having a MIC > 1 mg/L and CIP^{DS} isolates as having a MIC comprised between 0.125 and 1.0 mg/L (Accou-Demartin et al., 2011; Hassing et al., 2013). MICs of these antibiotics were also determined in the presence of the efflux pump inhibitor Phe-Arg-β-naphthylamide (PAβN, Sigma) at the following concentrations: 10, 20, 30, 40, 50, and 60 mg/L.

ASSESSMENT OF TARGET-AFFECTING MECHANISMS

Mutations in the QRDRs of *gyrA*, *gyrB*, *parC*, and *parE* genes were detected as described previously (Le et al., 2007; Song et al., 2010; Accou-Demartin et al., 2011).

The search of plasmid-mediated quinolone resistances genes, *qnrA*, *qnrB*, *qnrS*, *qnrD*, *aac*(6')-Ib-cr, and *qepA* was performed as described previously (Accou-Demartin et al., 2011).

ASSESSMENT OF EFFLUX MECHANISMS

Efflux pump production was assessed by dot blot using an anti-AcrA polyclonal antibody as described previously (Abouzeed et al., 2008). Occurrence of mutations affecting *acrAB*, *acrEF*, and *tolC* expression was determined by PCR and sequencing the regulatory regions *ramR-ramA*, *acrR-acrA*, *marC*-marO-*marR-marA*, *soxS-soxR*, and *acrS-acrE* using primers listed in (**Table 2**).

Table 2 | Primers used for PCRs.

Primer used and target region	Primer	Nucleotide position relative to the LT2 strain genome sequence*	Oligonucleotide sequence(s) (5'–3')	Size (bp)	Annealing temp (°C)	Reference
DETECTION OF MUTATIONS						
ramR-ramA	ram5	638085	TCGGTAAAAGGCAGTTCCAG	958	60	Baucheron et al., 2013
	ramA6	639042	GTCGATAACCTGAGCGGAAA			
acrR-acrA	acrR1	533463	CAGTGGTTCCGTTTTTAGTG	992	58	Olliver et al., 2005
	acrR2	534454	ACAGAATAGCGACACAGAAA			
marC-marO-*marR-marA*	marR1	1597459	CAGTGTTGCGTCTGGACATC	787	60	Baucheron et al., 2013
	marR2	1598245	GCTAACGGGAGCAGTACGAC			
soxS-soxR	sox1	4503970	CTACAGGCGGTGACGGTAAT	915	60	Baucheron et al., 2013
	sox2	4504884	CGGCGCTTTAGTTTTAGGTG			
acrS-acrE	acrS3	3559106	AAAACGAACGGGAACTGATG	2874 ***	58	This study
	acrS4	3561978	ACAAACATACCGGGAAGCAG			
qRT-PCR						
gmk	gmk-f	3933294	TTGGCAGGGAGGCGTTT	62	60	Baucheron et al., 2012
	gmk-r	3933355	GCGCGAAGTGCCGTAGTAAT			
gyrB	gyrB-f	4040275	TCTCCTCACAGACCAAAGATAAGCT	81	60	Baucheron et al., 2012
	gyrB-r	4040195	CGCTCAGCAGTTCGTTCATC			
rrs	rrs-f	NA**	CCAGCAGCCGCGGTAAT	57	60	Baucheron et al., 2012
	rrs-r	NA**	TTTACGCCCAGTAATTCCGATT			
ramA	ramA-f	639180	GCGTGAACGGAAGCTAAAAC	167	60	Baucheron et al., 2012
	ramA-r	639346	GGCCATGCTTTTCTTTACGA			
ramR	ramR-f	638623	TAACGCAGGTGTTGCAGAAG	192	64	Baucheron et al., 2012
	ramR-r	638432	TGGTTCAGACCCCAACTGAT			
acrA	acrA-f	533120	GAAACCGCACGTATCAACCT	220	60	Baucheron et al., 2012
	acrA-r	532901	CCTGTTTCAGCGAACCATTT			
acrB	acrB-f	531348	TCGTGTTCCTGGTGATGTACCT	68	66	Baucheron et al., 2012
	acrB-r	531281	AACCGCAATAGTCGGAATCAA			
acrF	acrF-f	3563042	GCTCTGTCGTCCATCTCAAAGA	70	66	This study
	acrF-r	3563111	CGCGCTACAACGTTATAGTTTTCA			
tolC	tolC-f	3349107	GCCCGTGCGCAATATGAT	67	60	Baucheron et al., 2012
	tolC-r	3349173	CCGCGTTATCCAGGTTGTTG			

**GenBank NC_003197.1.*

***NA: Not Applicable due to the number of copies of this gene in Salmonella.*

****2874 bp for S. Typhimurium or S. Paratyphi A and 539 bp for S. Typhi (see **Figure 1**).*

Transcription levels of efflux related genes *acrA*, *acrB*, *acrF*, *tolC*, *ramA*, and *ramR* were done by quantitative reverse transcription-PCR (qRT-PCR) as described previously (Baucheron et al., 2012; Giraud et al., 2013). Primers used for qRT-PCR are listed in (**Table 2**).

RESULTS AND DISCUSSION

RESISTANCE PHENOTYPES AND TARGET-AFFECTING MECHANISMS

The twenty one *S.* Typhi and *S.* Paratyphi A strains of this study were isolated in France but acquired abroad, mainly in Asia and Africa (**Table 1**). Among the *S.* Typhi strains, all but two were NAL^R (MIC > 16 mg/L). One of the two strains was pansusceptible and the second was CIP^{DS} but only categorized as intermediate for NAL (NAL^I, MIC 16 mg/L). Of the 14 NAL^R strains, one was CIP^R, 12 were CIP^{DS} and one was CIP^S (MIC 0.03 mg/L). Eight NAL^R *S.* Typhi strains were also multidrug resistant. The majority of the NAL^R *S.* Typhi strains belonged to haplotype H58 which had emerged in Southern Asia during the mid 1990s (Roumagnac et al., 2006; Le et al., 2007). Among the *S.* Paratyphi A strains, all but two were NAL^R. One of the two strains was pansusceptible and the second was NAL^I-CIP^{DS}. The three others were NAL^R- CIP^{DS}.

As shown in **Table 1**, both NAL^I-CIP^{DS} had a mutation resulting in an amino acid substitution at position 464 of GyrB: serine to tyrosine for the *S.* Typhi isolate and serine to phenylalanine for the *S.* Paratyphi A isolate. The most frequent mechanism of resistance of NAL^R-CIP^{DS} ($n = 17$) and NAL^R-CIP^S ($n = 1$) strains, whatever the serovar, was a substitution at position 83 (serine to phenylalanine, $n = 12$, 66.6%) of GyrA. Other GyrA modifications were observed at position 83 (serine to tyrosine) in two isolates or at position 87 (aspartic acid to glycine, aspartic acid to asparagine) in one isolate for each. As described previously, a single substitution in GyrA was associated with resistance to nalidixic acid and decreased susceptibility to CIP (Bhan et al., 2005; Le et al., 2007; Gaborieau et al., 2010; Hassing et al., 2011). One exception was the *S.* Typhi strain 4 (02) MB, which was NAL^R-CIP^S (and not CIP^{DS}) despite a mutation in *gyrA* resulting in substitution serine to tyrosine at position 83.

Additional substitutions were found in ParE of 2 NAL^R-CIP^{DS} *S.* Typhi strains that led to amino acid substitution aspartic acid to asparagine at position 420. In both cases, a 2-fold increase of NAL MICs was observed.

In the CIP^R *S.* Typhi isolate, three mutations leading to a double substitution in GyrA at positions 83 (serine to phenylalanine) and 87 (aspartic acid to asparagine) and one substitution at the position 80 of ParC (serine to isoleucine), as observed in previous studies (Renuka et al., 2005; Gaind et al., 2006; Lee et al., 2013).

The NAL^R and CIP^{DS} *S.* Typhi and *S.* Paratyphi A strains harboring a single substitution in GyrA showed various values for NAL (64–1024 mg/L) and CIP (0.03–0.5 mg/L) MICs which suggested the presence of other mechanisms of resistance. Since the plasmid-mediated quinolone resistance-conferring genes *qnrA*, *qnrB*, *qnrD* or *qnrS*, *qepA*, *and aac(6')-Ib-cr* were not detected, we investigated the role of the AcrAB-TolC efflux system.

INVOLVEMENT OF EFFLUX

None of the *S.* Typhi strains showed significant AcrA overproduction by dot blot, but nevertheless all *S.* Paratyphi A isolates showed a 2 or 3-fold increased AcrA production relative to the susceptible *S.* Typhi isolate (**Table 1**). Thus, overproduction of AcrA seems not to be involved in CIP^{DS} isolates compared with the susceptible isolates of *S.* Typhi or *S.* Paratyphi A. In presence of the efflux pump inhibitor PAβN (20 or 40 mg/L), the CIP MICs similarly decreased (4 or 8-fold) in CIP^{DS} and in susceptible strains (**Table 3** and data not shown), which is in accordance with previous studies on *S.* Typhimurium and corresponds to

Table 3 | Study of efflux in a subset of *Salmonella enterica* serovars Typhi and Paratyphi A strains.

Strain	Antimicrobial resistance pattern[a]	MIC (mg/L)[b]		Substitution(s) in the QRDR of[c]:				*acrSE* sequencing	Transcription level of:					
		NAL	CIP	GyrA	GyrB	ParC	ParE		*acrA*	*acrF*	*acrB*	*tolC*	*ramA*	*ramR*
***SALMONELLA* TYPHI**														
06–423	Pansusceptible	4	0.015 [0.004]	WT	WT	WT	WT	Deletion[d]	1.0	1.0	1.0	1.0	1.0	1.0
02–1180	NALCIP^{DS}	64	0.125 [0.015]	D87G	WT	WT	WT	Deletion[d]	1.5	0.7	0.5	0.8	0.9	1.4
05–3275	NALCIP^{DS}	64	0.125 [0.030]	D87N	WT	WT	WT	Deletion[d]	0.5	1.4	0.2	0.5	0.3	0.7
97–2307	NALCIP^{DS}	256	0.125 [0.030]	S83F	WT	WT	WT	Deletion[d]	1.7	0.8	0.8	0.7	1.9	2.2
04–2176	SSpSulTmpTeNALCIP	1024	8 [2]	S83F; A87N	WT	S80I	WT	Deletion[d]	1.5	0.8	1.3	0.9	1.2	2.2
***SALMONELLA* PARATYPHI A**														
08–8903	Pansusceptible	8	0.030 [0.008]	WT	WT	WT	WT	WT	1.0	1.0	1.0	1.0	1.0	1.0
07–6329	CIP^{DS}	16	0.25 [0.060]	WT	S464F	WT	WT	WT	1.6	1.4	1.0	1.0	1.0	1.2
05–208	NALCIP^{DS}	256	0.50 [0.030]	S83F	WT	WT	WT	WT	1.3	0.9	1.4	1.0	1.1	1.0
08–4271	NALCIP^{DS}	1024	1 [0.25]	S83F	WT	WT	WT	WT	1.2	1.1	0.7	1.4	1.3	1.3
08–2580	NALCIP^{DS}	1024	1 [0.25]	S83F	WT	WT	WT	WT	2.0	1.6	1.4	1.4	2.0	1.3

[a] *S, streptomycin; Sp, spectinomycin; Sul, sulfamethoxazole; Tmp, trimethoprim; Te, tetracycline; NAL, nalidixic acid; CIP, ciprofloxacin; CIP^{DS}, decreased susceptibility to ciprofloxacin.*

[b] *Values in brackets are MICs in the presence of the efflux pump inhibitor PAβN at 40 mg/L.*

[c] *WT, wild type; D, aspartic acid; F, phenylalanine; G, glycine; I, isoleucine; N, asparagine; S, serine.*

[d] *2334 bp deleted.*

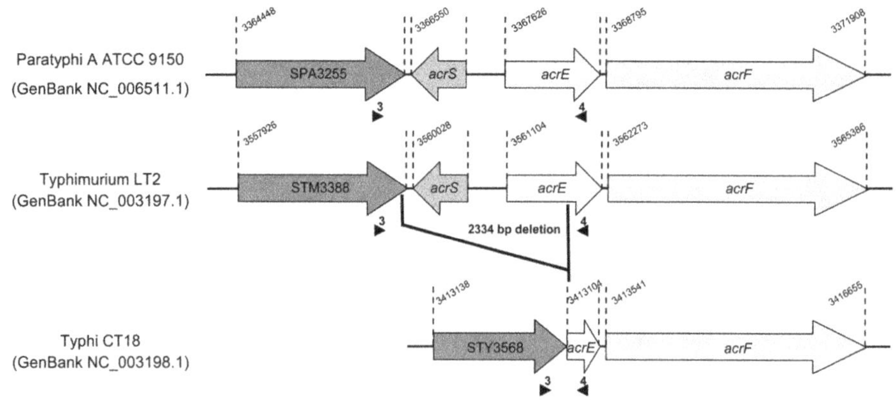

FIGURE 1 | Deletion identified in the *acrSE* region relative to the genome sequence of *S.* Typhi strain CT18 (GenBank NC_003198.1). The sequence of the *acrSE* region of *S.* Typhi strain CT18 is compared to those of *S.* Paratyphi A strain ATCC9150 (GenBank NC_006511.1) and *S.* Typhi strain LT2 (GenBank NC_003197.1). Small black arrows indicate primers positions used for PCR to amplify and sequence the *acrSE* region. The 2334 bp chromosomal deletion was found in all *S.* Typhi strains studied.

a decrease of resistance level observed for *acrB* or *tolC* deletion mutants (Baucheron et al., 2002, 2004b).

Despite a lack of evidence of increased efflux in the resistance phenotype, we measured by qRT-PCR the transcription levels of efflux related genes *acrA*, *acrF*, *acrB*, *tolC*, *ramA*, and *ramR* in CIP^{DS} non-MDR strains and in the CIP^{R} strain. No differences were detected in the transcription levels of these genes, between susceptible, CIP^{DS} and CIP^{R} strains, whatever the serovar (**Table 3**). In addition, no mutations were detected in the regulatory regions of the AcrAB-TolC efflux system. However, during the screening of the regulatory regions, we identified a single large deletion of 2334 bp in the *acrS-acrE* region of all *S.* Typhi strains, including the susceptible one (**Table 3**). This deletion encompassed the *acrS* gene, that encodes a transcriptional repressor, and a large part of the *acrE* gene that encodes the AcrE periplasmic lipoprotein, which is homologous to AcrA (Olliver et al., 2005). This 2334 bp deletion was also observed in the *acrS-acrE* region of sequenced genomes of MDR *S.* Typhi CT18 strain (Parkhill et al., 2001) and pansusceptible TY2 strain (Deng et al., 2003) (**Figure 1**). Previously, it has been shown that *acrS* deletion in *S.* Typhimurium does not affect *acrEF* expression (Olliver et al., 2005). Similarly the natural *acrSE* deletion detected in *S.* Typhi had no impact on the *acrF* transcription level as observed in this study. To our knowledge, this is the first description of such a natural *acrS-acrE* chromosomal deletion and seems specific to *S.* Typhi since it was not detected in all currently sequenced genomes of the other serovars (not shown).

CONCLUSIONS

The main mechanisms involved in quinolone or FQ resistance in both *S.* Typhi and *S.* Paratyphi A are target modifications. In contrast to what is seen in enteric pathogenic serovars, such as Typhimurium or the emerging CIP^{R} Kentucky ST198 clone (Baucheron et al., 2013), increased efflux pump production-mediated mechanisms seem to be totally absent in both *S.* Typhi and *S.* Paratyphi A. The deletion identified in the *acrSEF* region, although not involved in the resistance phenotype, may be helpful for the specific detection of *S.* Typhi.

ACKNOWLEDGMENTS

We are grateful to Dr. Hong Le for providing some of the studied strains and to Laëtitia Fabre for excellent technical assistance. We would like to thank all corresponding laboratories of the French National Reference Center for *E. coli*, *Shigella*, and *Salmonella*. The French National Reference Center for *E. coli*, *Shigella*, and *Salmonella* is funded by the Institut Pasteur and the Institut de Veille Sanitaire. The "Unité des Bactéries Pathogènes Entériques" belongs to the "Integrative Biology of Emerging Infectious Diseases" Laboratory of Excellence funded by the French Government "Investissement d'Avenir" programme (grant no. ANR-10-LABX-62-IBEID).

REFERENCES

Abouzeed, Y. M., Baucheron, S., and Cloeckaert, A. (2008). *ramR* mutations involved in efflux-mediated multidrug resistance in *Salmonella enterica* serovar Typhimurium. *Antimicrob. Agents Chemother.* 52, 2428–2434. doi: 10.1128/ AAC.00084-08

Accou-Demartin, M., Gaborieau, V., Song, Y., Roumagnac, P., Marchou, B., Achtman, M., et al. (2011). *Salmonella enterica* Serotype Typhi with nonclassical quinolone resistance phenotype. *Emerg. Infect. Dis.* 17, 1091–1094. doi: 10.3201/ eid/1706.101242

Akiyama, T., and Khan, A. A. (2012). Molecular characterization of strains of fluoroquinolone-resistant *Salmonella enterica* serovar Schwarzengrund carrying multidrug resistance isolated from imported foods. *J. Antimicrob. Chemother.* 67, 101–110. doi: 10.1093/jac/dkr414

Bailey, A. M., Ivens, A., Kingsley, R., Cottell, J. L., Wain, J., and Piddock, L. J. V. (2010). RamA, a member of the AraC/XylS family, influences both virulence and efflux in *Salmonella enterica* serovar Typhimurium. *J. Bacteriol.* 192, 1607–1616. doi: 10.1128/ JB.01517-09

Baucheron, S., Chaslus-Dancla, E., and Cloeckaert, A. (2004a). Role of TolC and *parC* mutation in high-level fluoroquinolone resistance in *Salmonella enter- ica* serotype Typhimurium DT204. *J. Antimicrob. Chemother.* 53, 657–659. doi: 10.1093/jac/dkh122

Baucheron, S., Tyler, S., Boyd, D., Mulvey, M. R., Chaslus-Dancla, E., and Cloeckaert A. (2004b). AcrAB-TolC directs efflux-mediated multidrug resis- tance in *Salmonella enterica* serovar Typhimurium DT104. *Antimicrob. Agents Chemother.* 48, 3729–3735. doi: 10.1128/AAC.48.10.3729-3735.2004

Baucheron, S., Coste, F., Canepa, S., Maurel, M. C., Giraud, E., Culard, F., et al. (2012). Binding of the RamR repressor to wild-type and mutated promoters of the RamA gene involved in efflux-mediated multidrug resistance in *Salmonella enterica* serovar Typhimurium. *Antimicrob. Agents Chemother.* 56, 942–948. doi: 10.1128/AAC.05444-11

Baucheron, S., Imberechts, H., Chaslus-Dancla, E., and Cloeckaert, A. (2002). The AcrB multidrug transporter plays a major role in high-level fluoroquinolone resistance in *Salmonella enterica* serovar Typhimurium phage type DT204. *Microb. Drug Resist.* 8, 281–289. doi: 10.1089/10766290260469543

Baucheron, S., Le Hello, S., Doublet, B., Giraud, E., Weill, F. X., and Cloeckaert, A. (2013). *ramR* mutations affecting fluoroquinolone susceptibility in epi- demic multidrug-resistant *Salmonella enterica* serovar Kentucky ST198. *Front. Microbiol.* 4:213. doi: 10.3389/fmicb.2013.00213

Bhan, M. K., Bahl, R., and Bhatnagar, S. (2005). Typhoid and paratyphoid fever. *Lancet* 366, 749–762. doi: 10.1016/S0140-6736(05)67181-4

Cloeckaert, A., and Chaslus-Dancla, E. (2001). Mechanisms of quinolone resistance in *Salmonella*. *Vet. Res.* 32, 291–300. doi: 10.1051/vetres:2001105

Connor, B. A., and Schwartz, E. (2005). Typhoid and paratyphoid fever in travellers. *Lancet Infect. Dis.* 5, 623–628. doi: 10.1016/S1473-3099(05)70239-5

Crump, J. A., Luby, S. P., and Mintz, E. D. (2004). The global burden of typhoid fever. *Bull. World Health Organ.* 82, 346–353.

Crump, J. A., and Mintz, E. D. (2010). Global trends in typhoid and paratyphoid Fever. *Clin. Infect. Dis.* 50, 241–246. doi: 10.1086/649541

Deng, W., Liou, S. R., Plunkett, G. 3rd., Mayhew, G. F., Rose, D. J., Burland, V., et al. (2003). Comparative genomics of *Salmonella enterica* serovar Typhi strains Ty2 and CT18. *J. Bacteriol.* 185, 2330–2337. doi: 10.1128/JB.185.7.2330-2337.2003

Gaborieau, V., Weill, F. X., and Marchou, B. (2010). A case of *Salmonella enterica* serovar Typhi with decreased susceptibility to ciprofloxacin. *Med. Mal. Infect.* 40, 691–695. doi: 10.1016/j.medmal.2010.06.009

Gaind, R., Paglietti, B., Murgia, M., Dawar, R., Uzzau, S., Cappuccinelli, P., et al. (2006). Molecular characterization of ciprofloxacin-resistant *Salmonella enter- ica* serovar Typhi and Paratyphi A causing enteric fever in India. *J. Antimicrob. Chemother.* 58, 1139–1144. doi: 10.1093/jac/dkl391

Giraud, E., Baucheron, S., and Cloeckaert, A. (2006). Resistance to fluoro- quinolones in *Salmonella*: emerging mechanisms and resistance prevention strategies. *Microbes Infect.* 8, 1937–1944. doi: 10.1016/j.micinf.2005.12.025

Giraud, E., Baucheron, S., Virlogeux-Payant, I., Nishino, K., and Cloeckaert, A. (2013). Effects of natural mutations in the *ramRA* locus on invasiveness of epidemic fluoroquinolone-resistant *Salmonella enterica* serovar Typhimurium isolates. *J. Infect. Dis.* 207, 794–802. doi: 10.1093/infdis/jis755

Giraud, E., Cloeckaert, A., Kerboeuf, D., and Chaslus-Dancla, E. (2000). Evidence for active efflux as the primary mechanism of resistance to ciprofloxacin in *Salmonella enterica* serovar Typhimurium. *Antimicrob. Agents Chemother.* 44, 1223–1228. doi: 10.1128/AAC.44.5.1223-1228.2000

Hassing, R. J., Goessens, W. H., Mevius, D. J., van Pelt, W., Mouton, J. W., Verbon, A., et al. (2013). Decreased ciprofloxacin susceptibility in *Salmonella* Typhi and Paratyphi infections in ill-returned travellers: the impact on clinical outcome and future treatment options. *Eur. J. Clin. Microbiol. Infect. Dis.* 32, 1295–1301. doi: 10.1007/s10096-013-1878-9

Hassing, R. J., Menezes, G. A., van Pelt, W., Petit, P. L., van Genderen, P. J., and Goessens, W. H. (2011). Analysis of mechanisms involved in reduced suscepti- bility to ciprofloxacin in *Salmonella enterica* serotypes Typhi and Paratyphi A isolates from travellers to Southeast Asia. *Int. J. Antimicrob. Agents* 37, 240–243. doi: 10.1016/j.ijantimicag.2010.10.026

Hentschke, M., Christner, M., Sobottka, I., Aepfelbacher, M., and Rohde, H. (2010). Combined *ramR* mutation and presence of a Tn1721-associated tet(A) variant in a clinical isolate of *Salmonella enterica* serovar Hadar resistant to tigecycline. *Antimicrob. Agents Chemother.* 54, 1319–1322. doi: 10.1128/AAC.00993-09

Kehrenberg, C., Cloeckaert, A., Klein, G., and Schwarz, S. (2009). Decreased fluoroquinolone susceptibility in mutants of *Salmonella* serovars other than Typhimurium: detection of novel mutations involved in modulated expression of *ramA* and *soxS*. *J. Antimicrob. Chemother.* 64, 1175–1180. doi: 10.1093/jac/ dkp347

Le, T. A., Fabre, L., Roumagnac, P., Grimont, P. A., Scavizzi, M. R., and Weill, F. X. (2007). Clonal expansion and microevolution of quinolone-resistant *Salmonella enterica* serotype Typhi in Vietnam from 1996 to 2004. *J. Clin. Microbiol.* 45, 3485–3492. doi: 10.1128/JCM.00948-07

Lee, C. J., Su, L. H., Huang, Y. C., and Chiu, C. H. (2013). First isolation of ciprofloxacin-resistant *Salmonella enterica* serovar Typhi in Taiwan. *J. Microbiol. Immunol. Infect.* 46, 469–473. doi: 10.1016/j.jmii.2013.01.002

Nikaido, E., Yamaguchi, A., and Nishino, K. (2008). AcrAB multidrug efflux pump regulation in *Salmonella enterica* serovar Typhimurium by RamA in response to environmental signals. *J. Biol. Chem.* 283, 24245–24253. doi: 10.1074/jbc. M804544200

Ochiai, R. L., Wang, X., von Seidlein, L., Yang, J., Bhutta, Z. A., Bhattacharya, S. K., et al. (2005). *Salmonella* paratyphi A rates, Asia. *Emerg. Infect. Dis.* 11, 1764–1766. doi: 10.3201/eid1111.050168

Olliver, A., Valle, M., Chaslus-Dancla, E., and Cloeckaert, A. (2005). Overexpression of the multidrug efflux operon *acrEF* by insertional acti- vation with IS1 or IS10 elements in *Salmonella enterica* serovar typhimurium DT204 *acrB* mutants selected with fluoroquinolones. *Antimicrob. Agents Chemother.* 49, 289–301. doi: 10.1128/AAC.49.1.289-301.2005

Parkhill, J., Dougan, G., James, K. D., Thomson, N. R., Pickard, D., Wain, J., et al. (2001). Complete genome sequence of a multiple drug resistant *Salmonella enterica* serovar Typhi CT18. *Nature* 413, 848–852. doi: 10.1038/35101607

Piddock, L. J. V. (2002). Fluoroquinolone resistance in *Salmonella* serovars isolated from humans and food animals. *FEMS Microbiol. Rev.* 26, 3–16. doi: 10.1016/S0168-6445(01)00076-6

Piddock, L. J. V. (2006). Clinically relevant chromosomally encoded multidrug resistance efflux pumps in bacteria. *Clin. Microbiol. Rev.* 19, 382–402. doi: 10.1128/CMR.19.2.382-402.2006

Renuka, K., Sood, S., Das, B. K., and Kapil, A. (2005). High-level ciprofloxacin resistance in *Salmonella enterica* serotype Typhi in India. *J. Med. Microbiol.* 54, 999–1000. doi: 10.1099/jmm.0.45966-0

Roumagnac, P., Weill, F. X., Dolecek, C., Baker, S., Brisse, S., Chinh, N. T., et al. (2006). Evolutionary history of *Salmonella* Typhi. *Science* 314, 1301–1304. doi: 10.1126/science.1134933

Song, Y., Roumagnac, P., Weill, F. X., Wain, J., Dolecek, C., Mazzoni, C. J., et al. (2010). A multiplex single nucleotide polymorphism typing assay for detecting mutations that result in decreased fluoroquinolone susceptibility in *Salmonella enterica* serovars Typhi and Paratyphi A. *J. Antimicrob. Chemother.* 65, 1631–1641. doi: 10.1093/jac/dkq175

Velge, P., Cloeckaert, A., and Barrow, P. (2005). Emergence of *Salmonella* epi- demics: the problems related to *Salmonella enterica* serotype Enteritidis and multiple antibiotic resistance in other major serotypes. *Vet. Res.* 36, 267–288. doi: 10.1051/vetres:2005005

24

Rise and dissemination of aminoglycoside resistance: the *aac(6')-Ib* paradigm

María S. Ramirez, Nikolas Nikolaidis and Marcelo E. Tolmasky*

Department of Biological Science, Center for Applied Biotechnology Studies, College of Natural Sciences and Mathematics, California State University Fullerton, Fullerton, CA, USA

Edited by:
Marilyn C. Roberts, University of Washington, USA

Reviewed by:
Karen J. Shaw, Trius, USA
Thomas F. O'Brien, Brigham and Women's Hospital, USA

Correspondence:
Marcelo E. Tolmasky, Department of Biological Science, Center for Applied Biotechnology Studies, College of Natural Sciences and Mathematics, California State University Fullerton, 800 N State College Boulevard, Fullerton, CA 92831, USA.
e-mail: mtolmasky@fullerton.edu

Enzymatic modification is a prevalent mechanism by which bacteria defeat the action of antibiotics. Aminoglycosides are often inactivated by aminoglycoside modifying enzymes encoded by genes present in the chromosome, plasmids, and other genetic elements. The AAC(6')-Ib (aminoglycoside 6'-*N*-acetyltransferase type Ib) is an enzyme of clinical importance found in a wide variety of gram-negative pathogens. The AAC(6')-Ib enzyme is of interest not only because of his ubiquity but also because of other characteristics, it presents significant microheterogeneity at the N-termini and the *aac(6')-Ib* gene is often present in integrons, transposons, plasmids, genomic islands, and other genetic structures. Excluding the highly heterogeneous N-termini, there are 45 non-identical AAC(6')-Ib related entries in the NCBI database, 32 of which have identical name in spite of not having identical amino acid sequence. While some variants conserved similar properties, others show dramatic differences in specificity, including the case of AAC(6')-Ib-cr that mediates acetylation of ciprofloxacin representing a rare case where a resistance enzyme acquires the ability to utilize an antibiotic of a different class as substrate. Efforts to utilize antisense technologies to turn off expression of the gene or to identify enzymatic inhibitors to induce phenotypic conversion to susceptibility are under way.

Keywords: antibiotic resistance, aminoglycoside, inhibition, acetyltransferase, mobile elements, integron, transposon

AMINOGLYCOSIDES AND RESISTANCE

Aminoglycosides are bactericidal antibiotics that affect translation fidelity and, according to recent data, they may also stimulate the production of highly deleterious hydroxyl radicals (Vakulenko and Mobashery, 2003; Magnet and Blanchard, 2005; Jana and Deb, 2006; Kohanski et al., 2007; Majumder et al., 2007). Aminoglycosides are used to treat infections caused by gram-negative bacilli and, in combination with β-lactams or vancomycin, to treat some gram-positive pathogens, mainly staphylococci (Yao and Moellering, 2007). Since a step in the uptake process requires functional respiration, the spectrum of action of aminoglycosides is limited to aerobic bacteria (Muir et al., 1984). In addition to their most common uses, aminoglycosides can be utilized to treat diseases such as tuberculosis (Menzies et al., 2009; Brossier et al., 2010), plague, tularemia, brucellosis, endocarditis caused by enterococci, and others (Vakulenko and Mobashery, 2003; Yao and Moellering, 2007; Ramirez and Tolmasky, 2010). The fact that aminoglycosides also cause a decrease in eukaryotic translational fidelity permitted to initiate efforts to developed them as drugs to treat nonsense mutation related genetic disorders such as cystic fibrosis and Duchenne muscular dystrophy (Rich et al., 1990; Kellermayer, 2006; Hermann, 2007; Kondo et al., 2007; Zingman et al., 2007; Bidou et al., 2012; Kandasamy et al., 2012). A chemical labyrinthectomy using intratympanic injection of aminoglycosides is used when most treatments of Ménière's disease fail (Huon et al., 2012; Pacheu-Grau et al., 2012). Aminoglycoside-based drugs are also inhibitors of reproduction of the HIV virus, a property that could result in their utilization in the treatment of AIDS patients (Houghton et al., 2010).

The basic chemical structure of aminoglycosides is characterized by the presence of an aminocyclitol nucleus (streptamine, 2-deoxystreptamine, or streptidine) linked to amino sugars through glycosidic bonds. However, other compounds with different basic structures are also included within the aminoglycosides family, e.g., spectinomycin, an aminocyclitol not linked to amino sugars or compounds containing the aminocyclitol fortamine (Bryskier, 2005). They reach the cytoplasm of the bacterial cell in a three-step process, of which the first one is energy-independent and the following two are energy-dependent (Taber et al., 1987; Vakulenko and Mobashery, 2003; Ramirez and Tolmasky, 2010). At the molecular level, the action of aminoglycosides is characterized by interactions between the antibiotic molecule and the 16S rRNA. Although for all aminoglycosides the effect of this interaction is a change of conformation of the decoding A site producing one that resembles the closed state induced by interaction between cognate tRNA and mRNA, it must be noted that not all aminoglycosides seem to bind the same sites of the 16S rRNA. The consequence of the conformational change induced by the interaction 16S rRNA-aminoglycoside is the reduction of the proofreading capabilities of the ribosome, which in turns results in high levels of mistranslation (Bakker, 1992; Busse et al., 1992; Vakulenko and Mobashery, 2003; Vicens and Westhof, 2003; Magnet and Blanchard, 2005; Majumder et al., 2007; Zaher and Green, 2009; Ramirez and Tolmasky, 2010). Other molecular effects of some aminoglycosides have been described but it is not clear if some of them are not secondary to protein mistranslation. They include inhibition of 30S ribosomal subunit assembly, induction of RNA cleavage, or interference with the action of RNase P (Mikkelsen et al., 1999; Mehta and Champney, 2003; Belousoff et al., 2009).

Aminoglycosides are powerful tools against infections (Labaune et al., 2001; Avent et al., 2011) but unfortunately the levels of resistance are growing and in consequence failure of treatments with aminoglycosides is becoming more common (Galani et al., 2002; van 't Veen et al., 2005; Tolmasky, 2007a; Soler Bistue et al., 2008). Bacteria have developed numerous mechanisms to resist the action of aminoglycosides and cells can possess the genetic determinants for several of them enhancing the levels of resistance and making it very difficult to overcome all of them. Enzymatic inactivation by acetylation, adenylylation, or phosphorylation at different locations of the aminoglycoside molecule is among the most clinically relevant strategies bacteria use to resist the action of these antibiotics (Shaw et al., 1993; Vakulenko and Mobashery, 2003; Tolmasky, 2007a; Ramirez and Tolmasky, 2010; Chen et al., 2011; Chiang et al., 2013). The enzymes that catalyze these reactions are collectively known as aminoglycoside modifying enzymes. Other well studied mechanisms are: (1) mutation of the 16S rRNA or ribosomal proteins modify the target eliminating or reducing the interaction with the antibiotic molecule (O'Connor et al., 1991); (2) methylation of 16S rRNA, a mechanism found in most aminoglycoside-producing organisms and in clinical strains (Schmitt et al., 2009; Wachino and Arakawa, 2012); (3) reduced permeability to the antibiotic molecule by modification of the permeability of the outer membrane or diminished inner membrane transport (Hancock, 1981; Taber et al., 1987; Macleod et al., 2000; Over et al., 2001); (4) export outside the cell by active efflux pumps (Hocquet et al., 2003; Morita et al., 2012; Wachino and Arakawa, 2012); (5) sequestration by tight binding to a low active aminoglycoside acetyltransferase (Magnet et al., 2003); and (6) extracellular DNA shielding in biofilms (Chiang et al., 2013).

The general characteristics of all known aminoglycoside modifying enzymes have been recently reviewed (Ramirez and Tolmasky, 2010). This review will focus on the aminoglycoside 6'-*N*-acetyltransferase type Ib [AAC(6')-Ib], which is of great clinical relevance and it is found in over 70% of AAC(6')-I-producing gram-negative clinical isolates (Vakulenko and Mobashery, 2003), and has been the subject of numerous studies (Tolmasky, 2007a; Cambray and Mazel, 2008; Ramirez and Tolmasky, 2010).

THE AAC(6')-Ib PROTEIN

The aminoglycoside *N*-acetyltransferases (AAC) belong to the GCN5-related N-acetyltransferase superfamily, also known as GNAT. This is a large group of enzymes that includes about 10,000 proteins from all kinds of organisms that share the property to catalyze the acetylation of a primary amine in numerous acceptor molecules using acetyl CoA as donor substrate (Neuwald and Landsman, 1997; Dyda et al., 2000; Vetting et al., 2005). The AACs are subdivided in groups based on the position where the acetyl group is transferred in the acceptor aminoglycoside molecule. Known AACs catalyze acetylation at the 1 [AAC(1)], 3 [AAC(3)], 2' [AAC(2')], or 6' [AAC(6')] positions (Shaw et al., 1993; De Pascale and Wright, 2010; Ramirez and Tolmasky, 2010). AAC(6') enzymes are the most numerous group of AACs, more than 40 have been described, and can be found in gram-negatives as well as gram-positives (Shaw et al., 1993; Miller et al., 1997; Wright, 1999; Tolmasky, 2007a; Ramirez and Tolmasky, 2010). AAC(6') enzymes are subdivided in two groups, AAC(6')-I and AAC(6')-II, which are differentiated by the profile of the aminoglycosides inactivated. With a few exceptions, AAC(6')-I enzymes specify resistance to several aminoglycosides plus amikacin and gentamicin C1a and C2 but not to gentamicin C1 (Shaw et al., 1993). On the other hand, AAC(6')-II enzymes catalyze acetylation of all forms of gentamicin but not of amikacin (Rather et al., 1992). In addition, enzymes with extended spectrum that may merit addition of new subclasses of AAC(6')-I enzymes have been recently described (Casin et al., 2003; Robicsek et al., 2006; Strahilevitz et al., 2009). Phylogenetic analyses divided the AAC(6') enzymes into three clades. However, with the information available it is still not clear if all AAC(6') enzymes evolved from a single origin or the three groups are less related and the 6' acetylating activity has evolved independently at least three times (Salipante and Hall, 2003). According to the phylogenetic analyses recently communicated by Salipante and Hall (Salipante and Hall, 2003) the AAC(6')-Ib is most closely related to AAC(6')-IIa AAC(6')-IIb, AAC(6')-IIc, and AAC(6')-IId.

There are numerous variants of AAC(6')-Ib, many of them identified by modifications in the name of the enzyme such as the addition of subscripts or a prime symbol superscript (Cambray and Mazel, 2008; Ramirez and Tolmasky, 2010). However, a large number of versions of the protein, or predicted protein, have all been named AAC(6')-Ib, which can be a source of confusion or indetermination. These variants mainly differ at the N-terminus, however one should be careful when considering these differences because not in all of them the N-terminus has been experimentally determined (Dery et al., 1997; Casin et al., 2003; Soler Bistue et al., 2006; Maurice et al., 2008). **Table 1** shows a list of the *aac(6')-Ib* gene versions found in different genetic environments and bacterial species. Some variants differing at the N-termini such as AAC(6')-Ib$_3$, AAC(6')-Ib$_4$, AAC(6')-Ib$_6$, and AAC(6')-Ib$_7$ have been compared and it was found that they have similar behavior (Casin et al., 1998) but variations as small as one or two amino acids at key positions proved to be of high relevance (**Table 2**). For example, the AAC(6')-Ib$_{11}$ found in *S. Typhimurium* has L and S residues at positions 118 and 119 as opposed to Q and L or Q and S, the amino acids present at these positions in all previously described enzymes, acquired an extended resistance spectrum that includes all three gentamicin forms (Casin et al., 2003). (Amino acid numbers throughout the text are based on the sequence corresponding to accession number AF479774.) Another example worth mentioning is the AAC(6')-Ib', originally found in *Pseudomonas fluorescens* BM2687, but previously generated by site-directed mutagenesis in the laboratory (**Table 1**). This protein has a L to S substitution at amino acid 119 that confers the enzyme an AAC(6')-II profile, i.e., the enzyme confers resistance to gentamicin but

Table 1 | AAC(6′)-Ib variants.

Number	AAC(6′)-Ib enzyme	Gene allele	Genetic localization	Species	Reference
1	NP_608307	*aac(6′)-Ib*	pJHCMW1::Tn*1331*, pKPN4, pMET1::Tn*1331.2*, pKlebpneu15S, pR23::Tn*1331*, pAAC154::ΔTn*1331*, pColEST258, pJHC-MW1, Tn*1332*, class 1 integron, pRMH712::Tn*1331*, SGI1-V::class 1 integron	*K. pneumoniae*, *En.* spp., *Pseudomonas putida*, *Proteus mirabilis*	NP_608307, YP_001338668, YP_001928078, YP_001928081, YP_002286819, YP_004455304, YP_006958960, YP_006959190, ZP_14492679 (contig), ZP_14498301 (contig), ZP_14503930 (contig), ZP_14509538 (contig), ZP_14515174 (contig), ZP_14520767 (contig), ZP_14526392 (contig), ZP_14531781 (contig), ZP_14537604 (contig), ZP_14543183 (contig), ZP_14548764 (contig), ZP_14554292 (contig), ZP_14559831 (contig), ZP_14565429 (contig), ZP_14571055 (contig), ZP_14576504 (contig), ZP_14581777 (contig), ZP_14587733 (contig), ZP_14593028 (contig), ZP_14598930 (contig), ZP_19010829 (contig), AAC6_KLEPN, AF479774_5, AAA69747, AAA98404, ABA54975, ABR80438, ACB55476, ACB55479, ACI63081, ACL36604, ADK35766, AED98720, AED99555, AEG74535, AEW43367, EJJ31842 (contig), EJJ31842 (contig), EJJ31884 (contig), EJJ31888 (contig), EJJ48672 (contig), EJJ48714 (contig), EJJ49532 (contig), EJJ65671 (contig), EJJ65889 (contig), EJJ68295 (contig), EJJ79581 (contig), EJJ81436 (contig), EJJ85464 (contig), EJJ96302 (contig), EJJ96595 (contig), EJK03278 (contig), EJK13161 (contig), EJK16025 (contig), EJK18863 (contig), EJK30890 (contig),

(Continued)

Table 1 | Continued

Number	AAC(6′)-Ib enzyme	Gene allele	Genetic localization	Species	Reference
					EJK33635 (contig), EKV58688 (contig)
2	YP_002286969	*aac(6′)-Ib*	p12::Tn*1331*	*K. pneumoniae, E. coli*	YP_002286969, ZP_16459764 (genomic scaffold), ZP_19016755 (contig), ACI63027, EGB78408 (contig), EKV58524 (contig)
3	AAA26550	*aac(6′)-Ib*	pAZ007	*Serratia marcescens*	AAA26550
4	AAR18814	*aac(6′)-Ib*	pKP31::class 1 integron	*K. pneumoniae*	AAR18814
5	CBI63199	*aac(6′)-Ib*	Class 1 integron	*P. aeruginosa*	CBI63199
6	CBI63201	*aac(6′)-Ib*	Class 1 integron	*P. aeruginosa*	CBI63201
7	CBI63203	*aac(6′)-Ib*	Class 1 integron	*P. aeruginosa*	CBI63203
8	ABG77519	*aac(6′)-Ib*	Class 1 integron	*P. aeruginosa*	ABG77519
9	CBL95252	*aac(6′)-Ib*	Class 1 integron	*P. aeruginosa*	CBL95252
10	CBL95256	*aac(6′)-Ib*	Class 1 integron	*P. aeruginosa*	CBL95256
11	CBI63204	*aac(6′)-Ib*	Class 1 integron	*P. aeruginosa*	CBI63204
12	CBI63202	*aac(6′)-Ib*	Class 1 integron	*P. aeruginosa*	CBI63202
13	YP_003937697	*aac(6′)-Ib*	pETN48::Δclass 1 integron	*E. coli*	YP_003937697, CBX36023
14	ADC80806	*aac(6′)-Ib*	pRYC103T24::class 1 integron In4-like, pKSP212::class 1 integron	*E. coli*, uncultured bacterium	ADC80806, AFR44153
15	YP_005797131	*aac(6′)-Ib*	Class 1 integron (Chromosome)	*A. baumannii*	YP_005797131, AEN92376
16	YP_005525242	*aac(6′)-Ib*	Class 1 integron (Chromosome)	*A. baumannii*	YP_005525242, YP_006289231, YP_006848983, ZP_11603605 (contig), ZP_16142456 (contig), ZP_16146111 (contig), EGK45756 (seq0044), AEP05746, AFI94936, EKE64317 (contig), EKE64588 (contig), AFU38752
17	NP_863005	*aac(6′)-Ib*	p1658/97::class 1 integron, class 1 integron (Chromosome), class 1 integron, plasmid In238a	*E. coli, A. baumannii, K. pneumoniae, K. oxytoca, En. cloacae*	NP_863005, YP_001844882, AAO49600, ACZ55927, ACZ64698, AFS33307
18	ADC80825	*aac(6′)-Ib*	pRYC103T24::class 1 integron	*E. coli*	ADC80825

(Continued)

Table 1 | Continued

Number	AAC(6′)-Ib enzyme	Gene allele	Genetic localization	Species	Reference
19	YP_002791392	*aac(6′)-Ib*	pEC-IMP::class 1 integron, pEC-IMPQ::class 1 integron, pb1004::class 1 integron, class 1 integron	*En. cloacae, Salmonella enterica subsp. enterica* serovar *Bredeney, P. aeruginosa*	YP_002791392, YP_002791702, ACF59628, ACO54016, ACO54326, ADF47469
20	AEO50496	*aac(6′)-Ib*	Class 1 integron	*Se. marcescens*	AEO50496
21	ACB41759	*aac(6′)-Ib*	Class 1 integron	*E. coli*	ACB41759
22	BAL45797	*aac(6′)-Ib*	pKPI-6::class 1 integron	*K. pneumoniae*	BAL45797
23	AAC46343	*aac(6′)-Ib*	Class 1 integron	*P. aeruginosa*	AAC46343
24	AAD02244	*aac(6′)-Ib9*	Class 1 integron	*P. aeruginosa*	AAD02244
25	YP_003108195	*aac(6′)-Ib-cr*	pEK516, pEK499, pEC_L8, pUUH239.2	*E. coli, K. pneumoniae*	YP_003108195, YP_003108338, YP_003829182, YP_005351453, ACQ41894, ACQ42045, ADL14076, AET17280
26	ZP_18354173	*aac(6′)-Ib-cr*		*K. pneumoniae*	ZP_18354173 (genomic scaffold), EKF76226
27	ACD56150	*aac(6′)-Ib-cr*	pHS1387::class 1 integron	*Escherichia coli*	ACD56150
28	ADY02579	*aac(6′)-Ib-cr*	Class 1 integron	*Aeromonas media*	ADY02579
29	NP_957555	*aac(6′)-Ib-cr*	pC15-1a, pKP96::class 1 integron, pNDM-MAR, pGUE-NDM, pKDO1, pHe96, pKas96, pECZ6-1::class 1 integron, Class 1 integron, pLC108::class 1 integron, pJIE101,	*Escherichia coli, K. pneumoniae, Kluyvera ascorbata,* mixed culture bacterium, *K. oxytoca, Se. rubidaea, En. cloacae, Aeromonas allosaccharophila, Providencia* spp., *Shigella* spp., *En. aerogenes*	NP_957555, YP_002332851, YP_005352168, YP_006953881, YP_006973732, AAR25030, ABC17627, ABM47029, ABY74389, ACD03312, ACD03322, ACM24788, ACT97328, ACT97332, ACT97345, ACT97681, ACV60575, ADA60222, ADE44336, ADP30789, ADU16107, ADU16118, ADY02556, AEC49701, AEC49704, AEL33522, AEO45791, AEO79936, AEO79967, AEP16466, AER36609, AEU10750, AEU10754, AFB82784, AFC38861, AFI72862, AFV52812, AFV70394
30	1V0C_A	*aac(6′)-Ib*		*Escherichia coli* Chain A, Structure	1V0C_A, 2BUE_A, 2VQY_A
31	YP_006501621		pKOX_R1::class 1 integron, class 1 integorn,	*K. oxytoca, K. pneumoniae*	YP_006501621, AFM57748, AFN35014

(Continued)

Table 1 | Continued

Number	AAC(6′)-Ib enzyme	Gene allele	Genetic localization	Species	Reference
32	ABC54722	*aac(6′)-Ib*	pAS1::InVC117	*Vibrio cholerae*	ABC54722
33	BAE66666	*aac(6′)-Ib*	Class 1 integron	*Vibrio cholerae* O1	BAE66666
34	YP_007232190	*aac(6′)-Ib*	pPC9	*P. putida*	YP_007232190
35	ZP_16084267	*aac(6′)-Ib*	Class 1 integron (Chromosome)	*A. baumannii*	ZP_16084267 (contig), ZP_16086960 (contig), ZP_16140385 (contig), EKA73751 (contig), EKK08901 (contig), EKK18976 (contig)
36	AFS51540	*aac(6′)-Ib9*	pKS208::class 1 integron	Uncultured bacterium	AFS51540
37	YP_006957899	*aac(6′)-Ib-cr4*	pMdT	*SS. enterica* subsp. *enterica serovar* Typhimurium	YP_006957899, AFU63391
38	ADZ96942	*aac(6′)-Ib-cr*	Plasmid	*K. pneumoniae*	ADZ96942
39	CAA42873	*aac(6′)-Ib3, aac(6′)-Ib5*	plasmid pCFF04	*P. aeruginosa*	CAA42873
40	AAB24284	*aac(6′)-Ib4*	pSP21::class 1 integron, pEI1573::class 1 integron	*Se.* spp., uncultured bacterium, *En. cloacae*	AAB24284, YP_006941442, YP_006965430
41	AAN41403	*aac(6′)-Ib11*	pSTI1::class 1 integron	*SS. enterica* subsp. *enterica* serovar Typhimurium	AAN41403
42	YP_006903338	*aac(6′)-Ib*	pNDM102337::class 1 integron, pNDM10505::class 1 integron	*Escherichia coli*	YP_006903338, YP_006953195
43	YP_006959139	*aac(6′)-Ib*	pNDM10469::class 1 integron	*K. pneumoniae*	YP_006959139
44		*aac(6′)-Ib7*	Plasmid	*En. cloacae, Citrobacter freundii*	Not available
45		*aac(6′)-Ib8*	Plasmid	*En. cloacae*	Not available

The pJHCMW1-encoded AAC(6′)-Ib variant (accession number NP_608307) was subjected to BLASTP and the identical proteins were identified. Those that were closely related but not identical were identified by numbers. The names given in the publications or GenBank entries are shown. Those that were named aacA4 were named aac(6′)-Ib here.

not amikacin (Rather et al., 1992; Lambert et al., 1994). A highly surprising effect occurred in the natural variant known as AAC(6′)-Ib-cr, which has the modifications W104R and N181Y (**Tables 1, 2**). The substrate spectrum was expanded to include quinolone antibiotics, crossing the barrier from the aminoglycosides (Robicsek et al., 2006). Since the first detection of the AAC(6′)-Ib-cr variant there have been numerous reports of its presence, and variants of it, across the world in different genetic environments suggesting an extraordinary ability to disseminate (Quiroga et al., 2007; Cattoir and Nordmann, 2009; Strahilevitz et al., 2009; Rodriguez-Martinez et al., 2011; Ruiz et al., 2012; De Toro et al., 2013). Furthermore, there have been cases where a strain was found to simultaneously include genes coding for AAC(6′)-Ib and AAC(6′)-Ib-cr (Kim et al., 2011). AAC(6′)-Ib is also found fused to the C-terminal end of AAC(3)-Ib protein within a class I integron found in a *Pseudomonas aeruginosa* strain (Dubois et al., 2002) and to the C-terminus of the AAC(6′)-30 also within a *P. aeruginosa* class I integron (Mendes et al., 2004).

Subcellular localization studies of the AAC(6′)-Ib enzyme encoded by Tn*1331* showed that the enzyme is homogeneously distributed in the cytoplasmic compartment (Dery et al., 2003).

Table 2 | Phenotypes of representative mutants of AAC(6′)-Ib.

Mutation[a]	AAC(6′)-Ib variant name	Phenotype	References
Y80C		S	Panaite and Tolmasky, 1998
D117A		S	Pourreza et al., 2005
L119S	AAC(6′)-Ib′, AAC(6′)-Ib_7, AAC(6′)-Ib_8^b	Specificity, Gm^r Ak^s	Rather et al., 1992; Lambert et al., 1994; Casin et al., 2003
Q118L, L119S	AAC(6′)-Ib_{11}	Specificity, Gm^r Ak^r	Casin et al., 2003
L120A		S	Pourreza et al., 2005
Y166A		Specificity, Ak^S Km^r	Shmara et al., 2001
E167A		S	Shmara et al., 2001
F171A		S	Shmara et al., 2001
F171L		Thermosensitive for Ak and Nm	Panaite and Tolmasky, 1998; Shmara et al., 2001
W104R, D181Y	AAC(6′)-Ib-cr	Expanded substrate spectrum including quinolones	Robicsek et al., 2006

S, susceptible.
[a] Numbering from sequence in accession number AF479774.
[b] The proteins differ at the amino terminus.

AAC(6′)-Ib was one of three aminoglycoside modifying enzymes used in a study consisting of molecular dynamics simulations of the enzymes and aminoglycoside ribosomal RNA binding site, unliganded, and complexed with an aminoglycoside, kanamycin A. These studies concluded that the enzymes efficiently mimic the nucleic acid environment of the ribosomal RNA binding cleft (Romanowska et al., 2013). Extensive studies using mutagenesis showed some interesting phenotypes such as modifications in specificity, enhanced activity, or selective thermosensitivity (**Table 2**) (Panaite and Tolmasky, 1998; Chavideh et al., 1999; Shmara et al., 2001; Casin et al., 2003; Pourreza et al., 2005; Kim et al., 2007; Maurice et al., 2008). In addition, alanine scanning showed that several amino acid substitutions by A had minor effects. These mutagenesis studies together with structural and enzymatic analyses led to a deep understanding of features and characteristics of AAC(6′)-Ib proteins (Rather et al., 1992; Vetting et al., 2004; Maurice et al., 2008; Vetting et al., 2008; Ramirez and Tolmasky, 2010). The three dimensional structure of AAC(6′)-Ib and AAC(6′)-Ib_{11} have been experimentally determined in various conditions. AAC(6′)-Ib was crystallized in complex with coenzyme A and also in complex with both coenzyme A and kanamycin. The structures were solved to 1.8 Å and 2.4 Å resolution, respectively (Maurice et al., 2008). The broad spectrum variant AAC(6′)-Ib_{11} was crystallized in the absence of substrate and the structure was solved to 2.1 Å resolution (Maurice et al., 2008). These studies concluded that AAC(6′)-Ib exists as a monomer while AAC(6′)-Ib_{11} shows monomer/dimer equilibrium (Maurice et al., 2008). This was a somewhat surprising finding considering that previous studies had shown that two other acetyltransferases, AAC(6′)-Ii and AAC(6′)-Iy, exist as dimers (Wright and Ladak, 1997; Wybenga-Groot et al., 1999; Draker et al., 2003; Vetting et al., 2004; Wright and Berghuis, 2007; Vong et al., 2012). Interestingly, analysis of these crystal structures showed the presence of a flexible flap in AAC(6′)-Ib_{11} that may be the basis for its ability to utilize amikacin as well as gentamicin as substrates (Maurice et al., 2008). In another study a molecular model of AAC(6′)-Ib-cr has been generated (Maurice et al., 2008; Vetting et al., 2008), which led to postulate that the D181Y substitution is mainly responsible for modification in the strength of binding of the antibiotic substrate and that the substitution W104R stabilizes the positioning of Y181 (Robicsek et al., 2006; Strahilevitz et al., 2009).

Table 1 shows that there are 45 non-identical AAC(6′)-Ib related entries in the NCBI database, 32 of which have identical name in spite of not having identical amino acid sequence. The N-termini of these proteins show the highest degree of heterogeneity with high variations in length stretching up to 60 amino acids, but these differences were suggested to be irrelevant (Casin et al., 1998; Maurice et al., 2008). Therefore, we defined a highly conserved central region composed of 181 amino acids shared by all proteins, which were compared using the MAFFT alignment algorithm (Katoh and Standley, 2013). Pairwise comparisons show that the sequences have 1 to 8 amino acid differences and a total of 24 positions showed amino acid variations. Moreover, clustering using the UPGMA algorithm (Sneath and Sokal, 1973) defined 18 sequence clusters, 14 of which consist of a singleton, and 4 of which include 2–16 proteins (**Figure 1**). Different clusters can exhibit similar properties while others show substantial differences in their characteristics such as those cases in which there are significant specificity variations like extended substrate spectrum as described in the above paragraphs.

THE *aac(6′)-Ib* GENE

The *aac(6′)-Ib* genes are usually found as fully functional or deficient gene cassettes associated to class 1 integrons, insertion sequences such as IS*26*, and truncated or disrupted integrons (**Figure 2** and **Table 1**) (Sarno et al., 2002; Woodford et al., 2009; Ramirez and Tolmasky, 2010). These genetic elements may be part of plasmids, transposons, genomic islands, or other structures such as the KQ element (Rice et al., 2008), which together contribute to the gene's ability to disseminate at the cellular and molecular levels (Tolmasky, 2007b). When present in integrons, *aac(6′)-Ib* gene cassettes can be found located adjacent to the 5′-conserved region, i.e., flanked by *attI* and *attC*, or internal to the variable portion containing *attC* loci at both ends (**Figure 2**). In both cases, as expected, the gene cassette can be mobilized by the integrase IntI1 (**Figure 2**) (Cambray et al., 2010; Hall, 2012). In addition, a gene cassette-like structure containing *aac(6′)-Ib*, composed of a copy of *attI1** at

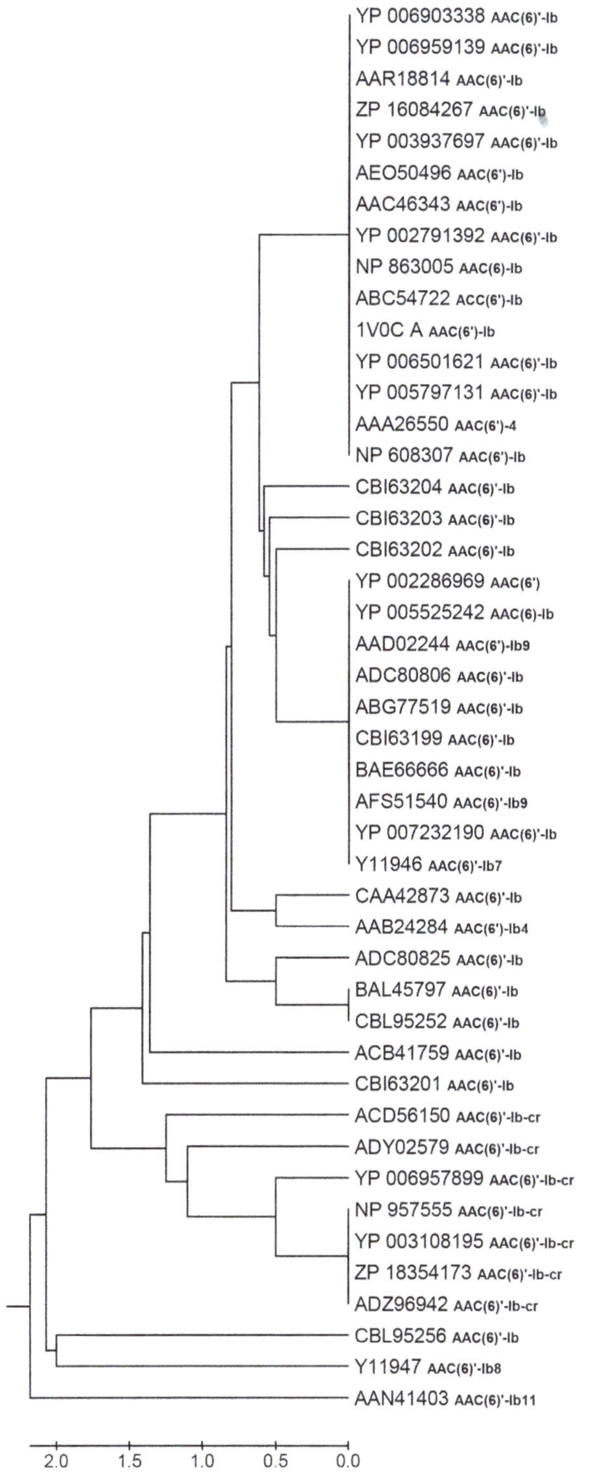

FIGURE 1 | UPGMA clustering analyses of 45 AAC(6′)-Ib protein sequences. The optimal tree with the sum of branch length = 20.70628249 is shown. The evolutionary distances were computed using the number of differences method and are in the units of the number of amino acid differences per sequence. All positions containing gaps and missing data were eliminated. There were a total of 181 positions in the final dataset. Evolutionary analyses were conducted in MEGA5.

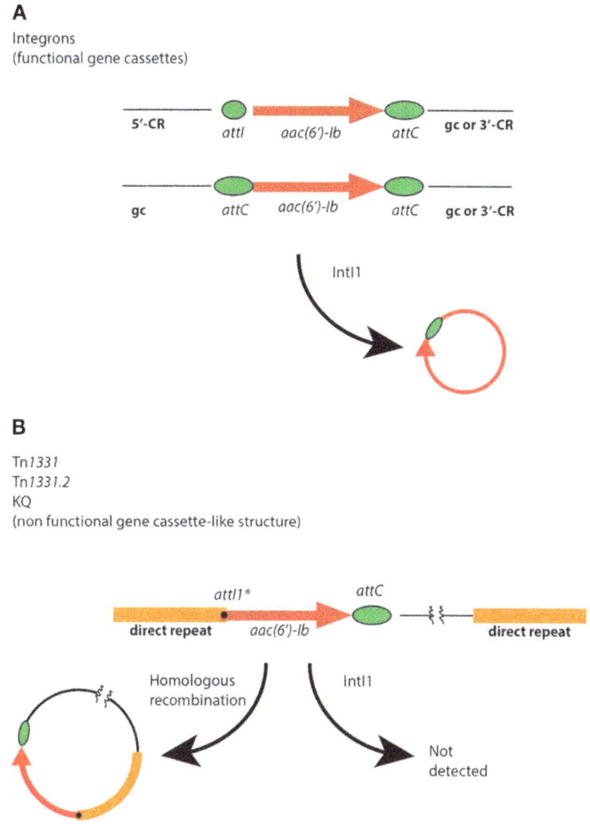

FIGURE 2 | Mobilization of *aac(6′)-Ib*. (A) Generic genetic maps of integrons in which an *aac(6′)-Ib* gene cassette is located immediately following the 5′ conserved region (5′-CR) (top map) or following one or more gene cassettes (gc) inside the variable portion, and followed by other gene cassettes or the 3′ conserved region (3′-CR) (bottom map). The small green ellipse represents *attI* and the big green ellipses represent *attC*. **(B)** Relevant portion of the Tn*1331*, Tn*1331.2*, and KQ elements (Tolmasky and Crosa, 1987; Tolmasky et al., 1988; Sarno et al., 2002; Rice et al., 2008). For clarity Tn*1332*, which has a more complicated structure in its direct repeats (Poirel et al., 2006), is not shown, but it could experience mobilization by homologous recombination as shown. The black dot represents *attI1**. The homologous recombination pathway for generation of an *aac(6′)-Ib*-containing circular molecule has been proposed by Zong et al. (2009).

the beginning of the structural gene and a regular *attC* downstream of it (see **Figure 2**), was found as part of a region resembling the variable portion of integrons in Tn*1331* (Woloj et al., 1986; Tolmasky et al., 1988; Tolmasky, 1990; Tolmasky and Crosa, 1993; Sarno et al., 2002), Tn*1331.2* (Tolmasky and Crosa, 1991), Tn*1332* (Poirel et al., 2006), the KQ element (Rice et al., 2008), a Tn*1331* derivative recently isolated from a clinical *Klebsiella pneumoniae* strain belonging to the ST512, which derived from the ST258, known to be spread worldwide (Chen et al., 2012; Garcia-Fernandez et al., 2012; Warburg et al., 2012), and a complex mosaic region present in the chromosome of *Proteus mirabilis* JIE273 (Zong et al., 2009). Assays overexpressing IntI1 in cells containing Tn*1331* were unable to detect any excision of the *aac(6′)-Ib* gene cassette-like structure, suggesting that it is nonfunctional or it excises at an extremely low efficiency (Ramirez et al., 2008). Interestingly, despite the IntI1-mediated lack of mobility of this DNA region, the gene could be mobilized by means of a mechanism recently proposed by Zong et al. that occurs through homologous recombination between 520-bp direct repeats located upstream and downstream of the gene cassette-like structure (**Figure 2**) (Zong et al., 2009).

These multiple locations taken together with the ability of the genetic elements to spread at the molecular and cellular level provide *aac(6′)-Ib* genes with the capability to reach virtually all gram-negatives and other undetermined bacteria such as those that are still unculturable. The gene has also been found in plasmids harboring resistance genes of high importance such as the recently described *ndm-1* (Yong et al., 2009; Bonnin et al., 2012; Villa et al., 2012).

INHIBITION

The rise in drug resistance affects all known antibiotics and has been identified as one of the greatest threats to human health. Therefore, there is an immediate need for new agents with activity against multiresistant bacteria and at the present moment there is no evidence that this need will be fully met in the near future (Boucher et al., 2009). A group of pathogens that cause the majority of hospital infections, named ESKAPE (*Enterococcus faecium, Staphylococcus aureus, K. pneumoniae, Acinetobacter baumannii, P aeruginosa,* and *Enterobacter*), is becoming highly resistant to antibiotics including aminoglycosides (Rice, 2008). They carry aminoglycoside modifying enzymes genes, and one of the most common in the gram-negative members is *aac(6′)-Ib* (Ramirez and Tolmasky, 2010; Shaul et al., 2011; Herzog et al., 2012). An obvious solution to this problem would be the development of new aminoglycosides, a strategy that is being pursued using numerous approaches (Green et al., 2010, 2011; Houghton et al., 2010). A variety of new aminoglycoside derivatives including chemical modification of existing aminoglycosides, aminoglycoside dimers, or aminoglycoside-small molecule conjugated are being produced and tested (reviewed in Houghton et al., 2010). In particular plazomicin (ACHN-490), a novel neoglycoside derived from sisomicin that carries a hydroxymethyl group at position 6′, has shown enhanced activity against multiresistance gram-negatives and gram-positives including strains carrying *aac(6′)-Ib* (Endimiani et al., 2009; Landman et al., 2011).

Others are approaching the problem in such a way that the existing aminoglycosides continue to be effective by designing enzymatic inhibitors that can act in combination with the antibiotic, mimicking the strategy successfully used to curb resistance to β-lactams (Williams and Northrop, 1979; Daigle et al., 1997; Haddad et al., 1999; Liu et al., 2000; Burk and Berghuis, 2002; Boehr et al., 2003; Draker et al., 2003; Gao et al., 2005, 2006; Welch et al., 2005; Lombes et al., 2008; Magalhaes et al., 2008; De Pascale and Wright, 2010; Drawz and Bonomo, 2010; Green et al., 2012; Vong et al., 2012). However, these efforts are still scarce when one compares them to those invested to discover and design β-lactamase inhibitors. Furthermore, the attempts to find inhibitors of AAC(6′)-Ib have only yielded a compound, synthesized using non-aminoglycoside-like fragments, with a rather modest level of inhibition of AAC(6′)-Ib (Lombes et al., 2008).

An alternative approach that is being explored is silencing expression of the resistance gene. Early attempts at interfering with expression of *aac(6′)-Ib* consisted of identifying regions available for interaction with antisense oligonucleotides in a monocistronic *in vitro* synthesized mRNA by RNase H mapping in combination with computer prediction of its secondary structure (Sarno et al., 2003). The selected sites were used as targets for a collection of oligodeoxynucleotides, of which some had the ability to induce RNase H-mediated *in vitro* degradation of the mRNA, inhibited *in vitro* synthesis of the enzyme in coupled transcription/translation assays, and upon delivery by electroporation significantly reduced the number of cells surviving after exposure to amikacin (Sarno et al., 2003). The mechanism of this *in vivo* inhibition is most probably through RNase H digestion of the mRNA, but other possibilities such as steric hindrance cannot be discarded at this time. Alternatively, modest but significant inhibition of expression of *aac(6′)-Ib* was achieved by applying EGS technology, in which short antisense RNA molecules, known as external guide sequences, are used to elicit RNase P-mediated degradation of a target mRNA (Guerrier-Takada et al., 1997; Lundblad and Altman, 2010). Initially, *E. coli* harboring *aac(6′)-Ib* were transformed with recombinant clones specifying the appropriate RNA oligonucleotide sequences under an inducible promoter. The transformed derivatives were then cultured in the presence of amikacin under conditions of expression of the external guide sequences. The results showed that in a few cases the external guide sequences induced a reduction of the minimal inhibitory concentration of amikacin (Soler Bistue et al., 2007). These results were considered proof of concept, but the strategy was not viable because antisense oligonucleotides must be added from the milieu and find their way inside the cells without being degraded. Thus, nuclease resistant oligonucleotide analogs that still induce inhibition of gene expression by RNase P activation had to be found. Out of a variety of oligoribonucleotide analogs including 2′-*O*-methyl oligoribonucleotides, phosphorodiamidate morpholino oligomers, phosphorothioate oligodeoxynucleotides, or locked nucleic acids (LNA)/DNA co-oligomers that were tested, LNA/DNA co-oligomers with certain configurations were found to be capable of eliciting RNase P-mediated cleavage of mRNA *in vitro* (Soler Bistue et al., 2009). Following this finding, a selected LNA/DNA co-oligomer was added to the hyperpermeable *E. coli* AS19 harboring *aac(6′)-Ib* and it was found that growth was inhibited in the presence of amikacin, indicating that the compound may have induced RNase P-mediated inhibition of expression of the gene (Soler Bistue et al., 2009). These results were encouraging but it must be noted that inhibition of expression of *aac(6′)-Ib* is still far from being a viable option to overcome aminoglycoside resistance in the clinical setting. Several problems remain to be solved like inducing penetration of the oligonucleotide analogs inside wild type cells in enough quantities to exert the biological activity or achieve enough inhibition levels in spite of the usual presence of multiple copies of the gene due to its inclusion in high copy number plasmids. Toward finding solutions to these problems, recent experiments suggest that LNA/DNA co-oligomers may be able to reach the cytoplasm of untreated cells at low efficiency (Traglia et al., 2012). Strategies will have to be developed to increase the efficiency of delivery inside bacterial cells.

ACKNOWLEDGMENTS

The authors' work cited in this review article was funded by Public Health Service grant 2R15AI047115 (to Marcelo E. Tolmasky) from the National Institutes of Health. María S. Ramirez is a research career member of C.O.N.I.C.E.T.

REFERENCES

Avent, M. L., Rogers, B. A., Cheng, A. C., and Paterson, D. L. (2011). Current use of aminoglycosides: indications, pharmacokinetics and monitoring for toxicity. *Intern. Med. J.* 41, 441–449.

Bakker, E. P. (1992). Aminoglycoside and aminocyclitol antibiotics: hygromycin B is an atypical bactericidal compound that exerts effects on cells of *Escherichia coli* characteristics for bacteriostatic aminocyclitols. *J. Gen. Microbiol.* 138, 563–569.

Belousoff, M. J., Graham, B., Spiccia, L., and Tor, Y. (2009). Cleavage of RNA oligonucleotides by aminoglycosides. *Org. Biomol. Chem.* 7, 30–33.

Bidou, L., Allamand, V., Rousset, J. P., and Namy, O. (2012). Sense from nonsense: therapies for premature stop codon diseases. *Trends Mol. Med.* 18, 679–688.

Boehr, D. D., Draker, K. A., Koteva, K., Bains, M., Hancock, R. E., and Wright, G. D. (2003). Broad-spectrum peptide inhibitors of aminoglycoside antibiotic resistance enzymes. *Chem. Biol.* 10, 189–196.

Bonnin, R. A., Poirel, L., Carattoli, A., and Nordmann, P. (2012). Characterization of an IncFII plasmid encoding NDM-1 from *Escherichia coli* ST131. *PLoS ONE* 7:e34752. doi: 10.1371/journal.pone.0034752

Boucher, H. W., Talbot, G. H., Bradley, J. S., Edwards, J. E., Gilbert, D., Rice, L. B., et al. (2009). Bad bugs, no drugs: no ESKAPE! An update from the Infectious Diseases Society of America. *Clin. Infect. Dis.* 48, 1–12.

Brossier, F., Veziris, N., Aubry, A., Jarlier, V., and Sougakoff, W. (2010). Detection by Geno- type MTBDRsl test of complex resistance mechanisms to second-line drugs and ethambutol in multidrug-resistant *Mycobacterium tuberculosis* complex isolates. *J. Clin. Microbiol.* 48, 1683–1689.

Bryskier, A. (2005). "Antibiotics and antibacterial agents: classifications and structure- activity relationships," in *Antimicrobial Agents*, ed A. Bryskier (Washington, DC: ASM Press), 13–38.

Burk, D. L., and Berghuis, A. M. (2002). Protein kinase inhibitors and antibiotic resistance. *Pharmacol. Ther.* 93, 283–292.

Busse, H. J., Wostmann, C., and Bakker, E. P. (1992). The bactericidal action of streptomycin: membrane permeabilization caused by the insertion of mistranslated proteins into the cytoplasmic membrane of *Escherichia coli* and subsequent caging of the antibiotic inside the cells due to degradation of these proteins. *J. Gen. Microbiol.* 138, 551–561.

Cambray, G., Guerout, A. M., and Mazel, D. (2010). Integrons. *Annu. Rev. Genet.* 44, 141–166.

Cambray, G., and Mazel, D. (2008). Synonymous genes explore different evolutionary landscapes. *PLoS Genet.* 4:e1000256. doi: 10.1371/journal.pgen.1000256

Casin, I., Bordon, F., Bertin, P., Coutrot, A., Podglajen, I., Brasseur, R., et al. (1998). Aminoglycoside 6′-*N*-acetyltransferase variants of the Ib type with altered substrate profile in clinical isolates of *Enterobacter cloacae* and *Citrobacter freundii*. *Antimicrob. Agents Chemother.* 42, 209–215.

Casin, I., Hanau-Bercot, B., Podglajen, I., Vahaboglu, H., and Collatz, E. (2003). *Salmonella enterica* serovar Typhimurium *bla*(PER-1)-carrying plasmid pSTI1 encodes an extended-spectrum aminoglycoside 6′-*N*-acetyltransferase of type Ib. *Antimicrob. Agents Chemother.* 47, 697–703.

Cattoir, V., and Nordmann, P. (2009). Plasmid-mediated quinolone resistance in gram-negative bacterial species: an update. *Curr. Med. Chem.* 16, 1028–1046.

Chavideh, R., Sholly, S., Panaite, D., and Tolmasky, M. E. (1999). Effects of F171 mutations in the 6′-*N*-acetyltransferase type Ib [AAC(6′)-Ib] enzyme on susceptibility to aminoglycosides. *Antimicrob. Agents Chemother.* 43, 2811–2812.

Chen, L., Chavda, K. D., Mediavilla, J. R., Zhao, Y., Fraimow, H. S., Jenkins, S. G., et al. (2012). Multiplex real-time PCR for detection of an epidemic KPC-producing *Klebsiella pneumoniae* ST258 clone. *Antimicrob. Agents Chemother.* 56, 3444–3447.

Chen, W., Biswas, T., Porter, V. R., Tsodikov, O. V., and Garneau-Tsodikova, S. (2011). Unusual regioversatility of acetyltransferase Eis, a cause of drug resistance in XDR-TB. *Proc. Natl. Acad. Sci. U.S.A.* 108, 9804–9808.

Chiang, W. C., Nilsson, M., Jensen, P. O., Hoiby, N., Nielsen, T. E., Givskov, M., et al. (2013). Extracellular DNA shields against aminoglycosides in *Pseudomonas aeruginosa* biofilms. *Antimicrob. Agents Chemother.* 57, 2352–2361.

Daigle, D. M., McKay, G. A., and Wright, G. D. (1997). Inhibition of aminoglycoside antibiotic resistance enzymes by protein kinase inhibitors. *J. Biol. Chem.* 272, 24755–24758.

De Pascale, G., and Wright, G. D. (2010). Antibiotic resistance by enzyme inactivation: from mechanisms to solutions. *Chembiochem* 11, 1325–1334.

Dery, K. J., Chavideh, R., Waters, V., Chamorro, R., Tolmasky, L. S., and Tolmasky, M. E. (1997). Characterization of the replication and mobilization regions of the multiresistance *Klebsiella pneumoniae* plasmid pJHCMW1. *Plasmid* 38, 97–105.

Dery, K. J., Soballe, B., Witherspoon, M. S., Bui, D., Koch, R., Sherratt, D. J., et al. (2003). The aminoglycoside 6′-N-acetyltransferase type Ib encoded by Tn*1331* is evenly distributed within the cell's cytoplasm. *Antimicrob. Agents Chemother.* 47, 2897–2902.

De Toro, M., Rodriguez, I., Rojo-Bezares, B., Helmuth, R., Torres, C., Guerra, B., et al. (2013). pMdT1, a small ColE1-like plasmid mobilizing a new variant of the *aac(6′)-Ib-cr* gene in *Salmonella enterica* serovar Typhimurium. *J. Antimicrob. Chemother.* doi: 10.1093/jac/dkt001. [Epub ahead of print].

Draker, K. A., Northrop, D. B., and Wright, G. D. (2003). Kinetic mechanism of the GCN5-related chromosomal aminoglycoside acetyltransferase AAC(6′)-Ii from *Enterococcus faecium*: evidence of dimer subunit cooperativity. *Biochemistry* 42, 6565–6574.

Drawz, S. M., and Bonomo, R. A. (2010). Three decades of beta-lactamase inhibitors. *Clin. Microbiol. Rev.* 23, 160–201.

Dubois, V., Poirel, L., Marie, C., Arpin, C., Nordmann, P., and Quentin, C. (2002). Molecular characterization of a novel class 1 integron containing *bla*(GES-1) and a fused product of *aac3-Ib/aac6′-Ib′* gene cassettes in *Pseudomonas aeruginosa*. *Antimicrob. Agents Chemother.* 46, 638–645.

Dyda, F., Klein, D. C., and Hickman, A. B. (2000). GCN5-related N-acetyltransferases: a structural overview. *Annu. Rev. Biophys. Biomol. Struct.* 29, 81–103.

Endimiani, A., Hujer, K. M., Hujer, A. M., Armstrong, E. S., Choudhary, Y., Aggen, J. B., et al. (2009). ACHN-490, a neoglycoside with potent *in vitro* activity against multidrug-resistant *Klebsiella pneumoniae* isolates. *Antimicrob. Agents Chemother.* 53, 4504–4507.

Galani, I., Xirouchaki, E., Kanellakopoulou, K., Petrikkos, G., and Giamarellou, H. (2002). Transferable plasmid mediating resistance to multiple antimicrobial agents in *Klebsiella pneumoniae* isolates in Greece. *Clin. Microbiol. Infect.* 8, 579–588.

Gao, F., Yan, X., Baettig, O. M., Berghuis, A. M., and Auclair, K. (2005). Regio- and chemoselective 6′-*N*-derivatization of aminoglycosides: bisubstrate inhibitors as probes to study aminoglycoside 6′-*N*-acetyltransferases. *Angew. Chem. Int. Ed. Engl.* 44, 6859–6862.

Gao, F., Yan, X., Shakya, T., Baettig, O. M., Ait-Mohand-Brunet, S., Berghuis, A. M., et al. (2006). Synthesis and structure-activity relationships of truncated bisubstrate inhibitors of aminoglycoside 6′-*N*-acetyltransferases. *J. Med. Chem.* 49, 5273–5281.

Garcia-Fernandez, A., Villa, L., Carta, C., Venditti, C., Giordano, A., Venditti, M., et al. (2012). *Klebsiella pneumoniae* ST258 producing KPC-3 identified in italy carries novel plasmids and OmpK36/OmpK35 porin variants. *Antimicrob. Agents Chemother.* 56, 2143–2145.

Green, K. D., Chen, W., and Garneau-Tsodikova, S. (2011). Effects of altering aminoglycoside structures on bacterial resistance enzyme activities. *Antimicrob. Agents Chemother.* 55, 3207–3213.

Green, K. D., Chen, W., and Garneau-Tsodikova, S. (2012). Identification and characterization of inhibitors of the aminoglycoside resistance acetyltransferase Eis from *Mycobacterium tuberculosis. ChemMedChem* 7, 73–77.

Green, K. D., Chen, W., Houghton, J. L., Fridman, M., and Garneau-Tsodikova, S. (2010). Exploring the substrate promiscuity of drug-modifying enzymes for the chemoenzymatic generation of N-acylated aminoglycosides. *Chembiochem* 11, 119–126.

Guerrier-Takada, C., Salavati, R., and Altman, S. (1997). Phenotypic conversion of drug-resistant bacteria to drug sensitivity. *Proc. Natl. Acad. Sci. U.S.A.* 94, 8468–8472.

Haddad, J., Vakulenko, S. B., and Mobashery, S. (1999). An antibiotic cloaked by its own resistance enzyme. *J. Am. Chem. Soc.* 121, 11922–11923.

Hall, R. M. (2012). Integrons and gene cassettes: hotspots of diversity in bacterial genomes. *Ann. N.Y. Acad. Sci.* 1267, 71–78.

Hancock, R. E. (1981). Aminoglycoside uptake and mode of action–with special reference to streptomycin and gentamicin. I. Antagonists and mutants. *J. Antimicrob. Chemother.* 8, 249–276.

Hermann, T. (2007). Aminoglycoside antibiotics: old drugs and new therapeutic approaches. *Cell. Mol. Life Sci.* 64, 1841–1852.

Herzog, I. M., Green, K. D., Berkov-Zrihen, Y., Feldman, M., Vidavski, R. R., Eldar-Boock, A., et al. (2012). 6′-Thioether tobramycin analogues: towards selective targeting of bacterial membranes. *Angew. Chem. Int. Ed. Engl.* 51, 5652–5656.

Hocquet, D., Vogne, C., El Garch, F., Vejux, A., Gotoh, N., Lee, A., et al. (2003). MexXY-OprM efflux pump is necessary for a adaptive resistance of *Pseudomonas aeruginosa* to aminoglycosides. *Antimicrob. Agents Chemother.* 47, 1371–1375.

Houghton, J. L., Green, K. D., Chen, W., and Garneau-Tsodikova, S. (2010). The future of aminoglycosides: the end or renaissance? *Chembiochem* 11, 880–902.

Huon, L. K., Fang, T. Y., and Wang, P. C. (2012). Outcomes of intratympanic gentamicin injection to treat Meniere's disease. *Otol. Neurotol.* 33, 706–714.

Jana, S., and Deb, J. K. (2006). Molecular understanding of aminoglycoside action and resistance. *Appl. Microbiol. Biotechnol.* 70, 140–150.

Kandasamy, J., Atia-Glikin, D., Shulman, E., Shapira, K., Shavit, M., Belakhov, V., et al. (2012). Increased selectivity toward cytoplasmic versus mitochondrial ribosome confers improved efficiency of synthetic aminoglycosides in fixing damaged genes: a strategy for treatment of genetic diseases caused by nonsense mutations. *J. Med. Chem.* 55, 10630–10643.

Katoh, K., and Standley, D. (2013). MAFFT multiple sequence alignment software version 7: improvements in performance and usability. *Mol. Biol. Evol.* 30, 772–780.

Kellermayer, R. (2006). Translational readthrough induction of pathogenic nonsense mutations. *Eur. J. Med. Genet.* 49, 445–450.

Kim, C., Villegas-Estrada, A., Hesek, D., and Mobashery, S. (2007). Mechanistic characterization of the bifunctional aminoglycoside-modifying enzyme AAC(3)-Ib/AAC(6′)-Ib′ from *Pseudomonas aeruginosa. Biochemistry* 46, 5270–5282.

Kim, Y. T., Jang, J. H., Kim, H. C., Kim, H., Lee, K. R., Park, K. S., et al. (2011). Identification of strain harboring both *aac(6′)-Ib* and *aac(6′)-Ib-cr* variant simultaneously in *Escherichia coli* and *Klebsiella pneumoniae. BMB Rep.* 44, 262–266.

Kohanski, M. A., Dwyer, D. J., Hayete, B., Lawrence, C. A., and Collins, J. J. (2007). A common mechanism of cellular death induced by bactericidal antibiotics. *Cell* 130, 797–810.

Kondo, J., Hainrichson, M., Nudelman, I., Shallom-Shezifi, D., Barbieri, C. M., Pilch, D. S., et al. (2007). Differential selectivity of natural and synthetic aminoglycosides towards the eukaryotic and prokaryotic decoding A sites. *Chembiochem* 8, 1700–1709.

Labaune, J. M., Bleyzac, N., Maire, P., Jelliffe, R. W., Boutroy, M. J., Aulagner, G., et al. (2001). Once-a-day individualized amikacin dosing for suspected infection at birth based on population pharmacokinetic models. *Biol. Neonate* 80, 142–147.

Lambert, T., Ploy, M. C., and Courvalin, P. (1994). A spontaneous point mutation in the *aac(6′)-Ib*′ gene results in altered substrate specificity of aminoglycoside 6′-*N*-acetyltransferase of a *Pseudomonas fluorescens* strain. *FEMS Microbiol. Lett.* 115, 297–304.

Landman, D., Kelly, P., Backer, M., Babu, E., Shah, N., Bratu, S., et al. (2011). Antimicrobial activity of a novel aminoglycoside, ACHN-490, against *Acinetobacter baumannii* and *Pseudomonas aeruginosa* from New York City. *J. Antimicrob. Chemother.* 66, 332–334.

Liu, M., Haddad, J., Azucena, E., Kotra, L. P., Kirzhner, M., and Mobashery, S. (2000). Tethered bisubstrate derivatives as probes for mechanism and as inhibitors of aminoglycoside 3′-phosphotransferases. *J. Org. Chem.* 65, 7422–7431.

Lombes, T., Begis, G., Maurice, F., Turcaud, S., Lecourt, T., Dardel, F., et al. (2008). NMR-guided fragment-based approach for the design of AAC(6′)-Ib ligands. *Chembiochem* 9, 1368–1371.

Lundblad, E. W., and Altman, S. (2010). Inhibition of gene expression by RNase P. *N. Biotechnol.* 27, 212–221.

Macleod, D. L., Nelson, L. E., Shawar, R. M., Lin, B. B., Lockwood, L. G., Dirk, J. E., et al. (2000). Aminoglycoside-resistance mechanisms for cystic fibrosis *Pseudomonas aeruginosa* isolates are unchanged by long-term, intermittent, inhaled tobramycin treatment. *J. Infect. Dis.* 181, 1180–1184.

Magalhaes, M. L., Vetting, M. W., Gao, F., Freiburger, L., Auclair, K., and Blanchard, J. S. (2008). Kinetic and structural analysis of bisubstrate inhibition of the Salmonella enterica aminoglycoside 6′-*N*-acetyltransferase. *Biochemistry* 47, 579–584.

Magnet, S., and Blanchard, J. S. (2005). Molecular insights into aminoglycoside action and resistance. *Chem. Rev.* 105, 477–498.

Magnet, S., Smith, T. A., Zheng, R., Nordmann, P., and Blanchard, J. S. (2003). Aminoglycoside resistance resulting from tight drug binding to an altered aminoglycoside acetyltransferase. *Antimicrob. Agents Chemother.* 47, 1577–1583.

Majumder, K., Wei, L., Annedi, S., and Kotra, L. P. (2007). "Aminoglycoside antibiotics," in *Enzyme-Mediated Resistance to Antibiotics: Mechanisms, Dissemination, and Prospects for Inhibition*, eds R. A. Bonomo and M. E. Tolmasky (Washington, DC: ASM Press), 7–20.

Maurice, F., Broutin, I., Podglajen, I., Benas, P., Collatz, E., and Dardel, F. (2008). Enzyme structural plasticity and the emergence of broad-spectrum antibiotic resistance. *EMBO Rep.* 9, 344–349.

Mehta, R., and Champney, W. S. (2003). Neomycin and paromomycin inhibit 30S ribosomal subunit assembly in *Staphylococcus aureus. Curr. Microbiol.* 47, 237–243.

Mendes, R., Toleman, M., Ribeiro, J., Sader, H., Jones, R., and Walsh, T. (2004). Integron carrying a novel metallo-b-lactamase gene, bla_{IMP-16}, and a fused form of aminoglycoside-resistance gene *aac(6′)-30/aac(6′)-Ib*: report from the SENTRY antimicrobial surveillance program. *Antimicrob. Agents Chemother.* 48, 4693–4702.

Menzies, D., Benedetti, A., Paydar, A., Martin, I., Royce, S., Pai, M., et al. (2009). Effect of duration and intermittency of rifampin on tuberculosis treatment outcomes: a systematic review and meta-analysis. *PLoS Med.* 6:e1000146. doi: 10.1371/journal.pmed.1000146

Mikkelsen, N. E., Brannvall, M., Virtanen, A., and Kirsebom, L. A. (1999). Inhibition of RNase P RNA cleavage by aminoglycosides. *Proc. Natl. Acad. Sci. U.S.A.* 96, 6155–6160.

Miller, G. H., Sabatelli, F. J., Hare, R. S., Glupczynski, Y., Mackey, P., Shlaes, D., et al. (1997). The most frequent aminoglycoside resistance mechanisms–changes with time and geographic area: a reflection of aminoglycoside usage patterns? Aminoglycoside Resistance Study Groups. *Clin. Infect. Dis.* 24(Suppl. 1), S46–S62.

Morita, Y., Tomida, J., and Kawamura, Y. (2012). MexXY multidrug efflux system of *Pseudomonas aeruginosa. Front. Microbiol.* 3:408. doi: 10.3389/fmicb.2012.00408

Muir, M. E., Van Heeswyck, R. S., and Wallace, B. J. (1984). Effect of growth rate on streptomycin accumulation by *Escherichia coli* and *Bacillus megaterium. J. Gen. Microbiol.* 130, 2015–2022.

Neuwald, A. F., and Landsman, D. (1997). GCN5-related histone *N*-acetyltransferases belong to a diverse superfamily that includes the yeast SPT10 protein. *Trends Biochem. Sci.* 22, 154–155.

O'Connor, M., De Stasio, E. A., and Dahlberg, A. E. (1991). Interaction between 16S ribosomal RNA and ribosomal protein S12: differential effects of paromomycin and streptomycin. *Biochimie* 73, 1493–1500.

Over, U., Gur, D., Unal, S., Miller, G. H., and Aminoglycoside Resistance Study Group. (2001). The changing nature of aminoglycoside resistance mechanisms and prevalence of

newly recognized resistance mechanisms in Turkey. *Clin. Microbiol. Infect.* 7, 470–478.
Pacheu-Grau, D., Perez-Delgado, L., Gomez-Diaz, C., Fraile-Rodrigo, J., Montoya, J., and Ruiz-Pesini, E. (2012). Mitochondrial ribosome and Meniere's disease: a pilot study. *Eur. Arch. Otorhinolaryngol.* 269, 2003–2008.
Panaite, D. M., and Tolmasky, M. E. (1998). Characterization of mutants of the 6′-*N*-acetyltransferase encoded by the multiresistance transposon Tn*1331*: effect of Phen171-to-Leu171 and Tyr80-to-Cys80 substitutions. *Plasmid* 39, 123–133.
Poirel, L., Cabanne, L., Collet, L., and Nordmann, P. (2006). Class II transposon-borne structure harboring metallo-beta-lactamase gene *bla*VIM-2 in *Pseudomonas putida*. *Antimicrob. Agents Chemother.* 50, 2889–2891.
Pourreza, A., Witherspoon, M., Fox, J., Newmark, J., Bui, D., and Tolmasky, M. E. (2005). Mutagenesis analysis of a conserved region involved in acetyl coenzyme A binding in the aminoglycoside 6′-*N*-acetyltransferase type Ib encoded by plasmid pJHCMW1. *Antimicrob. Agents Chemother.* 49, 2979–2982.
Quiroga, M. P., Andres, P., Petroni, A., Soler Bistue, A. J., Guerriero, L., Vargas, L. J., et al. (2007). Complex class 1 integrons with diverse variable regions, including *aac(6′)-Ib-cr*, and a novel allele, *qnrB10*, associated with IS*CR1* in clinical enterobacterial isolates from Argentina. *Antimicrob. Agents Chemother.* 51, 4466–4470.
Ramirez, M. S., Parenteau, T. R., Centron, D., and Tolmasky, M. E. (2008). Functional characterization of Tn1331 gene cassettes. *J. Antimicrob. Chemother.* 62, 669–673.
Ramirez, M. S., and Tolmasky, M. E. (2010). Aminoglycoside modifying enzymes. *Drug Resist. Updat.* 13, 151–171.
Rather, P. N., Munayyer, H., Mann, P. A., Hare, R. S., Miller, G. H., and Shaw, K. J. (1992). Genetic analysis of bacterial acetyltransferases: identification of amino acids determining the specificities of the aminoglycoside 6′-*N*-acetyltransferase Ib and IIa proteins. *J. Bacteriol.* 174, 3196–3203.
Rice, L. B. (2008). Federal funding for the study of antimicrobial resistance in nosocomial pathogens: no ESKAPE. *J. Infect. Dis.* 197, 1079–1081.
Rice, L. B., Carias, L. L., Hutton, R. A., Rudin, S. D., Endimiani, A., and Bonomo, R. A. (2008). The KQ element, a complex genetic region conferring transferable resistance to carbapenems, aminoglycosides, and fluoroquinolones in *Klebsiella pneumoniae*. *Anti-microb. Agents Chemother.* 52, 3427–3429.
Rich, D. P., Anderson, M. P., Gregory, R. J., Cheng, S. H., Paul, S., Jefferson, D. M., et al. (1990). Expression of cystic fibrosis transmembrane conductance regulator corrects defective chloride channel regulation in cystic fibrosis airway epithelial cells. *Nature* 347, 358–363.
Robicsek, A., Strahilevitz, J., Jacoby, G. A., Macielag, M., Abbanat, D., Park, C. H., et al. (2006). Fluoroquinolone-modifying enzyme: a new adaptation of a common aminoglycoside acetyltransferase. *Nat. Med.* 12, 83–88.
Rodriguez-Martinez, J. M., Cano, M. E., Velasco, C., Martinez-Martinez, L., and Pascual, A. (2011). Plasmid-mediated quinolone resistance: an update. *J. Infect. Chemother.* 17, 149–182.
Romanowska, J., Reuter, N., and Trylska, J. (2013). Comparing aminoglycoside binding sites in bacterial ribosomal RNA and aminoglycoside modifying enzymes. *Proteins* 81, 63–80.
Ruiz, J., Pons, M. J., and Gomes, C. (2012). Transferable mechanisms of quinolone resistance. *Int. J. Antimicrob. Agents* 40, 196–203.
Salipante, S. J., and Hall, B. G. (2003). Determining the limits of the evolutionary potential of an antibiotic resistance gene. *Mol. Biol. Evol.* 20, 653–659.
Sarno, R., Ha, H., Weinsetel, N., and Tolmasky, M. E. (2003). Inhibition of aminoglycoside 6′-*N*-acetyltransferase type Ib-mediated amikacin resistance by antisense oligodeoxynucleotides. *Antimicrob. Agents Chemother.* 47, 3296–3304.
Sarno, R., McGillivary, G., Sherratt, D. J., Actis, L. A., and Tolmasky, M. E. (2002). Complete nucleotide sequence of *Klebsiella pneumoniae* multiresistance plasmid pJHCMW1. *Antimicrob. Agents Chemother.* 46, 3422–3427.
Schmitt, E., Galimand, M., Panvert, M., Courvalin, P., and Mechulam, Y. (2009). Structural bases for 16s rRNA methylation catalyzed by ArmA and RmtB methyltransferases. *J. Mol. Biol.* 388, 570–582.
Shaul, P., Green, K. D., Rutenberg, R., Kramer, M., Berkov-Zrihen, Y., Breiner-Goldstein, E., et al. (2011). Assessment of 6′- and 6‴-N-acylation of aminoglycosides as a strategy to overcome bacterial resistance. *Org. Biomol. Chem.* 9, 4057–4063.
Shaw, K. J., Rather, P. N., Hare, R. S., and Miller, G. H. (1993). Molecular genetics of aminoglycoside resistance genes and familial relationships of the aminoglycoside-modifying enzymes. *Microbiol. Rev.* 57, 138–163.
Shmara, A., Weinsetel, N., Dery, K. J., Chavideh, R., and Tolmasky, M. E. (2001). Systematic analysis of a conserved region of the aminoglycoside 6′-*N*-acetyltransferase type Ib. *Antimicrob. Agents Chemother.* 45, 3287–3292.
Sneath, P. H., and Sokal, R. R. (1973). *Numerical Taxonomy. The Principles and Practice of Numerical Classification.* San Francisco, CA: W. H. Freeman.
Soler Bistue, A. J., Birshan, D., Tomaras, A. P., Dandekar, M., Tran, T., Newmark, J., et al. (2008). *Klebsiella pneumoniae* multiresistance plasmid pMET1: similarity with the *Yersinia pestis* plasmid pCRY and integrative conjugative elements. *PLoS ONE* 3:e1800. doi: 10.1371/journal.pone.0001800
Soler Bistue, A. J., Ha, H., Sarno, R., Don, M., Zorreguieta, A., and Tolmasky, M. E. (2007). External guide sequences targeting the *aac(6′)-Ib* mRNA induce inhibition of amikacin resistance. *Antimicrob. Agents Chemother.* 51, 1918–1925.
Soler Bistue, A. J., Martin, F. A., Petroni, A., Faccone, D., Galas, M., Tolmasky, M. E., et al. (2006). *Vibrio cholerae* InV117, a class 1 integron harboring *aac(6′)-Ib* and *bla*CTX-M-2, is linked to transposition genes. *Antimicrob. Agents Chemother.* 50, 1903–1907.
Soler Bistue, A. J., Martin, F. A., Vozza, N., Ha, H., Joaquin, J. C., Zorreguieta, A., et al. (2009). Inhibition of *aac(6′)-Ib*-mediated amikacin resistance by nuclease-resistant external guide sequences in bacteria. *Proc. Natl. Acad. Sci. U.S.A.* 106, 13230–13235.
Strahilevitz, J., Jacoby, G. A., Hooper, D. C., and Robicsek, A. (2009). Plasmid-mediated quinolone resistance: a multifaceted threat. *Clin. Microbiol. Rev.* 22, 664–689.
Taber, H. W., Mueller, J. P., Miller, P. F., and Arrow, A. S. (1987). Bacterial uptake of aminoglycoside antibiotics. *Microbiol. Rev.* 51, 439–457.
Tolmasky, M. (2007a). "Aminogylcoside-modifying enzymes: characteristics, localization, and dissemination," in *Enzyme-Mediated Resistance to Antibiotics: Mechanisms, Dissemination, and Prospects for Inhibition*, eds R. Bonomo and M. Tolmasky (Washington, DC: ASM Press), 35–52.
Tolmasky, M. E. (2007b). "Overview of dissemination mechanisms of genes coding for resistance to antibiotics," in *Enzyme-Mediated Resistance to Antibiotics: Mechanisms, Dissemination, and Prospects for Inhibition*, eds R. Bonomo and M. E. Tolmasky (Washington, DC: ASM Press), 267–270.
Tolmasky, M. E. (1990). Sequencing and expression of *aadA*, *bla*, and *tnpR* from the multiresistance transposon Tn*1331*. *Plasmid* 24, 218–226.
Tolmasky, M. E., Chamorro, R. M., Crosa, J. H., and Marini, P. M. (1988). Transposon-mediated amikacin resistance in *Klebsiella pneumoniae*. *Antimicrob. Agents Chemother.* 32, 1416–1420.
Tolmasky, M. E., and Crosa, J. H. (1987). Tn*1331*, a novel multiresistance transposon encoding resistance to amikacin and ampicillin in *Klebsiella pneumoniae*. *Antimicrob. Agents Chemother.* 31, 1955–1960.
Tolmasky, M. E., and Crosa, J. H. (1991). Regulation of plasmid-mediated iron transport and virulence in *Vibrio anguillarum*. *Biol. Met.* 4, 33–35.
Tolmasky, M. E., and Crosa, J. H. (1993). Genetic organization of antibiotic resistance genes (*aac(6′)-Ib*, *aadA*, and *oxa9*) in the multiresistance transposon Tn*1331*. *Plasmid* 29, 31–40.
Traglia, G., Davies Sala, C., Fuxman Bass, J., Soler Bistué, A., Zorreguieta, A., Ramirez, M. S., et al. (2012). Internalization of locked nucleic acids/DNA hybrid oligomers into *Escherichia coli*. *Biores. Open Access* 1, 260–263.
Vakulenko, S. B., and Mobashery, S. (2003). Versatility of aminoglycosides and prospects for their future. *Clin. Microbiol. Rev.* 16, 430–450.
van 't Veen, A., Van Der Zee, A., Nelson, J., Speelberg, B., Kluytmans, J. A., and Buiting, A. G. (2005). Outbreak of infection with a multiresistant *Klebsiella pneumoniae* strain associated with contaminated roll boards in operating rooms. *J. Clin. Microbiol.* 43, 4961–4967.
Vetting, M. W., Lp, S. D. C., Yu, M., Hegde, S. S., Magnet, S., Roderick, S. L., et al. (2005). Structure and functions of the GNAT superfamily

of acetyltransferases. *Arch. Biochem. Biophys.* 433, 212–226.

Vetting, M. W., Magnet, S., Nieves, E., Roderick, S. L., and Blanchard, J. S. (2004). A bacterial acetyltransferase capable of regioselective N-acetylation of antibiotics and histones. *Chem. Biol.* 11, 565–573.

Vetting, M. W., Park, C. H., Hegde, S. S., Jacoby, G. A., Hooper, D. C., and Blanchard, J. S. (2008). Mechanistic and structural analysis of aminoglycoside *N*-acetyltransferase AAC(6′)-Ib and its bifunctional, fluoroquinolone-active AAC(6′)-Ib-cr variant. *Biochemistry* 47, 9825–9835.

Vicens, Q., and Westhof, E. (2003). Molecular recognition of aminoglycoside antibiotics by ribosomal RNA and resistance enzymes: an analysis of x-ray crystal structures. *Biopolymers* 70, 42–57.

Villa, L., Poirel, L., Nordmann, P., Carta, C., and Carattoli, A. (2012). Complete sequencing of an IncH plasmid carrying the *bla*NDM-1, *bla*CTX-M-15 and *qnrB1* genes. *J. Antimicrob. Chemother.* 67, 1645–1650.

Vong, K., Tam, I. S., Yan, X., and Auclair, K. (2012). Inhibitors of aminoglycoside resistance activated in cells. *ACS Chem. Biol.* 7, 470–475.

Wachino, J., and Arakawa, Y. (2012). Exogenously acquired 16S rRNA methyltransferases found in aminoglycoside-resistant pathogenic Gram-negative bacteria: an update. *Drug Resist. Updat.* 15, 133–148.

Warburg, G., Hidalgo-Grass, C., Partridge, S. R., Tolmasky, M. E., Temper, V., Moses, A. E., et al. (2012). A carbapenem-resistant *Klebsiella pneumoniae* epidemic clone in Jerusalem: sequence type 512 carrying a plasmid encoding *aac(6′)-Ib*. *J. Antimicrob. Chemother.* 67, 898–901.

Welch, K. T., Virga, K. G., Whittemore, N. A., Ozen, C., Wright, E., Brown, C. L., et al. (2005). Discovery of non-carbohydrate inhibitors of aminoglycoside-modifying enzymes. *Bioorg. Med. Chem.* 13, 6252–6263.

Williams, J. W., and Northrop, D. B. (1979). Synthesis of a tight-binding, multisubstrate analog inhibitor of gentamicin acetyltransferase I. *J. Antibiot.* 32, 1147–1154.

Woloj, M., Tolmasky, M. E., Roberts, M. C., and Crosa, J. H. (1986). Plasmid-encoded amikacin resistance in multiresistant strains of *Klebsiella pneumoniae* isolated from neonates with meningitis. *Antimicrob. Agents Chemother.* 29, 315–319.

Woodford, N., Carattoli, A., Karisik, E., Underwood, A., Ellington, M. J., and Livermore, D. M. (2009). Complete nucleotide sequences of plasmids pEK204, pEK499, and pEK516, encoding CTX-M enzymes in three major *Escherichia coli* lineages from the United Kingdom, all belonging to the international O25:H4-ST131 clone. *Antimicrob. Agents Chemother.* 53, 4472–4482.

Wright, G. D. (1999). Aminoglycoside-modifying enzymes. *Curr. Opin. Microbiol.* 2, 499–503.

Wright, G. D., and Berghuis, A. M. (2007). "Structural aspects of aminoglycoside modifying enzymes," in *Enzyme-Mediated Resistance to Antibiotics: Mechanisms, Dissemination, and Prospects for Inhibition*, eds R. Bonomo and M. Tolmasky (Washington, DC: ASM Press), 21–33.

Wright, G. D., and Ladak, P. (1997). Overexpression and characterization of the chromosomal aminoglycoside 6′-*N*-acetyltransferase from *Enterococcus faecium*. *Antimicrob. Agents Chemother.* 41, 956–960.

Wybenga-Groot, L. E., Draker, K., Wright, G. D., and Berghuis, A. M. (1999). Crystal structure of an aminoglycoside 6′-*N*-acetyltransferase: defining the GCN5-related N-acetyltransferase superfamily fold. *Structure* 7, 497–507.

Yao, J., and Moellering, R. (2007). "Antibacterial agents," in *Manual of Clinical Microbiology*, eds P. Murray, E. Baron, J. Jorgensen, M. Landry, and M. Pfaller (Washington, DC: American Society for Microbiology Press), 1077–1113.

Yong, D., Toleman, M. A., Giske, C. G., Cho, H. S., Sundman, K., Lee, K., et al. (2009). Characterization of a new metallo-beta-lactamase gene, *bla*(NDM-1), and a novel erythromycin esterase gene carried on a unique genetic structure in *Klebsiella pneumoniae* sequence type 14 from India. *Antimicrob. Agents Chemother.* 53, 5046–5054.

Zaher, H. S., and Green, R. (2009). Fidelity at the molecular level: lessons from protein synthesis. *Cell* 136, 746–762.

Zingman, L. V., Park, S., Olson, T. M., Alekseev, A. E., and Terzic, A. (2007). Aminoglycoside-induced translational read-through in disease: overcoming nonsense mutations by pharmacogenetic therapy. *Clin. Pharmacol. Ther.* 81, 99–103.

Zong, Z., Partridge, S. R., and Iredell, J. R. (2009). A *bla*VEB-1 variant, *bla*VEB-6, associated with repeated elements in a complex genetic structure. *Antimicrob. Agents Chemother.* 53, 1693–1697.

Permissions

All chapters in this book were first published in MAR, by Frontiers; hereby published with permission under the Creative Commons Attribution License or equivalent. Every chapter published in this book has been scrutinized by our experts. Their significance has been extensively debated. The topics covered herein carry significant findings which will fuel the growth of the discipline. They may even be implemented as practical applications or may be referred to as a beginning point for another development.

The contributors of this book come from diverse backgrounds, making this book a truly international effort. This book will bring forth new frontiers with its revolutionizing research information and detailed analysis of the nascent developments around the world.

We would like to thank all the contributing authors for lending their expertise to make the book truly unique. They have played a crucial role in the development of this book. Without their invaluable contributions this book wouldn't have been possible. They have made vital efforts to compile up to date information on the varied aspects of this subject to make this book a valuable addition to the collection of many professionals and students.

This book was conceptualized with the vision of imparting up-to-date information and advanced data in this field. To ensure the same, a matchless editorial board was set up. Every individual on the board went through rigorous rounds of assessment to prove their worth. After which they invested a large part of their time researching and compiling the most relevant data for our readers.

The editorial board has been involved in producing this book since its inception. They have spent rigorous hours researching and exploring the diverse topics which have resulted in the successful publishing of this book. They have passed on their knowledge of decades through this book. To expedite this challenging task, the publisher supported the team at every step. A small team of assistant editors was also appointed to further simplify the editing procedure and attain best results for the readers.

Apart from the editorial board, the designing team has also invested a significant amount of their time in understanding the subject and creating the most relevant covers. They scrutinized every image to scout for the most suitable representation of the subject and create an appropriate cover for the book.

The publishing team has been an ardent support to the editorial, designing and production team. Their endless efforts to recruit the best for this project, has resulted in the accomplishment of this book. They are a veteran in the field of academics and their pool of knowledge is as vast as their experience in printing. Their expertise and guidance has proved useful at every step. Their uncompromising quality standards have made this book an exceptional effort. Their encouragement from time to time has been an inspiration for everyone.

The publisher and the editorial board hope that this book will prove to be a valuable piece of knowledge for researchers, students, practitioners and scholars across the globe.

List of Contributors

Hidetaka Nagai, Mototaka Hiki and Tetsuo Asai
National Veterinary Assay Laboratory, Ministry of Agriculture, Forestry and Fisheries, Kokubunji, Tokyo, Japan

Yutaka Tamura
School of Veterinary Medicine, Rakuno Gakuen University, Ebetsu, Hokkaido, Japan

Masaru Usui
National Veterinary Assay Laboratory, Ministry of Agriculture, Forestry and Fisheries, Kokubunji, Tokyo, Japan
School of Veterinary Medicine, Rakuno Gakuen University, Ebetsu, Hokkaido, Japan

Agnese Lupo and Thomas Ulrich Berendonk
Institute of Hydrobiology, Department of Hydrosciences, Technical University Dresden, Dresden, Germany

Sébastien Coyne
Department of Biomolecular Chemistry, Leibniz Institute for Natural Product Research and Infection Biology - Hans Knöll Institute, Jena, Germany

Yuji Morita, Junko Tomida and Yoshiaki Kawamura
Department of Microbiology, School of Pharmacy, Aichi Gakuin University, Nagoya, Japan

Marilyn C. Roberts and David No
Department of Environmental and Occupational Health Sciences, University of Washington, Seattle, WA, USA

Olusegun O.Soge
Department of Global Health, University of Washington, Seattle, WA, USA

Ana P. Tedim
Department of Microbiology, Hospital Universitario Ramón y Cajal, Instituto Ramón y Cajal de Investigación Sanitaria, Madrid, Spain
Centros de Investigación Biomédica en Red de Epidemiología y Salud Pública, Madrid, Spain

Fernando Baquero and Teresa M.Coque
Department of Microbiology, Hospital Universitario Ramón y Cajal, Instituto Ramón y Cajal de Investigación Sanitaria, Madrid, Spain
Centros de Investigación Biomédica en Red de Epidemiología y Salud Pública, Madrid, Spain
Unidad de Resistencia a Antibióticos y Virulencia Bacteriana asociada al Consejo Superior de Investigaciones Científicas, Madrid, Spain

RyotaIino and Hiroyuki Noji
Department of Applied Chemistry, Graduate School of Engineering, The University of Tokyo, Tokyo, Japan
Core Research for Evolutional Science and Technology, Japan Science and Technology Agency, Tokyo, Japan

Yoshimi Matsumoto and Kunihiko Nishino
Laboratory of Microbiology and Infectious Diseases, Institute of Scientific and Industrial Research, Osaka University, Osaka, Japan

Akihito Yamaguchi
Department of Cell Membrane Biology, Institute of Scientific and Industrial Research, Osaka University, Osaka, Japan
Graduate School of Pharmaceutical Sciences, Osaka University, Osaka, Japan

Xianyun Sun,Wenzhao Wang, Kangji Wang and Shaojie Li
State Key Laboratory of Mycology, Institute of Microbiology, Chinese Academy of Sciences, Beijing, China

Xinxu Yu and Baogui Xie
Mycological Research Center, College of Life Sciences, Fujian Agriculture and Forestry University, Fuzhou, China

Jie Liu and Fucai Zhou
College of Bioscience and Biotechnology, Yangzhou University, Yangzhou, China

Erica C. Pehrsson, Kevin J. Forsberg and Molly K. Gibson
Center for Genome Sciences and Systems Biology, Washington University School of Medicine, St. Louis, MO, USA

Sara Ahmadi
Center for Genome Sciences and Systems Biology, Washington University School of Medicine, St. Louis, MO, USA
Department of Pathology and Immunology, Washington University School of Medicine, St. Louis, MO, USA

Gautam Dantas
Center for Genome Sciences and Systems Biology, Washington University School of Medicine, St. Louis, MO, USA
Department of Pathology and Immunology, Washington University School of Medicine, St. Louis, MO, USA
Department of Biomedical Engineering, Washington University, St. Louis, MO, USA

Tucker R. Burch
Department of Civil Engineering, University of Minnesota, Minneapolis, MN, USA

Michael J. Sadowsky
Biotechnology Institute, University of Minnesota, St. Paul, MN, USA

Timothy M. La Para
Department of Civil Engineering, University of Minnesota, Minneapolis, MN, USA
Biotechnology Institute, University of Minnesota, St. Paul, MN, USA

Takehisa Chuma, Daisuke Miyasako, Tomoko Takayama, Yuko Nakamoto and Karoku Okamoto
Laboratory of Veterinary Public Health, Department of Veterinary Medicine, Joint Faculty of Veterinary Medicine, Kagoshima University, Kagoshima, Japan

Hesham Dahshan
Laboratory of Veterinary Public Health, Department of Veterinary Medicine, Joint Faculty of Veterinary Medicine, Kagoshima University, Kagoshima, Japan
Department of Veterinary Public Health, Faculty of Veterinary Medicine, Zagazig University, Zagazig, Egypt

Francis Shahada and Masato Akiba
Safety Research Team, National Institute of Animal Health, Tsukuba, Japan

Satoru Suzuki, Mitsuko Ogo and Todd W. Miller
Center for Marine Environmental Studies, Ehime University, Matsuyama, Japan

Akiko Shimizu and Hideshige Takada
Laboratory of Organic Geochemistry, Tokyo University of Agriculture and Technology, Fuchu, Japan

Maria Auxilia T. Siringan
Microbiological Research and Services Laboratory, Natural Sciences Research Institute, College of Science, University of the Philippines Diliman, Manila, Philippines

Ziqing Deng, Yue Shan, Qing Pan, Xiang Gao and Aixin Yan
School of Biological Sciences, The University of Hong Kong, Hong Kong, China

Nicole Fahrenfeld,Yanjun Ma and Amy Pruden
Department of Civil and Environmental Engineering, Virginia Tech, Blacksburg, VA, USA

MaureenO'Brien
Department of Civil and Environmental Engineering, Colorado School of Mines, Golden, CO, USA

Keith D. Green and Sylvie Garneau- Tsodikova
Department of Pharmaceutical Sciences, University of Kentucky, Lexington, KY, USA

Richard R. Watkins
Department of Internal Medicine, North east Ohio Medical University, Rootstown, OH, USA
Division of Infectious Diseases, Akron General Medical Center, Akron, OH, USA

Krisztina M. Papp-Wallace
Research Service, Louis Stokes Cleveland Department of Veterans Affairs Medical Center, Cleveland, OH, USA
Department of Medicine, Case Western Reserve University, Cleveland, OH, USA

Sarah M. Drawz
Department of Lab Medicine and Pathology, University of Minnesota, Minneapolis, MN, USA

Robert A. Bonomo
Research Service, Louis Stokes Cleveland Department of Veterans Affairs Medical Center, Cleveland, OH, USA
Department of Medicine, Case Western Reserve University, Cleveland, OH, USA
Pharmacology, Case Western Reserve University, Cleveland, OH, USA
Molecular Biology and Microbiology, Case Western Reserve University, Cleveland, OH, USA

Julie A. Perry and Gerard D. Wright
M. G.DeGroote Institute for Infectious Disease Research, McMaster University, Hamilton, ON, Canada
Department of Biochemistry and Biomedical Sciences, McMaster University, Hamilton, ON, Canad

Elena N. Ilina, Maya V. Malakhova, Ivan N. Bodoev, Nina Y. Oparina, Alla V. Filimonova and Vadim M. Govorun
Research Institute of Physico-Chemical Medicine, Moscow, Russia

Rahat Zaheer, Shaun R. Cook, Cassidy L. Klima, Trevor Alexander and Tim A. McAllister
Lethbridge Research Centre, Agriculture and Agri-Food Canada, Lethbridge, AB, Canada

Kim Stanford
Alberta Agriculture and Rural Development, Lethbridge, AB, Canada

Edward Topp
Southern Crop Protection and Food Research Centre, Agriculture and Agri-Food Canada, London, ON, Canada

Ron R. Read
Faculty of Medicine, University of Calgary, Calgary, AB, Canada

Eddie Cytryn
Department of Soil Chemistry, Plant Nutrition and Microbiology, Institute of Soil, Water and Environmental Sciences, The Volcani Center, Agricultural Research Organization, Beit Dagan, Israel

Edouard Jurkevitch
Department of Agroecology and Plant Health, The Robert H.Smith Faculty of Agriculture, Food and Environment, The Hebrew University of Jerusalem, Jerusalem, Israel

Ella Kaplan and Maya Ofek
Department of Soil Chemistry, Plant Nutrition and Microbiology, Institute of Soil, Water and Environmental Sciences, The Volcani Center, Agricultural Research Organization, Beit Dagan, Israel
Department of Agroecology and Plant Health, The Robert H.Smith Faculty of Agriculture, Food and Environment, The Hebrew University of Jerusalem, Jerusalem, Israel

Claudio D. Miranda
Department of Aquaculture, Universidad Católica del Norte, Coquimbo, Chile

Alfredo Tello
Instituto Tecnológico del Salmón, INTESAL de SalmonChile, Puerto Montt, Chile

Patricia L. Keen
Department of Civil Engineering, University of British Columbia, Vancouver, BC, Canada

Ximin ZengandJunLin
Department of Animal Science, The University of Tennessee, Knoxville, TN, USA

Jorge Olivares, Alejandra Bernardini, Guillermo Garcia-Leon, Fernando Corona, Maria B. Sanchez and Jose L. Martinez
Centro Nacional de Biotecnología, Consejo Superior de Investigaciones Científicas, Madrid, Spain

Sylvie Baucheron, Isabelle Monchaux and Axel Cloeckaert
UMR1282 Infectiologie et Santé Publique, Institut National de la Recherche Agronomique, Nouzilly, France
UMR1282 Infectiologie et Santé Publique, Université François Rabelais de Tours, Tours, France

Simon Le Hello and François-Xavier Weill
Institut Pasteur, Unité des Bactéries Pathogènes Entériques, Centre National de Référence des Escherichia coli, Shigella et Salmonella, Paris, France

María S. Ramirez, Nikolas Nikolaidis and Marcelo E. Tolmasky
Department of Biological Science, Center for Applied Biotechnology Studies, College of Natural Sciences and Mathematics, California State University Fullerton, Fullerton, CA, USA

Index

CPSIA information can be obtained
at www.ICGtesting.com
Printed in the USA
LVHW061719120222
711000LV00002B/54

9 781639 890507